Giovanni Pierluigi da Palestrina

ROUTLEDGE MUSICAL BIBLIOGRAPHIES
Series Editor: Brad Eden

Composers

Isaac Albéniz (1998)
Walter A. Clark

C. P. E. Bach (2002)
Doris Powers

Samuel Barber (2001)
Wayne C. Wentzel

Béla Bartók (1997)
Second Edition
Elliott Antokoletz

Vincenzo Bellini (2002)
Stephen A. Willier

Alban Berg (1996)
Bryan R. Simms

Leonard Bernstein (2001)
Paul F. Laird

Benjamin Britten (1996)
Peter J. Hodgson

Elliott Carter (2000)
John F. Link

Carlos Chávez (1998)
Robert Parker

Frédéric Chopin (1999)
William Smialek

Aaron Copland (2001)
Marta Robertson and Robin Armstrong

Gaetano Donizetti (2000)
James P. Cassaro

Edward Elgar (1993)
Christopher Kent

Gabriel Fauré (1999)
Edward R. Phillips

Charles Ives (2002)
Gayle Sherwood

Scott Joplin (1998)
Nancy R. Ping-Robbins

Zoltán Kodály (1998)
Mícheál Houlahan and Philip Tacka

Guillaume de Machaut (1995)
Lawrence Earp

Felix Mendelssohn (2001)
John Michael Cooper

Giovanni Battista Pergolesi (2001)
Clara Marvin

Giacomo Puccini (1999)
Linda B. Fairtile

Alessandro and Domenico Scarlatti (1993)
Carole F. Vidali

Jean Sibelius (1998)
Glenda D. Goss

Giuseppe Verdi (1998)
Gregory Harwood

Tomás Luis de Victoria (1998)
Eugene Casjen Cramer

Richard Wagner (2002)
Michael Saffle

Genres

Central European Folk Music (1996)
Philip V. Bohlman

Choral Music (2001)
Avery T. Sharp and James Michael Floyd

Jazz Research and Performance Materials, (1995)
Second edition
Eddie S. Meadows

Music in Canada (1997)
Carl Morey

North American Indian Music (1997)
Richard Keeling

Opera, Second edition (2001)
Guy Marco

Serial Music and Serialism (2001)
Johns D. Vander Weg

Giovanni Pierluigi da Palestrina

A Guide to Research

Clara Marvin

Routledge
New York and London

Published in 2002 by
Routledge Publishing, Inc.
29 West 35th Street
New York, NY 10001

An Imprint of the Taylor & Francis Group

10 9 8 7 6 5 4 3 2 1

Library of Congress Cataloging-in-Publication Data

Marvin, Clara.
Giovanni Pierluigi da Palestrina : a guide to research / Clara Marvin.
p. cm. — (Composer resource manuals ; v. 56)
Includes discography (p. 383) and indexes.
ISBN 0-8153-2351-4 (acid-free paper)
1. Palestrina, Giovanni Pierluigi da, 1525?–1594—Bibliography. I. Title. II. Series.
ML134.P2 M37 2001
016.7822'2'092—dc21
00-068435

Printed on acid-free, 250–year-life paper
Manufactured in the United States of America

Contents

Introduction

It has been justly said that the reputation of Giovanni Pierluigi da Palestrina (c.1525–1594) is unlike that of any other musician. He is the oldest composer who has been present continuously in the consciousness of the Western art tradition since his death over four centuries ago. For many historians writing from the seventeenth century to well into the early twentieth, Palestrina was *the* pivotal figure in the progressive development of music. Musical historiography was rich with metaphorical language emphasizing the composer's role both as an originator of "true" polyphony and as a foundation for the organic development of the art of his professional successors. Not only did many histories divide music into "before and after Palestrina" phases, but they established the composer as a new musical foundation, the mighty root out of which subsequent music had its growth and flower. Palestrina was also the linchpin in many genealogies of music: not only did the lines of musical descent, improving the musical heritage from one generation to another, converge on and culminate in him, but those who came after him were true followers only insofar as they continued to project qualities epitomized in his style. Palestrina was the musical Everest, the flagship on the sea of harmony, the virtual Counter-Reformation saint, complete with a miracle—the "salvation" of polyphony—to his credit. To Baini, his worshipful biographer, he was *amanuensis Dei*, "God's secretary."

But Palestrina's reputation evolved in a series of shifting phases. Although he has not needed reviving by modern scholarship, his historical image has undergone a remarkable series of changes and colorations, perhaps none more radical than in the twentieth century. Even more than being regarded as a perfect model for the contrapuntal technique of the late Renaissance, his name and style early became a metaphor for an ideal of pious devotion in ecclesiastical music, the semidivine purity of which vanquished the indecorous and the inept. Associated with these featured qualities were a cluster of distinct but intricately connected ideas whose links and historical crosscurrents have not always been fully understood. Many agendas have been at work in the history of Palestrina reception which reach far beyond the specific assessment of the quality of his music. In turns his fame was caught up in Roman Church history and reform, music theory and technique, politics, poetics and aesthetics, rationalist revision, antiquarianism, spiritual and religious revival movements, nationalist pride, and sociological and scientific study.

Unquestionably Palestrina was greatly esteemed by his contemporaries. As an incumbent of some of the most prestigious musical posts in Europe, he was described by a diplomat in 1575 as "now considered the very first musician in the world." Late in his life he was even presented with a printed collection of compositions by students and friends dedicated to his honor—an early *Festschrift*, as it were. His own works continued to be printed until well after his death, and some of them were perpetuated in copies that were well-used through not only the seventeenth but the eighteenth centuries. Yet there is a difference between lasting regard, however strong, and becoming a "legend," the real particulars of which in Palestrina's case did not evolve fully until well into the seventeenth century.

This elevation in status was brought about by the intersection of several factors. Musically, it came about in part because in the theory of style in baroque music, the canons of generic propriety for compositional technique became increasingly severe, especially for certain kinds of church music. The theory and practice of this strict style came to be regarded as the criterion by which quality and refinement of music for the church were to be judged. Not only technical skill but conceptual insight into the contrapuntal foundations of the tradition was the *sine qua non* for a truly learned and sophisticated *musicus*. Producing effective exemplars of the style was not only a matter of spiritual loyalty but an issue of professional dignity and pride.

Powerful cultural and political factors played a role in establishing Palestrina as a major role model for composers in the seventeenth century. As Jean Lionnet and Arnaldo Morelli have established, direct evidence that Palestrina's music was cited as an ideal model for emulation in the Sistine Chapel is not readily available before the 1660s. In the mid-seventeenth century, however, as the papacy ceased to play a critical role in European political affairs and lost much of its ideological hegemony, it continued to assert its spiritual primacy in other ways. It presented itself as the *fons et origo* and epicenter of a "true" religious culture as exhibited in the institutional traditions that it held should be transmitted to the rest of the world. It was during this period that Palestrina, the "prince of musicians" who had once reigned over the pope's own musical chapels, was increasingly heralded as the great restorer of the music of the Roman Catholic tradition.

Transmitted to the eighteenth century by such writers as Antimo Liberati and Adami da Bolsena, this "tradition" was disseminated through such theorists as Fux and his successors in methods of species counterpoint, and by composers who continued to emulate the *osservato* or *stile antico* schools, with greater or lesser intensity depending on their religious and stylistic orientation. While this era tended to emphasize Palestrina's technical mastery and elegance, insofar as they had experienced it, by the later part of the century a romanticized version of the "legendary" image began to reassert itself. Emerging with the nascent Romantic movement was a search for an aesthetic sense of spiritual exaltation, as well as for a kind of noble and archaic simplicity—for "origins"—that led to a revival of active interest in the composer. In 1814, E.T.A. Hoffmann predicated in a famous essay a restoration of church music based on the transcendent purity of the Palestrina style, asserting that for sublimity it was the vocal counterpart of the absolute symphonic style. To a startling extent, Giuseppe Baini's landmark biography of the composer, published in 1828, reflected the romantic program of the composer as the archetypically solitary, afflicted genius, one whose manner was at once grandly religious and sublimely simple. In Ian Bent's words, Palestrina's style was perceived to be one "in which all antitheses are resolved: nature is wed to art, rhetoric and philosophy are reconciled, and art and science join forces." But also thanks to the pioneering Baini, Palestrina was also the first of the pre-1600 composers whose biography and works were addressed in detail with some of the tools of documentary scholarship. While Baini could not interview his subject, he was surrounded at the Vatican by a wealth of manuscript and archival materials. He sought both to know something of Palestrina's personality and to make a serious attempt to describe the composer's stylistic methods over time as a series of phases in a stylistic development.

The resurgence of devoted interest in Palestrina in the nineteenth century was part of a general revival of older music, which was in itself a function of the period's aestheticized nostalgia for the past. This was especially true within the Roman Catholic community, many of whose European institutions, both monastic and secular, had been destroyed or attenuated during the last decades of the eighteenth century. The church music restoration movement was closely related to a general Catholic renewal in France, and in central and southern Germany a strong continuity existed between the Romantic revival and the various artistic, philosophical, and religious programs of the Cecilians. By the 1880s there were also some in Italy who were reacting against the hegemony of the current operatic style, and they looked to the *stile alla Palestrina* as a potential model for a restoration of church music to spiritual simplicity. Although the papacy itself retreated politically into the Vatican after 1848, it continued to be powerfully concerned with musical religious reform, and even during the most visible phase of the movement for the recovery of Gregorian chant, it was recognized that there was a practical liturgical place for polyphony based on Palestrinian models. But interest in Palestrina was by no means exclusively associated with Roman Catholicism. His historical prestige as spiritual musician and contrapuntist *par excellence* was such that many High Church Anglican and Lutheran circles in particular increasingly sought the music of the older Roman school for their antiquarian and musicological studies, choral societies, and liturgies through much of the nineteenth century.

Palestrina's music was also indirectly drawn into national and political issues. The second modern edition of his music, announced by Monsignor Casimiri in 1934, was in part a monument to the Italian striving at that time to recover the magnificent cultural heritage of its own more remote past. To a number of early-twentieth-century Italians, it then appeared that the continuity of their historical musical culture—seemingly swallowed up by the great maw of nineteenth-century opera on the one hand and an apparent German hegemony in instrumental music on the other—needed to be reasserted. While the *fascista* mentality may have capitalized upon such thinking to some extent, these stirrings had in fact been present virtually since Italy's birth as a united nation in the 1860s and '70s. Casimiri's edition was by his own admission meant not only to take advantage of the tools of modern scholarship but to provide a particular kind of native sensibility and commitment, both of which would act as a corrective to Haberl's treatment of Latin and Italian prosody and text underlay.

Twentieth-century musicology has tempered some of the past extravagances addressed to Palestrina. The hagiographies of the nineteenth century, with their imaginary conversations with the composer and their sometimes treacly religious sentiment, have been largely superseded, but the modified picture that has emerged, particularly since 1960, is rich and various on its own terms. The composer's image has been put on a more scientific and sociological footing. Palestrina has been discovered to be not only for the ages, but also a man and citizen of his own time: a sophisticated working artist among others in an energetic musical marketplace, a craftsman, a businessman, and a family man, as well as a spiritual being. Renewed studies of his music are being made with a much more extensive knowledge of both his contemporaries and the structures and practices of the cultures in which he lived. As a result, not only the "timeless" but the modern and forward-looking qualities of his personal style have been rediscovered and celebrated: his attention to sonority and color, his interest in vertical as well as linear sound, his use of large-scale sonic groupings and contrasts and polychorality, his elegant "finish"—the seemingly effortless art that conceals study, that quality so prized by Renaissance culture—and his sophisticated attention to text setting.

In a postmodern era dominated by unpredictability, unceasing change, continuous readjustment, and overwhelming cultural irony, Palestrina's music retains an immutable quality that may be one of its great current attractions. It seems to possess a magical combination of exquisite technical comprehensibility and a certain indefinable "otherness." Perhaps, in the wave of the 'new age' phenomenon, some of the present attraction of Palestrina's music may be due less to the association of his name with certain traditions than to the sense of its *differentness*—to the sense that it is not really of our time. How else to explain *Sicut cervus* being played on the boombox as "cooled-out" mood music for Generation Xers while they throw steaks on the barbecue of a summer evening? Perhaps it is the case, as James Erb has suggested, that notwithstanding the magnificent range and breathtaking technique of even an Orlando di Lasso, Palestrina has managed to keep an image of posthumous preeminence (whether deserved or not) over Lasso, among many others, precisely because Palestrina's music is less turbulent and more predictable in its parameters. *These* qualities, surely, seem to be different from the life of our time. Indeed, the minutest aspects of Palestrina's technique have been pondered, literally, for centuries. But the precise relationship between Palestrina's personality and his music remains elusive, and that very elusiveness has created a defense against final deconstruction and postmodern fatigue.

One of the recent remarkable discoveries about Palestrina is that, for a composer whose entire *oeuvre*, more or less, has been available in collected editions for a century, the range of prospective research options and projects yet to be done is remarkably wide. Over the course of his research Noel O'Regan has pointed out the challenges in the area of source work alone, where there is an ongoing need to establish manuscript and print traditions of music and to review documents. In her dissertation on a group of Palestrina's imitation masses, Veronica Franke has pointed out the need to address the difficult problems of establishing a proper chronology of the composer's works: "The problem [of mass chronology] . . . remains almost entirely unresolved. The dates of few masses can be ascertained. The majority were published posthumously and had been in manuscript for many years. Stylistic elements in certain masses as well as comments in some of the composer's formal letters of dedication would seem to indicate that a fair number of the masses published during Palestrina's lifetime were composed well before their appearance in print" [Item E0232].

There have been excellent studies since 1975 of aspects of Palestrina's compositional process, although much remains to be done with respect to his imitation technique, his recomposition of model material, and parody procedures—not only those in masses but in other genres cultivated in his time. In recent years several scholars have explored the liturgical and paraliturgical use of particular genres, notably spiritual madrigals as well as motets in nonchurch contexts. Some notable work has been done with Palestrina's activity for confraternities and devotional processions that has expanded understanding of the cultural uses of music in a variety of social contexts. For that matter, knowledge of the practical liturgical uses of Palestrina's motets might benefit from further investigation. In addition, it would be profitable to build upon some of the recent work on performance practice in this repertory—its resources, vocal techniques, and ornamentation—not only to enhance performances in our time, but to understand better how the execution of Palestrina's music has been understood in the past.

The present Composer Resource Manual is meant to facilitate some of the preliminary steps required for general or more specialized research in any of these suggested directions. It presents a picture of primary sources, modern editions, current secondary literature, and the history of recordings of Palestrina's music. It is also designed in part to provide a digest of the secondary literature, much of which is in languages other than English, in order to assist researchers with acquiring some control over a wide-ranging body of material. It is intended for use by students, researchers, and scholars as well as practical musicians (primarily choral directors) involved in the preparation of performances of Palestrina's music. Items are identified by unique sigla that are identified and explained in the List of Abbreviations, page xv, and cross-listed in the indexes.

Chapter 1 contains a biographical outline of the composer's life and activities in chronological order, based primarily on documentary sources. For researchers desiring a more integrated or comprehensive biography, full studies can be located in the "Biographical Literature" section of the annotated bibliography in chapter 6.

Chapter 2 lists primary printed sources for Palestrina's music dating approximately from before 1700. A remarkably large proportion of the composer's *oeuvre* was printed during his lifetime, sometimes clearly under his supervision, or within a few years of his death by his immediate heirs. A number of these prints, particularly those associated with Dorico, can be considered as reliable representations of the composer's text, as he himself is believed to have had an editorial or supervisory function in their preparation. The list is based on RISM, the collection and examination of individual prints, and library catalogues. The lists in this chapter include prints in anthologies dating from before 1700, as well as prints and significant printed examples found in published theoretical treatises and in studies of counterpoint or of musical style dating from before 1800. Here, and throughout the text, irregularities in Latin and Italian spellings in the primary sources have been preserved unless otherwise indicated.

Chapter 3 is a provisional checklist of primary manuscript sources for Palestrina's music. It includes works that circulated and remained in manuscript; manuscript copies of prints that were used usually for local ferial liturgical practice, when this can be determined, and works attributed to the composer but that, on examination of available evidence, are doubtful or questionable. I have not separated manuscript copies of printed material from copies that belong distinctly to a circulating manuscript tradition. This area is very problematic and yet it clearly holds important evidence on chronology and performance tradition. Generally speaking, I have attempted to include significant manuscript music clearly datable up to about 1700 and some post-1700 manuscript material associated with certain relatively well-documented and catalogued traditions such as that of the Sistine itself. I have excluded most later eighteenth- and nineteenth-century manuscript material, including scorings and arrangements made of the composer's music by amateurs and scholars. This includes most of the indisputably important material by Martini, Santini, Proske, and others, unless it represents otherwise undocumented or poorly documented music possibly associated with Palestrina. Explanations are provided as necessary.

Chapters 4 and 5 present listings of modern printed editions of Palestrina's music that have been published since approximately 1770. Chapter 4 is essentially a register of the "Haberl" and "Casimiri" comprehensive editions, including a complete list of their contents with page numbers and information on reprintings. It also includes descriptions of the presently available volumes in the series of primary-source photoreproductions that the Palestrina Foundation began to publish in 1975. Chapter 5 is in two sections, the first listing items from collected editions, sets, and anthologies, while the second is a selective list of individual publications. Whenever possible, disposition, performance indications, and special remarks are added. Included here are a number of pedagogical works on classical vocal polyphony, because they may contain extensive musical examples; there is some overlap in this case with material in the annotated bibliography in chapter 6. A number of unusual nineteenth-century arrangements of works are included here as evidence of performance traditions (either of a place or of a performer) that in very recent years have been the subject of articles in the secondary literature. These materials are often of genuine scholarly interest, even if they would not be recognized as "editions of choice" for present-day performing groups.

Chapter 6 is an annotated bibliography of secondary literature. This contains citations from sources in English, German, Italian, French, Spanish, and Latin, together with occasional entries in other languages if a translation or summary in one of the listed languages is provided. It deals primarily with books, journal articles or articles in compendia or *Festschriften*, and doctoral dissertations. A more general book is included if it is dedicated to a clearly Palestrina-related topic or contains a substantial portion of relevant material or a passage of importance for reception history. Items from newspapers and reviews of books or other items such as recordings have been omitted unless a review contains significant independent writing or presents new information that annotates another source. The listing originated in the collation of a number of shorter and/or unannotated bibliographies, plus an independent general search for literature after 1950. General bibliographies consulted include Lino Bianchi's "Bibliografia brevis" in his *Palestrina nella vita, nelle opere, nel tempo* (Palestrina, 1996, pp. 911–913); Michael Heinemann's in his *Giovanni Pierluigi da Palestrina und seine Zeit* (Laaber, 1994, pp. 285–309); Knud Jeppesen's in his article on Palestrina in the first edition of *Die Musik in Geschichte und Gegenwart* (1962); Lewis Lockwood's in his article on Palestrina for *The New Grove Dictionary of Music and Musicians* (1980); Peter Lüttig's in his *Der Palestrina-Stil als Satzideal* (Tützing, 1994); and Giancarlo Rostirolla's dedicated "Bibliografia palestriniana" in *La casa di Giovanni Pierluigi da Palestrina* (Palestrina, 1986, pp. 213–259), as well as its amplified and updated version, *Bibliografia degli scritti su Giovanni Pierluigi da Palestrina (1568–1996)* (Palestrina, 1997). Searches for literature after 1950 were performed in RILM, *The Music Index,* the *Social Sciences and Humanities Index*, OCLC, National Union Catalog, British Union Catalogue, and *Doctoral Dissertations in Musicology*. The bibliography represents a significant percentage of the available literature, but it remains selective. Needless to say, given the specified research parameters, a sizable amount of material was disqualified that may be of interest to some serious researchers, who are encouraged to consult some of the additional bibliographies listed here. Some judgment calls also had to be made, of course. Items which in the present author's opinion were clearly peripheral, unoriginal, poorly written, repetitive, or factually insubstantial, or did not contribute usefully to Palestrina reception history were eliminated, save for a few peculiar items included—with an explanation—because they seemed representative of a type. I apologize in advance for inconvenience caused by the absence of any more important items that may have escaped my notice or did not fall within my parameters for inclusion.

This bibliography is divided into four primary sections: 1) Selected studies offering historical background on musical, social, and cultural life in sixteenth-century Italy that offer useful information or insight into the contexts of Palestrina's creative, intellectual, social, and personal life; 2) Biographical literature, consisting of full-length works and selected source studies, documents, and iconographical items. The citations of full-length biographical studies can be profitably examined in association with those for reception history, with careful attention to publication dates and milieux of origin; 3)

Studies of sources, music, and style, involving citations of works dealing with aspects of individual works, characteristics of genres, works of style analysis, music history, or music history as applied to Palestrina's *oeuvre*. This section also contains historical research on performance conditions and practices as they would have applied in Palestrina's time; 4) Reception history, embracing how Palestrina influenced, and how his influence has been assessed by, others. These items have been sorted roughly by date of origin or the time frame they address, although there are inevitably items that overlap, and a certain fogginess in the boundaries between subsections. They are divided roughly into the periods dating from Palestrina's lifetime to about 1750; from about 1750 to about 1914; from 1914 to the present. Included in this last category, in addition to assessments as such, are items dealing with questions concerning the performance of Palestrina's music in a late-twentieth-century context.

With respect to nineteenth-century reception history, the present author has had to treat two topics with great selectivity. The personalities and activities of the Cecilian movement form a major topic in themselves. I have included literature if the item was directly relevant to image-making about Palestrina; the recovery, editing, and performance of his music; if his music was used as a direct model for the work of another composer; or if the item provided contemporary critical insight into the relevance of the actual style to the musical or cultural life of the period. Items such as full-length biographical studies of ecclesiastics nominally associated with Cecilianism, for instance, have not been included, even if Palestrina is mentioned at times. The other topic involves the literature about Hans Pfitzner's "musical legend," the opera *Palestrina*. The bibliography does not survey the literature on this work. I have, however, included a few items that deal with quotations or reworkings of Palestrina's music within the opera or that discuss how the image of Palestrina was refracted through nineteenth-century issues of solitary genius, integrity, the defense of art, and so forth, as found in Pfitzner's work. This material—especially Pfitzner's own comments on these subjects—falls clearly within the topic of Palestrina reception.

Chapter 7 contains a discography of Palestrina's music, providing coverage of European and North American recordings made since 1900. It has often been said how rapidly a discography can become outdated, how full of erroneous information, and how confusing the history of a recorded performance can be in the retelling. I can only hope that this doubtless incomplete discography is not a monument to the truth of those observations. It is arranged in alphabetical order according to the name of the recording company, beneath which are provided citations as complete as my direct examination of discs and information resources allowed, including a list of the Palestrina works recorded. The reader is directed to search the title index for the work for which a recording is sought, and to follow the sigla cited there back to the main discography. As I have not been able to hear all of these recordings personally, I have annotated a few post-1960 recordings as well as certain older ones of particular historical interest, for choral directors desiring to gain ideas of style in performance, or for students and instructors who wish to document and study aspects of music and style.

However one regards this particular effort at discography, careful study of the Palestrina recorded repertory has its own fascinations. Through recordings alone, the history of various national performing traditions for Palestrina's music can readily be followed and analyzed—Italian, German, and British especially. Performance practices can be traced not only nationally but chronologically, even to the very beginning of the twentieth century, right to the very heart of the tradition: the Sistine Chapel itself. Apparently the very earliest extant and available recording of Palestrina's music is (to present sensibilities) the rather strange—and yet historically priceless—performance from 1904 of Palestrina's madrigal *La cruda mia nemica*, which included Alessandro Moreschi, the only true castrato known to have been recorded in the West.

In the preparation of this guide, I have had the great good fortune to benefit from the assistance and advice of many people and numerous institutions. For their kindness I would like to acknowledge the Edward Johnson Library of the University of Toronto, where much of the initial research for this project was carried out, with special thanks to Kathleen McMorrow, John Fodi, Suzanne Meyers Sawa, and all the other members of the staff; to my gracious colleague Vivien Taylor, of the Music Library and Special Collections at Queen's University, Kingston, for her generous help and advice on organizing and accessing the information in this manual. My gratitude also goes to the staff of the Queen's University Music Library, especially Susan Chan and Paula Werden, for their constant cheerful help and their kindness and patience with a very demanding client; and to the music libraries and staff of the Loeb Music Library of Harvard University; the Sterling Music Library, Beinecke Rare Book and Manuscript Library, and the Seeley W. Mudd Library, all of Yale University; and the Library of Congress, Washington, DC.

Additional thanks to the numerous libraries in Europe where I made my initial first-hand acquaintance with much primary and secondary material referenced in this volume, especially to the Biblioteca Apostolica Vaticana, Rome, the Civico Museo Bibliografico Musicale, Bologna, and the British Library, London; to Professor Noel O'Regan of the University of Edinburgh, for responding to several queries and for his kind encouragement; to Ms. Susan Rosenstein and the Hispanic Society of America for providing me with information on several manuscripts of Hispanic provenance; to Leo Balk of Garland Publishing, who initially agreed to this project, and to my editors at Garland and Routledge, who helped me in many ways, showed much patience, and probably saved me from many a folly. All have my heartfelt thanks.

To Tim Berners-Lee and the world of electronic communications, and to Chester Carlson, inventor of photocopying, my thanks for their indispensible aid and comfort to me as a researcher.

Finally, whatever is good in this work is dedicated with gratitude and affection to three people:

To Professor Mary Ann Parker of the University of Toronto for her encouragement, and whose ongoing friendship and mentorship I cherish; to the memory of Al Raskin, a wise and able man of boundless generosity who always expressed a genuine interest in whatever I was doing (or said I was doing); and, as always, to Lawrie Raskin, who continues somehow to put up with household chaos and my long hours and has offered constant good-humored support to this project. By now, he *sure* knows who Palestrina is.

CLARA MARVIN
Queen's University, Kingston, Ontario

Abbreviations

Guide to the Enumeration Classes Used in this Volume

A Early printed editions of music: dedicated prints, anthologies, collections, theoretical or didactic works (chapter 2)
B Manuscript sources (chapter 3)
C Comprehensive editions (chapter 4)
D Modern editions of printed music: sets, anthologies, series, and individual items (chapter 5)
E Bibliography (chapter 6)
F Discography (chapter 7)

The siglum letter is followed by a number pertaining to the individual item, thereby indicating both its unique identity and conveying general information about its type (printed, manuscript, sound recording, etc.). It is also designed to offer more immediate recognition of a type of source referenced in an Index listing.

Abbreviations

4to	quarto
5	quintus, quinta pars, quinto, fifth part
6	sextus, sesta pars, sesto, sixth part
8vo	octavo, ottavo
A, a, alt	alto
arr	arranged by, arrangement
B, b, bas	bass
Bar, bar	baritone
bc	basso continuo
Cas	*Palestrina Works*, ed. Raffaele Casimiri, et al. (1939–present)
c, ca.	circa
ed	edition, edited by
Eitner	Robert Eitner, *Quellen-Lexicon* (repr. Graz 1959)
facs	facsimile
Hab	Palestrina *Works*, ed. Haberl, et al. (1862–1907)
MGG	*Die Musik in Geschichte und Gegenwart* (first edition)
MS, ms	manuscript
mot	motet
NdA	*Note d'Archivio* (journal)
p, pp	page, pages
repr	reprint, reprinted
rev	revised, revised edition

RILM	*Répertoire Internationale de la Littérature Musicale*
RISM	*Répertoire Internationale des Sources Musicales*
S, s, sop	soprano
SATB	soprano, alto, tenor, bass
SATB56	soprano, alto, tenor, bass, quinto, sesto
T, t, ten	tenor
trans	translation, translated by
treb	treble

Giovanni Pierluigi da Palestrina

Chapter 1

Chronology and Biographical Outline

Part I: 1525–1544

Giovanni Pierluigi is born, probably between February 3, 1525 and February 2, 1526, either in the town of Palestrina or in Rome, to Santo (also spelled Sante) Pierluigi and his wife, Palma. The precise date of the child's birth remains unknown, but the obituary written by Melchior Major describes him as having lived sixty-eight years. It has been suggested that his birthday might have been December 27, the feast day of the composer's name saint, John (Heinemann 1994). In a Roman census in early 1527, one "Santo de Prenestino" is listed as head of a household of twelve in the rione Monti, a neighborhood near the church of St. John Lateran (Casimiri 1918–1922).

The first documentary evidence of his life is in the form of a will made on October 22, 1527 by his paternal grandmother, Jacobella (Cametti 1903). In the will she divided her estate among her four children, two sisters, a daughter-in-law Palma (Santo's wife), and "il piccolo Giovanni," her grandson. The particular mention of Giovanni suggests that he may have been a firstborn grandchild (Bianchi 1995 [E0079]).

On January 16, 1536, the composer's mother, Palma Pierluigi dies.

A contract dated October 25, 1537 lists "Giovanni da Palestrina" as the second of six *pueri chorialis* at Santa Maria Maggiore (Casimiri 1918–1922) entitled to receive musical instruction and an education as well as clothing and care. Hypothetically, he may have entered the basilica as early as 1533, for the typical age of admission for such children was around six to eight years of age. The music masters at the basilica in the period 1538–1540 included Rubino Mallapert (1538–1539), "Robert" (perhaps Robert de Fevin), and Firmin Le Bel (1540).

On May 11, 1540, Santo Pierluigi, Giovanni's widowed father, married Maria Gismondi. Five children were eventually born of the marriage.

Part II: 1544–1571

1544–1549 A contract dated October 28, 1544 indicates that "Giovanni figlio di Sante Pietro Aloisio da Palestrina" has been engaged as an organist at the church of San Agapito in Palestrina. He was required to play the organ on feast days and to lead the choir at mass, vespers, and compline. He was also expected to instruct the clergy in plainchant or else to undertake the musical education of some of the choirboys (Casimiri 1924; see item E0105). Further documentation of Giovanni's professional activities in Palestrina is lacking until 1551.

On December 13, 1545, the Council of Trent (the Nineteenth General Council of the church) is opened.

On June 12, 1547, Palestrina marries Lucrezia Gori, the daughter of the deceased Francesco de Goris. On November 7, the couple receive a dowry of 130 florins from the estate of Lucrezia's father, while on November 16 the division of property is made, and Lucrezia receives various household items from her family inheritance. Sancta Gori, Lucrezia's mother, dies on December 13.

In Rome, Philip Neri with Persiano Rosa founds the confraternity of SS. Trinità dei Pellegrini in 1548, while Marcello Cervini (afterwards pope) becomes head of the Vatican Library.

Lucrezia and Giovanni's son Rodolfo is born sometime in 1549 or 1550 (and dies in 1572).

1550 On February 8, after an extended conclave due to political conditions, Cardinal Giovanni Maria Ciocchi del Monte (bishop of Palestrina) is elected Pope Julius III. The new pope's successor in the bishopric of Palestrina, Cardinal Luigi Borbone, names Giovanni Pierluigi as organist and *maestro di cappella* at San Agapito.

1551–1553 Palestrina's second son Angelo is born (dies 1571). On September 1, Pope Julius III appoints the composer *maestro di cappella* at the Cappella Giulia (San Pietro). He receives a salary of 10 scudi per month, plus four more for the maintenance of two choirboys. Mallapert meanwhile leaves the Vatican to assume another position at Santa Maria Maggiore. Together with the chapel choir, Palestrina probably also participates in confraternity, processional, and other extramural activities. Some Magnificat and other works are datable to this early Vatican period, around 1552.

1554 Palestrina publishes *Missarum liber primus* [Dorico] with a dedication to Pope Julius III (Giovanni Maria del Monte). This is the first single publication of masses issued in Rome by a native Italian composer. In the same year, the madrigal *Con dolce altiero* appears in a Venetian anthology published by Gardano.

1555 On January 13, Palestrina is admitted to the Sistine Chapel at the command of Pope Julius, in spite of being married and without being examined or with the consent of the singers. As he was not considered to have a particularly good voice, he was most likely admitted on the basis of already demonstrated compositional skill (Sherr 1994). On March 23, however, Julius III dies, and on April 9 he is succeeded by the humanist cardinal Marcello Cervini, who takes the name Marcellus II. On April 12, three days after his election, as reported in the diary of Angelo Massarelli, the new pope's private secretary, Marcellus admonishes the papal singers to sing the divine services "with properly modulated voices, and . . . in such a way that everything could be heard and understood." However, after a pontificate of only three weeks, Marcellus dies (April 30). He is succeeded on May 23 by Giovanni Pietro Caraffa, Pope Paul IV.

Beginning in mid-July, the composer apparently suffers from a serious illness for several weeks.

On July 30, a decretal is issued forbidding the presence of married singers in the chapel membership. In September, Palestrina and two other married singers are dismissed from the Cappella Sistina as the chapel's rule requiring celibacy of its members is enforced. He receives a pension, however. But on

October 1, he is named *maestro di cappella* of St. John Lateran, the pope's episcopal seat, where he remains until 1560. His payment is 6 scudi per month.

During this year, *Il primo libro di madrigali a quattro voci* is published by Dorico.

1556 Between 1556 and 1561, Palestrina composes versions of the Improperia and Lamentations (MS Lateran 59). In 1556, the town of Palestrina is sacked by troops of the duke of Alba, enemy of the Caraffa, the current pope's family. The tragedy is apparently compounded by devastation caused by weather conditions. It is possible that early documentation of the Pierluigi family is lost at this time.

1557 On May 30, the composer, together with his sons Rodolfo and Angelo, receives the rights of Roman citizens.

In July, another sack of the town of Palestrina occurs, this time by troops of Marcantonio Colonna, an ally of the duke of Alba. The destruction continues for three weeks. Some of Palestrina's relatives, including his father, are in the town or have fled from it.

1558 The composer's son Iginio is born (dies 1610).

In addition to his other duties, Palestrina imports wine from his hometown to the Lateran.

1559 Palestrina's father, Santo, apparently dies around this time, for a cross is noted next to his name on a list of members of the Compagnia del Corpo di Cristo in Palestrina.

Pope Paul IV dies; as he was feared as the founder of the Inquisition, the news of his death is received joyously. In December, Giovanni Angelo Medici is elected as Pope Pius IV.

1560 Near the end of July, Palestrina is in disagreement with the chapter of St. John Lateran over salaries and over the costs of instructing the *pueri*, and on August 3, he abruptly leaves the post. His son Rodolfo, a choirboy, leaves with him.

Cardinal Carlo Borromeo (nephew of Pope Pius IV) is appointed papal secretary of state and archbishop of Milan.

1561 On March 1, Palestrina enters employment at Santa Maria Maggiore. He receives 16 scudi per month for his services and for the upkeep of four of the chapel's choirboys.

The composer has legal dealings with officials in the town of Palestrina, apparently connected with the settlement and distribution of his father's estate.

1562 In the town of Palestrina, Palma Pierluigi, the composer's sister, marries Giovanni di Tommaso Bovis, and the composer provides a dowry for the marriage. This may be more indirect evidence that the composer was an eldest son who effectively became head of the family on his father's death.

During this year, there is an exchange of music between Rome and

Munich, involving cardinals Borromeo and Vitelli in Rome and Duke Albrecht V of Bavaria. In November, Palestrina's music, particularly a *Missa Benedicta*, is sent to Munich through agency of Cardinal Truchsess von Waldburg.

1563 In addition to his other duties, the composer takes part in processional activities outside Santa Maria Maggiore.

On September 17, the twenty-third session of the Council of Trent addresses music in church: "*Ab ecclesiis vero musicas, ubi sive organo sive cantu lascivum aut impurum aliquid misceatur, arceant (ordinarii locorum) ut domus Dei vere domus orationis esse videatur ac dici possit.*" In the twenty-fourth council session on November 11, decisions regarding the implementation of the decretal of September 17 are expressly referred to the discretion of bishops within their own respective dioceses.

Formal adjournment of the Council of Trent.

1564 Palestrina's *Motecta festorum* is published with a dedication to Cardinal Rodolfo Pio Carpi. In his prefatory remarks, Palestrina describes his use of antiphons and his avoidance of all secular or questionable melodic content as the basis for his motet material.

From July to September, Palestrina works for Cardinal Ippolito II d'Este as *maestro dei concerti*, receiving an honorarium of 6 scudi.

In October, the composer's recently married sister Palma dies. He travels to Palestrina, where on October 26 he makes a formal declaration that Palma's dowry has reverted to him.

Appointment of commission of cardinals by Pope Pius IV (including Cardinals Borromeo and Vitelli) to carry out decrees of Trent within Rome.

1565 Between January and August, a commission of cardinals, including Carlo Borommeo and Vitellozzi Vitelli, negotiates with the singers of the papal chapel on size of its membership, salaries, and regulations. In September, Borromeo leaves Rome permanently for Milan.

On January 20, Cardinal Borromeo orders his vicar in Milan "to reform the singing so that the words may be as intelligible as possible."

On February 1, the Seminario Romano (for the formation of priests) is opened by Francesco Borgia. Palestrina does some work for the institution.

On March 10, Borromeo sends an order to Vincenzo Ruffo, *maestro di cappella* at the Milan Cathedral, for a mass "that should be as clear as possible and send it to me here [in Rome]."

The Sistine diaries record that on April 28, the singers of the papal chapel "were assembled in the home of Cardinal [Vitelli] to sing some masses and test whether the words could be understood, as their Eminences desire." It is possible, although uncertain, that the *Missa Papae Marcelli* was among the music performed.

The diaries also record that on June 6, 3 scudi, 13 baiocchi were paid to Palestrina for the composition and preparation of several works for the use of the chapel musicians. The pope also bestows on Palestrina the title *modulator pontificus* (papal composer). Records of the Sistine Chapel indicate that Palestrina's pension is increased "owing to certain compositions he has written and is to write for the use of the chapel." He now receives 9 scudi per month and has a position among the active singers. (Jeppesen MGG 1962). In October, Palestrina is paid by the papal chapel for "various musical compositions that he has had copied for the chapel and is to have copied."

1566 Palestrina teaches music at the Seminario Romano (Casimiri 1935; see E0013) until 1571. On April 17, his two older sons, Rodolfo and Angelo, enter the seminary as students, probably for the next five years, to receive instruction in music, Latin and Greek, logic, and philosophy, and probably as partial recompense for the composer's services. (After Rodolfo's early death, he is described as accomplished in all these areas and could also play "all sorts of instruments.")

At the death of Pope Pius IV, Michele Ghislieri is elected as Pius V. He pursues seriously the ongoing reformation of the liturgy. Revisions of the catechism and breviary appear.

Palestrina's portrait is painted in this year; it currently survives in a private collection and is known as the "Gorga–de Rensis" portrait.

1567 During Holy Week (April), Palestrina is involved in music for services at St. John Lateran, suggesting that he may no longer be working at Santa Maria Maggiore (although documentation for this is lacking).

On August 1, Palestrina enters the full-time service of Cardinal Ippolito II d'Este, which continues until March 1571.

On November 8, Palestrina is approached by agents of Emperor Maximilian II of Austria with an offer to become *maestro* of the imperial chapel in Vienna. Palestrina makes a counteroffer asking for a salary of 400 scudi per annum. Negotiations eventually break down when Palestrina's terms are found to be too high. (In May of the following year, Philippe de Monte, who was being considered before Palestrina entered the negotiations, is hired at a salary of 300 scudi plus some payments in kind.)

In this year Dorico publishes Palestrina's second book of masses. In the preface dedicating these works to Philip II of Spain, the composer stresses their new method of composition.

1568 In this year, a remarkable exchange of correspondence begins between Palestrina and Duke Guglielmo Gonzaga of Mantua, which continues until Guglielmo's death in 1587.

On February 2, by way of the Mantuan agent Annibale Capello, Palestrina sends Duke Guglielmo some masses commissioned for the private use of his chapel, noting "I beg you to let me know how you prefer it: whether long or short or composed so that the words may be understood." The masses use an *alternatim* technique, with chant specially composed for the Mantuan liturgy alternating with Palestrina's polyphonic sections.

In a letter dated May 1, Duke Guglielmo sends an honorarium of 50 ducats for the masses.

On July 31, Cardinal Scipio Gonzaga, titular bishop of Jerusalem and the brother of Duke Guglielmo, sends to Mantua copies of some motets by Palestrina which he has heard in Rome. The composer receives a commission for new works on texts selected by the duke, which due to illness are not dispatched to Mantua until December.

In *Fronimo* (published in Venice by Scotto), Vincenzo Galilei publishes an intabulation of Palestrina's madrigal *Io son ferito*, citing the work for its skillful expression of text through musical means.

1569 The first book of motets for five to seven voices, dedicated to Cardinal Ippolito d'Este, is published by Dorico with a preface dated May 7 of this year.

On May 8, Palestrina signs a contract with the brothers Marzio and Vincenzo Ceci for the purchase of a house at Via dei Giubbonari in Rome for 725 scudi. He probably lived there from 1566, and some part of the purchase price may have been paid in the intervening years.

1570 Sometime before March 3, Duke Guglielmo sends Palestrina some motets and a madrigal of his composition with a request for a critique by the composer.

On March 3, in response to Guglielmo's request, Palestrina gives his opinion and suggestions, in the course of which he discusses matters of voice-leading as well as the challenges of making a text set to polyphony audible to the listener.

In this year, the third book of masses is published by Dorico with a dedication to Philip II of Spain, whose daughter has just married Maximilian II of Austria. Heinemann suggests that this might have been a move on the composer's part to attract the renewed bounty of a previously generous patron at a time when Palestrina's personal financial situation may have been strained.

Part III: 1571–1594 and Aftermath

1571 In April, after the death of Animuccia on March 25, Palestrina returns to the post of *maestro di cappella* in the Cappella Sistina, then under the patronage of the chapel's patron director Cardinal Alessandro Farnese. The composer is contracted to receive 100 scudi per annum (8 scudi, 33 baiocchi per month), plus 12 scudi for the use of his house for the care of four choirboys. Cardinal Alessandro Farnese becomes patron director of the Capella Giulia.

On December 4, a triumphal procession is held in Rome to mark the victory at Lepanto on October 7. Palestrina probably writes the madrigal *Le selv'avea* (pub. 1574) for this event.

In this year, there is the possible, although unproved, development of a relationship with Filippo Neri. Palestrina may have composed some works for Neri's oratory.

The composer, his wife, and their children, as well as other persons living in the household, are mentioned in the Roman census taken this year.

1572 Guglielmo Gonzaga visits Rome and meets Palestrina.

In September, Palestrina's second book of motets (published by Scotto in Venice) appears with a dedication to Guglielmo Gonzaga. It contains works for the special Mantuan liturgy as well as music by Palestrina's sons Rodolfo and Angelo and his brother Silla. Duke Guglielmo in return sends a gift of 25 scudi.

On November 20, Palestrina's apparently gifted son Rodolfo dies.

Pope Pius V dies, and Ugo Buoncompagni is elected Pope Gregory XIII.

1573 On January 1, the composer's brother Silla dies.

Angelo Pierluigi marries Doralice Uberti, the niece of a neighbor of Palestrina's, Giacomo Uberti. She brings a dowry of 1,000 scudi to be paid in installments. Palestrina apparently invests this dowry money in property.

During the summer the composer visits the town of Palestrina.

1574 In a letter dated April 7, Palestrina mentions that he is writing Lamentations for the use of the papal chapel.

On April 17, Palestrina returns to Guglielmo Gonzaga a mass composed by the duke and sent to the composer for a critical review.

In a letter of June 5, he describes payments for and the purchase of a house in Rome.

On November 7, Aurelia, the first child of Doralice Uberti and Angelo Pierluigi, is born.

Late in the year, the composer writes the motet *Jubilate Deo à 8* for the opening of the Holy Door, which inaugurates the Holy Year 1575. The work is published in 1576.

1575 In diplomatic correspondence of this year, the agent of the duke of Ferrara writes that Palestrina is "now considered the very first musician in the world."

On February 9, Palestrina informs Duke Guglielmo by letter that some texts for which he has requested settings have been completed.

On April 14, the payment records of the Cappella Giulia indicate that Lamentations by Palestrina were copied for the use of the chapel.

On December 11, the composer's son Angelo dies during an epidemic of influenza that began in July and killed about 10,000 people in Rome.

In this year, Palestrina's salary at St. Peter's is increased to 240 scudi per annum, possibly to prevent his transferring to Santa Maria Maggiore.

Palestrina also dedicates a third book of motets (published in Venice by Scotto) to Alfonso d'Este, brother of his now-deceased patron Cardinal Ippolito.

1576 On January 14, Doralice Uberti, the widow of Angelo Pierluigi, gives birth to a posthumous son, Angelo.

1577 Doralice Uberti remarries and requires restitution of the dowry payments contracted for her first marriage to Palestrina's late son. Palestrina apparently has some liquidation difficulties and has a mortgage on the ground floor of his house, but the matter is resolved on July 3, when his eighteen-year-old son Iginio contracts to marry Virginia Guarnacci, who brings with her a dowry of 1,500 scudi. The wedding takes place on August 15.

On October 25, Palestrina and Annibale Zoilo are entrusted with the revisions of the plainchant of the Roman Gradual and Antiphoner by Pope Gregory XIII (Ugo Buoncompagni). Palestrina was responsible for work on the *proprium de tempore*, while Zoilo addressed the feasts of the saints. They were charged with removal of the "superfluities . . . barbarisms and obscurities" from these books. Palestrina evidently worked earnestly at this task for a few years, but then his activity apparently diminished. The revisions were eventually completed by Francesco Soriano and Felice Anerio in 1614 to 1615 and published as the *Editio Medicea*.

1578 Duke Guglielmo commissions Palestrina to write a series of masses based on chant which had been specially composed for the Mantuan liturgy. Completion is delayed when Palestrina suffers from a serious illness in October, but the first mass is delivered by way of the Mantuan commissioner for Rome, Annibale Capello, on November 1. Two weeks later another is sent, and in December four settings are sung in Mantua.

Gregory XIII reorganizes the Sistine Chapel into two choirs of twelve singers each. Although the regulation stipulating that singers must be unmarried remains in place, Palestrina's position as composer for the papal chapel is confirmed.

On November 5, in a letter to Duke Guglielmo, Palestrina mentions his work on the revision of the Gradual and purgation of the chant of "barbarisms and bad sounds."

On November 23, Tommaso Pierluigi, the first child of Iginio Pierluigi and Virginia Guarnacci (who together would eventually have ten children), is baptized. Palestrina's patron, Cardinal Guglielmo Sirleto, is the boy's godfather.

In this year, Palestrina receives a payment of 80 scudi (partially payments in kind or produce) for musical services to the Confraternità della Trinità dei Pellegrini.

1579 In a letter of March 21, Palestrina thanks Duke Guglielmo for receipt of 100 scudi, and with the letter sends three more masses to Mantua.

1580 On June 16, Gregorio, son of Iginio Pierluigi and Virginia Guarnacci, is born.

On August 2, Lucrezia Gori, Palestrina's wife, dies suddenly during an epidemic. She is buried in the Cappella Nova in St. Peter's.

On November 13, Pope Gregory XIII receives Palestrina's petition for ordination to the priesthood. On December 7, the composer receives minor orders and the tonsure in San Silvestro al Quirinale, whose patron is his friend Cardinal Sirleto.

1581 On January 18, Palestrina, still apparently planning to enter the priesthood, is named *chierico perpetuo beneficiato* at the cathedral of Santa Maria Maggiore. The prebend, which carries with it no duties, provides an annual income of 24 scudi.

On February 24 and 26 and March 5, however, banns are published indicating that the composer is contemplating remarriage. On March 28, with little advance warning, Palestrina marries Virginia Dormoli, the widow of the papal fur merchant Giuliano Guerrazzi, who had died in 1576 at the age of thirty-six. The marriage takes place in the Dormoli house (rather than a church) by special permission, and the couple settle in their own house on via Armellino. It is evidently an advantageous match for both parties and finally provides the composer economic security. Virginia brings to her marriage with the now internationally renowned Palestrina a dowry of 1,500 scudi, and he in turn will play an important role in the management of her fur and wine businesses.

Gregorio Pierluigi, the year-old son of Iginio, dies on June 21 and is buried in the Cappella Nova with other members of his family.

Aurelia Pierluigi and Angelo Pierluigi, the composer's two grandchildren by Doralice Uberti and his late son Angelo, also die within a short period of one another in August and September.

1582 On September 25, Palestrina buys a parcel of land in the town of Palestrina from Pietro Paolo Appolloni.

In October, Pope Gregory XIII's calendar reform is implemented; eleven days are added, and October 4 is followed the next day by October 15.

1583 The Mantuan ambassador to Rome indicates that Duke Guglielmo is looking for a new *maestro di cappella*. After considering alternative candidates, Palestrina enters into discussion with Guglielmo in March about the possibility of transferring to Mantua himself as *maestro*. The composer may have seriously considered the move but ultimately found the inducement to leave Rome insufficient.

A letter to Mantua states that Francesco Soriano is among his pupils, and it states that Marenzio is "not greater than Soriano, either in knowledge or in managing musicians."

1584 Formation of the Vertuosa Compagnia de i Musici di Roma, founded under papal auspices for the purposes of fraternal association, the performance of music, and probable job networking. Palestrina becomes one of the members.

At the end of 1583 and beginning of 1584, the composer publishes the fourth book of motets (*Canticum canticorum*) with a dedication to Gregory XIII. Palestrina hastens to send a copy to Guglielmo Gonzaga in April with an inscription.

On July 11, Virginia Dormoli makes a new will, increasing the value of what she plans to leave to her second husband.

1585 Early in the year Palestrina edits and corrects some compositions by Duke Guglielmo. In a letter of March 23, he thanks the duke for the privilege of being allowed to advise him, "even at his advanced age."

On April 10, Pope Gregory XIII dies.

On April 24, Felice Peretti is elected pope, and takes the name Sixtus V.

At this time Palestrina is involved for several months in some conflict with the other papal choirmaster, Antonio Boccapaduli, over privileges. Eventually some singers are expelled from the chapel over this matter.

1586 By September 1, the papal chapel is reorganized: the leader of the chapel will be chosen yearly from among the more senior members. Palestrina remains composer to the chapel while also serving as head of the Cappella Giulia.

The composer takes a partner, Annibale Gagliardi, into his wife's fur business.

1587 On July 6, Palestrina writes his last letter to Duke Guglielmo, who dies on August 14. At the duke's request, the composer has found a Roman bass singer to serve at the Mantuan establishment.

1588 The composer has *Lamentationes* printed. Its dedicatory preface suggests an elegiac, even depressed turn of mind, but he also asserts that "not even under the most difficult circumstances have I neglected the study of music."

1589 The anthology *Le gioie*, a collection of madrigals by members of the Vertuosa Compagnia de i Musici di Roma, assembled by Felice Anerio, is published. Palestrina contributes the madrigal *Dunque perfido amante*.

In the dedication of the volume of hymns published in this year, Palestrina writes: "Nothing . . . is so congenial to me, as to be able to give myself to that study of music . . . when I can abide by my purpose of embracing topics which most fully show forth God's praise, and which, pondered in all their weightiness and dignity of word and idea, and embellished with some amount of musical art, may well move the heart of man to devotion."

1590 A large number of reprints of Palestrina's music are issued from presses in Venice and Milan.

On August 20, Pope Sixtus V dies; Cardinal Giambattista Castagna is named Pope Urban VII, but dies only a few weeks later; Cardinal Niccola Sfondrato becomes Pope Gregory XIV.

1591 On October 15, Pope Gregory XIV dies; Cardinal Antonio Facchinetti is elected Pope Innocent IX and crowned on November 3, but he dies on December 30.

1592 Palestrina receives the dedication of an anthology of vespers psalms for five voices edited by G. M. Asola and containing works by Baccusi, Croce, Gastoldi, and Costanzo Porta.

In *Prattica di musica*, published in Venice in this year, Lodovico Zacconi cites passages from Palestrina's masses *Virtute magna, Ad coenam agni providi*, and *L'homme armé* as valuable studies in compositional problems of proportion and rhythm.

After the death of Pope Innocent IX, Cardinal Ippolito Aldobrandini is elected Pope Clement VIII on January 30 (dies 1605).

1593 Palestrina makes plans to transfer to the post of *maestro di cappella* at San Agapito, the cathedral at Palestrina, the original home of the Pierluigi family.

1594 In the first weeks of January appear the last publications by the composer to be published during his lifetime, the sixth book of masses for four and five voices and the second book of spiritual madrigals.

On February 2, Palestrina dies in Rome. In the records of the Cappella Giulia it is noted: "Giovanni da Palestrina died 2 February and was buried in our basilica." The *puntatore* of the Cappella Sistina recorded: "Wednesday on the 2nd. This morning Sig. Giovanni Pierloisci, the most excellent musician our colleague and master of the Chapel in St. Peter's, passed from this life to a better one. . . . At 24 hours he was borne to the said church, accompanied not only by all the musicians of Rome but also by a multitude of people and, according to our custom, in accord with our constitution, we sang the responsory *Libera me Domine*. . . ." He is buried in the crypt in which lie his first wife, his predeceased sons Rodolfo and Angelo, and other family members. The Sistine diaries note a memorial service held in his honor on February 14. Ruggiero Giovanelli is elected in his place as *maestro di cappella* of the Cappella Giulia, while Felice Anerio takes his place as the papal composer.

As the composer apparently dies intestate (rather surprisingly; his final illness must have been sudden and rapid), Iginio, the sole surviving son, spends the next several months concluding his father's business affairs.

Shortly after the composer's death, Pope Clement VIII indicates interest in having some of Palestrina's unpublished music printed for use in churches. For Palestrina's seventh book of masses, the pope underwrites the publication to the amount of 100 scudi. Most of the posthumous printing of the composer's music, however, does not occur under Clement's direct auspices; but Iginio Pierluigi continues to publish his father's music for several subsequent years.

On March 14, Iginio signs a contract with Raimondi to publish the books of Gregorian chant on which his father worked. This relationship is unsuccessful and devolves into a series of lawsuits. The so-called Medicean edition does not appear until 1614.

On May 30, Gregorio (a younger brother of the Gregorio who died in 1581) and Olimpia, children of Iginio and Virginia, are confirmed in St. Peter's.

1595–1678 Two more children are eventually born to Iginio and Virginia Pierluigi: Caterina in 1597 and Margherita on October 30, 1600 in Palestrina. Late in 1599, with Iginio's agreement, his stepmother Virginia Dormoli has her dowry returned to her. On June 12, 1605, his daughter Caterina is confirmed in St. Peter's.

In 1608, Iginio's wife dies in Palestrina, and after her death, Iginio takes holy orders, becoming a priest in 1609. However, he does not long enjoy his clerical estate; Iginio dies on October 9, 1610. Two months later, on December 10, Virginia Dormoli, the composer's widow, dies and is buried next to her first husband in San Girolamo della Carità.

Immediate descendants of the composer live on in the town of Palestrina until late in the seventeenth century. Iginio's son Tommaso (born 1578), also a priest, becomes a canon of the cathedral there from 1621 until his death in 1633. Tommaso's brother Gregorio marries Maddalena Sepia, and together they have seven children. The fifth child, Agapito, in his turn becomes a priest and canon in Palestrina, where he dies on April 26, 1677, the last direct male survivor in the family, although descendants in the female line survive until circa 1880. The family house in Palestrina remains in the family's possession until 1678. Since the 1960s it has undergone restoration, and it is presently the seat of the Palestrina Foundation.

Chapter 2

Primary Sources: Printed Music

I. Early Editions of Printed Music by Palestrina as Sole Composer

Masses

A0001 [RISM P655] *Missarum liber primus.* Rome: Valerio & Aloysio Dorico, 1554 [choirbook].

1. *Missa Ecce sacerdos magnus a 4* (f.2v)
2. *Missa O regem coeli a 4* (f.21v)
3. *Missa Virtute magna a 4* (f.39v)
4. *Missa Gabriel Archangelus a 4* (f.56v)
5. *Missa Ad cenam Agni providi a 5* (f.74v)

Reprint History

A0002 [RISM P656] *Missarum liber primus.* Rome: heirs of Aloysio Dorico, 1572 [choirbook].

A0003 [RISM P657] *Missarum liber primus quatuor vocum.* Brescia: Tomaso Bozzola, 1581 [shortened version, partbooks].

A0004 [RISM P658] *Missarum cum quatuor, quinque, ac sex vocibus, liber primus.* Rome: Alessandro Gardano ("*impensis Jacobi Tornerij*"), 1591 [enlarged version, partbooks]:

1. *Missa Ecce sacerdos magnus a 4* (p.1)
2. *Missa Virtute magna a 4* (p.7)
3. *Missa O regem coeli a 4* (p.12)
4. *Missa Gabriel Arcangelus a 4* (p.18)
5. *Missa Ad cenam Agni providi a 5* (p.25)
6. *Missa Pro defunctis a 5* (p.29)
7. *Missa sine nomine a 6* (p.32)

A0005 [RISM P659] *Missarum cum quatuor, quinque ac sex vocibus . . . liber primus.* Venice: Angelo Gardano, 1596 [partbooks].

Print Locations

[A0001] Vienna, Österreiches Nationalbibliothek, Musiksammlung [incomplete, with manuscript supplement]; Berlin, Staatsbibliothek; Bologna, Civico Museo Bibliografico Musicale; Cambrai, Bibliothèque municipale; Florence, Biblioteca Nazionale Centrale; Gubbio, Biblioteca Vescovile Fonti e

Archivio; Pesaro, Biblioteca capitolare della Cattedrale Archivio del Duomo; Rome, Biblioteca Musicale governativa del Conservatorio di Santa Cecilia [incomplete, with manuscript supplement]; Rome, Archivio di San Giovanni in Laterano; Vatican City, Biblioteca Apostolica Vaticana, *fondo* Cappella Giulia; Spoleto, Archivio del Duomo; Turin, Archivio capitolare del Duomo [incomplete]; Venice, Biblioteca nazionale Marciana.

[A0002] Brussels, Bibliothèque Royale Albert I; Berlin, Staatsbibliothek; Saragossa, Archivo di música del Cabildo; London, British Library [three exemplars]; Assisi, Biblioteca comunale; Bologna, Civico Museo Bibliografico Musicale; Bergamo, Biblioteca civico “Angelo Maj”; Florence, Biblioteca del Conservatorio di Musica “Luigi Cherubini”; Ferrara, Biblioteca comunale Ariostea; Lucca, Biblioteca del seminario archivescovile; Loreto, Archivio Storico della Cappella Lauretana; Milan, Biblioteca del Conservatorio “Giuseppe Verdi”; Orvieto, Archivio musicale del Duomo; Rome, Biblioteca dell'Accademia nazionale dei Lincei e Corsiniana; Rome, Biblioteca Musicale governativa del Conservatorio di Santa Cecilia; Rome, Archivio capitolare di Santa Maria Maggiore (housed in Biblioteca Apostolica Vaticana); Vatican City, Biblioteca Apostolica Vaticana, *fondo* Cappella Giulia [three exemplars], *ibid.*, *fondo* Cappella Sistina; Reggio Emilia, Biblioteca municipale [two exemplars, one of which lacks title page]; Reggio Emilia, Archivio capitolare di San Prospero [incomplete]; Turin, Archivio capitolare del Duomo; Terni, Istituto Musicale “G. Briccialdi”; Treviso, Archivio della Cappella del Duomo; Urbino, Biblioteca Universitaria; Chicago, Newberry Library; Washington, DC, Library of Congress, Music Division.

[A0003] Munich, Bayerische Staatsbibliothek, Musiksammlung [S,A,T,B]; Rome, Biblioteca Casanatense [S,A,T,B]; Hälsingborg, Fryklund Collection [in care of Stockholm, Kunglinga Musikaliska Akademiens Bibliotek] [S,A].

[A0004] Vienna, Österreiches Nationalbibliothek, Musiksammlung [S,A,T,B,5/6]; Berlin, Staatsbibliothek [S,T]; Münster, Bibliothek des Bischöflichen Priesterseminars und Santini-Sammlung; Regensburg, Bischöfliche Zentralbibliothek (Proske-Musikbibliothek) [S]; London, Royal College of Music [S,A]; Bologna, Civico Museo Bibliografico Musicale; Macerata, Biblioteca comunale “Mozzi-Borgetti” [S,A,5/6]; Rome, Biblioteca dell'Accademia nazionale dei Lincei e Corsiniana; Rome, Biblioteca Musicale governativa del Conservatorio di Santa Cecilia; Rome, Archivio di San Giovanni in Laterano; Vatican City, Biblioteca Apostolica Vaticana, *fondo* Cappella Giulia [four exemplars], *ibid.*, *fondo* Cappella Sistina; Rochester, NY, Sibley Music Library, University of Rochester [5/6].

[A0005] Regensburg, Bischöfliche Zentralbibliothek (Proske-Musikbibliothek) [A,T,B]; Bologna, Civico Museo Bibliografico Musicale [complete: S,A,T,B,5/6]; Bologna, Archivio di San Petronio; Vatican City, Biblioteca Apostolica Vaticana; Gdansk, Biblioteka Polskiej Akademii Nauk [T,B]; Rochester, NY, Sibley Music Library, University of Rochester [S,A,T,B].

A0006 [RISM P660] *Missarum liber secundus.* Rome: heirs of Valerio and Aloysio Dorico, 1567 [choirbook].

1. *Missa De beata Virgine a* (f.2v)
2. *Missa Inviolata a 4* (f.16v)
3. *Missa Sine nomine a 4* (f.30v)
4. *Missa Ad fugam a 4* (f.40v)
5. *Missa Aspice domine a 5* (f.45v)
6. *Missa Salvum me fac a 5* (f.63v)
7. *Missa Papae Marcelli a 6* (f.82v)

Reprint History

A0007 [RISM P661] *Missarum cum quattuor, quinque ac sex vocibus . . . liber secundus.* Venice: Angelo Gardano, 1598 [partbooks].

A0008 [RISM P662] *Missarum cum quatuor, quinque & sex vocum.* Rome: Nicolo Mutii, 1599 [choirbook].

A0009 [RISM P663] *Missarum cum quaternis, quinis ac senis vocibus.* Rome: Nicolo Mutii, 1600 [choirbook].

Print Locations

[A0006] Brno, Moravské múseum, Ústav dejin hudby [incomplete]; Berlin, Staatsbibliothek; Granada, Archivio capitular de la Catedral; Segorbe, Archivo de la Catedral; Cambrai, Bibliothèque municipale; London, British Library [two copies]; Assisi, Biblioteca comunale [two copies]; Bologna, Civico Museo Bibliografico Musicale; Bergamo, Civico Instituto musicale "G. Donizetti"; Città di Castello, Archivio del Duomo (lacks title page); Florence, Biblioteca del Conservatorio di Musica "Luigi Cherubini"; Gubbio, Biblioteca Vescovile Fonti e Archivio; Loreto, Archivio Storico della Cappella Lauretana; Milan, Biblioteca del Conservatorio "Giuseppe Verdi"; Padua, Biblioteca capitolare; Palermo, Archivio del Duomo; Rome, Biblioteca Musicale governativa del Conservatorio di Santa Cecilia; Rome, Archivio di San Giovanni in Laterano; Vatican City, Biblioteca Apostolica Vaticana, *fondo* Cappella Sistina; Reggio Emilia, Archivio capitolare di San Prospero [incomplete, with manuscript supplement]; Terni, Istituto Musicale "G. Briccialdi"; Treviso, Archivio della Cappella del Duomo [incomplete]; Coimbra, Biblioteca Geral da Universidade; Chapel Hill, NC, University of North Carolina Music Library [incomplete]; New York, James J. Fuld private collection.

[A0007] Brussels, Bibliothèque Royale Albert I [complete: S,A,T,B,5/6]; Münster, Bibliothek des Bischöflichen Priesterseminars und Santini-Sammlung; Regensburg, Bischöfliche Zentralbibliothek (Proske-Musikbibliothek) [A,T,B]; Brescia, Archivio del Duomo; Milan, Biblioteca del Conservatorio "Giuseppe Verdi" [A,T,5]; Piacenza, Archivio del Duomo; Vatican City, Biblioteca Apostolica Vaticana, *fondo* Cappella Giulia, *ibid.*, *fondo* Cappella Sistina; Siena, Archivio musicale dell'opera del Duomo; Spello, Collegiata di Santa Maria Maggiore, Archivio [T].

[A0008] Ljubljana, University Library.

[A0009] Bologna, Civico Museo Bibliografico Musicale; Florence, Archivio musicale dell'opera di Santa Maria del Fiore; Lucca, Biblioteca del seminario arcivescovile; Rome, Biblioteca Musicale governativa del Conservatorio di Santa Cecilia; Vatican City, Biblioteca Apostolica Vaticana, *fondo* Cappella Giulia.

A0010 [RISM P664] *Missarum liber tertius*. Rome: heirs of Valerio and Aloysio Dorico, 1570 [choirbook].

1. *Missa Spem in alium a 4* (f.1v)
2. *Missa Primi toni a 4* (f.18v)
3. *Missa Brevis a 4* (p.36v)
4. *Missa De feria a 4* (f.46v)
5. *Missa L'homme armé a 5* (f.52v)
6. *Missa Repleatur os meum a 5* (f.71v)
7. *Missa de Beata Virgine a 6* (f.87v)
8. *Missa Ut re mi fa sol la a 6* (f.105v)

Reprint History

A0011 [RISM P665] *Missarum cum quatuor, quinque, ac sex vocibus . . . liber tertius*. Venice: Angelo Gardano, 1598 [partbooks].

A0012 [RISM P666] *Missarum cum quatuor, quinque, ac sex vocibus . . . liber tertius*. Venice: Angelo Gardano, 1599 [shortened edition, partbooks].

Print Locations

[A0010] Berlin, Staatsbibliothek; Munich, Bayerische Staatsbibliothek, Musiksammlung; Regensburg, Bischöfliche Zentralbibliothek (Proske-Musikbibliothek) [incomplete, with manuscript supplement]; London, British Library; Albenga, Cattedrale di San Michele, Biblioteca e Archivio Capitolari; Assisi, Biblioteca comunale; Bologna, Civico Museo Bibliografico Musicale; Città di Castello, Archivio del Duomo (imperfect copy); Fabriano, Biblioteca comunale; Florence, Archivio musicale dell'opera di S. Maria del Fiore; Gubbio, Biblioteca Vescovile Fonti e Archivio; Paris, Bibliothèque nationale (ancien fonds du Conservatoire nationale de musique); Milan, Biblioteca del Conservatorio "Giuseppe Verdi"; Palermo, Archivio del Duomo (Biblioteca capitolare); Rome, Bibioteca Casanatense; Rome, Biblioteca dell'Accademia nazionale dei Lincei e Corsiniana; Rome, Biblioteca Musicale governativa del Conservatorio di Santa Cecilia [two exemplars]; Rome, Archivio capitolare di Santa Maria Maggiore (housed in Biblioteca Apostolica Vaticana); Vatican City, Biblioteca Apostolica Vaticana, *fondo* Cappella Giulia; *ibid.*, *fondo* Cappella Sistina; Reggio Emilia, Archivio capitolare di San Prospero;

Spoleto, Archivio del Duomo; Terni, Istituto Musicale "G. Briccialdi"; Treviso, Archivio della Cappella del Duomo; Coimbra, Biblioteca Geral da Universidade; Berkeley, University of California Music Library [incomplete].

[A0011] Vienna, Österreiches Nationalbibliothek, Musiksammlung [complete: S,A,T,B, 5/6 (incomplete)].

[A0012] Regensburg, Bischöfliche Zentralbibliothek (Proske-Musikbibliothek) [A,T,B]; Dresden, Sächsische Landesbibliothek, Musikabteilung [S,A,T,B, 5/6]; Cuenca, Archivo capitular de Cuenca [5/6 (incomplete)]; Bologna, Civico Museo Bibliografico Musicale [S,T,5]; Milan, Biblioteca del Conservatorio "Giuseppe Verdi"; Vatican City, Biblioteca Apostolica Vaticana, *fondo* Cappella Giulia; *ibid.*, *fondo* Cappella Sistina.

A0013 RISM P667] *Missarum cum quatuor et quinque vocibus, liber quartus.* Venice: Angelo Gardano, 1582 [partbooks].

1. *Missa Prima a 4* (p.1)
2. *Missa Secunda a 4* (p.7)
3. *Missa Tertia a 4* (p.13)
4. *Missa Quarta a 4* (p.20)
5. *Missa Prima a 5* (p.26)
6. *Missa Secunda a 5* (p.35)
7. *Missa Tertia a 5* (p.43)

Reprint History

A0014 [RISM P668] *Missarum cum quatuor et quinque vocibus, liber quartus.* Milan: Francesco and heirs of Simon Tini, 1590 [partbooks].

A0015 [RISM P669] *Basso principale co' l soprano del quarto libro delle messe a 4 e 5 v. . . . novamente fatto d'Alessandro Nuvoloni organista.* Milan: heirs of Simon Tini and Francesco Lomazzo, 1610 [one vol].

Print Locations

[A0013] Vienna, Österreiches Nationalbibliothek, Musiksammlung [exemplar 1=S,A,T,B,5; exemplar 2=A,B]; Berlin, Staatsbibliothek [T]; Regensburg, Bischöfliche Zentralbibliothek (Proske-Musikbibliothek) [A,T,B]; Tudela, Archivo capitular; Paris, Bibliothèque nationale (ancien fonds du Conservatoire nationale de musique) [S,A,T,B]; London, British Library [A,T,B,5]; Assisi, Biblioteca comunale [S,A,T,B (incomplete), 5]; Bologna, Civico Museo Bibliografico Musicale; Brescia, Archivio del Duomo [S,A,T,B]; Faenza, Archivio capitolare [5]; Pistoia, Archivio capitolare della Cattedrale [S,A,T,B]; Vatican City, Biblioteca Apostolica Vaticana, *fondo* Cappella Giulia [5], *ibid.*, *fondo* Cappella Sistina; Gdansk, Biblioteka Polskiej Akademii Nauk.

[A0014] Brussels, Bibliothèque Royale Albert I [S,5]; Aosta, Cattedrale, Biblioteca capitolare [S,T,B]; Como, Archivio musicale storico del Duomo [S,A,T,B,5]; Rome, Archivio di San Luigi de' Francesi [T]; Vatican City, Biblioteca Apostolica Vaticana, *fondo* Cappella Giulia [S,A,T,B].

[A0015] Bologna, Civico Museo Bibliografico Musicale.

A0016 [RISM P670] *Missarum liber quintus, quatuor, quinque, ac sex vocibus concinendarum.* Rome: Francesco Coattino ("*sumptibus Iacobi Berichiae*"), 1590 [choirbook]

1. *Missa Aeterna Christi munera a 4* (p.1)
2. *Missa Iam Christus ad astra ascenderat a 4* (f.12)
3. *Missa Panis quem ego dabo a 4* (p.28)
4. *Missa Iste Confessor a 4* (p.45)
5. *Missa Nigra sum a 5* (p.57)
6. *Missa Sicut lilium inter spinas a 5* (p.84)
7. *Missa Nasce la gioia mia a 6* (p.106)
8. *Missa Sine nomine a 6* (p.128)

Reprint History

A0017 [RISM P671] *Missarum cum quatuor, quinque, et sex vocibus, liber quintus.* Venice: heir of Girolamo Scotto, 1591 [partbooks].

A0018 [RISM P672] *Missarum cum quatuor, quinque, et sex vocibus, liber quintus.* Rome: Nicolo Mutii, 1599 [partbooks].

Print Locations

[A0016] Cologny, Fondation Martin Bodmer, Bibliotheca Bodmeriana; Prague, Národní knihovna (dríve Universitní knihovna); Berlin, Staatsbibliothek; Munich, Bayerische Staatsbibliothek, Musiksammlung; Tarazona, Archivo capitular [incomplete]; Paris, Bibliothèque nationale (ancien fonds du Conservatoire nationale de musique); London, British Library [incomplete]; Assisi, Biblioteca comunale; Ferrara, Biblioteca comunale Ariostea; Florence, Archivio musicale dell'opera di Santa Maria del Fiore; Fermo, Archivio della Metropolitana, Duomo; Modena, Archivio capitolare (Duomo); Loreto, Archivio Storico della Cappella Lauretana; Orvieto, Archivio musicale del Duomo; Pesaro, Biblioteca capitolare della Cattedrale Archivio del Duomo; Rome, Biblioteca Musicale governativa del Conservatorio di Santa Cecilia; Rome, Archivio dell'Archiconfraternita di San Giovanni de' Fiorentini; Rome, Archivio capitolare di Santa Maria Maggiore (housed in Biblioteca Apostolica Vaticana); Vatican City, Biblioteca Apostolica Vaticana, *fondo* Cappella Giulia [two exemplars], *ibid.*, *fondo* Cappella Sistina; Venice, Museo Civico Correr; Coimbra, Biblioteca Geral da Universidade; Lamego, Arquivo da Sé.

[A0017] Berlin, Staatsbibliothek [complete: S,A,T (two copies), B,5/6, with manuscript b.c. part]; Regensburg, Bischöfliche Zentralbibliothek (Proske-Musikbibliothek) [A,T,B]; Madrid, Biblioteca nacional [T]; Paris, Bibliothèque nationale [S,B]; Bologna, Civico Museo Bibliografico Musicale; Milan, Biblioteca del Conservatorio di Musica "Giuseppe Verdi"; Siena, Bibioteca dell'Accademia Musicale Chigiana [A]; Vatican City, Biblioteca Apostolica Vaticana, *fondo* Cappella Giulia [two exemplars, one of which lacks T part]; *ibid., fondo* Cappella Sistina; Spello, Archivio di Santa Maria Maggiore [T, 5/6]; Stockholm, Statens musikbibliotek [A]; Berkeley, CA, University of California Music Library; Cambridge, MA, Harvard University Music Libraries [A,T,B (incomplete), 5].

[A0018] Rome, Biblioteca Musicale governativa del Conservatorio di Santa Cecilia [complete].

A0019 [RISM P673] *Missarum cum quatuor vocibus, liber primus.* Venice: Giacomo Vincenti, 1590 [partbooks, containing two masses from Book II and one from Book III; *Missa Papae Marcelli* from Book II is a four-part arrangement here].

1. *Missa Papae Marcelli a 4* [anonymous four-part arrangement of mass *a 6* from Book II]
2. *Missa Sine nomine a 4* [from Book II (1567)]
3. *Missa Brevis a 4* [from Book III (1570)]

Reprint History

A0020 [RISM P674] *Missarum cum quatuor vocibus, liber primus.* Milan: Francesco and heirs of Simon Tini, 1590 [partbooks].

A0021 [RISM P675] *Missarum cum quatuor vocibus, liber primus.* Venice: Giacomo Vincenti, 1605 [partbooks].

A0022 [RISM P675a] *Missarum cum quatuor vocibus, liber primus.* Venice: Giacomo Vincenti, 1608 [partbooks].

Print Locations

[A0019] Brescia, Archivio del Duomo [S,A,B]; Brescia, Biblioteca Queriniana [T]; Milan, Biblioteca del Conservatorio "Giuseppe Verdi" [complete: S,A,T,B]; Moscow, Rossijskaja Gosudarstvennaja Biblioteka [S,A,T].

[A0020] Berlin, Staatsbibliothek [complete: S,A,T,B]; Bologna, Civico Museo Bibliografico Musicale [T,B]; Vercelli, Archivio del Duomo (Biblioteca capitolare) [A].

[A0021] Bologna, Civico Museo Bibliografico Musicale [T,B].

[A0022] Bologna, Civico Museo Bibliografico Musicale [complete: S,A,T,B].

A0023 [RISM P676] *Missae quinque, quatuor ac quinque vocibus concinendae . . .*

liber sextus. Rome: Francesco Coattino, 1594 [partbooks]
1. *Missa Dies sanctificatus a 4*
2. *Missa In te Domine speravi a 4*
3. *Missa Sine nomine a 4*
4. *Missa Quam pulchra es a 4*
5. *Missa Dilexi quoniam a 5*

Reprint History

A0024 [RISM P677] *Missae cum quatuor, quinque, ac sex vocibus . . . liber sextus.* Venice: Angelo Gardano, 1596 [enlarged edition, partbooks]:
1. *Missa Dies sanctificatus a 4* (p.2)
2. *Missa In te Domine speravi a 4* (p.10)
3. *Missa Sine nomine a 4* (p.18)
4. *Missa Quam pulchra es a 4* (p.25)
5. *Missa Dilexi quoniam a 5* (p.34)
6. *Missa Ave Maria a 6* (p.42)

Print Locations

[A0023] Bologna, Civico Museo Bibliografico Musicale [S]; Rome, Biblioteca dell' Accademia nazionale dei Lincei e Corsiniana [complete: S,A,T,B,5]; Vatican City, Biblioteca Apostolica Vaticana, *fondo* Cappella Giulia; *ibid., fondo* Cappella Sistina.

[A0024] Vienna, Österreiches Nationalbibliothek, Musiksammlung [complete: S,A,T,B, 5/6]; Regensburg, Bischöfliche Zentralbibliothek (Proske-Musikbibliothek) [S,A,T,B]; Bologna, Civico Museo Bibliografico Musicale; Milan, Biblioteca del Conservatorio di Musica "Giuseppe Verdi"; Siena, Biblioteca dell'Accademia Musicale Chigiana [S,A]; Spello, Archivio di Santa Maria Maggiore [T]; Vatican City, Biblioteca Apostolica Vaticana, *fondo* Cappella Sistina; Venice, Biblioteca nazionale Marciana; Amsterdam, Toonkunst-Bibliotheek [T]; Warsaw, Bibliotecka Uniwersytecka [S,A,B,5/6].

A0025 [RISM P678] *Missae quinque, quatuor ac quinque vocibus concinendae . . . liber septimus*. Rome: Francesco Coattino, 1594 [partbooks]
1. *Missa Ave Maria a 4* (p.3)
2. *Missa Sanctorum meritis a 4* (p.12)
3. *Missa Emendemus a 4* (p.21)
4. *Missa Sacerdos et Pontifex a 5* (p.27)
5. *Missa Tu es Pastor ovium a* 5 (p.35)

Reprint History

A0026 [RISM P679] *Missae cum quatuor, quinque, ac sex vocibus . . . liber septimus*. Venice: Angelo Gardano, 1605 [enlarged edition, partbooks].

A0027 [RISM P680] *Missae cum quatuor, quinque, & sex vocibus, liber septimus.*

Venice: heirs of Girolamo Scotto, 1609 [enlarged edition, partbooks]:
1. *Missa Ave Maria a 4* (p.2)
2. *Missa Sanctorum meritis a 4* (p.11)
3. *Missa Emendemus a 4* (p.20)
4. *Missa Sacerdos et Pontifex a 5* (p.26)
5. *Missa Tu es Pastor ovium a 5* (p.34)
6. *Missa ad Beneplacitum a 6* (p.44)

Print Locations

[A0025] Berlin, Staatsbibliothek [T]; Regensburg, Bischöfliche Zentralbibliothek (Proske-Musikbibliothek) [A,T,B]; London, British Library [complete: S,A,T,B,5]; Bologna, Civico Museo Bibliografico Musicale [A,T,B,5]; Vatican City, Biblioteca Apostolica Vaticana,*fondo* Cappella Giulia; *ibid.*, *fondo* Cappella Sistina.

[A0026] Oxford, Bodleian Library [complete: S,A,T,B,5/6]; Vatican City, Biblioteca Apostolica Vaticana, *fondo* Cappella Sistina; Siena, Archivio musicale dell'-opera del Duomo; Chicago, Newberry Library.

[A0027] Vienna, Österreiches Nationalbibliothek, Musiksammlung [complete: S,A,T,B,5/6]; Münster, Bibliothek des Bischöflichen Priesterseminars und Santini-Sammlung [S,B,5/6]; London, Royal College of Music [T]; Vatican City, Biblioteca Apostolica Vaticana, *fondo* Cappella Sistina; Venice, Biblioteca nazionale Marciana.

A0028 [RISM P681] *Missarum cum quatuor, quinque, & sex vocibus, liber octavus.* Venice: Heir of Girolamo Scotto, 1599 [partbooks]
1. *Missa Quem dicunt homines a 4* (p.3)
2. *Missa Dum esset Summus Pontifex a 4* (p.12)
3. *Missa O admirabile commercium a 5* (p.19)
4. *Missa Memor esto a 5* (p.27)
5. *Missa Dum complerentur a 6* (p.34)
6. *Missa Sacerdotes Domini a 6* (p.42)

Reprint History

A0029 [RISM P682] *Missarum cum quatuor, quinque, & sex vocibus, liber octavus.* Venice: heir of Girolamo Scotto, 1609 [partbooks].

Print Locations

[A0028] Regensburg, Bischöfliche Zentralbibliothek (Proske-Musikbibliothek) [A,T,B]; Cuenca, Archivo capitular de Cuenca [S (incomplete)]; Bologna, Civico Museo Bibliografico Musicale [complete: S,A,T,B,5/6]; Lucca, Biblioteca del seminario arcivescovile; Milan, Biblioteca del Conservatorio "Giuseppe Verdi"; Vatican City, Biblioteca Apostolica Vaticana, *fondo* Cappella Sistina; Gdansk, Biblioteka Polskiej Akademii Nauk [S,T,B,5/6].

[A0029] Vienna, Österreiches Nationalbibliothek, Musiksammlung [complete: S,A,T,B,5/6]; Vatican City, Biblioteca Apostolica Vaticana, *fondo* Cappella Giulia; *ibid.*, *fondo*, Cappella Sistina [two exemplars]; Venice, Biblioteca nazionale Marciana.

A0030 [RISM P683] *Missarum cum quatuor, quinque, & sex vocibus, liber nonus.* Venice: Heir of Girolamo Scotto, 1599 [partbooks]

1. *Missa Ave regina coelorum a 4* (p.3)
2. *Missa Veni sponsa Christi a 4* (p.12)
3. *Missa Vestiva i colli a 5* (p.20)
4. *Missa Sine nomine a 5* (p.28)
5. *Missa In te Domine speravi a 6* (p.36)
6. *Missa Te Deum laudamus a 6* (p.45)

Reprint History

A0031 [RISM P684] *Missarum cum quatuor, quinque, & sex vocibus, liber nonus.* Venice: heir of Girolamo Scotto, 1608 [partbooks].

Print Locations

[A0030] Regensburg, Bischöfliche Zentralbibliothek (Proske-Musikbibliothek) [A,T,B]; Bologna, Civico Museo Bibliografico Musicale [complete: S,A,T,B,5/6]; Vatican City, Biblioteca Apostolica Vaticana, *fondo* Cappella Sistina; Gdansk, Biblioteka Polskiej Akademii Nauk [S,T,B,5]; Washington, DC, Library of Congress, Music Division.

[A0031] Vienna, Österreiches Nationalbibliothek, Musiksammlung [complete: S,A,T,B,5/6]; Brussels, Bibliothèque Royale Albert I; Vatican City, Biblioteca Apostolica Vaticana, *fondo* Cappella Giulia; *ibid., fondo,* Cappella Sistina; Venice, Biblioteca nazionale Marciana.

A0032 [RISM P685] *Missarum cum quatuor, quinque, & sex vocibus, liber decimus.* Venice: heir of Girolamo Scotto, 1600 [partbooks]

1. *Missa In illo tempore a 4* (p.3)
2. *Missa Già fù chi m'ebbe cara a 4* (p.12
3. *Missa Pietra sancta a 5* (p.19)
4. *Missa O virgo simul et mater a 5* (p.27)
5. *Missa Quinti toni a 6* (p.35)
6. *Missa Illumina oculos meos a 6* (p.44)

Print Locations

[A0032] Vienna, Österreiches Nationalbibliothek, Musiksammlung [complete: S,A,T,B,5/6]; Regensburg, Bischöfliche Zentralbibliothek (Proske-Musikbibliothek) [A,T,B]; Cuenca, Archivo capitular de Cuenca [B]; Lucca, Biblioteca del seminario arcivescovile [complete set, with S and A parts incomplete]; Milan, Biblioteca del Conservatorio "Giuseppe Verdi"; Pistoia, Archivio capitolare della Cattedrale; Vatican City, Biblioteca Apostolica Vaticana, *fondo* Cappella Giulia; *ibid., fondo,* Cappella Sistina [three copies].

A0033 [RISM P686] *Missarum cum quatuor, quinque, & sex vocibus, liber undecimus*. Venice: Heir of Girolamo Scotto, 1600 [partbooks]

1. *Missa Descendit angelus a 4* (p.3)
2. *Missa Regina coeli a 5* (p.12: print says 22)
3. *Missa Quando lieta sperai a 5* (p.21)
4. *Missa Octavi toni a 6* (p.29)
5. *Missa Alma Redemptoris a* 6 (p.39)

Print Locations

[A0033] Vienna, Österreiches Nationalbibliothek, Musiksammlung [complete: S,A,T,B,5/6]; Regensburg, Bischöfliche Zentralbibliothek (Proske-Musikbibliothek) [A,T,B]; Lucca, Biblioteca del seminario arcivescovile [A,T,B,5]; Vatican City, Biblioteca Apostolica Vaticana, *fondo* Cappella Giulia; *ibid., fondo* Cappella Sistina [three copies]; Berkeley, CA, University of California Music Library.

A0034 [RISM P687] *Missarum cum quatuor, quinque, et sex vocibus, liber duodecimus*. Venice: heir of Girolamo Scotto, 1601 [partbooks]

1. *Missa regina coeli a 4* (p.3)
2. *Missa O rex gloriae a 4* (p.12)
3. *Missa Ascendo ad patrem a 5* (p.20)
4. *Missa Qual è il più grand'amor a 5* (p.29)
5. *Missa Tu es Petrus a 6* (p.37)
6. *Missa Viri Galilaei a 6* (p.45)

Print Locations

[A0034] Brussels, Bibliothèque Royale Albert I [complete: S,A,T,B,5/6]; Regensburg, Bischöfliche Zentralbibliothek (Proske-Musikbibliothek) [A,T,B]; Vatican City, Biblioteca Apostolica Vaticana, *fondo* Cappella Giulia; *ibid., fondo* Cappella Sistina [two exemplars]; Berkeley, CA, University of California Music Library.

A0035 [RISM 688] *Missae quatuor octonis vocibus concinendae*. Venice: Ricciardo Amadino, 1601 [partbooks]

1. *Missa Laudate Dominum omnes gentes a 8* (p.1)
2. *Missa Hodie Christus natus est a 8* (p.8)
3. *Missa Fratres ego enim accepi a 8* (p.14)
4. *Missa Confitebor tibi Domine a 8* (p.22)

Print Locations

[A0035] Vienna, Österreiches Nationalbibliothek, Musiksammlung [I: S,A,T,B; II: A]; Regensburg, Bischöfliche Zentralbibliothek (Proske-Musikbibliothek) [I: A,B; II: S]; Tarazona, Archivo capitular [complete: I: S,A,T,B; II: S,A,T,B]; Bologna, Civico Museo Bibliografico Musicale [I: S,A,T,B]; Milan, Biblioteca del Conservatorio di Musica "Giuseppe Verdi"; Vatican City, Biblioteca Apostolica Vaticana, *fondo* Cappella Sistina [II: S].

Motets

A0036 [RISM P689] *Motecta festorum totius anni cum Communi sanctorum . . . quarternis vocibus . . . liber primus.* Venice: Antonio Gardano, 1564 [partbooks] [see A0040 for contents].

Reprint History

A0037 [RISM P690] *Motecta festorum totius anni cum Communi sanctorum . . . quarternis vocibus . . . liber primus.* Venice: sons of Antonio Gardano, 1571 [partbooks].

A0038 [RISM P691] *Motecta festorum totius anni cum Communi sanctorum . . . quarternis vocibus . . . liber primus.* Venice: sons of Antonio Gardano, 1574 [partbooks].

A0039 [RISM P692] *Motecta festorum totius anni cum Communi sanctorum . . . quarternis vocibus . . . liber primus.* Venice: Angelo Gardano, 1579 [partbooks].

A0040 [RISM P693] *Motecta festorum totius anni cum Communi sanctorum . . . quarternis vocibus . . . liber primus.* Venice: Angelo Gardano, 1585 [partbooks]:

1. In die Natalis Domini, *Dies sanctificatus* (p.1)
2. In Sancti Stephani, *Lapidabant Stephanum* (p.2)
3. In Sancti Io. Evang., *Valde honorandus est* (p.3)
4. In die Circumcisionis Domini, *Magnum hereditatis* (p.4)
5. In Epiphania, *Tribus miraculis* (p.5)
6. In Purificatione B. M., *Hodie beata virgo Maria* (p.6)
7. In Annuntiatione, *Ave Maria* (p.7)
8. In Resurrectione Domini, *Iesus iunxit se* (p.8)
9. In Ascensione Domini, *O Rex gloriae* (p.9)
10. In die Pentecostes, *Loquebantur in variis linguis* (p.10)
11. In festo Sanct. Trin., *Benedicta sit sancta Trinitas* (p.11)
12. In die Corporis Christi, *Lauda Syon* (p.12)
13. In Nativitate Ioan. Bap., *Fuit homo missus a Deo* (p.13)
14. In Sancti Petri Apost., *Tu es pastor ovium* (p.14)
15. In Sancti Pauli, *Magnus Sanctus Paulus* (p.15)
16. In Visitatione B. Mariae, *Surge propera* (p.16)
17. In Sancte Mariae Mag., *In diebus illis* (p.17)
18. In Sancti Laurentii, *Beatus Laurentius* (p.18)
19. In Assumptione B. Mariae, *Quae est ista* (p.19)
20. In Decollatione Io. Bap., *Misso Herodes spiculatore* (p.20)
21. In Nativitate B. Mariae, *Nativitas tua* (p.21)
22. In festo Sanctae Crucis, *Nos autem gloriari* (p.22)
23. In festo Omnium Sanctorum, *Salvator mundi* (p.23)
24. In S. Martini episc., *O quantus luctus* (p.24)
25. In Presentatione B. M., *Congratulamini mihi* (p.25)
26. In Sancte Caecilie, *Dum aurora finem* (p.26)
27. In Sancti Andree, *Doctor bonus* (p.27)

28. In conceptione B. M., *Quam pulchri sunt* (p.28)

Common of saints:

29. In festo Apostolorum, *Tollite iugum* (p.29)
30. In festo Evangelistarum, *Isti sunt viri* (p.30)
31. In festo unius martiris, *Hic est vere martyr* (p.31)
32. In festo plur. Mart., *Gaudent in celis* (p.32)
33. In festo confess. pont., *Iste est qui ante Deum* (p.33)
34. In festo confess. non pont., *Beatus vir qui suffert* (p.34)
35. In festo virginum, *Veni sponsa* (p.35)
36. In dedicatione templi, *Exaudi domine* (p.36)

A0041 [RISM P694] *Motecta festorum totius anni cum Communi sanctorum . . . quarternis vocibus . . . liber primus.* Milan: Francesco and heirs of Simon Tini, 1587 [partbooks].

A0042 [RISM P695] *Motecta festorum totius anni cum Communi sanctorum . . . quarternis vocibus . . . liber primus.* Rome: Francesco Coattino, 1590 [partbooks].

A0043 [RISM P696] *Cantiones sacrae quatuor vocum pro festis totius anni et Communi sanctorum.* Antwerp: Pierre Phalèse, 1613 [partbooks].

A0044 [RISM P697] *Motecta festorum totius anni cum Communi sanctorum . . . quarternis vocibus . . . liber primus.* Venice: heirs of Girolamo Scotto, 1595 [partbooks].

A0045 [RISM P698] *Motecta festorum totius anni cum Communi sanctorum . . . quarternis vocibus . . . liber primus.* Venice: Angelo Gardano, 1601 [partbooks].

A0046 [RISM P699] *Motecta festorum totius anni cum Communi sanctorum . . . quarternis vocibus . . . liber primus.* Rome: Luca Antonio Soldi, 1622.

Print Locations

[A0036] Naples, Biblioteca del Conservatorio di Musica S. Pietro a Maiella [T].

[A0037] Bologna, Civico Museo Bibliografico Musicale [complete: S,A,T,B]; Castell'Arquato, Archivio capitolare (parrocchiale), Archivio della Chiesa Collegiata [A,T,B]; Treviso, Archivio della Cappella del Duomo.

[A0038] Vienna, Österreiches Nationalbibliothek, Musiksammlung [S]; Regensburg, Bischöfliche Zentralbibliothek (Proske-Musikbibliothek) [S,B]; Treviso, Archivio della Cappella del Duomo [complete: S,A,T,B].

[A0039] Berlin, Staatsbibliothek [A,B]; Paris, Bibliothèque de l'Arsenal [T]; Assisi, Biblioteca comunale [complete: S,A,T,B]; Bologna, Civico Museo Bibliografico Musicale [T].

[A0040] London, Royal College of Music [complete: S,A,T (manuscript copy), B]; Vatican City, Biblioteca Apostolica Vaticana, *fondo* Cappella Sistina; Coimbra, Biblioteca Geral da Universidade [B].

[A0041] Cuenca, Archivo capitular de Cuenca [complete: S,A,T,B]; Tudela, Archivo capitular.

[A0042] Rome: Biblioteca Musicale governativa del Conservatorio di Santa Cecilia [complete: S,A,T (lacking title page), B].

[A0043] Regensburg, Bischöfliche Zentralbibliothek (Proske-Musikbibliothek) [complete: S,A,T,B].

[A0044] Münster, Bibliothek des Bischöflichen Priesterseminars und Santini-Sammlung [complete: S,A,T,B]; Regensburg, Bischöfliche Zentralbibliothek (Proske-Musikbibliothek) [A,T]; Madrid, Biblioteca nacional [T].

[A0045] Chapel Hill, NC, University of North Carolina Music Library [complete: S,A,T,B].

[A0046] Odense, Odense Universitetsbibliotek, Musikafdelingen; Oxford, Christ Church Library [complete: S,A,T,B]; Vatican City, Biblioteca Apostolica Vaticana, *fondo* Chigi [S,A].

A0047 [RISM P700] *Liber primus . . . mottettorum, quae partim quinis, partim senis, partim septenis vocibus concinantur*. Rome: heirs of Valerio and Aloysio Dorico, 1569 [partbooks; see A049 for contents]

Reprint History

A0048 [RISM P701] *Liber primus . . . mottettorum, quae partim quinis, partim senis, partim septenis vocibus concinantur.* Venice: Angelo Gardano, 1579 [partbooks].

A0049 [RISM P702] *Liber primus . . . motettorum, quae partim quinis, partim senis, partim septenis vocibus concinantur.* Venice: heir of Girolamo Scotto, 1586 [partbooks]:

Five voices:

1. *O admirabile commercium* (p.2)
2. *Stella quam viderant Magi* (p.3)
3. *O Antoni eremita* (p.4)
4. *Senex puerum portabat* (p.5); *Hodie beata virgo Maria* [secunda pars] (p.6)
5. *Suscipe verbum virgo Maria* (p.7); *Paries quidem filium* [secunda pars] (p.8)
6. *Alleluia! tulerunt Dominum* (p.9)
7. *Crucem sanctam subiit* (p.10)
8. *O beata et benedicta et gloriosa Trinitas* (p.11); *O vera summa* [secunda pars] (p.12)

9. *Ego sum panis vivus* (p.13); *Panis quem ego dabo* [secunda pars] (p.14)
10. *Puer qui natus est* (p.15)
11. *Beatae Mariae Magdalenae* (p.16)
12. *Sancte Paule apostole* (p.17)
13. *Beatus Laurentius* (p.18)
14. *Hodie nata est beata virgo* (p.19)
15. *O beatum virum* (p.20)
16. *Venit Michael archangelus* (p.21)
17. *O beatum pontificem* (p.22)
18. *Deus qui dedisti legem* (p.23)
19. *Lapidabant Stephanum* (p.24)
20. *Hic est discipulus ille* (p.25)
21. *Sicut lilium inter spinas* (p.26)
22. *Quam pulchri sunt gressus* (p.27)
23. *Unus ex duobus* (p.28)
24. *Cum pervenisset beatus Andreas* (p.29)

Six voices:

25. *Viri Galilaei quid statis* (p.30); *Ascendit Deus in iubilatione* [secunda pars] (p.31)
26. *Dum complerentur dies Pentecostes* (p.32); *Dum ergo essent in unum* [secunda pars] (p.33)
27. *Pulchra es, o virgo Maria* (p.34)
28. *Solve jubente Deo* (p.35); *Quodcumque ligaveris* [secunda pars] (p.36)
29. *Vidi turbam magnam* (p.37); *Et omnes angeli stabant* [secunda pars] (p.38)
30. *O magnum mysterium* (p.39); *Quem vidistis pastores* [secunda pars] (p.40)
31. *O Domine Jesu Christe* (p.41)

Seven voices:

32. *Tu es Petrus* (p.42)
33. *Virgo prudentissima* (p.43); *Maria Virgo* [secunda pars] (p.44)

A0050 [RISM P703] *Liber primus . . . mottettorum, quae partim quinis, partim senis, partim septenis vocibus concinantur.* Venice: Angelo Gardano, 1590 [partbooks].

A0051 [RISM P704] *Liber primus . . . mottettorum, quae partim quinis, partim senis, partim septenis vocibus concinantur.* Venice: heir of Girolamo Scotto, 1600 [partbooks].

Print Locations

[A0047] Berlin, Staatsbibliothek [complete: S,A,T,B,5,6]; Hamburg, Staats- und Universitätsbibiothek Carl von Ossietzky, Musikabteilung [S,T,B,5,6 (lacking A)]; Regensburg, Bischöfliche Zentralbibliothek (Proske-Musikbibliothek) [A,B]; Valladolid, Archivo musical de la Catedral [T,B]; London, British Library [S]; Bologna, Civico Museo Bibliografico Musicale; Coimbra, Biblioteca Geral da Universidade [A, 6 (incomplete)]; Stockholm, Stiftelsen Musikkulturens främjande [S]; Rochester, NY, Sibley Music Library, Eastman School of Music, University of Rochester.

[A0048] Munich, Bayerische Staatsbibliothek [complete: S,A,T,B,5,6]; Cuenca, Archivo capitular de Cuenca [A]; Paris, Bibliothèque nationale; Bologna, Civico Museo Bibliografico Musicale; Gubbio, Biblioteca Vescovile Fonti e Archivio [A,5,6]; Lucca, Biblioteca del seminario arcivescovile; Treviso, Archivio della Cappella del Duomo [incomplete]; Legnica (Liegnitz), Biblioteka Towarzystwa Przjaciól Nauk [B]; Warsaw, Biblioteka Narodowa [T,5,6]; Bloomington, IN, Indiana University School of Music Library.

[A0049] Berlin, Staatsbibliothek [A,B]; Hamburg, Staats- und Universitätsbibiothek Carl von Ossietzky, Musikabteilung [6]; Regensburg, Bischöfliche Zentralbibliothek (Proske-Musikbibliothek) [5]; Tudela, Archivo capitular [complete: S,A,T,B,5,6]; Tarazona, Archivo capitular [T]; Saragossa, Archivo de música del Cabildo [A,6]; Paris, Bibliothèque nationale [S,B,6]; Assisi, Biblioteca comunale [A,T,B,5,6 (lacks S)]; Bologna, Civico Museo Bibliografico Musicale; Bologna, Archivio di San Petronio; Vatican City, Biblioteca Apostolica Vaticana, *fondo* Cappella Giulia [A,T,B,5,6 (lacks S); *ibid., fondo* Cappella Sistina; Berkeley, CA, University of California Music Library.

[A0050] Berlin, Staatsbibliothek [complete: S,A,T,B,5,6,]; Hamburg, Staats- und Universitätsbibiothek Carl von Ossietzky, Musikabteilung [5]; Regensburg, Bischöfliche Zentralbibliothek (Proske-Musikbibliothek) [S,T,5]; Cuenca, Archivo capitular de Cuenca [A,B]; Montserrat, Monasterio di Montserrat [A]; Valencia, Colegio y capilla del Corpus Christi; London, British Library [6 (two copies)]; Assisi, Biblioteca comunale [complete, with two copies of B]; Bologna, Civico Museo Bibliografico Musicale [S,B]; Ferrara, Biblioteca comunale Ariostea; Rome, Biblioteca Musicale governativa del Conservatorio di Santa Cecilia [A]; Vatican City, Biblioteca Apostolica Vaticana, *fondo* Cappella Giulia [A,T,B,5,6 (lacks S)]; Coimbra, Biblioteca Geral da Universidade [A (incomplete)]; Stockholm, Statens musikbibliotek [5].

[A0051] Regensburg, Bischöfliche Zentralbibliothek (Proske-Musikbibliothek)[6]; Cambridge, University Library [6]; London, British Library [T]; Rome, Archivio di San Giovanni in Laterano [complete: S,A,T,B,5,6]; Vatican City, Biblioteca Apostolica Vaticana, *fondo* Cappella Giulia [S]; *ibid., fondo* Cappella Sistina; Lisbon, Biblioteca do Palácio nacional da Ajuda; Berkeley CA, University of California, Music Library [S,A,T (incomplete), 5]; Washington, DC, Library of Congress, Music Division.

A0052 [RISM P705] *Motettorum quae partim quinis, partim senis, partim octonis vocibus concinantur, liber secundus.* Venice: Girolamo Scotto, 1572 [partbooks; see A056 for contents]

Reprint History

A0053 [RISM P706] *Motettorum quae partim quinis, partim senis, partim octonis vocibus concinantur, liber secundus.* Venice: Girolamo Scotto, 1573 [partbooks].

A0054 [RISM P707] *Motettorum quae partim quinis, partim senis, partim octonis vocibus concinantur, liber secundus.* Venice: Heir of Girolamo Scotto, 1577 [partbooks].

A0055 [RISM P708] *Motettorum quae partim quinis, partim senis, partim octonis vocibus concinantur, liber secundus.* Venice: Heir of Girolamo Scotto, 1580 [partbooks].

A0056 [RISM P709] *Motettorum quae partim quinis, partim senis, partim octonis vocibus concinantur, liber secundus.* Venice: Heir of Girolamo Scotto, 1588 [partbooks]

Five voices:

1. *O virgo simul et mater* (p.3)
2. *Memor esto verbi tui* (p.4)
3. *Corona aurea* (p.5); *Domine praevenisti eum* [secunda pars] (p.6)
4. *In illo tempore egressus* (p.7)
5. *Coenantibus illis* (p.9)
6. *Derelinquat impius* (p.10)
7. *Ascendo ad patrem meum* (p.11); *Ego rogabo patrem* [secunda pars] (p.12)
8. *Canite tuba in Sion* (p.14); *Rorate coeli* [secunda pars] (p.15)
9. *Exi cito in plateas* (p.16)
10. *Circuire possum* (p.17); *In hac cruce te invenit* [secunda pars] (p.18) [Angelo Pierluigi]
11. *Gaude Barbara beata* (p.19); *Gaude quia meruisti* [secunda pars] (p.20)
12. *Domine Pater* (p.21) [Silla Pierluigi]
13. *Confitebor tibi Domine* (p.22) [Rodolfo Pierluigi]
14. *Peccantem me quotidie* (p.23)
15. *Domine Jesus in qua nocte* (p.24)

Six voices:

16. *Tribularer si nescirem* (p.25); *Secundum multitudinem dolorum* [secunda pars] (p.26)
17. *Veni Domine et noli tardare* (p.27); *Excita Domine* [secunda pars] (p.28)
18. *Hierusalem, cito veniet salus tua* (p.29); *Ego enim sum Dominus* [secunda pars] (p.30)
19. *Beata Barbara* (p.31); *Gloriosa mortem* [secunda pars] (p.32)
20. *Sancta et immaculata virginitas* (p.33); *Benedicta tu* [secunda pars] (p.34)
21. *Cantabo Domino in vita mea* (p.35); *Deficiant peccatores* [secunda pars] (p.36)

22. *Tu es Petrus et super hanc petram* (p.37); *Quodcumque ligaveris* [secunda pars] (p.38)
23. *Nunc dimittis* (p.40) [Silla Pierluigi]

Eight voices:

24. *Confitebor tibi Domine* (p.40); *Notas facite in populis* [secunda pars] (p.41)
25. *Laudate pueri Dominum* (p.42); *Quis sicut Dominus Deus* [secunda pars] (p.44)
26. *Domine in virtuta tua* (p.46); *Magna est gloria eius* [secunda pars] (p.47)
27. *Laudate Dominum omnes gentes* (p.48)

A0057 [RISM P710] *Motettorum quae partim quinis, partim senis, partim octonis vocibus concinantur, liber secundus.* Venice: Angelo Gardano, 1594 [partbooks].

Print Locations

[A0052] Regensburg, Bischöfliche Zentralbibliothek (Proske-Musikbibliothek) [A,B]; Bologna, Civico Museo Bibliografico Musicale [lacks T part]; Castell'Arquato, Archivio capitolare (parrocchiale) [6]; Milan, Conservatorio di Musica "Giuseppe Verdi" [complete: S,A,T,B, 5, 6 (two copies of this part)]; Rome, Biblioteca Musicale governativa del Conservatorio di Santa Cecilia [A]; Coimbra, Biblioteca Geral da Universidade [A].

[A0053] London, British Library [S, incomplete]; Assisi, Biblioteca comunale [S,A,T,5,6]; Bologna, Civico Museo Bibliografico Musicale [B]; Piacenza, Archivio del Duomo [A,T,B,5,6 (two copies), lacks S]; Spello, Collegiata di Santa Maria Maggiore, Archivio [T,5 (both incomplete)].

[A0054] Munich, Bayerische Staatsbibliothek; Valladolid, Archivo musical de la Catedral [B]; Paris, Bibliothèque nationale [A]; Assisi, Biblioteca comunale [6]; Bologna, Civico Museo Bibliografico Musicale [complete: S,A,T,B,5,6]; Vatican City, Biblioteca Apostolica Vaticana, *fondo* Cappella Giulia [S]; Siena, Biblioteca dell'Accademia Musicale Chigiana [S (incomplete), A,B]; Spoleto, Archivio del Duomo [A,T,5,6]; Treviso, Archivio della Cappella del Duomo [S,A,B,5,6 (lacks T)]; Legnica (Liegnitz), Biblioteka Towarzystwa Przjaciól Nauk [B]; Warsaw, Biblioteka Narodowa [T,5,6]; Rochester, NY, Sibley Music Library, University of Rochester.

[A0055] Brussels, Bibliothèque Royale Albert I; Hamburg, Staats- und Universitätsbibliothek, Musikabteilung [6]; Tarazona, Archivo capitular [T]; Bologna, Civico Museo Bibliografico Musicale [complete: S,A,T,B,5,6]; Bologna, Archivio di San Petronio [S,A,T,B,5 (lacking 6)]; Lucca, Biblioteca del seminario arcivescovile; Modena, Biblioteca Estense [A,5,6]; Modena, Duomo, Biblioteca e Archivio capitolare [T]; Piacenza, Archivio del Duomo [S,A,T,B,5 (lacking 6)]; Treviso, Archivio della Cappella del Duomo [A,B,5]; Rochester, NY, Sibley Music Library, Eastman School of Music, University of Rochester.

[A0056] Berlin, Staatsbibliothek [S]; Regensburg, Bischöfliche Zentralbibliothek (Proske-Musikbibliothek) [5,6]; Valencia, Colegio y capilla del Corpus Christi [S,A,T,B]; Saragossa, Archivo di música del Cabildo [A,6]; Paris, Bibliothèque nationale [S,B,6]; Cambridge, UK, University Library [6]; Glasgow, Euing Music Library [S,A,B,5,6 (lacks T)]; London, British Library [T]; London, Royal College of Music [A,T,5]; Bologna, Civico Museo Bibliografico Musicale [complete: S,A,T,B,5,6]; Rome, Biblioteca Musicale governativa del Conservatorio di Santa Cecilia [S,A]; Vatican City, Biblioteca Apostolica Vaticana, *fondo* Cappella Sistina [complete, in 2 exemplars]; Lisbon, Biblioteca do Palácio nacional da Ajuda; Berkeley CA, University of California, Music Library [A,5]; Cambridge, MA, Harvard University Music Libraries [A,T,5 (incomplete), 6]; Oberlin, OH, Oberlin College Conservatory of Music, Mary M. Vail Library; Washington, DC, Library of Congress, Music Division.

[A0057] Berlin, Staatsbibliothek [S,A,T,B,5 (lacks 6)]; Hamburg, Staats- und Universitätsbibiothek Carl von Ossietzky, Musikabteilung [5]; Regensburg, Bischöfliche Zentralbibliothek (Proske-Musikbibliothek) [S,T]; London, British Library [6]; Assisi, Biblioteca comunale [complete: S,A,T,B,5,6]; Milan, Biblioteca nazionale Braidense [A,T,B,5,6 (lacks S)]; Vatican City, Biblioteca Apostolica Vaticana, *fondo* Cappella Giulia [three exemplars: one and two lack S part, three lacks S, 6 parts]; *ibid., fondo* Cappella Sistina [6]; Amsterdam, Toonkunst-Bibliotheek [5]; Coimbra, Biblioteca Geral da Universidade [A]; Stockholm, Statens musikbibliotek [5]; Cambridge, MA, Harvard University Music Libraries [5].

A0058 [RISM P711] *Motettorum quae partim quinis partim senis, partim octonis vocibus coincinantur, liber tertius.* Venice: heir of Girolamo Scotto, 1575 [list of contents from A059, below].

Reprint History

A0059 [RISM P712] *Motettorum quae partim quinis partim senis, partim octonis vocibus coincinantur, liber tertius.* Venice: heir of Girolamo Scotto, 1581 [partbooks]:

Five voices:

1. *Pater noster* (p.3)
2. *Ave Maria gratia plena* (p.4)
3. *Cantantibus organis Caecilia* (p.5); *Biduanis et triduanis* [secunda pars] (p.6)
4. *Caro mea vere est cibus* (p.7)
5. *Angelus Dominus descendit* (p.8); *Et introeuntes* [secunda pars] (p.9)
6. *Congrega Domine* (p.12); *Afflige opprimentes nos* [secunda pars] (p.14)
7. *Inclytae sanctae virginis Catherinae* (p.16)
8. *Fuit homo missus a Deo* (p.17); *Erat Ioannes in deserto* [secunda pars] (p.18)
9. *O lux et decus hispaniae* (p.19); *O singulare praesidium* [secunda pars] (p.20)

10. *Quid habes Ester* (p.21); *Vidi te Domine* [secunda pars] (p.22)
11. *Tradent enim vos* (p.23)
12. *Sanctificavit Dominus* (p.24)
13. *O quam metuendus* (p.25)
14. *Iubilate Deo omnis terra* (p.26); *Laudate nomen eius* [secunda pars] (p.27)
15. *Omnipotens sempiterne Deus* (p.28)
16. *O sancte praesul Nicolae* (p.29); *Gaude praesul optime* [secunda pars] (p.30)
17. *Domine Deus qui conteris* (p.31); *Tu Domine cui humilium* [secunda pars] (p.32)
18. *Manifesto vobis* (p.33)
19. *Pax vobis noli timere* (p.34)

Six voices:

20. *Susanna ab improbis* (p.35); *Postquam autem* [secunda pars] (p.36)
21. *Cum mortuus fuerit* [sic; *recte* Cum ortus fuerit] (p.37)
22. *Rex pacificus* (p.38)
23. *Haec dies quam fecit Dominus* (p.39)
24. *Columna es immobilis* (p.40)
25. *Iudica me Deus* (p.41)
26. *Accepit Iesus calicem* (p42)
27. *O bone Iesu exaudi me* (p.43)
28. *Deus qui ecclesiam tuam* (p.44)

Eight voices:

29. *Surge illuminare Hierusalem* (p.46)
30. *Lauda Syon* (p.47)
31. *Veni sancte spiritus* (p.48)
32. *Ave regina coelorum* (p.49)
33. *Hodie Christus natus est* (p.50)
34. *Iubilate Deo* (p.51)

A0060 [RISM P713] *Liber III. motectorum quinque vocum.* Milan: Francesco and heirs of Simon Tini, 1587 [partbooks].

A0061 [RISM P714] *Liber III. motectorum quinque vocum.* Venice: heir of Girolamo Scotto, 1589 [partbooks].

A0062 [RISM P715] *Liber III. motectorum quinque vocum.* Venice: Angelo Gardano, 1594 [partbooks].

Print Locations

[A0058] Berlin, Staatsbibliothek [B]; Munich, Bayerische Staatsbibliothek [complete: S,A,T,B,5,6, with manuscript supplement to S]; Regensburg, Bischöfliche Zentralbibliothek (Proske-Musikbibliothek) [A,B]; Paris, Bibliothèque nationale [A]; London, British Library; Assisi, Biblioteca comunale; Bologna, Civico Museo Bibliografico Musicale; Castell'Arquato, Archivio capitolare (parrocchiale) [6]; Milan, Biblioteca del Conservatorio "Giueppe Verdi"; Spello, Collegiata di Santa Maria Maggiore, Archivio [5]; Treviso, Archivio della Cappella del Duomo [S,A,T,B,6 (lacks 5)]; Venice, Archivio della Procuratoria di San Marco; Amsterdam, Toonkunst-Bibliotheek [5]; Legnica (Liegnitz), Biblioteka Towarzystwa Przjaciól Nauk [B]; Warsaw, Biblioteka Narodowa [T,5,6;]; Rochester, NY, Sibley Music Library, Eastman School of Music, University of Rochester.

[A0059] Berlin, Staatsbibliothek [complete: S,A,T,B,5,6]; Hamburg, Staats- und Universitätsbibiothek Carl von Ossietzky, Musikabteilung [6]; Tarazona, Archivo capitular [T]; Saragossa, Archivo de música del Cabildo [A,6]; London, British Library [6]; Ancona, Biblioteca comunale Luciano Benincasa [A,5]; Bologna, Civico Museo Bibliografico Musicale; Modena, Biblioteca Estense [A,5,6]; Vatican City, Biblioteca Apostolica Vaticana, *fondo* Cappella Sistina [two exemplars, both complete]; Treviso, Archivio della Cappella del Duomo [A,B,5]; Stockholm, Statens musikbibliotek [6]; Cambridge, MA, Harvard University Music Libraries [A,T,5,6].

[A0060] Milan, Archivio della Veneranda Fabbrica, Cappella Musicale del Duomo [complete: S,A,T,B,5].

[A0061] Berlin, Staatsbibliothek [S,A]; Regensburg, Bischöfliche Zentralbibliothek (Proske-Musikbibliothek) [6]; Jaca, Archivo musical de la Catedral [B,6]; Valencia, Colegio y capilla del Corpus Christi [complete: S,A,T,B,5,6]; Paris, Bibliothèque nationale [S,B,6]; Cambridge, UK, University Library [6]; London, Royal College of Music [T]; Bologna, Civico Museo Bibliografico Musicale; Vatican City, Biblioteca Apostolica Vaticana, *fondo* Cappella Giulia [two exemplars: one complete, one incomplete (lacks 6)]; *ibid., fondo* Cappella Sistina; Lisbon, Biblioteca do Palácio nacional da Ajuda; Washington, DC, Library of Congress, Music Division.

[A0062] Berlin, Staatsbibliothek [complete: S,A,T,B,5,6];]; Hamburg, Staats- und Universitätsbibiothek Carl von Ossietzky, Musikabteilung [5]; Regensburg, Bischöfliche Zentralbibliothek (Proske-Musikbibliothek) [S,T,5 (two copies)]; London, British Library [6]; Assisi, Biblioteca comunale; Milan, Biblioteca nazionale Braidense [A,T,B,5,6]; Rome: Biblioteca Musicale governativa del Conservatorio di Santa Cecilia [A]; Vatican City, Biblioteca Apostolica Vaticana, *fondo* Cappella Giulia [lacks S]; *ibid., fondo* Cappella Sistina [A,6]; Coimbra, Biblioteca Geral da Universidade [A]; Berkeley, CA, University of California, Music Library [A,5].

A0063 [RISM P716] *Motettorum quinque vocibus liber quartus*. Rome: Alessandro Gardano, 1583 [tenor and bassus partbooks dated 1583; superius, altus, and quintus partbooks dated 1584]

1. *Osculetur me* (p.1)
2. *Trahe me post te* (p.2)
3. *Nigra sum sed formosa* (p.3)
4. *Vineam meam* (p.4)

5. *Si ignoras te* (p.5)
6. *Pulchri sunt* (p.6)
7. *Fasciculus mirrae* (p.7)
8. *Ecce tu pulcher es* (p.8)
9. *Tota pulchra es* (p.9)
10. *Vulnerasti cor meum* (p.10)
11. *Sicut lilium* (p.11)
12. *Introduxit me* (p.12)
13. *Leva eius* (p.13)
14. *Vox dilecti* (p.14)
15. *Surge propera* (p.15)
16. *Surge amica mea* (p.16)
17. *Dilectus meus* (p.17)
18. *Surgam et circuibo* (p.18)
19. *Adiuro vos* (p.19)
20. *Caput eius* (p.20)
21. *Dilectus meus* (p.21)
22. *Pulchra es amica mea* (p.22)
23. *Quae est ista* (p.23)
24. *Descendit in hortum meum* (p.24)
25. *Quam pulchri sunt* (p.25)
26. *Collum tuum* (p26)
27. *Quam pulchra es* (p.27)
28. *Guttur tuus* (p.28)
29. *Veni veni dilecti mei* (p.29)

Reprint History

A0064 [RISM P717] *Motettorum quinque vocibus liber quartusex canticis Salomonis*. Venice: Angelo Gardano, 1587 [partbooks].

A0065 [RISM P718] *Liber IIII motectorum quinque vocum*. Milan: Francesco and heirs of Simon Tini, 1587 [partbooks].

A0066 [RISM P719] *Motectorum quinque vocibus liber quartus*. Venice: Giacomo Vincenti, 1588 [partbooks].

A0067 [RISM P720] *Motectorum quinque vocibus liber quartus ex canticis Salomonis*. Milan: heirs of Francesco and Simon Tini, 1593 [partbooks].

A0068 [RISM P721] *Mottetorum cum quinque vocibus liber quartus, ex canticis Salomonis.* Venice: Heir of Girolamo Scotto, 1596 [partbooks].

A0069 [RISM P722] *Motectorum cum quinque vocibus liber quartus, ex canticis Salomonis.* Venice: Angelo Gardano, 1601[partbooks].

A0070 [RISM P723] *Mottetorum cum quinque vocibus liber quartus, ex canticis Salomonis.* Venice: Heir of Girolamo Scotto, 1603 [partbooks].

A0071 [RISM P724] *Cantiones sacrae quinque vocum ex cantico canticarum.* Antwerp: Pierre Phalèse, 1605 [expanded edition, partbooks].

A0072 [RISM P725] *Motectorum . . . addita parte infima pro pulsatoris organi comoditate.* Venice: Alessandro Raverii, 1608 [partbooks].

A0073 [RISM P726] *Organum pro libro quarto motectorum ex canticis Salomonis . . . quinque vocibus.* Venice: Angelo Gardano and brothers, 1608.

A0074 [RISM P727] *Cantica Salomonis quinque vocum . . . liber quartus, bassus ad organum.* Venice: heirs of Bartolomei Magni, 1613 [partbooks].

Print Locations

[A0063] Berlin, Staatsbibliothek [complete: S,A,T,B,5]; Regensburg, Bischöfliche Zentralbibliothek (Proske-Musikbibliothek) [A,B]; Rome, Biblioteca Casanatense; Treviso, Archivio della Cappella del Duomo [A,B,5]; Rochester, NY, Sibley Music Library, Eastman School of Music, University of Rochester.

[A0064] Berlin, Staatsbibliothek [complete: S,A,T,B,5]; Munich, Bayerische Staatsbibliothek; Valencia, Colegio y capilla del Corpus Christi; Bologna, Civico Museo Bibliografico Musicale; Vatican City, Biblioteca Apostolica Vaticana, *fondo* Cappella Giulia [two copies: one complete, one lacks S part]; Gdansk, Biblioteka Polskiej Akademii Nauk [S,A,T,5].

[A0065] Milan, Archivio della Veneranda Fabbrica, Cappella musicale del Duomo [complete: S,A,T,B,5].

[A0066] Nuremberg, Bibliothek des Germanischen National-Museum [A]; Tudela, Archivo capitular [complete: S,A,T,B,5]; Tarazona, Archivo capitular [T]; Assisi, Biblioteca comunale [complete, two copies]; Rome, Biblioteca Musicale governativa del Conservatorio di Santa Cecilia [S,T,B]; Gdansk, Biblioteka Polskiej Akademii Nauk [T,B]; Cambridge, MA, Harvard University Music Libraries [A,T,5].

[A0067] Aosta, Cattedrale, Biblioteca capitolare; Lodi, Biblioteca comunale Laudense [5]; Piacenza, Archivio del Duomo [A,T,5]; Trento, Biblioteca comunale [S].

[A0068] Brussels, Bibliothèque Royale Albert I [complete: S,A,T,B,5]; Valladolid, Archivo musical de la Catedral [T,5]; Paris, Bibliothèque nationale [S,B]; London, Royal College of Music [S,A]; Bologna, Civico Museo Bibliografico Musicale [S]; Ferrara, Biblioteca comunale Ariostea; Washington, DC, Library of Congress, Music Division.

[A0069] Hamburg, Staats- und Universitätsbibiothek Carl von Ossietzky, Musikabteilung [5]; Cuenca, Archivo capitular de Cuenca [S,B]; Saragossa,

Archivo de música de Cabildo [A]; London, Royal College of Music [T]; Bologna, Civico Museo Bibliografico Musicale [complete: S,A,T,B,5]; Bologna, Archivio di San Petronio; Vatican City, Biblioteca Apostolica Vaticana, *fondo* Cappella Sistina [T,B,5]; Coimbra, Biblioteca Geral da Universidade [A].

[A0070] Regensburg, Bischöfliche Zentralbibliothek (Proske-Musikbibliothek) [S,T,5]; Gerona, Archivo musical de la Catedral [A]; Vatican City, Biblioteca Apostolica Vaticana, *fondo* Cappella Sistina [A].

[A0071] Oxford, Bodleian Library [complete: S,A,T,B,5].

[A0072] Aosta, Cattedrale, Biblioteca capitolare; Bologna, Civico Museo Bibliografico Musicale [complete: S,A,T,B,5, organ]; Vatican City, Biblioteca Apostolica Vaticana, *fondo* Cappella Sistina [S].

[A0073] Bologna, Civico Museo Bibliografico Musicale.

[A0074] Regensburg, Bischöfliche Zentralbibliothek (Proske-Musikbibliothek) [5]; London, British Library [complete: S,A,T,B,5, organ]; Bologna, Civico Museo Bibliografico Musicale [organ]; Pistoia, Archivio capitolare della Cattedrale [organ]; Rome, Biblioteca Musicale governativa del Conservatorio di Santa Cecilia [A]; Vatican City, Biblioteca Apostolica Vaticana, *fondo* Cappella Sistina [A,T,B].

A0075 [RISM P728] *Motettorum quinque vocibus liber quintus.* Rome: Alessandro Gardano, 1584 [partbooks]

1. *Laetus Hyperboream* (p.1); *O patruo* [secunda pars] (p.2)
2. *Paucitas dierum* (p.3); *Manus tuae Domine* [secunda pars] (p.4)
3. *Tempus est ut revertar* (p.5); *Nisi ego abiero* [secunda pars] (p.6)
4. *Domine secundum actum meum* (p.7); *Ave mundum sanctuarium* [Ave Trinitas sanctuarium] [secunda pars] (p.8)
5. *Parce mihi Domine* (p.9); *Peccavi peccavi* [secunda pars] (p.10)
6. *Orietur stella* (p.11)
7. *Egipte noli flere* [Aegypte noli flere] (p.12)
8. *Ardens est cor meum* (p.13)
9. *Sic Deus dilexit mundum* (p.14)
10. *Surge Petre* (p.15)
11. *Apparuit caro suo* (p.16)
12. *Ecce mercer sanctorum* (p.17)
13. *Ideus secundus* [Videns secundus] (p.18)
14. *Rex Melchior* (p.19)
15. *Ave regina coelorum* (p.20)
16. *Gaude gloriosa* (p.21)
17. *Exultate Deo* (p.24)
18. *Tribulationes civitatum* (p.23); *Peccavimus* [secunda pars] (p.24)
19. *Surge sancte Dei* (p.25); *Ambula sancte Dei* [secunda pars] (p.26)
20. *Salve Regina* (p.27)

Reprint History

A0076 [RISM P729] *Motettorum quinque vocibus liber quintus.* Venice: heir of Girolamo Scotto, 1588 [partbooks].

A0077 [RISM P730] *Motettorum quinque vocibus liber quintus.* Venice: heir of Girolamo Scotto, 1593 [partbooks].

A0078 [RISM P731] *Motettorum quinque vocibus liber quintus.* Venice: Angelo Gardano, 1595 [partbooks].

A0079 [RISM P732] *Motettorum quinque vocibus liber quintus.* Venice: heir of Girolamo Scotto, 1601 [partbooks].

Print Locations

[A0075] Munich, Bayerische Staatsbibliothek [complete: S,A,T,B,5]; Regensburg, Bischöfliche Zentralbibliothek (Proske-Musikbibliothek) [A,B]; Tudela, Archivo capitular; Bologna, Civico Museo Bibliografico Musicale [S]; Rome, Biblioteca Casanatense; Vatican City, Biblioteca Apostolica Vaticana, *fondo* Cappella Sistina; Spoleto, Archivio del Duomo; Treviso, Archivio della Cappella del Duomo [A,B,5]; Gdansk, Biblioteka Polskiej Akademii Nauk [S,A,T,5 (lacks B)]; Berkeley, CA, University of California Music Library [A,T,B,5, all parts incomplete]; Rochester, NY, Sibley Music Library, Eastman School of Music, University of Rochester.

[A0076] Berlin, Staatsbibliothek [A]; Tarazona, Biblioteca capitular [T]; Saragossa, Archivo di música del Cabildo [A]; Bologna, Civico Museo Bibliografico Musicale [complete: S,A,T,B,5]; Rome, Biblioteca Musicale governativa del Conservatorio di Santa Cecilia; Vatican City, Biblioteca Apostolica Vaticana, *fondo* Cappella Sistina; Gdansk, Biblioteka Polskiej Akademii Nauk [T,B]; Cambridge, MA, Harvard University Music Libraries [A,T,B (incomplete), 5]; Washington, DC, Library of Congress, Music Division.

[A0077] Paris, Bibliothèque nationale [S,B].

[A0078] Berlin, Staatsbibliothek [complete: S,A,T,B,5]; Hamburg, Staats- und Universitätsbibiothek Carl von Ossietzky, Musikabteilung [5]; Regensburg, Bischöfliche Zentralbibliothek (Proske-Musikbibliothek) [S,T,5 (2 copies)]; Cuenca, Archivio capitular de Cuenca [B]; London, Royal College of Music [T]; Rome, Biblioteca Musicale governativa del Conservatorio di Santa Cecilia [A]; Vatican City, Biblioteca Apostolica Vaticana, *fondo* Cappella Giulia [two copies: one complete, one lacks S part]; *ibid., fondo* Cappella Sistina; Coimbra, Biblioteca Geral da Universidade [A].

[A0079] Oxford, Bodleian Library [complete: S,A,T,B,5]; Assisi, Biblioteca comunale [B]; Vatican City, Biblioteca Apostolica Vaticana, *fondo* Cappella Sistina [A]; Lisbon, Biblioteca do Palácio nacional da Ajuda; San Francisco,

CA, San Francisco State College, Col. Frank V. de Bellis Collection [5]; Washington, DC, Library of Congress, Music Division; Wellesley, MA, Wellesley College Library [S].

A0080 [RISM P733] *Liber secundum motectorum quatuor vocum.* Milan: Francesco and heirs of Simon Tini, 1587 [partbooks]

1. *Domine, quando veneris*; *Commisso mea* [secunda pars]
2. *Heu mihi Domine*; *Anima mea turbata est* [secunda pars]
3. *Super flumina Babilonis*
4. *Ecce nunc benedicite Dominum*
5. *Ad te levavi oculos meos*; *Miserere nostri Domine* [secunda pars]
6. *Ad Dominum cum tribularer*; *Sagittae potentis* [secunda pars]
7. *Fundamenta eius*; *Numquid Sion dicet* [secunda pars]
8. *Quia vidisti me Thoma*
9. *Ego sum panis vivus*
10. *Sicut cervus desiderat*; *Sitivit anima mea* [secunda pars]
11. *Ave regina coelorum*; *Gaude gloriosa* [secunda pars]
12. *Alma redemptoris mater*; *Tu quae genuisti natura mirante* [secunda pars]
13. *Salve regina*; *Eja ergo advocata nostra* [secunda pars]
14. *Ave Maria gratia plena*
15. *Haec dies quam fecit Dominus*
16. *Confitemini Domino*
17. *Pueri Hebraeorum*
18. *Sub tuum praesidium*
19. *Adoramus te Christe*
20. *Surrexit pastor bonus*
21. *Gloriosi principes*

Reprint History

A0081 [RISM P733a] *Motettorum quatuor vocibus, liber secundus.* Venice: heir of Girolamo Scotto, 1588 [partbooks].

A0082 [RISM P734] *Motettorum quatuor vocibus, partim plena voce, et partim paribus vocibus, liber secundus.* Venice: heir of Girolamo Scotto, 1596 [partbooks].

A0083 [RISM P735] *Motettorum quatuor vocibus, liber secundus*. Venice: Heir of Girolamo Scotto, 1596 [partbooks].

A0084 [RISM P736] *Motectorum quatuor vocibus, partim plena voce et partim paribus vocibus, liber secundus*. Venice: Angelo Gardano, 1604.

Print Locations

[A0080] Milan, Archivio della Veneranda Fabbrica, Cappella musicale del Duomo [A,T,B (lacks S)]; Coimbra, Biblioteca Geral da Universidade [T].

[A0081] Valencia, Real Colegio-Seminario del Corpus Christi (Patriarca), Archivio [complete].

[A0082] Regensburg, Bischöfliche Zentralbibliothek (Proske-Musikbibliothek) [S,A]; London, British Library [S,A,B (lacks T)]; Treviso, Archivio della Cappella del Duomo [complete: S,A,T,B].

[A0083] Regensburg, Bischöfliche Zentralbibliothek (Proske-Musikbibliothek) [A,T,B]; Madrid, Biblioteca nacional [T]; Paris, Bibliothèque nationale [S,B]; Florence, Biblioteca Ricciardiana [S,T]; San Francisco, CA, San Francisco State College Library, Col. Frank V. de Bellis Collection [T].

[A0084] London, Royal College of Music [S,A,T]; Assisi, Biblioteca comunale [complete: S,A,T,B]; Fabriano, Biblioteca comunale [T]; Rome, Biblioteca Musicale governativa del Conservatorio di Santa Cecilia; Chapel Hill, NC, University of North Carolina Music Library.

Hymns

A0085 [RISM P737] *Hymni totius anni, secundum Sanctae Romanae Ecclesiae consuetudinem, quattuor vocibus concinendi, necnon hymni religionum.* Rome: Giacomo Torniero and Bernardo Donangelo (Francesco Coattino), 1589 [choirbook]

1. *Conditor alme siderum* (p.1)
2. *Vergente mundi vespere* (p.2)
3. *Te deprecamur agie* (p.3)
4. *Laus honor virtus gloria* (p.4)
5. *Christe Redemptor omnium* (p.6)
6. *Memento salutis auctor* (p.7)
7. *Hunc coelum terra* (p.8)
8. *Gloria tibi Domine* (p.9)
9. *A solis ortus cardine* (p.10)
10. *Castae parentis* (p.11)
11. *Enixa est puerpera* (p.13)
12. *Gaudent chorus coelestium* (p.14)
13. *Salvete flos martyrum* (p.15)
14. *Gloria tibi Domine* (p.16)
15. *Hostes Herodes impie* (p.17)
16. *Lavacra puri gurgitis* (p.18)
17. *Gloria tibi Domine* (p.19)
18. *Lucis Creator optime* (p.21)
19. *Ne mens gravata crimine* (p.22)
20. *Praesta pater piissime* (p.23)
21. *O lux beata Trinitas* (p.25)
22. *Deo Patris sit gloria* (p.26)
23. *Ad praeces nostras* (p.28)
24. *Crimina laxa* (p.29)
25. *Christe lux vera* (p.30)

26. *Tu nobis dona* (p.31)
27. *Gloria Deo* (p.32)
28. *Vexilla regis prodeunt* (p.33)
29. *Impleta sunt* (p.34)
30. *Beata cuius brachiis* (p.35)
31. *O crux ave spes unica* (p.36)
32. *Te summa Deus Trinitas* (p.37)
33. *Ad coenam Agni providi* (p.39)
34. *Protecti Paschae vespere* (p.40)
35. *O vere digna hostia* (p.41)
36. *Quaesumus auctor omnium* (p.42)
37. *Iesu nostra redemptio* (p.44)
38. *Inferni claustra penetrans* (p.45)
39. *Tu esto nostrum gaudium* (p.46)
40. *Veni Creator Spiritus* (p.48)
41. *Tu septiformis munere* (p.49)
42. *Hostes repellas longius* (p.50)
43. *Gloria patri Domino* (p.52)
44. *Pange lingua gloriosi* (p.54)
45. *In supreme nocte coene* (p.55)
46. *Tantum ergo sacramentum* (p.56)
47. *Quodcumque vinclis* (p.58)
48. *Doctor egregie* (p.60)
49. *Ave maris stella* (p.62)
50. *Solve vincla reis* (p.63)
51. *Virgo singularis* (p.64)
52. *Sit laus Deo Patri* (p.65)
53. *Quo vulneratus insuper* (p.66)
54. *Arbor decora* (p.67)
55. *O crux ave* (p.68)
56. *Ut queant laxis* (p.69)
57. *Illi promissi* (p.70)
58. *Gloria Patri* (p.72)
59. *Aurea luce* (p.74)
60. *O felix Roma* (p.76)
61. *Lauda mater Ecclesia* (p.78)
62. *Post fluxa carnis* (p.79)
63. *Surgentem cum victoria* (p.80)
64. *Petrus beatus* (p.81)
65. *Quicumque Christum quaeritis* (p.83)
66. *Hic ille rex* (p.84)
67. *Gloria tibi Domine* (p.85)
68. *Tibi Christe* (p.86)
69. *Quo custode procul* (p.87)
70. *Christe Redemptor omnium* (p.88)
71. *Vates aeterni iudicis* (p.89)
72. *Chori sanctarum virginum* (p.90)
73. *Gloria patri ingenito* (p.91)

In communi Apostolorum:

74. *Exultet coelum laudibus* (p.93)
75. *Qui coelum verbo* (p.94)
76. *Ut cum iudex* (p.95)
77. *Tristes erant Apostoli* (p.96)
78. *Illae dum pergunt* (p.97)
79. *Quaesumus auctor* (p.98)
80. *Deus tuorum militum* (p.99)
81. *Poenas cucurrit* (p.100)
82. *Laus et perennis gloria* (p.101)
83. *Deus tuorum militum* (p.103)
84. *Poenas cucurrit* (p.104)
85. *Gloria tibi Domine* (p.105)
86. *Sanctorum meritis* (p.106)
87. *Hi pro te furias* (p.107)
88. *Quae vox quae poterit* (p.108)
89. *Rex gloriose martyrum* (p.110)
90. *Tu vincis in martyribus* (p.111)
91. *Iste confessor* (p.112)
92. *Ad sacrum cuius* (p.113)
93. *Sit salus illi* (p.114)
94. *Iesu corona virginum* (p.116)
95. *Quodcumque pergis* (p.117)
96. *Laus honor* (p.118)
97. *Iesu corona virginum* (p.119)
98. *Quodcumque pergis* (p.120)
99. *Gloria tibi Domine* (p.121)
100. *Huius obtentu* (p.122)
101. *Urbs beata Ierusalem* (p.123)
102. *Portae nitent* (p.123)
103. *Gloria et honor Deo* (p.124)
104. *Magne pater Augustine* (p.125)
105. *Quae obscura* (p.129)
106. *Regi regem salus* (p.130)
107. *Laudibus summis* (p.132)
108. *Ex suo te nunc* (p.133)
109. *Dive celestique* (p.134)
110. *En gratulemur* (p.136)
111. *Longe lateque* (p.137)
112. *Sub tanto duci* (p.138)
113. *Prestet hoc nati* (p.139)
114. *Proles de coelo* (p.140)
115. *Assumptus cum apostolis* (p.141)
116. *Legi prophete gratiae* (p.142)
117. *Domum portam* (p.143)
118. *Franciscus tenens* (p.144)
119. *Demptum solo* (p.145)
120. *Hunc sequantur huic* (p.146)

121. *Est dux fidus* (p.147)
122. *Christe qui lux est* (p.148)
123. *Ne gravis somnus* (p.149)
124. *Defensor noster* (p.150)
125. *Deo patri sit gloria* (p.151)
126. *Prima lux surgens* (p.152)
127. *Palio visi* (p.153)
128. *Ac tuo nuctu* (p.154)
129. *Nunc iuvat celsi* (p.156)
130. *Dum fames terram* (p.157)
131. *Claudis et nubes* (p.158)
132. *Mensis augusti* (p.159)
133. *Candido velans* (p.160)
134. *Vicit altricem* (p.161)

A0086 [RISM 738] *Hymni totius anni, secundum Sanctae Romanae Ecclesiae consuetudinem, quattuor vocibus concinendi, necnon hymni religionum.* Venice: Angelo Gardano, 1589 [partbooks]:

1. *Conditor alme siderum* (p.2)
2. *Christe Redemptor omnium* (p.2)
3. *A solis ortu cardine* (p.6)
4. *Salvete flos Martyrum* (p.8)
5. *Hostes Herodes impie* (p.9)
6. *Lucis Creator optime* (p.11)
7. *O lux beata Trinitas* (p.13)
8. *Ad preces nostras* (p.14)
9. *Vexilla regis prodeunt* (p.16)
10. *Ad coenam Agni providi* (p.19)
11. *Jesu nostra redemptio* (p.21)
12. *Veni Creator Spiritus* (p.23)
13. *Pange lingua gloriosi* (p.26)
14. *Quodcumque vinclis* (p.28)
15. *Doctor egregie* (p.29)
16. *Ave maris stella* (p.30)
17. *Quo vulneratus insuper* (p.32)
18. *Ut queant laxis* (p.34)
19. *Aurea luce* (p.36)
20. *Lauda mater Ecclesia* (p.37)
21. *Petrus beatus* (p.39)
22. *Quicumque Christus quaeritis* (p.40)
23. *Tibi Christe splendor Patris* (p.41)
24. *Christe Redemptor omnium* (p.42)

In communi Apostolorum:

25. *Exultet coelum laudibus* (p.44)
26. *Tristes erant Apostoli* (p.46)
27. *Deus tuorum militum* (p.48)
28. *Deus tuorum militum* (p.50)
29. *Sanctorum meritis* (p.51)
30. *Rex gloriose Martyrum* (p.53)

31. *Iste confessor* (p.54)
32. *Iesu corona virginum* (p.56)
33. *Iesu corona virginum* (p.57)
34. *Huius obtentu* (p.59)
35. *Urbs beata Ierusalem* (p.59)
36. *Magne pater Augustine* (p.62)
37. *Laudibus summis* (p.64)
38. *En gratulemur hodie* (p.66)
39. *Proles de coelo prodiit* (p.68)
40. *Decus morum* (p.70)
41. *Christe qui lux es* (p.72)
42. *Prima lux surgens* (p.74)
43. *Dum fames terras* (p.76)
44. *Mensis augusti* (p.77)
45. *Hymnis canoris* (p.79)

Reprint History

A0087 [RISM P739] *Hymni totius anni, secundum Sanctae Romanae Ecclesiae consuetudinem, quattuor, quinque et sex vocibus concinendi, necnon hymni religionum.* Venice: heir of Girolamo Scotto, 1590 [partbooks].

A0088 [RISM P740] *Hymni totius anni secundum Sanctae Romanae Ecclesiae consuetudinem, cum basso ad organum, necnon hymni religionum quatuor vocibus concinendi.* Rome: Luca Antonio Soldi, 1625 [partbooks].

A0089 [RISM P741] *Hymni sacri in Breviario Romano . . . cantu musico pro praecipuis anni festivitatibus expressi.* Antwerp: "ex officina Platiniana, Baltasaris Moreti," 1644 [choirbook].

Print Locations

[A0085] Güssing, Franziskaner-Kloster; Vienna, Österreiches Nationalbibliothek, Musiksammlung; Brussels, Bibliothèque Royale Albert I; Augsburg, Staats- und Stadtbibliothek; Berlin, Staatsbibliothek; Munich, Bayerische Staatsbibliothek; Paris, Bibliothèque nationale (ancien fonds du Conservatoire nationale de musique); London, British Library (with manuscript supplement); Assisi, Biblioteca comunale; Bologna, Civico Museo Bibliografico Musicale; Florence, Biblioteca del Conservatorio di Musica "L. Cherubini"; Florence, Archivio del Duomo, Archivio musicale dell'opera di Santa Maria Maggiore; Gubbio, Biblioteca Vescovile Fonti e Archivio; Modena, Archivio capitolare (Duomo); Modena, Biblioteca Estense; Naples, Archivio musicale della Communità Oratoriana del Padri Filippini; Orvieto, Archivio musicale del Duomo (lacks title page); Padua, Biblioteca capitolare; Piacenza, Archivio del Duomo; Rome, Biblioteca Musicale governativa del Conservatorio di Santa Cecilia; Rome, Archivio di San Giovanni in Laterano; Rome, Archivio dell'Arciconfraternita di San Giovanni de'Fiorentini; Vatican City, Biblioteca Apostolica Vaticana, *fondo* Cappella Giulia; *ibid., fondo* Cappella Sistina; Spoleto, Archivio del Duomo; Terni, Istituto Musicale "G.Briccialdi"; Urbino, Biblioteca universitaria; Venice, Biblioteca del Conservatorio "Benedetto Marcello"; Venice: Museo Civico Correr; Coimbra, Biblioteca Geral da Universidade.

[A0086] Regensburg, Bischöfliche Zentralbibliothek (Proske-Musikbibliothek) [S,B]; London, Royal College of Music [complete: S,A,T,B]; Bologna, Civico Museo Bibliografico Musicale; Bologna, Archivio di San Petronio; Vatican City, Biblioteca Apostolica Vaticana, *fondo* Cappella Sistina; Treviso, Archivio della Cappella del Duomo; Princeton, NJ, Princeton University Library.

[A0087] Paris, Bibliothèque nationale [S,B]; London, British Library [B]; Lucca, Biblioteca del seminario arcivescovile [complete: S,A,T,B,5]; Cambridge, MA, Harvard University Music Libraries [A,T,B (lacking title page), 5].

[A0088] Hannover, Niedersächsische Landesbibliothek [S,A,TB,5, with fragmentary manuscript basso continuo part]; Rome, Biblioteca dell'Accademia nazionale dei Lincei e Corsiniana [S,A,T,B]; Vatican City, Biblioteca Apostolica Vaticana, *fondo* Cappella Giulia [S,A,T,B (two copies of part)].

[A0089] Munich, Bayerische Staatsbibliothek; Assisi, Biblioteca comunale; Bologna, Civico Museo Bibliografico Musicale; Loreto, Archivio Storico della Cappella Lauretana (incomplete); Rome, Archivio di San Giovanni in Laterano (lacks title page); Vatican City, Biblioteca Apostolica Vaticana, *fondo* Cappella Sistina.

Lamentations

A0090 [RISM P742] *Lamentationum Hieremiae prophetae, liber primus.* Rome: Alessandro Gardano, 1588 [partbooks]

Feria V. In coena Domini

1. Lectio I [Incipit Lamentatio . . . *Aleph. Quomodo sedet*]
2. Lectio II [*Vau. Et egreesus est*]
3. Lectio III [*Jod. Manum suam*]

Feria VI. In Parasceve

4. Lectio I [De lamentatione . . . *Cogitavit*]
5. Lectio II [*Lamed. Matribus suis*]
6. Lectio III [*Aleph. Ego vir videns*]

Sabbato sancto.

7. Lectio I [De lamentatione . . . *Heth. Misericordiae Domini*]
8. Lectio II [Aleph. *Quomodo obscuratum est*]
9. Lectio III [Incipit oratio . . . *Recordare Domine*]
10. *Benedictus Dominus Deus Israel*

Reprint History

A0091 [RISM P743] *Lamentationum Hieremiae prophetae cum quatuor vocibus, liber primus*. Venice: Heir of Girolamo Scotto, 1589 [partbooks].

Print Locations

[A0090] Regensburg, Bischöfliche Zentralbibliothek (Proske-Musikbibliothek) [complete: S,A,T,B]; London, British Library [B].

[A0091] Regensburg, Bischöfliche Zentralbibliothek (Proske-Musikbibliothek) [T]; Wolfenbüttel, Herzog-August-Bibliothek [complete: S,A,T,B]; Lucca, Biblioteca del seminario arcivescovile; Padua, Biblioteca del seminario vescovile; Vatican City, Biblioteca Apostolica Vaticana, *fondo* Cappella Sistina [S].

Litanies

A0092 [RISM P744] *Litaniae Deiparae Virginis . . . cum quatuor vocibus; additae litaniae, quae in sancta ecclesia Lauretana utuntur, auctore Orlando Lasso.* Venice: Angelo Gardano, 1600

1. *Litaniae Deiparae Virginis*. Prima parte: Kyrie eleison . . . Virgo mater audi nos. Ave Maria gratia plena. Seconda parte: Kyrie eleison . . . Maria Mater gratiae. Terza parte: Kyrie eleison . . . Virgo Maria respice nos. Quarta parte: Kyrie eleison . . . Ave de coelis. Quinta parte: Kyrie eleison . . . Ab omni malo. (pp.1–10)
2. [new title page:] *Litaniae Liber Secundus.* Prima parte: Kyrie eleison . . . Virgo mater audi nos. Ave Maria gratia plena. Seconda parte: Kyrie eleison . . . Maria Mater gratiae. Terza parte: Kyrie eleison . . . Virgo Maria respice in nos, Virgo virginum, defende nos. Quarta parte: Kyrie eleison . . . Ave de coelis. Quinta parte: Kyrie eleison . . . Ab omni malo. (pp.11–20)

Print Locations

[A0092] Bologna, Civico Museo Bibliografico Musicale [complete: S,A,T,B]; London, British Library.

Magnificat

A0093 [RISM P745] *Magnificat octo tonum.* Venice: Angelo Gardano, 1591 [partbooks].

Anima mea Dominum ["odd" verses]	Et exultavit spiritum meum ["even" verses]
1. *Primi toni* (p.2)	9. *Primi toni* (p.18)
2. *Secundi toni* (p.5 [recte 4])	10. *Secundi toni* (p.20)
3. *Tertii toni* (p.6)	11. *Tertii toni* (p.22)
4. *Quarti toni* (p.7)	12. *Quarti toni* (p.24)
5. *Quinti toni* (p.10)	13. *Quinti toni* (p.26)
6. *Sexti toni* (p.12)	14. *Sexti toni* (p.28)
7. *Septimi toni* (p.14)	15. *Septimi toni* (p.29)
8. *Octavi toni* (p.16)	16. *Octavi toni* (p.31)

Reprint History

A0094 [RISM P745a] *Magnificat octo tonum. Liber primus . . . nunc recens in lucem editus.* Rome: Alessandro Gardano, 1591 [partbooks].

Print Locations

[A0093] Brussels, Bibliothèque Royale Albert I [B]; Kassel, Murhard'sche Bibliothek der Stadt Kassel und Landesbibliothek [complete: S,A,T,B]; Regensburg, Bischöfliche Zentralbibliothek (Proske-Musikbibliothek) [B]; Bologna, Civico Museo Bibliografico Musicale; Brescia, Archivio e Biblioteca capitolare; Brescia, Biblioteca Queriniana [A]; Milan, Biblioteca del Conservatorio di Musica "Giuseppe Verdi"; Siena, Biblioteca dell'Accademia Musicale Chigiana; Vatican City, Biblioteca Apostolica Vaticana, *fondo* Cappella Sistina [S,T]; Treviso, Archivio della Cappella del Duomo; Venice, Biblioteca nazionale Marciana; Lisbon, Arquivo da Fabrica da Sé; Moscow, Rossijskaja Gosudarstvennaja Biblioteka [S,A,T]; Berkeley, CA, University of California Music Library.

[A0094] Bologna, Civico Museo Bibliografico Musicale; Pistoia, Biblioteca dell'Archivio capitolare [S]; Vatican City, Biblioteca Apostolica Vaticana, *fondo* Chigi [A].

Offertories

A0095 [RISM P746] *Offertoria totius anni, secundum Sanctae Romanae Ecclesiae consuetudinem, quinque vocibus concinenda . . . pars prima.* Rome: Francesco Coattino, 1593 [partbooks]

1. *Ad te levavi animam meam* (p.1)
2. *Deus tu conversus* (p.2)
3. *Benedixisti Domine* (p.3)
4. *Ave Maria* (p.4)
5. *Tui sunt coeli* (p.5)
6. *Elegerunt Apostoli Stephanum* (p.6)
7. *Iustus ut palma* (p.7)
8. *Anima nostra* (p.8)
9. *Posuisti Domine* (p.9)
10. *Deus enim firmavit* (p.10)
11. *Inveni David* (p.11)
12. *Reges Tarsis* (p.12)
13. *Iubilate Deo omnis terra* (p.13)
14. *Iubilate Deo universa terra* (p.14)
15. *Dextera Domini (p.15)*
16. *Bonum est confiteri* (p.16)
17. *Perfice gressus meos* (p.17)
18. *Benedictus Domine* (p.18)
19. *Scapulis suis* (p.19)
20. *Meditabor in mandatis* (p.20)

21. *Iustitiae Domini* (p.22)
22. *Laudate Dominum quia benignus* (p.22)
23. *Confitebor tibi Domine* (p.23)
24. *Improperium exspectavit* (p.24)
25. *Terra tremuit* (p.25)
26. *Angelus Domini* (p.26)
27. *Deus Deus meus* (p.27)
28. *Lauda anima mea* (p.28)
29. *Benedicta gentes* (p.29)
30. *Ascendit Deus* (p.30)
31. *Confirma hoc Deus* (p.31)
32. *Benedicta sit* (p.32)
33. *Sacerdotes Domini* (p.33)
34. *Domine convertere* (p.34)
35. *Sperent in te omnes* (p.35)
36. *Illumina oculos meos* (p.36)
37. *Benedicam Dominum* (p.37)
38. *Sicut in holocaustis* (p.38)
39. *Populem humilem* (p.39)
40. *Iustitiae Domini* (p.40)

Reprint History

A0096 [RISM P747] *Offertoria totius anni, secundum Sanctae Romanae Ecclesiae consuetudinem, quinque vocibus concinenda . . . pars prima.* Venice: Angelo Gardano, 1593 [partbooks].

A0097 [RISM P748] *Offertoria totius anni, secundum Sanctae Romanae Ecclesiae consuetudinem, quinque vocibus concinenda . . . pars prima.* Venice: Angelo Gardano, 1594 [partbooks].

Print Locations

[A0095] Berlin, Staatsbibliothek [complete: S,A,T,B,5]; Hannover, Niedersächsische Landesbibliothek [T,B,5, with manuscript S (fol.37–56) and bc]; Regensburg, Bischöfliche Zentralbibliothek (Proske-Musikbibliothek) [S,T]; Tarazona, Archivo capitular [S,T, B (lacks title page), 5]; London, British Library [S,T,B,5]; London, Royal College of Music; Lucca, Biblioteca del seminario arcivescovile; Florence, Biblioteca del Conservatorio di Musica "Luigi Cherubini"; Pistoia, Archivio capitolare della Cattedrale [with various fragments, both manuscript and printed]; Rome, Archivio di San Giovanni in Laterano; Vatican City, Biblioteca Apostolica Vaticana, *fondo* Cappella Giulia; *ibid., fondo* Cappella Sistina [T,B,5]; Vercelli, Archivio del Duomo (Biblioteca capitolare) [S,B,5].

[A0096] London, British Library [B].

[A0097] Hamburg, Staats- und Universitätsbibiothek Carl von Ossietzky, Musikabteilung [5]; Cuenca, Archivo capitular de Cuenca [S,A,T,5]; London, British Library [B]; Assisi, Biblioteca comunale [S,A,T,5]; Bologna, Civico Museo Bibliografico Musicale [complete: S,A,T,B,5]; Milan, Biblioteca del Conservatorio "Giuseppe Verdi"; Pistoia, Archivio capitolare della Cattedrale [A,T,b]; Vatican City, Biblioteca Apostolica Vaticana, *fondo* Cappella Sistina [T]; Treviso, Archivio della Cappella del Duomo; Rochester, NY, Sibley Music Library, Eastman School of Music, University of Rochester; Washington, DC, Library of Congress, Music Division.

A0098 [RISM P749] *Offertoria totius anni, secundum Sanctae Romanae Ecclesiae consuetudinem, quinque vocibus concinenda . . . pars secunda.* Rome: Francesco Coattino, 1593 [partbooks]

1. *Exaltabo te* (p.1)
2. *Precatus est Moyses* (p.2)
3. *In te speravi* (p.3)
4. *Immittit Angelus* (p.4)
5. *Exspectans exspectavi* (p.5)
6. *Domine in auxilium meum* (p.6)
7. *Oravi ad Dominum* (p.7)
8. *Sanctificavit Moyses* (p.8)
9. *Si ambulavero* (p.9)
10. *Super flumina* (p.10)
11. *Vir erat in terra* (p.11)
12. *Recordare mei* (p.12)
13. *De profundis clamavi* (p.13)
14. *Iustus ut palma* (p.14)
15. *Mihi autem nimis* (p.15)
16. *Confessio et pulchritudo* (p.16)
17. *Assumpta est Maria* (p.17)
18. *Stetit angelus* (p.18)
19. *Constituos eos principes* (p.19)
20. *Confitebuntur coeli* (p.20)
21. *In omnem terram* (p.21)
22. *Iustorum animae* (p.22)
23. *Veritas mea* (p.23)
24. *Laetamini in Domino* (p.24)
25. *Afferentur regi* (p.25)
26. *Domine Deus* (p.26)
27. *Diffusa est gratia* (p.27)
28. *Tu es Petrus* (p.28)

Reprint History

A0099 [RISM P750] *Offertoria totius anni, secundum Sanctae Romanae Ecclesiae consuetudinem, quinque vocibus concinenda . . . pars secunda.* Venice: Angelo Gardano, 1596.

A0100 [RISM P751] *Cantiones sacrae quinque vocum pro diebus dominicis & fes-*

tis totius anni. Antwerp: Pierre Phalèse, 1603 [parts 1 and 2] [partbooks].

Print Locations

[A0098] Hannover, Niedersächsische Landesbibliothek [complete: S,A,T,B,5]; Tarazona, Archivo capitular [S,T,B,5]; Valladolid, Archivo musical de la Catedral [T]; Aosta, Cattedrale, Biblioteca capitolare [S,A,5]; London, British Library [S,T,B,5]; London, Royal College of Music; Lucca, Biblioteca del seminario arcivescovile, Pistoia, Archivio capitolare della Cattedrale [with various fragments, both manuscript and printed]; Rome, Archivio di San Giovanni in Laterano; Vatican City, Biblioteca Apostolica Vaticana, *fondo* Cappella Giulia; *ibid., fondo* Cappella Sistina [T,B,5]; Vercelli, Archivio del Duomo (Biblioteca capitolare) [S,B,5 (two copies)].

[A0099] Brussels, Bibliothèque Royale Albert I [complete: S,A,T,B,5]; Hamburg, Staats- und Universitätsbibiothek Carl von Ossietzky, Musikabteilung [5]; Cuenca, Archivo capitular de Cuenca [T,B]; London, British Library [B]; Bologna, Civico Museo Bibliografico Musicale; Milan, Biblioteca di Conservatorio di Musica "Giuseppe Verdi"; Pistoia, Archivio capitolare della Cattedrale [A,T,b]; Treviso, Archivio della Cappella del Duomo; Venice, Biblioteca nazionale Marciana [T]; Rochester, NY, Sibley Music Library, Eastman School of Music, University of Rochester; Washington, DC, Library of Congress, Music Division.

[A0100] Oxford, Bodleian Library [complete: S,A,T,B,5].

Madrigals

A0101 [RISM P752] *Il primo libro di madrigali a quattro voci di Gio. Pierluigi da Palestrina cantore nella cappella di N.S.* Rome: Valerio and Aloisio Dorico, 1555 [partbooks]

1. *Deh hor foss'io col vago* (p.1) [Petrarch]
2. *S'il dissi mai, ch' io venga* (p.2) [Petrarch]
3. *Queste saranno ben lagrime* (p.3) [N. Armanio]
4. *Che non sia che già mai* (p.4) [N. Armanio]
5. *Rime dai sospir miei* (p.5)
6. *Lontan dalla mia diva* (p.6)
7. *Là ver l'aurora, che sì dolce l'aura* (p.7) [Petrarch]
8. *Chiara, sì chiar' è de' vostr'occhi* (p.8)
9. *Che estinguerà' l mio foco* (p.9) [L. Capilupi]
10. *Donna, vostra mercede ogni pietade* (p.10)
11. *Già fu chi m'hebbe cara* (p.11) [G. Boccaccio]
12. *Che debbo far, che mi consigli* (p.12) [Petrarch]
13. *Ovver de' sensi è priva* (p.13)
14. *Amor, fortun' et la mia mente schiva* (p.14) [Petrarch]
15. [seconda parte:] *Nè spero i dolci dì* (p.15) [Petrarch]
16. *Gitene, liete rime* (p.16)
17. *Mentre a le dolci et le purpuree labbia* (p.17)

18. *Amor, che mec'in quest'ombre* (p.18) [P. Bembo]
19. [seconda parte:] *Ecc'ove gionse prima* (p.19) [P. Bembo]
20. *Vaghi pensier, che così passo passo* (p.20) [Petrarch]
21. *Mentre ch'al mar descenderanno i fiumi* (p.21) [Petrarch]
22. *Qual rime fur sì chiare* (p.22)
23. *Ecc'oscurat'i chiari raggi al sole*. Sestina (p.23) [Cristiani]
24. [seconda parte:] *Rara beltà, non mai più vista* (p.24) [Cristiani]
25. [terza parte:] *Questo doglioso stil colmo* (p.25) [Cristiani]
26. [quarta parte:] *Mai fu più cruda, o più spietata morte* (p.26) [Cristiani]
27. [quinta parte:] *Privo di fed'oltra l'usato corso* (p.27) [Cristiani]
28. [sesta parte:] *Ma voi fiorit' et honorati colli* [a 5] (p.28) [Cristiani]

Reprint History

A0102 [RISM P753] *Il primo libro di madrigali a quattro voci di Gio. Pierluigi da Palestrina . . . nuovamente ristampato*. Venice: Claudio Merulo da Corregio, 1568 [partbooks].

A0103 [RISM P754] *Il primo libro di madrigali a quattro voci di Gio. Pierluigi da Palestrina . . . di nuova ristampato, et da M. Claudio Merulo da Corregio con ogni diligenza corretto*. Venice: Giorgio Anglieri, 1574 [partbooks].

A0104 [RISM P755] *Il primo libro di madrigali a quattro voci di Gioan Pierluigi da Palestina . . . novamente ristampati, & corretti*. Venice: Giacomo Vincenti and Ricciardo Amadino, 1583 [partbooks].

A0105 [RISM P756] *Il primo libro di madrigali a quattro voci di Gioan Pierluigi da Palestina . . . novamente ristampati, & corretti*. Venice: Ricciardo Amadino, 1587 [partbooks].

A0106 [RISM P757] *Il primo libro di madrigali a quattro voci di Gioan Pierluigi da Palestina . . . novamente ristampati & corretti*. Venice: Giacomo Vincenti, 1588 [partbooks].

A0107 [RISM P758] *Il primo libro di madrigali a quattro voci di Gioan Pierluigi da Palestina. . . .* Venice: Angelo Gardano, 1594 [enlarged edition]. [*Nesun visse giamai più di me lieto* [Petrarch] is added between nos. 5 and 6 of the 1555 Dorico ordering and is also listed as being on page 6.]

A0108 [RISM P759] *Il primo libro di madrigali a quattro voci di Gio. Pierluigi da Palestina . . . novamente ristampato*. Venice: Heir of Girolamo Scotto, 1596 [partbooks].

A0109 [RISM P760] *Il primo libro di madrigali a quattro voci di Gioan Pierluigi da Palestina . . . novamente ristampato*. Venice: Angelo Gardano, 1605 [partbooks].

Print Locations

[A0101] Rochester, NY, Sibley Music Library, Eastman School of Music, University of Rochester [S].

[A0102] Brussels, Bibliothèque Royale Albert I [S].

[A0103] London, British Library [S].

[A0104] Munich, Bayerische Staatsbibliothek [B].

[A0105] Brussels, Bibliothèque Royale Albert I [complete: S,A,T,B]; Munich, Bayerische Staatsbibliothek [S,A,T]; Bologna, Civico Museo Bibliografico Musicale [A,T,B]; Gdansk, Biblioteka Polskiej Akademii Nauk.

[A0106] Treviso, Archivio della Cappella del Duomo [B]; Vatican City, Biblioteca Apostolica Vaticana [S,T,B]; Coimbra, Biblioteca Geral da Universidade [B].

[A0107] Rome, Archivio Doria Pamphili [A].

[A0108] Bologna, Civico Museo Bibliografico Musicale [complete: S,A,T,B].

[A0109] Regensburg, Bischöfliche Zentralbibliothek (Proske-Musikbibliothek) [T]; Wolfenbüttel, Herzog-August-Bibliothek [complete: S,A,T,B]; Bologna, Civico Museo Bibliografico Musicale; Vatican City, Biblioteca Apostolica Vaticana, *fondo* Cappella Sistina [S,A].

A0110 [RISM P761] *Il primo libro di madrigali a cinque voci, di Gio. Petr'Alosio Prenestino novamenti composti et dati in luce.* Venice: Angelo Gardano, 1581 [partbooks]

1. *Vergine bella, che di sol vestita* (p.1) [Petrarch]
2. [seconda parte:] *Vergine saggia et del bel numer'una* (p.2) [Petrarch]
3. [terza parte:] *Vergine pura, d'ogni part'intera* (p.3) [Petrarch]
4. [quarta parte:] *Vergine santa, d'ogni gratia piena* (p.5) [Petrarch]
5. [quinta parte:] *Vergina sola al mondo senz'esempio* (p.6) [Petrarch]
6. [sesta parte:] *Vergine chiara e stabile in eterno* (p.8) [Petrarch]
7. [settima parte:] *Vergine, quante lagrime ho già sparte* (p.9) [Petrarch]
8. [ottava parte:] *Vergine, tale è terra e post'ha in doglia* (p.10) [Petrarch]
9. *Spirito santo, amore, consolator interno di quel lume superno* (p.12)
10. *O sol, incoronato di sette adorni lumi, o foco temperato* (p.13)
11. *O cibo di dolcezza, che pasci et non fastidi, fontana d' allegrezza* (p.14)
12. *O refrigerio acceso d'un nutricante foco, o leve et dolce peso* (p.15)
13. *Tu sei suave fiume de bei parlar profondi, tu sei mediante lume* (p.16)

14. *Paraclito amoroso, quando t'havrò io quando* (p.17)
15. *Amor, senza il tuo dono in van io m'affatico* (p.18)
16. *Dunque, divin spiracolo, inspira il mio cor vano* (p.19)
17. *O manna saporita, d'ogni dolcezza pieno* (p.20)
18. *Signor, dammi scientia, consiglio et intelletto* (p.21)
19. *O Iesù dolce, o infinito amore, inestimabile dono* (p.22)
20. *Giamai non resti a mille dolci modi* (p.23)
21. *Quanto più t'offendo'io, tanto più sei cortese* (p.24)
22. *Non basta ch'una volta, tu portasti sì vil morte* (p.25)
23. *S'io non ti cognoscessi in altre cose* (p.26)
24. *Ma so ben, signor mio, che ciò che fai è solo* (p.27)
25. *E tu, anima mia, fatta di Dio sì bella et sì gentile* (p.28)
26. *Per questo, signor mio, non ti stancare* (p.29)

Reprint History

A0111 [RISM P762] *Il primo libro di madrigali a cinque voci, di Gio. Petr'Alosio Prenestino . . . novamente ristampato.* Venice: Angelo Gardano, 1604 [partbooks].

Print Locations

[A0110] Vienna, Österreiches Nationalbibliothek, Musiksammlung [complete: S,A,T,B,5]; Brussels, Bibliothèque Royale Albert I [A]; Berlin, Staatsbibliothek; Kassel, Murhard'sche Bibliothek der Stadt Kassel und Landesbibliothek; Köln, Universitäts- und Stadtbibliothek [S,A,5]; Munich, Bayerische Staatsbibliothek; Regensburg, Bischöfliche Zentralbibliothek (Proske-Musikbibliothek) [S,T]; Valencia, Catedral, Archivio musical [S,A,T,B]; London, British Library [S]; Bologna, Civico Museo Bibliografico Musicale; Amsterdam, Toonkunst-Bibliotheek [S,T]; Gdansk, Biblioteka Polskiej Akademii Nauk [T,B,5]; New York, New York Public Library at Lincoln Center [5].

[A0111] Bologna, Civico Museo Bibliografico Musicale [complete: S,A,T,B,5]; Milan, Archivio della Veneranda Fabbrica, Cappella musicale del Duomo [A,T,B,5 (lacks S)].

A0112 [RISM P763] *Il secondo libro di madrigali a quatro voci.* Venice: heir of Girolamo Scotto, 1586 [partbooks]

1. *Così la fama scriva in sempiterni marmi* (p.3)
2. *S'un sguardo un fa beato* (p.4) [Alfonso d'Avalos]
3. *Amor, ben puoi tu hormai* (p.5)
4. *Partomi, donna, e teco lascio il core* (p.6)
5. *Veramente in amore* (p.7) [P. Bembo]
6. *Gioia m'abond'al cor tanta* (p.8) [P. Bembo]
7. *Donna gentil, quando tal'hor degnate* (p.9)
8. *Io dovea ben pensarmi* (p.10)
9. *Se'l pensier che mi strugge* (p.11) [Petrarch]

10. *Che dunque fia se voi donne* (p.12)
11. *Mirate altrove, vita mia* (p.13)
12. *Siè debole il filo* (p.14) [Petrarch]
13. *I vaghi fiori e l'amorose fronde* (p.15)
14. *Morì quasi il mio core* (p.16)
15. *A la riva del Tebro* (p.17)
16. *Amor, quando fioria mia speme* (p.18) [Petrarch]
17. *Beltà, se come in ment'io* (p.19)
18. *La cruda mia nemica* (p.20)
19. *O che splendor* (p.21)
20. *Io sento qui d'intorno spirarmi* (p.22)
21. *Deh foss'hor qui, madonna* (p.23)
22. *Se non fuss'il pensier crudel* (p.24) [P. Bembo]
23. *Perchè s'annida amore nelle luci* (p.25)
24. *Ogni beltà, madonna, ch'io veggio* (p.26)
25. *Ardo lungi et da presso* (p.27)

Print Locations

[A0112] Wolfenbüttel, Herzog-August-Bibliothek [complete: S,A,T,B]; Dresden, Sächsische Landesbibliothek [T (incomplete), B]; Paris, Bibliothèque nationale [T]; London, British Library; Oxford, Harding private collection [A]; Bologna, Civico Museo Bibliografico Musicale; Parma, Sezione Musicale della Biblioteca Palatina presso il Conservatorio "Arrigo Boito"; Gdansk, Biblioteka Polskiej Akademii Nauk [S,A,T]; Boston, MA, Boston Public Library, Music Department; Cambridge, MA, Harvard University Music Libraries [A,T].

A0113 [RISM P764] *Delle Madrigali spirituali a cinque voci di Gio. Pietro Luigi Prenestino, maestro di cappella di S. Pietro di Roma. Libro Secondo. . . .* Rome: Francesco Coattino, 1594 [partbooks]

1. *Figlio immortal d'immortal padre* (p.3)
2. *E se mai voci di qua giù son grate* (p.4)
3. *Hor tu sol, che di vivi, almi splendori* (p.5)
4. *Dammi, scala del ciel e del ciel porta* (p.6)
5. *E se fur già le mie mani immonde l'opre* (p.7)
6. *Dammi vermiglia rosa e bianco e puro giglio* (p.8)
7. *E se'l pensier de la futura morte* (p.9)
8. *Eletta Mirra, che suave odore doni* (p.10)
9. *Cedro gentil, da gli amorosi vermi* (p.11)
10. *Fà che con l'acque tue splendenti e vive* (p.12)
11. *Se amarissimo fele e mortal tosco cibo* (p.13)
12. *Horto, che sei sì chiuso e sì serrato* (p.14)
13. *E se nel foco di lascivie ardendo* (p.15)
14. *Vincitrice de l'empia hidra infernale* (p.16)
15. *Città di Dio, cui fà tempi e fortezze* (p.17)
16. *Santo altare, d'odor più veri e degni ardente* (p.18)
17. *Tu di fortezza torre e torre eburna* (p.19)

18. *Specchio, che fosti sì polito e terso sempre* (p.20)
19. *Vello di Gideon, cio Dio sì largo fu* (p.21)
20. *Novella aurora, che nascendo allegri il mondo* (p.22)
21. *E questo spirto, de la propria fede scacciato* (p.23)
22. *E dal letto di mille e mille colpe* (p.24)
23. *Et arda ogn'hor sopr'l lapideo altare* (p.25)
24. *E tua mercè, da così cieca e folta nebbia* (p.26)
25. *E quella certa speme e quella fede* (p.27)
26. *Anzi se foco e foco e se veleno* (p.28)
27. *E con i raggi tuoi, splendenti e chiari* (p.29)
28. *Regina de le vergini e di tutte le squadre beatissime* (p.30)
29. *Al fin, madre di Dio, che ne più bella cosa* (p.31)
30. *E tu, Signor, tu la tua gratia infondi al core* (p.32)

Print Locations

[A0113] Bologna, Civico Museo Bibliografico Musicale; Florence, Biblioteca nazionale; London, Royal College of Music [complete: S,A (in manuscript), T,B,5].

II. Printed Compositions in Musical Anthologies

Masses

A0114 [RISM 1585[5]] *Di M. Giovanni Pierluigi da Palestina una messa a otto voci sopra il suo Confitebor a due cori. Et di M. Bartholomeo lo Roi maestro di Capella di Vicere di Napoli una messa a quattro sopra Panis quem ego dabo tibi, de Lupo. Novamente poste in luce.* Venice: heirs of Girolamo Scotto, 1585.

Includes *MissaConfitebor tibi a 8.*

A0115 [RISM 1590[1]] *Missae quinque, quinis vocibus, a diversis et aetatis nostrae praestantissimus musicis compositae: ac in usum Ecclesiae DEI nuperrimé editae, studio et opera Friderici Lindeneri.* Nuremberg: Catharina Gerlach, 1590.

Includes *Missa Primi toni a 5; Missa Sine nomine a 5*; *Missa Secunda (Veni Sancte Spiritus) a 5.*

A0116 [RISM c.1590[2]][Missae 4 voc.]—(s.l. n.d.) 1 vol in fol, 31 f. [date uncertain; title page missing].

Includes *Missa Sine nomine a 4.*

A0117 [RISM 1592[1]] *Missae dominicales quinis vocibus diversorum auctorum a F. Iulio Pellino carmel. mant. collectae.* Milan: M.Tini, 1592.

Includes *Missa Dominicalis a 5.*

A0118 [RISM 1599[1]] *Selectissimarum missarum flores, ex praestantissimis nostrae aetatis autoribus quatuor, quinque, sex et plurimum vocum collecti: et ad ecclesiae catholicae usum ordine deceenti dispositi. Opera D. Matthiae Pot-*

tier cathedralis D. Mariae antverpiensis phonasci. . . . Antwerp: P. Phalèse, 1599.

Includes *Missa Sacerdotes et pontifex a 6.*

A0119 [RISM 1619[2]] *Messe a quattro voci. Le tre prime del Palestrina, cioè Iste Confessor, Sine nomine, & di papa Marcello, ridotta a quattro da Gio. Francesco Anerio, et la quarta della bataglia dell'istesso Gio. Francesco Anerio con il basso continuo per sonare.* Rome: L.A. Soldi, 1619 [repr. 1626, 1635, 1639].

Includes *Missa Iste confessor a 4; Missa sine nomine a 4*; *Missa Papae Marcelli a 4.*

A0120 [RISM 1626[1]] *Messe a quattro voci. Le tre prime del Palestrina cioè Iste Confessor, Sine nomine & di Papa Marcello ridotta a 4 da Gio. Francesco Anerio, & la quarta della Battaglia dell'istesso Gio. Francesco Anerio.* Rome: P. Masotti, 1626.

See item A119.

A0121 [RISM 1646[1]] *Messe a quattro voci le tre primi del Palestina cioè, di Papa Marcello ridotta a 4 da Gio. Francesco Anerio, Iste Confessor & Sine nomine & la quarta della Bataglia, dell'istesso Gio. Francesco Anerio con il Basso continuo per l'organo Di nuovo corrette con l'aggiunta di una messa di Pietro Heredia et un'altra per i Defonti del medessimo.* Rome: Lodovico Grignani 1646.

Includes *Missa Papae Marcelli* (arr. Anerio *a 4*); *Missa Iste Confessor a 4; Missa Sine nomine a 4.*

A0122 [RISM 1689[1]] *Messe a quattro voci del Palestina cioè, di Papa Marcello ridotta à quattro da Gio. Francesco Anerio, Iste Confessor, & Sine nomine; e la quarta della Battaglia à del istesso Gio, Francesco Anerio. Con il basso continuo per l'organo. Di novo diligentemente corretta da Francesco Gannini.* Rome: Mascardi, 1689 [partbooks, 5 vols in 8vo].

Includes *Missa Papae Marcelli* [*a 4*]; *Missa Iste Confessor a 4*; *Missa Sine nomine a 4.*

Motets

A0123 [RISM 1563[3]] *Liber primus Musarum cum quatuor vocibus sacrarum cantionum que vulgo mottetta vocantur ab Orlando di Lassus, Cipriano Rore, et aliis ecclesiasticis authoribus compositarum, et ab Antonio Barré collectarum et in lucem nunc primum editarum.* Venice: F. Rampazzetto, 1563.

Includes motets p.2, *O quam suavis est Dominus a 4*; p.14, *Nativitas tua Dei genetrix a 4.*

——— [RISM 1572[1]=RISM P705] *Iohannis Petraloysii praenestini Motettorum quae partim quinis, partim senis, partim octonis vocibus concinantur, liber secundus nunc primum in lucem aeditus.* Venice: Girolamo Scotto, 1572 [repr. 1573, 1577, 1580, 1588, and 1594].

See A052. Included here because the print contains music by members of Palestrina's family. Includes motets p.3, *O virgo simul et mater*; p.4, *Memor esto verbi tui*; p.5, *Corona aurea* [secunda pars *Domine prevenisti eum*]; p.7, *In illo tempore*; p.9, *O sacrum convivium*; p.10, *Coenantibus illis*; *Derelinquat impius* (pp.10–13); *Canite tuba in Sion* [secunda pars *Rorate coeli desuper*]; *Homo quidam* (p.14); *Ascendo ad patrem* [secunda pars *Ego rogabo*] (p.14); *Exi cito* (p.16); *Gaude Barbara beata* [secunda pars *Gaude quia meruisti*] (p.18–20); *Peccantem me quotidie* (p.23); *Dominus Jesus in qua nocte* (pp.24); *Tribularer si nescirem* [secunda pars *Secundum multitudinem*] (pp.25–26); *Veni Domine et non tardare* [secunda pars *Excita Domine*] (pp.27–28); *Hierusalem cito veniet* [secunda pars *Ego enim sum Dominus*] (pp.29–30) *Beata Barbara* [secunda pars *Gloriosum mortem magis*] (pp.30–31); *Sancta et immaculata virginitas* [secunda pars *Benedicta tu*] (pp.33–34); *Cantabo Domino* [secunda pars *Deficiant peccatores*] (pp.35–36); *Tu es Petrus* [secunda pars *Quodcumque ligaveris*] (pp.37–39); *Confitebor tibi* [secunda pars *Notas facite*] (pp.40–41); *Laudate pueri Dominum* [secunda pars *Quis sicut Dominus*] (pp.42–45); *Domine in virtuta tua* [secunda pars *Magna est gloria eius*] (pp.46–51); *Laudate Dominum omnes gentes* (p.52)

Publication also includes the following music by members of Palestrina's immediate family:

Angelo Pierluigi: p.17, *Circuire possum a 5* [secunda pars *In hac cruce*].

Rodolfo Pierluigi: p.22, *Confitebor tibi Domine a 5*.

Silla Pierluigi: p.21, *Domine Pater a 5*; p.40, *Nunc dimittis a 6*.

A0124 [RISM 1583[2]] *Harmoniae miscellae cantionum sacrarum, ab exquisitissimis aetatis nostrae musicis cum quinque & sex vocibus concinnatae, pleraque omnes novae, necdum in Germania typis scriptae nunc autem editae studio Leonardi Lechneri athesini*. Nuremberg: Gerlach, 1583.

Includes motets no.5, *Fuit homo missus a Deo a 5* [secunda pars *Erat Joannes in deserto*]; no.30, *Susanna ab improbis* [secunda pars *Postquam autem salso eorum*]; no.36, *Haec dies quam fecit Dominus a 6*.

A0125 [RISM 1585[1]] *Sacrae cantiones, cum anni, a praestantissimis Italiae musicis nuperrime concinnatae. Quarum quaedam antea Venetiis separatim editae sunt, quaedam verò planè novae, nec usquam excusae, at nunc in gratiam & usum scholarum atque ecclesiarum germanicarum in unum corpus redactae, studio & opera Friderici Lindneri, . . .* Nuremberg: Catharina Gerlach, 1585.

Includes motets no.1, *O magnum mysterium a 6* [secunda pars *Quem vidistis pastores*]; no.4, *O admirabile commercium*; no.7, *Stella quam viderunt magi*; no.12, *Suscipe verbum virgo Maria*; no.19, *Alleluia. Tulerunt Dominum*; no.24, *Viri Galilaei a 6* [secunda pars *Ascendit Deus*]; no.25, *Dum complerentur a 6* [secunda pars *Dum ergo essent*]; no.30, *Puer qui natus est nobis a 5*.

A0126 [1587] *Cantus ecclesiasticus officii maioris hebdomadae iuxta ritum Capellae Sanctissimi Domini nostri Papae ac Basilicae Vaticanae. . . .* ed. J. Giudetti. Rome: J. Tornerius, 1587.

Includes *falsibordoni* motets p.36, *Miserere mei a 4*; p.78, *Miserere mei a 5;* p.112, *Miserere mei a 6;* p.114, *Benedictus Dominus a 4* [anon; found in Lateran 59 autograph] [Jeppesen (1958) suggested that the following, all anonymous in the source, may also be by Palestrina: p.36–37, *Benedictus Dominus a 4*; p.78–79, *Benedictus Dominus a 4*; p.112–113, *Benedictus Dominus a 4*].

A0127 [RISM 1588^{3}] *Liber primus musarum cum quatuor vocibus, seu sacrae cantiones, quae vulgo motecta appellantur, ab Orlando Lasso, Cipriano Rore, & alijs ecclesiasticis authoribus compositae, et ab Antonio Barre collectae, & in lucem editae, addito nuper dialogo cum octo vocibus Orphei Vecchij.* Milan: Francesco and heirs of Simon Tini, 1588 [partbooks, four vols in 4to, 16f].

Includes motets p.2, *O quam suavis est Dominus a 4*; p.14, *Nativitas tua Dei genetrix a 4.*

A0128 [RISM 1590^{5}] *Corollarium cantionum sacrarum quinque, sex, septem, octo, et plurium vocum, de festis praecipuis anni. Quarum quaedam antea, a praestantissimis nostrae aetatis musicis, in Italia separatim editae sunt, quaedam vero nuperrime concinnatae, nec uspiam typis excusae, at nunc in unum quasi corpus redactae studio & opera Friderici Lindneri &c*. Nuremberg: Catharina Gerlach, 1590.

Includes motets no.14, *Senex puerum portabat* [secunda pars *Hodie beata Virgo*]; no.29, *Angelus Dominus descendit* [secunda pars *Et introeuntes*]; no.36, *Ascendo ad Patrem* [secunda pars *Ego te rogabo patrem*]; no.37, *Veni Sancte Spiritus*; no.48, *Tu es Petrus a 7*; no.49, *Solve jubente Deo* [secunda pars *Quodcumque ligaveris*]; no.50, *Tu es Petrus a 6* [secunda pars *Quodcumque ligaveris*]; no.61, *Hierusalem cito veniet* [secunda pars *Ego enim sum*]; no.62, *Veni Domine a 6* [secunda pars *Excita Domine*]; no.63, *Canite tuba* [secunda pars *Rorate coeli desuper*]; no.70, *Surge illuminare a 8.*

Also includes motet by Silla Pierluigi: no.19, *Nunc dimittis a 6.*

A0129 [RISM 1590^{6}] *Suavissimorum modulorum selectissimae cantiones sacrae, ex praestantissimis quibusdam musicis collectae, quatuor, quinque, sex et octo vocum, cum viva voce, tum omnis generis instrumentis cantatu commodissime. His adjuncta est missa eleganti artificio composita, sex vocum. Nunc demum summa diligentia in gratiam studiosorum Musices in lucem emissae*. Munich: Adam Berg, 1590 [six vols in 4to].

Includes motet *Surge propera amica mea a 4.*

A0130 [RISM 1592^{2}] *Psalmi Motecta, Magnificat, et antiphona, Salve Regina diversorum auctorum: octo vocibus concinenda, selecta a Jo. Luca Conforti.* Rome: F. Coattino, 1592 [four vols. in 8tvo, 28pp].

Includes motet p.25, *Vos amici mei estis a 8.*

A0131 [RISM 1596^{3}] *Responsoria antiphonae, et hymni in processionibus per annum, quinis, et quaternis vocibus concinenda. Auctore Joanne Matelarto* *flandren. Collegiatae Ecclesiae S. Laurentii in Damaso de Urbe Capellae magistro*. Rome: N. Mutii, 1596.

Includes motet *Sicut cervus a 4*; *Crucem sanctam a 5; Hodie beata Virgo a 4; Homo quidam fecit coenam a 5; Jesus junxit se a 4.*

A0132 [RISM 1598^{2}] *Sacrae symphoniae, diversorum excellentissimorum authorum. Quaternis, V. VI. VII. VIII. X. XII. & XVI. vocibus, tam vivis, quam instrumentalibus accomodatae. Editae studio & opera Casparis Hasleri S.P.Q. norimberg. organista.* Nuremberg: P. Kaufmann, 1598 [eight vols in 8vo] [repr. 1601/2].

Includes motets no.14, *Ave Maria gratia plena a 5*; no.15, *Elegerunt Apostoli Stephanum a 5*; no.16, *Ad te levavi animam meam a 5*; no.17, *Justorum animae in manu Dei a 5.*

A0133 [RISM 1599^{2}] *Motetti et salmi a otto voci composti da otto eccellentiss. autori, con la parte de i bassi, per poter sonarli nell'organo. . . .* Venice: Giacomo Vincenti, 1599 [nine vols in 8vo, 14pp].

Includes motet p.5, *Vos amici mei estis a 8.*

A0134 [RISM 1599^{4}] *Motetti di Orfeo Vecchi maestro di Capella di S. Maria della Scala, e d'altri eccellentiss. musici a cinque voci. Libro primo. Con diligenza revisti et ristampati*. Milan: heir of S. Tini and G. F. Besozzi, 1599 [five vols in 8vo, 21pp].

Includes motets p.2, *Surge propera amica mea a 5* [secunda pars *Veni dilecti mi*] [=*Vestiva i colli a 5*]; p.14, *Quanti mercenarii in domo patris mei* [=*Io son ferito ahi lasso a 5*].

A0135 [RISM 1600^{2}] *Sacrarum symphoniarum continuatio. Diversorum excellentissimorum authorum. Quaternis, V. VI. VII. VIII. X. et XII. vocibus tam vivis, quam instrumentalibus accomodata.* Nuremberg: P. Kaufmann, 1600 [eight vols in 8vo].

Includes motet *Justus ut palma a 5.*

A0136 [RISM 1600^{11}] *Della nova Metamorfosi dell'infrascritti autori. Opera del R.P.F. Geronimo Cavaglieri con alcuni motetti dell molt'ill. sig. Lucio Castelnovato*. Milan: A. Tradate, 1600 [six vols in 8vo, 21pp].

Includes motets p.1, *Repleatur os meum laude tua a 5* [secunda pars *Exsurge gloria*]; p.14, *Semper laudabo salvatorem meum* [secunda pars *Sana mea Domine et sanabor*] [questionable attribution].

A0137 [RISM 1603^{6}] *Motetti di Orfeo Vecchi maestro di Capella di S. Maria della Scala, e d'altri eccellentiss. auttori. A cinque voci. Libro primo. In questa terza impressione, aggiontovi un motetto, con diligenta revisti, et corretti.* Milan: heirs of S. Tini and F. Lomazzo, 1603. 1599 [five vols in 8vo, 12f].

Includes motets *Surge propera amica mea a 5* [secunda pars *Veni dilecti mi*] [=*Vestiva i colli a 5*]; *Quanti mercenarii in domo patris mei* [=*Io son ferito ahi lasso a 5*].

A0138 [RISM 1605^{1}] *Triodia sacra, sive modi musici ternis vocibus tam ad* *tironum, quam peritiorum usum facti, et partim ex lectis auctoribus delecti, partim recens conditi. Liber I, . . .* Dillingen: A. Meltzer, 1605.

Includes hymn *Monstra te esse a 4* [Hab. XXX].

A0139 [RISM 1605[6]] *Della nova Metamorfosi de diversi autori. Opera del R.P.F. Geronimo Cavaglieri dell'Ordine di S. Basilio dell'Armeni. Libro secondo a cinque voci.* Milan: A. Tradate, 1605.

Includes motet *Salve sancta facies a 5* [=*Pulchra es amica mea a 5*].

A0140 [RISM 1606[6]] *Hortus musicalis, variis antea diversorum authorum Italiae floribus consitus, jam vero latinos fructus, mira suavitate quinque vocibus concinendos, pie & artificiose germinans. Authore R.P. Michaele Herrerio, ad S. Nicolai Strasburgi praeposito. Liber primus.* Pavia: M. Nenninger, 1606.

Includes motets no.23, *Succurite ahi lasso vos sancti Dei* [=*Io son ferito a 5*]; no.25, *Festiva dies agitur/Solemnitas haec est* [=*Vestiva i colli a 5/Così le chiome mie*].

A0141 [RISM 1607[6]] *Musarum Sioniar: motectae et psalmi latini, Michaelis Praetorij C. apud sereniss. principem Henricum Julium ducem Brunsv. & Lunaeb., chori musici magistri, IV. V. VI. VII. VIII. IX. X. XII. XVI. vocum, choro et organis accommodatae. I. Pars.* Nuremberg: A. Wagenmann, 1607.

Includes motet no.39, *Laudate Dominum in sanctis a 8.*

A0142 [RISM 1609[1]] *Florilegium sacrum cantionum quinque vocum pro diebus dominicis & festis totius anni, e celeberrimis nostri temporis musicis, quorum nomina habentur in indice.* Antwerp: Pierre Phalèse, 1609.

Includes motets, all *a 5*: *O admirabile commercium; Stella quam viderant; Senex puerum portabat* [secunda pars *Hodie beata virgo*]; *Suscipe verbum virgo Maria; Angelus Domini descendit* [secunda pars *Et introeuntes*]; *Alleluia. Tulerunt Dominum; Ascendo ad patrem* [secunda pars *Ego rogabo patrem*]; *Misit me vivens Pater; Puer qui natus es; Canite tuba; Corona aurea* [secunda pars *Domine praevenisti eum*].

A0143 [1612 = RISM P1974] *Cantiones sacrae, pro praecipuis festis totius anni et communi sanctorum, quinis vocibus. . . .* Antwerp: Pierre Phalèse, 1612.

Includes motets p.30, *Surge propera amica mea a 5* [=*Vestiva i colli a 5*]; p.32, *Quanti mercenarii* [=*Io son ferito ahi lasso a 5*].

A0144 [RISM 1612[3]] *Promptuarii musici, sacras harmonias sive motetas V. VI. VII. & VIII. vocum, e diversis, clarissimis huius & superioris aetatis authoribus, in Germania nusquam editis collectas exhibentis. Pars altera: quae aestivi temporis festivitatibus dominicisque diebus selectiores concentus S.S. Ecclesiae usui inservientes continet. Collectore Abrahamo Schadaeo, senfftebergensi. Cui basin ad organa musicaque instrumenta accommodatum, vulgo generalem dictam adjecit. Caspar Vincentius, spirensium organicem.* Strasbourg: K. Kieffer, 1612.

Includes motet no.50, *Lauda Sion Salvatorem a 8.*

A0145 [RISM 1613^{1}] *Sacrae symphoniae, diversorum excellentissimorum autorum: quaternis, 5. 6. 7. 8. 10. 12. & 16 vocibus, tam vivis quam instrumentalibus, accomodatae: hac quidem forma nunquam editae, studio et opera Casparis Hasleri. . . .* Nuremberg: P. Kaufmann, 1613 [eight vols in 8vo].

Includes motets *Ad te levavi animam meam*; *Justorum animae.*

A0146 [RISM 1613^{2}] *Promptuarii musici, sacras harmonias sive motetas V. VI. VII. & VIII. vocum, e diversis, iisque clarissimis hujus et superioris aetatis authoribus collectas comprehendentis, pars tertia: quae exhibet Concentus varios selectioresque, qui solennioribus sc. SS. Trinitatis, . . . Collectore Abrahamo Schadaeo senfftebergensi . . .* Strasbourg: K. Kieffer, 1613 [nine vols in 4to].

Includes motet no.48, *Tradent enim vos a 5.*

A0147 [RISM 1614^{3}] *Selectae cantiones excellentissimorum auctorum octonis vocibus concinendae. A Fabio Constantino romano urbeveteranae cathedralis musicae praefecto in lucem editae. Cum basso ad organum.* Rome: B. Zannetti, 1614.

Includes motets *Sub tuum praesidium a 8*; *Fratres ego enim accepi a 8*; *Caro mea vere est cibus* [secunda pars *Hic est panis*] *a 8.*

A0148 [RISM 1616^{7} =RISM P1983, also =RISM 1621,^{10} 1631^{1}]. *Les rossignols spirituels, liguez en duo dont les meilleurs accords, nommément les bas, relevant du seigneur Pierre Philippes.* Valenciennes: J. Vervliet, 1616.

Includes *Hodie Maria virgo coelos a 4* [ascribed in source to "I.Palestine"].

A0149 [RISM 1617^{1}] *Promptuarii musici, sacras harmonias V. VI. VII. et VIII. vocum, e diversis, clarissimis huius et superioris aetatis authoribus, in Germania nusquam editis, collectas exhibentis. Pars quarta: quae exhibet Concentus varios selectioresque, qui omnibus a SS. Trinitatis Dominicis inclusive inserviunt: cum spiritualibus Canticis, & sylva harmonica Deiparae Virgini sacra. Collegit vero et basi generali accommodavit Caspar Vincentius S. Andreae wormatiensis organoedus.* Strasbourg: A. Bertram, 1617.

Includes motets *Homo quidam fecit coenam a 5; Fratres ego enim accepi a 8.*

A0150 [RISM 1621^{1}] *Sacrae cantiones excellentissimorum auctorum octonis vocibus collectae a Fabio Constantino urbevetanae cathedralis musicae prefecto. Cum basso continuo ad organum.* Antwerpen, P. Phalèse, 1621 [nine (?) vols in 4to, 31pp] [from cantus II choir].

Motets: p.3, *Sub tuum praesidium a 8*; p.4, *Fratres sobrii estote a 8* [=*Fratres ego enim accepi a 8*]; p.5, *Caro mea vere est cibus* [secunda pars *Hic est panis*].

A0151 [1628 =RISM P1988, under name of Peter Philips] *Paradisus sacris cantionibus consitus, una, duabus et tribus vocibus decantandis, cum basso generali ad organum . . . prima pars.* Antwerp: Pierre Phalèse, 1628 [repr. 1633, 1641].

Includes motet *Quanti mercenarii* [=*Io son ferito*].

A0152 [1631; not in RISM; see Eitner QIII/163] *Florilegium musicum Lib. I Joh. Degen. . . .* Bamberg: A. Baals, 1631.

Includes *Hierusalem, quare moerore comsumeris* [=*Privo de fede* (pt.5 of *Ecc'oscurati*)].

A0153 [RISM 1639[2]] *Psalmi, Magnificat e Motetti a otto voci. . . .* Orvieto: Ruuli, 1639.

Includes motet *Ave Maria a 8.*

A0154 [RISM 1641[1]] *Paradisus sacris cantionibus consitus, una, duabus et tribus vocibus decantandis. Cum basso generali ad organum. Auctore R.D. Petro Philippo anglo, ecclesiae collegiatae S.Vincenti. Editio tertia.* Antwerp: heirs of P. Phalèse, 1641.

Includes motet no.15, *Benignissime Jesu a 3* [with basso continuo, questionable attribution].

Lamentations

——— *Lamentationum Hieremiae prophetae, liber primus.* Rome: Alessandro Gardano, 1588.

See A0090. In addition to the Lamentations, this print also includes the motet *Benedictus Dominus Deus Israel.*

Litanies

A0155 [RISM 1596[2]] *Thesaurus litaniarum. Quae a praecipuis hoc aevo musicis, tam in laudem sanctiss. nominis Iesu, quam in honorem deiparae coelitumque omnium, quatuor, quinque, sex, plurium vocum compositae: ad communem vero Ecclesiae usum collectae, opera & studio Georgii Victorini in aede D. Michaëlis. . . .* Munich: Adam Berg, 1596 [eight vols in 8vo].

Includes ten litanies, in two parts of five each [=Hab. XXVI.1–64].

A0156 [RISM 1620[1]] *Scelta de Salmi a 8, Magnificat, Antifone, cioe, Regina caeli, Ave regina caelorum, Alma Redemptoris. Et Litaniae della Madonna. De diversi eccellentissimi autori. Post'in luce da Fabio Costantini romano maestro di Cappella dell' illustrissima citta d'Orvieto con il basso continuo per l'organo. Libro quinto. Opera seconda.* Orvieto: B. Zannetti, 1620.

Includes litany p.20, *Litaniae della Beata Virgine a 8* [=Hab. XXVI.95].

Madrigals

A0157 [RISM 1554[28]] *De diversi autori il quarto libro de madrigali a quattro voci a note bianche novamente dato in luce.* Venice: A. Gardane, 1554.

Includes madrigal p.2, *Con dolce, altiero ed amoroso cenno a 4.*

A0158 [RISM 1557[24]] *Di Cipriano de Rore il secondo libro de madregali a quatro voci con un canzon di Gianneto sopra di Pace non trovo con quatordeci* *stanze novamente per Antonio Gardano stampato et dato in luce.* Venice: A. Gardano, 1557 [four vols. in 8vo. repr. 1569, 1571].

Includes madrigal *stanze*, stanza 1 (p.10), *Da fuoco così bel*; stanza 2 (p.11), *Rapace'ingord'e venenosa fera*; stanza 3 (pp.11–12), *Amo'e non nacque del mi'amor*; stanza 4 (p.12), *Da l'empia gelosia nasce il tormento*; stanza 5 (p.13), *Si mi vince tal'hor l'aspro martire*; stanza 6 (p.14), *O effetto rio che'l più felice stato*; stanza 7 (p.15), *Amor non volev'io ch'el mio gioire*; stanza 8 (p.16), *Non mi sferr'il crude*; stanza 9 (p.17), *Poi che la vista del mio caro sole*; stanza 10 (p.18), *Io non ho lingua e senza gl'occhi*; stanza 11 (p.19), *L'alta cagion del mio fermo pensiero*; stanza 12 (p.20), *Misero stato de gl'amanti*; stanza 13 (p.21), *Fuggir devriassi se fuggir se puote*; stanza 14 (p.22), *Satio di tormentarm'amore stassi.*

A0159 [RISM 1558[13]] *Secondo libro delle muse, a quattro voci. Madrigali ariosi, de diversi eccell. mi autori, con doe canzoni di Giannetto, di nuovo raccolti et dati in luce.* Rome: A. Barré, 1558.

Includes madrigal p.4, *Se da i soav'accenti ch'i si dolce*; canzone in five parts pp.30–34, *Chiare, fresche e dolci acque* [seconda parte *S'egli è pur il mio destino;* terza parte *Tempo verrà ancor forse;* quarta parte *Da'be'rami scendea;* quinta parte *Quante volte diss'io*); canzone in four parts pp.28–30, *Voi mi poneste in foco* [seconda parte *Però che da l'ardore;* terza parte *Che se tant'a voi piace;* quarta parte *E di voi non mi doglio*].

A0160 [RISM 1559[16]] *Il secondo libro de le Muse a cinque voci composto da diversi eccellentissimi musici con uno madregale a sei di Giovan Nasco, et con doi dialoghi a otto, novamente stampato & dato in luce*. Venice: A. Gardano, 1559 [repr. 1561].

Includes madrigal p.5, *Ogni loco mi porge doglia e pianto a 5* [seconda parte p.6, *Poscia che per mio mal*] [anonymous in 1583 print].

A0161 [RISM 1559[17]] *Secondo libro delle muse a quattro voci, madrigali ariosi de diversi eccell. autori, con due canzone di Giannetto, di nuovo raccolti et dati in luce.* Venice: G. Scotto, 1559.

Includes madrigal *Se da soav'accenti ch'i si dolce*; canzone in four parts *Voi mi poneste in foco* [seconda parte *Però che da l'ardore*; terza parte *Che se tant'a voi piace;* quarta parte *E di voi non mi doglio*]; canzona in five parts *Chiare, fresche e dolci acque* [seconda parte *S'egli è pur il mio destino;* terza parte *Tempo verrà ancor forse;* quarta parte *Da'be'rami scendea*; quinta parte *Quante volte diss'io*].

A0162 [RISM 1560[10]] *Madregali ariosi a quatro voci composti da diversi eccellentissimi autori, novamente con somma diligentia stampatti. Libro secondo.* Venice: A. Gardano, 1560.

Includes canzone: [prima parte] *Chiare, fresche e dolci acque* (p.1); [seconda parte] *Se gli e pur mio destino* (p.2); [terza parte] *Tempo verr'anchor forse ch'al'usato* (p.3); [quarta parte] *Da bei rami scendea* (p.4). *Quante volte diss'io* (p.5); *Se da'soavi accenti* (p.6). Canzona: [prima parte] *Voi me ponest'in foco* (p.21); [seconda parte] *Però che da l'ardore* (pp.21–22);

[terza parte] *Che se tant'a voi piace veder* (p.22); [quarte parte] *Et di voi non mi doglio* (p.23).

A0163 [RISM 1560[23]] *Di Alessandro Striggio gentil'huomo mantovano servitore dell'illustriss. & eccellentiss. Cosmo de Medici. . . . Il primo libro de madregali a cinque voci novamente per Antonio Gardano con nova gionta ristampato.* Venice: A. Gardano, 1560 [repr. Gardano 1569 without Rore madrigal; repr. Scotto 1560, 1564, 1585].

Includes madrigal *Donna bell'e gentil* (p.36).

A0164 [RISM 1560[24]] *Madrigali a cinque voci d'Alessandro Striggio gentil'huomo mantovano servitore dell'illustr. & eccell. Cosmo de Medici duca di Firenze, & di Siena. Novamente con la gionta ristampato e coretto. Libro primo.* Venice: G. Scotto, 1560 [= 1560 (previous publication), 1585].

Includes madrigal *Donna bell'e gentil* (p.36).

A0165 [RISM 1561[10]] *Il terzo libro delle Muse a cinque voci composto da diversi eccellentissimi musici con uno madregale a sei, et uno dialogo a otto, novamente per Antonio Gardano stampato & dato in luce.* Venice: A. Gardano, 1561.

Includes madrigals *Com'in più negre tenebre e più folte* (p.5); *Se fra quest'erb'e fiore* (p.6); *Il dolce sonno in cui sepolto giace* (p.7); *Io son ferito* (p.9); *Se ben non veggon gl'occhi* (p.12) ; *Dolor non fu, ne sia* (p.16); *Struggomi, e mi disfaccio* (pp.18–19); *Se lamentar augelli* (pp.22–23).

A0166 [RISM 1562[7]] *Il terzo libro delle Muse a quattro voci. Madrigali ariosi, da diversi eccell. musici raccolti, et dati in luce.* Rome: A. Barré, 1562 [repr. 1563].

Includes madrigals *Da poi ch'io vidi nostra falsa fede* (p.16); *Perch'al viso d'amor portan'insegna* (pp.16–17); *Qual più crudel martire* (pp.21–22) [this last is anonymous in 1583[15]].

A0167 [RISM 1562[22]] *Di Francesco Rosselli il primo libro de madrigali a cinque voci, insieme de altri autori, novamente per Antonio Gardano stampato et dato in luce.* Venice: A. Gardano, 1562.

Includes madrigal *Soligno e vagh'augello* (p.16), [seconda parte] *Io viss'in gioia hor sol di pianto* (pp.16–17, parts incomplete).

A0168 [RISM 1566[3]] *Il Desiderio secondo libro de madrigali a cinque voci, de diversi auttori, novamente posti in luce, per Giulio Bonagionta da S. Genesi.* Venice: G. Scotto, 1566.

Includes madrigal *Vestiva i colli* (pp.8–9), [seconda parte] *Cosi le chiome mie* (pp.9–10).

A0169 [RISM 1566[17]] *Di Cipriano de Rore il quinto libro di madrigali a cinque voci insieme alcuni de diversi autori. Novamente . . . stampato & dato in luce.* Venice: A. Gardano, 1566 [enlarged repr. 1568, 1574].

Includes madrigal *Il tempo vola* (p.24), [seconda parte] *Ivi vedrai la gloria* (p.25).

A0170 [RISM 1568[16]] *Corona della morte dell' illustre signore, il sig. Comendator Anibal Caro. Al nobile e generoso cavaliero il signor Giovanni Ferro da Macerata. Di novo posta in luce per Giulio Bonagionta da S. Genesi.* Venice: G. Scotto, 1568.

Includes madrigal *Il caro è morto & pur lasso* (p.25); [seconda parte] *Hor che la nobil lingua fredda giace* (p.26).

A0171 [RISM 1568[19]] *Di Cipriano de Rore il quinto libro di madrigali a cinque voci insieme alcune de diversi autori novamente per Antonio Gardano con nova gionta ristampato.* Venice: A. Gardano, 1568 [repr. 1574].

Includes madrigal *Il tempo vola* (p.24) [seconda parte] *Ivi vedrai la gloria* (p.25).

A0172 [RISM 1569[18]] *Il terzo libro delle muse a cinque voci composto da diversi eccellentissimi musici con uno madregale a sei, et uno dialogo a sette, d'Orlando novamente per Antonio Gardano ristampato.* Venice: Antonio Gardano, 1569.

Includes madrigals *Com'in più negre tenebre* (attributed to Cartolaio); *Se fra quest'erb e fiori; Il dolce sonno in cui giace; Io son ferito ahi lasso; Se ben non veggon gl'occhi; Dolor non fu ne fia; Struggomi et mi disfaccio; Se lamentar augelli.*

A0173 [RISM 1569[35]] *Di Alessandro Striggio gentil'huomo mantovano servitore dell'illustriss. et eccellentiss. Cosimo de Medici. . . . Il primo libro de madregali a cinque voci novamente per Antonio Gardano con nova giunta ristampato. . . .* Venice: Antonio Gardano, 1569.

Includes madrigal *Donna bell'e gentil* (p.37).

A0174 [RISM 1570[15]] *I dolci frutti primo libro de vaghi et dilettevoli madrigali di diversi eccellentissimi auttori a cinque voci, novamente posti in luce per il R.P.F. Cornelio Antonelli da Rimini detto il Turturino.* Venice: G. Scotto, 1570.

Includes madrigal *Quand'ecco donn'il vostro braccio* (quinta stanza, p.13).

A0175 [RISM 1570[16]] *Prima Stella. De madrigali a cinque voci,di Orlando Lasso. Di Zanetto di Palestina. Di Giovan Nascho. Di Francesco Roscelli. Et altri eccellentissimi musici. Novamente posti in luce.* Venice: G. Scotto, 1570.

Includes madrigals *Se fra quest'erb'e fiori* (p.6); *Il dolce sonno* (p.7); *Io son ferito* (p.9); *Se ben non veggon gl'occhi* (p.13); *Dolor non fu* (p.15); *Struggomi, e mi disfaccio* (p.18); *Se lamentar augelli* (p.19).

A0176 [RISM 1573[16]] *Primo libro de madrigali a cinque voci, composti da diversi eccell. autori et raccolti da M. Francesco Antoniio Baseo maestro di Capella del Duomo della citta di Leccio, novamente posti in luce.* Venice: son of A. Gardano, 1573.

Includes madrigal *Io son ferito hai lasso* (p.13; cf. setting in 1593).

A0177 [RISM 1574[4]] *Il quarto libro delle muse a cinque voci composto da diversi eccellentissimi musici, insieme dui mad. a sei, novamente stampati et dati in luce, intitolati benigni spirti.* Venice: son of A. Gardano, 1574 [Palestrina works repr. in 1582 ed.].

Includes madrigals *Io felice sarei* (p.27) *Le selv'avea* [seconda parte *Quando fe'loro impallidir*]; *Saggio e santo pastor* [seconda parte *Onde seguendo*] (p.2); *Se di pianti e di stridi* (p.6). [Also includes madrigal by Rodolfo Pierluigi, *Ahi! letizia fugace* (p.17).]

A0178 [RISM 1576[5]] *Musica di XIII. autori illustri a cinque voci, novamenti per Angelo Gardano raccolta et data in luce. Nella quale si contengono i pu belli madrigali che hoggidi si cantino. . . .* Venice: Angelo Gardano, 1576.

Includes madrigals *Placide l'acqu', e placid'era il vento* (p.29); *Soave fia il morir* (p.30).

A0179 [RISM 1577[7]] *Il primo fiore della ghirlanda musicale a cinque voci con un dialogo a nove. Di diversi eccellentissimi musici novamente posto in luce.* Venice: heir of Girolamo Scotto, 1577.

Includes madrigal *Anima dove sei che pensi homai* (p.24; tenor, basso, quinto partbooks missing).

A0180 [RISM 1580[9]] *Il terzo libro delle muse a cinque voci composto da diversi eccellentissimi musici, novamente con ogni diligentia ristampato*. Venice: A. Gardano, 1580.

Includes madrigals *Com' in più negre tenebre* (p.5, here attributed to G. Cartolaio); *Se fra quest'erb e fiori; Il dolce sonno in cui giace; Io son ferito ahi lasso; Se ben non veggon gl'occhi; Dolor non fu ne fia; Struggomi et mi disfaccio; Se lamentar augelli.*

A0181 [RISM 1582[4]] *Dolci affetti madrigali a cinque voci de diversi eccellentissimi musici di Roma. Novamente posti in luce.* Venice: Heir of G. Scotto, 1582 [repr. 1585, 1590].

Includes madrigal *O bella Ninfa mia* (p.9).

A0182 [RISM 1582[6]] *Il quarto libro delle Muse a cinque voci composti da diversi eccellentissimi musici novamente ristampati, intitolati Benigni spirti.* Venice: Angelo Gardano, 1582.

Includes madrigals *Saggio Santo Pastor* (p.3); [seconda parte] *Onde seguendo l'honorat'impresa* (pp.3–4); *Se di pianti et di stridi* (p.4); *Le selv'avea* (p.8); [seconda parte] *Quando fe loro impalidir le fronti* (p.9); *Io felici sarei se gl'occhi ond'io* (p.26). [Also includes madrigal by Rodolfo Pierluigi *Ahi letitie fugace* (p.16).]

A0183 [RISM 1583[12]] *Li amorosi ardori di diversi eccellentissimi musici novamente composti, et dati in luce. Libro primo a cinque voci*. Venice: Angelo Gardano, 1583.

Includes madrigal *Febre, ond'or per le vene* (p.20).

A0184 [RISM 1583^{14}] *Harmonia celeste di diversi eccellentissimi musici a IIII. V. VI. VII. et VIII. voci, nuovamente raccolta per Andrea Pevernage, et data in luce. Nella quale si contiene una scielta di migliori madrigali che hoggidi si cantino.* Antwerp: P. Phalèse and J. Bellère, 1583 [repr. 1589].

Includes madrigal *O bella Ninfa mia* (f.20A).

A0185 [RISM 1583^{15}] *Musica divina di XIX. autori illustri, a IIII. V. VI. et VII. voci, nuovamente raccolta da Pietro Phalesio, et data in luce. Nella quale si contengono i più excellenti madrigali che hoggidi si cantino.* Antwerp: P. Phalèse and J. Bellère, 1583 [repr. 1588, 1591, 1595, 1606, 1614, 1623, 1634].

Includes madrigal *Vestiva i colli* [spelled "Festivi colli"] (f.16v), [seconda parte] *Così le chiome* (p.17).

A0186 [RISM 1584^{5}] *Spoglia amorosa. Madrigali a cinque voci di diversi eccellentissimi musici, nuovamente posti in luce.* Venice: heir of G. Scotto, 1584 [repr. in 1585, with ed. in slightly different state but same Palestrina material; this version reprinted 1588, 1590, 1602, 1607].

Includes madrigal *Vestiva i colli* [seconda parte *Così le chiome mie*].

A0187 [RISM 1585^{16}] *De floridi virtuosi d'Italia il secondo libro de madrigali à cinque voci, novamente composte, et dati in luce.* Venice: G. Vincenzi and R. Amadino, 1585.

Includes madrigals *Erano le vostre lagrime* (p.5); *Dido che giace entro* (p.15).

A0188 [RISM 1586^{9}] *De floridi virtuosi d'Italia, il terzo libro de madrigali a cinque voci, novamente composti et date in luce.* Venice: G. Vincenzi and R. Amadino, 1586.

Includes madrigal *Dido che giace entro quest'urna* (p.15).

A0189 [RISM 1586^{11}] *Corona di dodici sonetti di Gio. Battista Zuccarini alla Gran Duchessa di Toscana posta in musica da dodici eccellentiss. auttori a cinque voci.* Venice: A. Gardano, 1586.

Includes madrigal ["Sonetto"] *O felice hore* (pp.13–14), [seconda parte] *Per mostrar gioia del conubio vostro* (p.14).

A0190 [RISM 1587^{5}] *Il quarto libro delle Muse a cinque voci, composto da diversi eccellentiss. musici. Novamente coretto [e] ristampato.* Milan: Francesco and heir of S. Tini, 1587.

Includes madrigals *Saggio e santo Pastor* (p.3); [seconda parte] *Onde seguendo l'honorat'impresa* (pp.3–4); *Se di pianti et di stridi* (p.4); *Le selv'avea* (p.8); [seconda parte] *Quando fe loro impalidir le fronti* (p.9); *Io son ferito; Io felici sarei se gl'occhi ond'io* (p.26). [Also includes madrigal by Rodolfo Pierluigi, *Ahi letitie fugace* (p.16).]

A0191 [RISM 1588^{19}] *Giardinetto de madrigali et canzonette a tre voci. De diversi auttori. Novamente posti in luce. Libro primo.* Venice: R. Amadino, 1588.

Includes madrigal *Amor se pur sei Dio* (p.4; tenor and alto partbooks missing).

A0192 [RISM 1588^{21}] *Gemma musicalis: selectissimas varii stili cantiones (vulgo Italis madrigali et napolitane dicuntur) quatuor, quinque, sex et plurium vocum continens: quae ex diversis praestantissimorum musicorum libellis, in Italia excusis, decerptae, & in gratiam utriusque musicae studiosorum, uni quasi corpori insertae & in lucem editae sunt, studio & opera Friderici Lindneri lignicensis. Liber primus*. Nuremberg: Catharina Gerlach, 1588.

Includes madrigals no.27, *Vestiva i colli a 5* [seconda parte: *Così le chiome miei*]; no.46, *O bella Ninfa mia a 5*; no.47, *Io son ferito ahi lasso a 5*.

A0193 [RISM 1588^{29}] *Musica transalpina. Madrigales translated of foure, five and sixe parts, chosen out of divers excellent authors, with the first and second part of La Verginella, made by maister Byrd, upon two stanza's of Ariosto, and brought to speake English with the rest. Published by N. Yonge, in favour of such as take pleasure in musick of voices*. London: Thomas East, 1588.

Includes madrigals no.3, "Joy so delights my heart" [=*Gioia m'abond' al cor*]; no.4, "False Love now shoot and spare not" [=*Amor ben puoi*]; no.8, "What meaneth Love to nest him" [=*Perché s'annida Amore*]; no.9, "Sweet Love when hope was flowring" [=*Amor quando fioriva*]; no.30, "Sound out my voice" [=*Vestiva i colli*].

A0194 [RISM 1589^{6}] *Musica di tredici autori illustri a cinque voci, per Angelo Gardano raccolta & data in luce, & di novo ristampata, nella quale si contengono I più belli madrigali; che hoggidí si cantino, delli infrascritti autori. . . .* Venice: Angelo Gardano, 1589.

Includes madrigals *Placide l'acque* (p.29); *Soave fia il morir* (p.30).

A0195 [RISM 1589^{7}] *Le gioie. Madrigali a cinque voci di diversi eccel.mi musici della compagnia di Roma, novamente posti in luce. Libro primo*. Venice: R. Amadino, 1589 [repr. 1590].

Includes madrigal *Dunque perfido Amante* (p.2).

A0196 [RISM 1589^{11}] *Ghirlanda di fioretti musicali composta da diversi ecc.ti musici a 3 voci con l'intavolatura del cimbalo, et liuto*. Rome: Simone Verovio, 1589 [see also Section III, Arrangements].

Includes madrigal *Ahi che quest'occhi miei* (p.1); *Da così dotta man sei stato* (p.3).

A0197 [RISM 1589^{12}]*Musicale essercitio di Ludovico Balbi maestro di capella del Santo di Padoa a cinque voci*. Venice: A. Gardano, 1589.

Includes madrigal *Mentre ch'al mar a 5*.

A0198 [RISM 1591^{10}] *Melodia olympica di diversi eccellentissimi musici a IIII. V. VI. et VIII. voci, nuovamente raccolta da Pietro Phillippi inglese, et data in luce. Nella quale si contengono i piu eccellenti madrigali che hoggidi si can-*

tino. Antwerp: P. Phalèse and J. Bellère, 1591 [repr. 1594, 1611, 1630].

Includes madrigals *Mori quasi il mio core* (p.5); *Veramente in amore* (p.7); *Non son le vostri mani* (p.18).

A0199 [RISM 1592[11]] *Il trionfo di dori, descritto da diversi, et posto in musica, a sei voci, da altretanti autori.* Venice: Angelo Gardano, 1592 [repr. 1595, 1596, 1599, 1601, 1614, 1628].

Includes madrigal *Quando del terzo cielo* (p.29).

A0200 [RISM 1592[13]] *De'floridi virtuosi d'Italia. Il secondo libro de'madrigali a cinque voci. Nuovamente ristampati, et con diligenza corretti.* Venice: G. Vincenti, 1592.

Includes madrigal *Eran le vostre lagrime nel viso* (p.2).

A0201 [RISM 1592[15]] *Spoglia amorosa. Madrigali a cinque voci, de diversi eccellentissimi musici. Novamente ristampata.* Venice: Angelo Gardano, 1592 [repr. 1600].

Includes madrigal *Vestiva i colli a 5* [seconda parte *Così le chiome miei*].

A0202 [RISM 1593[3]] *Florindo, e Armilla canzon pastorale, ornata di musica da doversi de piu celebri compositori de tempi nostri, et con altri madrigali novamente posta in luce. A cinque voci.* Venice: R. Amadino, 1593.

Includes madrigal *Non son le vostre mani* (p.19).

A0203 [RISM 1593[4]] *Harmonia celeste di diversi eccellentissimi musici a IIII. V. VI. VII. et VIII. voci. Nuovamente raccolta per Andrea Pevernage et data in luce. Nella quale si contengono i piu eccellenti madrigali che hoggidi si cantino*. Antwerp: P. Phalèse and J. Bellère, 1593 [six vols in 8vo], [repr. 1605 (?), 1614, 1628].

Includes madrigal *O bella ninfa mia a 5* (f.20v).

A0204 [RISM 1593[5]] *Nuova spoglia amorosa nella quale si contengono madrigali a quattro, et cinque voci scielti dall'opere de'più famosi, et eccellenti musici nuovamente posta in luce*. Venice: Giacomo Vincenti, 1593.

Includes madrigals *Mori quasi il mio core a 4* (p.20); *Io son ferito ahi lasso a 5* (p.31, setting different from 1573); *Vestiva i colli a 5.*

A0205 [1594=RISM D3948] *Il quarto libro di madrigali a cinque voci di Giov. Andr. Dragoni. . . .* Venice: Giacomo Vincenti, 1594.

Includes madrigal *O pastor dove vai a 6.*

A0206 [RISM 1596[10]] *Paradiso musicale di madrigali et canzoni a cinque voci, di diversi eccellentissimi autori. Novamente raccolti da P. Phalesio et posti in luce*. Antwerp: P. Phalèse, 1596.

Includes madrigal *Io son ferito a 5.*

A0207 [RISM 1596[11]] *Vittoria amorosa de diversi authori a cinque voci nuovamente stampata*. Venice: Giacomo Vincenti, 1596.

Includes madrigal *Donna presso al cui viso* (p.6); *Non fu già suon di trombe* (p.14) [cantus and tenor partbooks missing].

A0208 [RISM 1597[14]] *Canzonette a quattro voci composte da diversi eccellenti musici. Nouvamente date in luce.* Venice: G. Vincenti, 1597.

Includes canzonette *Pose un gran foco nel mio petto* (p.11); *Vedrassi prima senza luce* (p.13).

A0209 [RISM 1597[15]] *Il vago alboreto di madrigali et canzoni a quattro voci, di diversi eccellentissimi autori. Novamente raccolti et posti in luce.* Antwerp: P. Phalèse, 1597.

Includes madrigals *O che splendor de luminosi radi* (p.19); *I vaghi fiori & l'amorose fromde* (p.24v).

A0210 [RISM 1600[8]] *De floridi virtuosi d'Italia madrigali a cinque voci ridotti in un corpo. Nuovamente con ogni diligentia stampati & seguendo l' ordine de suoi toni posti in luce.* Antwerp: P. Phalèse, 1600.

Includes madrigal *Donna presso al cui viso a 5.*

A0211 [RISM 1601[8]] *Canzonette alla romana de diversi eccellentiss. musici romani a tre voci, novamente composte, et date in luce.* Venice: Angelo Gardano, 1601 [three vols in 8vo, 12f].

Includes canzonette *Ahi che quest'occhi miei* (f.10); *Da così dotta man* (f.11).

A0212 [RISM 1604[11]] *Scielta de madrigali a'cinque voci de diversi eccel. musici, accommodati in motetti da Orfeo Vecchi con la partitura d'essi motetti. Nuovamente data in luce.* Milan: heirs of S. Tini and F. Lomazzo, 1604.

Includes *Domine in virtute a 5* [=*Io felice sarei a 5*].

A0213 [RISM 1605[9]] *Nervi d'Orfeo, di eccellentiss. autori a cinque et sei voci: nuovamente con ogni diligentia raccolti, & sequendo l'ordine de suoi toni posti in luce.* Leiden: H. L. de Haestens, 1605.

Includes madrigal no.77, *Quando dal terzo ciel a 6.*

A0214 [RISM 1607[14]] *Canzonette alla romana de diversi eccellentissimi musici romani a tre voci. Nuovamente raccolte & date in luce.* Antwerp: P. Phalèse, 1607.

Includes canzonette *Ahi che quest'occhi miei* (p.28); *Da così dotta man sei stato* (p.39).

A0215 [RISM 1608[22]] *Newe teutsche Canzonetten mit dreyen Stimmen, von den fürtrefflichsten italienischen Componisten auff ihre Sprach componiret, und hiebevor in Italia zusammen getruckt. An jetzo aber mit unser Sprach den teutschen Musicis, Instrumentisten, und andern der Music Liebhabern zu Gefallen unterlegt. Durch Andream Myllerum hammelburgensem seeligen.* Frankfurt am Main: W. Richter, 1608 [three vols in 4to, 26pp].

Includes canzonette *Als Piramus kam a 3* [=*Da cosi dotta man sei stato*]; *Soll ich denn meiden dich a 3* [=*Ahi che quest'occhi a 3*].

A0216 [RISM 1613[13]] *Rest musikalisches Streitkränzleins: hiebevorn von den allerfürtrefflichsten unnd berhümtesten Componisten, in welscher Sprach, pro certamine, mit sonderlichen Fleiss, und auffs künstlichst, mit 6. Stimmen auffgesetzt, und dannenhero Tromphi di Dori oder de Dorothea genennet . . . in Druck gefördert, durch Solomonem Engelhart, . . .* Nuremberg: B. Scherff, 1613 [six vols in 4to].

Includes madrigal no.14, *Sagt einer viel a 6* [=*Quando del terzo cielo*].

A0217 [RISM 1619[16]] *Triumphi de Dorothea, non illâ italico-prophanâ; sed angelico-coelesti & immortali, id est: musica, sive laus musicae; a praestantissimis musicorum italicorum coryphaeis, olim, quasi aliud agentibus; sub nomine Dorotheae cujusdam, 6. vocibus, decantata. Das ist geistliches musicalisches Triumph-Cräntzlein von der hochedlen und recht englischen Dorothea oder grossen Gottes Gabe der Fraw Musica; . . . Aus dem der aller vortrefflichsten italiänischen Componisten, certamine musico Triomphi de Dori entlehnet: . . . mit gantz newen deutschen geistlichen Texten exorniret durch M. Martinum Rinckhardum ilebergensem. . . .* Leipzig: L. Koeber (B. Voigt), 1619.

Includes madrigal *Wach auf mein Ehr a 6* [=*Quando del terzo cielo*].

III. Contemporary Arrangements of Palestrina's Works

[This section includes intabulations for various instruments, arrangements of compositions for voices together with lute or other instruments, and addition of *passeggiati* or ornamented versions of works.]

A0218 [1568] *Fronimo dialogo di Vincentio Galilei fiorentino, nel quale si contengono le vere, et necessarie regole del intavolare la musica nel liuto, posto nuovamente in luce & da ogni errore emendato.* Venice: Girolamo Scotto, 1568.

Includes madrigals *Vestiva i colli* (p.15; seconda parte *Così le chiome mie* p.16); *Se tra quest'herbe'e fiore* (p.31); *Io son ferito hai lasso* (p.146); *Se ben non veggion gl'occhi* (p.147) [lute intabulations].

A0219 [RISM 1574[14]] *Il primo libro di tabolatura di citthara di ricercari madrigali anzoni napolitane et saltarelli. Di Paolo Virchi Organista Bresciano . . . novamente posta in luce. . . .* Venice: heir of Girolamo Scotto, 1574.

Includes madrigal *Io son ferit'ahi lasso* (p.16) [intabulation for six-course cittern].

A0220 [RISM 1582[1]] *Novae tabulae musicae testudinariae hexachordae et heptachordae. Julii Caesaris Barbetti Paduani. Neu Lautenbuch auff sechs und Siben Chorseyten gestellt. . . .* Strasbourg: Bernhart Jobin, 1582.

Includes madrigal *Dolce fial mortir* [*sic*] (f. F3) ["P.A. penesstrina"] [lute intabulation].

A0221 [RISM 1583^{23}] *Ein schön nutz unnd gebreüchlich Orgel Tabulaturbuch. Darinnen etlich der berümbten Componisten, beste Moteten, mit 12. 8. 7. 6. 5. und 4. Stimmen ausserlesen. . . . Zu letzt auch allerhand der schönsten Lieder, Pass'e'mezzo, und Taentz, alle mit grossem Fleiss coloriert . . . in Truck verwilligt. Von Iacobo Paix ausgustano. . . .* Laugingen: L. Reinmichel, 1583.

Includes organ intabulations of twelve Palestrina motets: *Angelus Domini a 5* [secunda pars *Et introeuntes*] (fol. $B_1{}^1$–$C_1{}^1$, transposed down a fourth); *Viri Galilaei a 6* [secunda pars *Ascendit Deus in jubilatione*] (fol. $C_3{}^1$–$D_1{}^1$, transposed down a fourth); *Dum complerentur a 6* [secunda pars *Dum ergo essent*])fol. $E_3{}^1$–$F_1{}^1$, transposed down a fourth); *O beata et gloriosa Trinitatis a 5* [secunda pars *O vera summa sempiterne Trinitas*] (fol. $F_1{}^1$–$F_6{}^1$, transposed down a fourth); *Hodie Christus natus est* a 8 (fol. G_4–$G_6{}^1$, transposed down a fifth); *Haec dies quam fecit Dominus a 6* (fol. G_4–$G_6{}^1$, transposed down a fourth); *Lapidabant Stephanum a 5* (fol. $I_2{}^1$–$I_5{}^1$, transposed down a fourth); *Valde honorandus est a 4* (fol. $I_5{}^1$–$K_1{}^1$, transposed down a fifth); *Senex puerum portabat a 5* [secunda pars *Hodie beata virgo Maria*] (fol. $K_1{}^1$–$K_6{}^1$, untransposed); *Tribus miraculis a 4* (fol. $K_6{}^1$–L_3, transposed down a fourth); *Cantantibus organis a 5* [secunda pars *Biduanis ac tribuanis*] (fol. $M_3{}^1$–$N_1{}^1$, transposed down a fourth); *Pater noster a 5* (fol. $O_4{}^1$–P_1, transposed down a fourth).

A0222 [RISM 1584] *Il vero modo di diminuir, con tutte le sorte di stromenti di fiato, & corda, & di voce humana. . . . Girolamo dalla Casa. . . . Libro secondo.* Venice: Angelo Gardano, 1584.

Includes madrigal *Vestiva i colli* (book 2, p.36; with seconda parte *Così le chiome mie,* book 2, p.37).

A0223 [RISM 1584^{12}] *Pratum musicum longe amoenissimum, cuius spatiosissimo, eoque iucundissino ambitu, (praeter varii generis automata seu phantasias) comprehenduntur. . . . Omnia ad testudinis tabulaturam fideliter redacta, per . . . Emanuelem Hadrianium. . . . Adiuncta est singulis carminibus, in gratiam eorum, qui vivae vocis concentu oblectantur, distincta vocibus aliquot notularum discriptio. . . . Opus novum.* Antwerp: Pierre Phalèse, 1584 [one vol in 4to].

Includes madrigal no.30, *Vestiva i colli* (f.34v; seconda parte, *Così le chiome mie*, f.35v) [lute intabulation and mensural notation].

A0224 [RISM 1584^{5}] *Il Fronimo dialogo di Vincentio Galilei nobile fiorentino, sopra l'arte del bene intavolare, et rettamente sonare la musica. . . .* Venice: Girolamo Scotto, 1584 [2nd ed.].

Madrigals: p.26, *Vestiva i colli a 5* [seconda parte *Così le chiome mie*]; p.53, *Se tra quest'herbe e fiore a 5*; p.121, *Io son ferito hai lasso a 5*; p.122, *Il dolce sonno in cui sepolto giace a 5* [intabulations for solo lute].

A0225 [RISM 1585^{38}] *Ricercate passaggi et cadentiae, per potersi essercitar nel diminuir terminatamente con ogni sorte d'instrumento: & anco diversi passaggi per la semplice voce. . . .* Venice: Giacomo Vincenti and Ricciardo Amadino, 1585. See A0230.

A0226 [1586. *Il primo libro d'intavolatura d' arpicordo . . . Marco Facoli.*]
No copy extant; possible contents inferred from manuscript materials [Brown]. May include madrigal *Vestiva i colli* [keyboard intabulation].

A0227 [RISM 1586[2]] *Diletto spirituale canzonette a tre et e quatro voci composte da diversi ecc.mi musici. Raccolte et scritte da Simone Verovio. . . . Con l'intavolatura del Cimbalo.* Rome: M. van Buyten, 1586 [repr. 1590, 1592].
Includes hymns no.4, *Jesu rex admirabilis a 3*; no.9, *Tua Jesu dilectio a 3*, with *Tua Jesu dilectio* [intabulation]; no.13, *Jesu flos matris Virginis a 4*, with *Jesu flos matris Virginis* [intabulation]; *In Domino laetabitur a 4.*

A0228 [RISM 1589[7]] *Thesaurus motetarum. Newerlessner zwey und zweintzig herrlicher Moteten, rechte Kunst Stück: der aller berhümbsten Componisten, in der Ordnung wie sie nach einander gelebt: und jede Moteten zum ihrem gewissen Modo gesetzt. Mit sonderm hohen Fleiss und müh zusamen getragen und in diese breuchige Tabulatur gebracht von Jacobo Paix augustano, organico lavingano.* Strasbourg: Bernhart Jobin, 1589.
Includes motet no.18, *O sacrum convivium* (f.48v) [organ or keyboard intabulation].

A0229 [RISM 1589[11]] *Ghirlanda di fioretti musicali composta da diversi ecc.ti musici a 3 voci con l'intavolatura del cimbalo, et liuto. . . .* Rome: Simone Verovio, 1589.
Includes madrigals no.1, *Ahi che quest'occhi miei* (p.1); no.2, *Di così dotta man sei stato* (p.3).

A0230 [1591] *Motetti, madrigali et canzoni francese, di diversi Eccellentissimi Auttori à Quattro Cinque, & Sei Voci. Diminuiti per sonar con ogni sorte di stromenti, & anco per cantar con semplice Voce da Giovanni Bassano musico della Serenissima Signoria di Venetia. Novamente dati in luce.* Venice: Giacomo Vincenti, 1591.
Includes diminutions for motets no.1, *Benedicta sit sancta Trinitas* (p.6); no.2, *Ave Maria a 4* (p.8); no.3, *Hodie beata Virgo* (p.9); no.17, *Fuit homo missus a Deo* (p.25); no.18, *Benedicta sit sancta Trinitas* [same model as no.1] (p.26); no.44, *Tota pulchra es* (p.64); no.45, *Introduxit me* (p.66); no.46, *Pulchra es amica mea* (p.66); no.47, *Veni, veni dilecte mi* (p.68); diminutions for madrigals no.26, *Vestiva i colli* (p.36; seconda parte *Così le chiome mie* p.37); no.27, *Io son ferito ahi lasso* (p.38).

A0231 [RISM 1591[12]] *Canzonette a quattro voci, composte da diversi ecc.ti musici, con l'intavolatura del cimbalo et del liuto. . . .* Rome: Simone Verovio, 1591.
Includes madrigals no.8, *Pose un gran foco* (f.9v); no.10, *Vedrassi prima senza luce* (f.11v) [keyboard score with Italian lute tabulature].

A0232 [RISM 1591[14]] *Canzonette per cantar et sonar di liuto a tre voci, Composte da diversi auttori, et nuovamente date in luce. Libro primo.* Venice: Giacomo Vincenti, 1591.
Includes madrigals no.9, *Da così dotta man* (f.6); no.10, *Ahi che quest'occhi miei* (f.6v) [voice and lute intabulations].

A0233 [RISM 1592^{11}]*Diletto spirituale canzonette a tre e quattro voci composte da diversi ecc.mi Musici con L'intavolatura a del Cimbalo & Liuto.* Rome: Simone Verovio, 1592 [vocal settings on left side of opening; keyboard and lute intabulations on right side].

Includes spiritual canzonette *Jesu Rex admirabilis a 3* (f.12v); *Tua Jesu dilectio a 3* (f.13v); *Jesu flos matris a 4* (f.21v).

A0234 [RISM 1592^{22}] *Novum pratum musicum longo amoenissimum, cujus spatiosissimo, eoque iucundissimo ambitu (praeter varii generis aytomata, seu phantasias) comprehenduntur selectissimi diversorum autorum et idiomatum madrigales, cantiones, & moduli 4. 5 & 6 vocum. . . . Omnia ad testudinis fideliter redacta, per id genus verpiensum. . . . Tum etiam methodus ad omnes omnium tonorum cantiones, in gratiam illorum, qui in fac arte mediocriter versati. . . . Opus plane novum, nec hactenus editem.* Antwerp: P. Phalèse and J. Bellère, 1592.

Includes madrigals no.27, *Ogni beltà* (f.7v); no.40, *Vestiva i colli* (f.21v; seconda parte *Così le chiome mie*, f.22v).

A0235 [RISM 1593^{11}] *Di Gio. Antonio Terzi da Bergamo, intavolatura di liutto, accomodata con diversi passagi per suonar in concerti a duoi liutti, et solo. Libro primo. Il qual contiene, motetti, contraponti, canzoni italiane, et francese, madrigali, fantasie, et balli di diversi sorti, italiani, francese, et alemani.* Venice: R. Amadino, 1593 [facs. repr. Antiquae Musicae Italicae Monumenta Bergomensia 14. Bergamo, 1964].

Includes motets no.4, *Tu es pastor ovium* a 4 (p.7); no.5, *Angelus ad pastores* a 4 (p.9) [intabulations for solo lute]; madrigals no.10, *Vestiva i colli* (p.19); "Contraponto sopra Vestiva i colli per sonar a duoi liutti in quarta o in concerto" (p.20); [seconda parte] *Così le chiome mie* (p.24); "Contraponto sopra il predetto per suonar come di sopra" (p.25) [intabulations for two lutes or solo lute].

A0236 [1594; RISM B4029] *Regole, passaggi di musica, madrigali, e motteti passeggiati di Gio. Battista Bovicelli d' Assisi. . . .* Venice: Giacomo Vincenti, 1594 [facs. repr. ed. Nanie Bridgman. Documenta musicologica 1/12. Kassel: Bärenreiter-Verlag, 1957].

Includes diminution for madrigal *Io son ferito* (pp.38–42); diminution for *Ave verum corpus* [contrafactum of *Io son ferito*] (pp.42–46).

A0237 [RISM 1596^{3}] *Canzoni alla francese a quattro voci per sonare dentrovi, un Echo, & in fine una Battaglia a Otto, & dui Concerti fatti sopra Lieto godea. Di Adriano Banchieri Bolognese Organista in S. Michele in Bosco. Libro Secondo. . . .* Venice: Ricciardo Amadino, 1596.

Includes no.6, 'Canzon Sesta. L' Alcenagina. Sopra " 'Vestiva i colli' " (p.6); no.9. " 'Canzon Nona.' La Camerina. Sopra 'Veni dilecti mi' " (p.9) [organ intabulations].

A0238 [RISM 1599^{19}] *Il secondo libro de intavolatura di liuto di Gio. Antonio Terzi da Bergamo. Nella quale si contengono fantasie, motetti, canzoni, madrigali pass'e mezi, et balli di varie, et diverse sorti. Novamente da lui data in luce.* Venice: G. Vincenti, 1599.

Includes madrigal no.67, *O bella Ninfa mia* (p.86) [intabulation for solo lute].

A0239 [RISM 1600[5a]] *Flores musicae, hoc est, suavissimae et lepidissimae cantiones, madrigalia vulgus nominat, una cum variis pavanis, paduanis, galliardis, intradiis, fantasiis & choriis, ex quam plurimis autoribus italicis, gallicis & germanicis magna industria collectae, et nunc primum ita decriptae, ut testudinis fidibus cani possint, per Joannem Rudenium lipsiensem. . . . Una veneunt Matthaei Raymanni toronensis Noctes musicae perquam artificiose compositae, in quibus variata praeludia et passamezae,* . . . Heidelberg: Vegelin, 1600.

Includes *O bella Ninfa mia a 5; Vestiva i colli a 5* [seconda parte *Così le chiome mie*] [keyboard intabulation].

A0240 [RISM 1600[18]] *Pratum musicum longe amoenissimum, cuius spatiosissimo, eoque iucundissimo ambitu (praeter varii generis aytomata, seu phantasias) comprehenduntur. Selectissimi diversorum autorum et idiomatum madrigales, et cantiones 4. 5. 6. vocum, Balletti 5. vocum. Cantiones trium vocum . . . variae . . . modulationes. Omnis generis choreae, passomezo cum suis saltarellis, galliardae, alemandae, branslae, courantae, voltae, &c. Omnia ad testudinis tabulaturam fideliter redacta, per id genus musices . . . Emannelem Hadrianum, antverpiensem. . . . Editio nova priori locupletior.* Antwerp: P. Phalèse, 1600.

Includes intabulation of a Palestrina work [according to RISM].

A0241 [RISM 1601[18]] *Florida, sive cantiones, e quamplurimus praestantissimorum nostri aevi musicorum libris selectae. Ad testudinis usum accomodatae . . . I. van Hove, antverpiani. . . .* Utrecht: S. de Roy and J. G. de Rhenen, 1601.

Includes intabulations of two Palestrina works [according to RISM].

A0242 [1620; RISM R1942] *Selva di varii passaggi secondo l'uso moderno, per cantare, & sonare con ogni sorte de stromenti divisa in due parti . . . Francesco Rognoni Taegio. . . .* Milan: Filippo Lomazzo, 1620, and [1620; RISM R1942] *Selva di varii pasaggi parte seconda, ove si tratta dei pasaggi difficili, par gl'istromenti del dar l'archata, portar della lingua, diminuire di grado in grado, cadentie, finali, essempi, canti diminuiti. Con la maniera di suonar la Viola bastarda . . . di Francesco Rognoni. . . .* Milan: Filippo Lomazzo, 1620 [facs. repr. ed. Guglielmo Barblan. Bologna, 1970. (Biblioteca musica Bononensis II/153). MT80.R6554.1620a].

Parte prima includes diminutions for motet *Pulchra es amica mea* for soprano or tenor (pp.45–46) and for basso and for the viola bastarda (pp.46–47); diminutions for *Quanti mercenarii* [sacred contrafactum of *Io son ferito*] (pp.48–48). Parte seconda includes diminutions for madrigals *Io son ferito* (pp.55–57); *Vestiva i colli* (pp.59–61, 65–67).

A0243 [1638] *Canzoni fantasie et correnti da suonar ad una 2.3.4. con basso continuo. Del P.F. Bartolomeo de Selma et Salaverde Agostiniano Spagnolo, già* *musico & suonator di fagotto. . . .* Venice: Bartolomeo Magni, 1638.

Includes madrigal no.6, *Vestiva i colli* (book 1, pp.15–16; book 2, pp.11–12, 35–36).

IV. Prints in Books, Theoretical Treatises, Manuals of Instruction, and Similar Sources Dating from before 1800

——— Bassano, Giovanni. See item A0230.

——— Bovicelli, Giovanni Battista. See item A0236.

——— Burney, Charles. *A General History of Music from the Earliest Ages to the Present Period. To which is prefixed a Dissertation on the Music of the Ancients. By Charles Burney. . . . Volume the first [—the fourth].* London: T. Becket, J. Robson, G. Robinson, 1776–1789 [four vols.] [repr. ed. Frank Mercer. New York: Dover, 1935. Repr. 1957].

Original edition of 1776–1789 includes a print of the motet *Exaltabo te* a 5 (III, 191), as well as an excerpt from *Magnificat secundi toni (Deposuit potentes de sede a 3*, III, 170).

See item E0475 for main entry.

——— Dalla Casa, Girolamo. See item A0222.

——— Eximeno y Pujaver, Antonio. *Delle origini e delle regole della musica colla storia del suo progresso, decadenza, e rinnovazione.* Rome: Michel'Angelo Barbiellini, 1774 [466pp].

Plate 9 provides scored excerpts from the *Missa Papae Marcelli*: *Kyrie* (first part only, six voices and basso continuo); *Gloria* (beginning only, six voices and basso continuo).

See item E0482 for main entry.

——— Galilei, Vincenzo. See items A0218 and A0224.

——— Hawkins, Sir John. *A General History of the Science and Practice of Music, by Sir John Hawkins.* London, 1776.

In the 1853 reprint: vol.1: Motet *Sicut cervus a 4* [secunda pars *Sitivit anima mea*] (pp.423–426); spiritual madrigal *Credo gentil dagli amorosi vermi* (pp.427–429).

See item E0494 for main entry.

——— Kircher, Athanasius. *Athanasio Kircheri Musurgia universalis sive ars magni consoni et dissoni in X libros digesta. . . . Tomus I–II.* Romae, Haeredes Francisci Corbelletti; [deinde] Ludovicus Grignanus, 1650 [two vols, 10 fnc + 692pp.; 2 fnc + 462pp].

Crucifixus etiam pro nobis a 4 (vol.1, p.582 [i.e. 584]); *Quia amore langueo* [from motet *Introduxit me Rex a 5*] (vol.1, p.599 [i.e. 601]).

See item E0430 for main entry.

A0244 Martini, Giovanni Battista. *Esemplare o sia saggio fondamentale pratico di* *contrappunto sopra il canto fermo. . . . Parte prima.* Bologna: Lelio della Volpe Impressore dell'Instituto delle Scienze, 1774.

This outstanding work teaches the art of composition using a *cantus firmus* through a detailed study of models and representative examples for each of the eight church tones. Each example is heavily annotated with Martini's observations on use of the *cantus firmus*, dissonance treatment, and other aspects of contrapuntal technique. Palestrina is the most abundantly represented composer. All works are scored with original clefs and note values and are probably derived from Martini's collection of early Palestrina prints.

Introduction: "Deposuit potentes" a 3 (from *Magnificat secundi toni*, pp.xxx–xxxi).

Tone I: no.2, "Chori Sanctarum Virginum" a 4 (third strophe of a hymn for the feast of All Saints, pp.5–8); no.3, "Sit laus Deo Patri" a 5 (final strophe of hymn *Ave maris stella* a 5, pp.8–11); no.4, "Et exultavit" a 5 (transposed up a fourth, from *Magnificat primi toni* a 5, pp.12–14).

Tone II: no.2, "Post fluxae carnis scandala" a 4 (from hymn for St. Mary Magdalene, pp.19–21); no.3, "Sicut locutus est" a 5 (from *Magnificat secundi toni* a 5, pp.21–24).

Tone III: no.3, "Quae vox quae poterit" a 4 (fifth strophe of vespers hymn for several martyrs, pp.47–50); no.4, "Laus et perennis gloria" a 5 (last strophe of hymn for a martyr, pp.51–53); no.5, "Sicut locutus est" (from *Magnificat tertii toni* a 5, pp.54–56).

Tone IV: no.2, "Hic ille Rex est gentium" a 4 (third strophe of hymn for the Transfiguration, pp.70–72); no.4, "O felix Roma" a 5 (third strophe of hymn for saints Peter and Paul, pp.75–79); no.5, "Sicut erat in principio" a 7 (from *Magnificat quarti toni* a 5, pp.80–87).

Tone V: no.2, "Legi prophetae gratiae" a 4 *voci pari* (from hymn for St. Francis, pp.97–99); no.3, "Praestat hoc nati genitor" a 5 (from hymn for St. Anthony of Padua, pp.100–102); no.4, "Esurientes" a 5 (from *Magnificat quinti toni* a 5, pp.103–106).

Tone VI: no.3, "Gaudent in coelis" a 4 (antiphon for second vespers for several martyrs, pp.122–128).

Tone VII: no.2, "Veni sponsa Christi" a 4 (antiphon for the vespers on a feast of a virgin, pp.144–148); no.5, "Sicut erat in principio" a 6 (from *Magnificat septimi toni* a 5, pp.153–157); no.6, "Agnus Dei II" a 6 (from *Missa Tu es Petrus*, book 12 of masses, pp.158–162).

Tone VIII: no.2, "Hostem repellas longius" a 4 (from hymn for Pentecost, pp.166–169); no.3, "Beatus Laurentius" a 5 (motet from Book I for five voices, pp.170–177); no.6, "Quia fecit mihi magna" a 6 (from *Magnificat octavi toni* a 6, pp.186–189).

A0245 Martini, Giovanni Battista. *Esemplare o sia saggio fondamentale pratico di contrappunto fugato. . . . Parte seconda.* Bologna: Lelio della Volpe Impressore dell'Instituto delle Scienze, 1774.

The second volume of the *Esemplare* is devoted to the study of imitative writing and *fughe*. A majority of Martini's examples are drawn from composers of the seventeenth and eighteenth centuries, although there are a significant number by Marenzio and Palestrina.

Includes "Fuga a tre voci", that is, a "Pleni sunt coeli" from the *Missa tertia* a 5 [*Missa O magnum mysterium*] from Masses Book IV (pp.45–47); "Fuga a quattro voci," that is, the madrigal *Alla riva del Tebro* (pp.72–77); "Fuga a cinque voci," that is, the spiritual madrigal *Tu di fortezza torre* (pp.173–179).

——— Paolucci, Giuseppe. *Arte prattica di Contrappunto dimostrata con esempi di varj autori e con osservazioni di F. Giuseppe Paolucci minor Conventuale.* Venice: Antonio de Castro, 1765–1772 [three vols, xv+269pp., 315pp, vii+247pp].

Vol. 1 includes *Benedictus a 3* [from *Missa Emendemus*] (p.81); *Litaniae Beatae Maria Virginis a 4* [incomplete] (pp.175–183); *Sicut cervus a 4* [prima parte only].

Vol. 2 includes *Plange quasi virgo a 5* [ascribed then to Palestrina, now to Marc'Antonio Ingegneri].

See item E0530 for main entry.

——— Zacconi, Lodovico. *Prattica di musica. . . . Divisa in quattro libri. Ne i quali . . . si dichiara tutta la Messa del Palestrina titolo Lomè armè. . . .* Venezia: Girolamo Polo, 1592; Venice: Bartolomeo Carampello, 1596 [218pp]. Second part Venice: Alessandro Vincenti, 1622 [283pp].

Book II, chap. 38, ff. 115v–121v includes a discussion of notational questions and printed selections from *Missa L'homme armé a 5: Kyrie I* (115v–116); *Christe* (116v–117); *Kyrie II* (117v–118); *Gloria* (118v–119); *Osanna* (119v–120); *Agnus Dei* (120v–121).

See item E0459 for main entry.

Chapter 3

Primary Sources:
A Checklist of Manuscripts

B0001 Augsburg. Staats- und Stadtbibliothek. MS Tonkunst Schletterer 4 (olim Schletterer 23). Choirbook labeled "Farrago cantionum." Dates 1598 and 1610 in MS. Provenance Augsburg. 304ff.

Contains motet f.147, *Ascendo ad Patrem a 5.*

B0002 Augsburg. Staats- und Stadtbibliothek. MS Tonkunst Schletterer 18 (olim Schletterer 21). Choirbook. Dated 1595–1596. Provenance Benedictine Cloister SS Ulrich and Afra, Augsburg. 375ff.

Contains f.4v, *Missa Beata Dei genetrix* (also known as *Missa Sine nomine*) *a 6.*

B0003 Augsburg. Staats- und Stadtbibliothek. MS Tonkunst Schletterer 20 (olim Schletter 24). Choirbook. Dated 1602.

Contains f.67v, 8 *Magnificat* [(even-numbered verses) beginning *Et exultavit*, Tone 1–8] *a 4.*

B0004 Augsburg. Staats- und Stadtbibliothek. MSS Tonkunst Schletterer 273–278 (formerly Schletterer 452–454). Six partbooks. Dated 1570–1571, with additions ca. 1598.

Contains motet f.18, *Dum complerentur a 6.*

B0005 Barcelona. Biblioteca Central. MS 382 [Pedrell]. Choirbook. End 16th to beginning 17th century. In various hands.

Contains motet *Senex puerum portabat a 5.*

B0006 Barcelona. Biblioteca Central. MS 587 [=Pedrell 383]. Choirbook. Late 16th century. Provenance Spanish.

Contains mass f.20v, *Missa Lauda Sion (Missa Prima) a 4*; lamentations f.74v, *Aleph. Quomodo sedet a 4*; f.76v, *Heth. Cogitavit a 4*; f.78v, *Heth. Misericordiae a 4.*

B0007 Barcelona. Biblioteca Central. MS 682 [=Pedrell 385]. Choirbook. 16th century.

Contains motet f.63, *Valde honorandus est a 4;* f.67, *Lapidabant Stephanum a 4;* f.71, *Tu es pastor ovium a 4;* f.73, *Congratulamini mihi a 4*; f.86, *Dies sanctificatus a 4*; f.87, *Fuit homo missus a Deo a 4.*

B0008 Barcelona. Biblioteca Central. MS 394 [Pedrell]. Four partbooks. Mid-17th century.

Contains *Missa Papae Marcelli a 4* [not original *a 6*].

B0009 Barcelona. Biblioteca Central, MS 859. MS in three sections: I (2nd half 16th century); II (2nd half 17th century); III (late 16th century).

Reported to contain two works by Palestrina.

B0010 Barcelona. Biblioteca de l'Orfeo Català. MS 10. Late 17th or early 18th century.

Contains *Requiem a 4* attributed to Palestrina, arguably genuine.

B0011 Barcelona. Biblioteca de l'Orfeo Català. MS 11bis (shelf mark: 12–VII–27). Early 17th century. Spanish origin.

Reported to contain two works by Palestrina.

B0012 Berlin. Staatsbibliothek zu Berlin. Sammlung Bohn Mus.ms.3 [formerly Breslau, Stadtbibliothek. MS Mus. 3]. Volume of intabulated scores. Second half 16th century.

Contains motets no.10, *Veni sancte spiritus a 8;* no.11, *Dum complerentur a 6* [secunda pars *Dum ergo essent*]; no.50, *O beata et benedicta a 5* [secunda pars *O vera summa*]; no.59, *Lauda Sion a 8;* no.61, *Vidi turbam magnam a 6* [secunda pars *Et omnes angeli stabant*].

B0013 Berlin. Staatsbibliothek zu Berlin. Sammlung Bohn Mus.ms.4 [formerly Breslau, Stadtbibliothek. MS Mus. 4]. Volume of intabulated scores. Dated circa 1575.

Contains motets no.65, *In illo tempore egressus Jesu a 5;* no.69, *Homo quidam fecit a 5;* no.70, *Exi cito in plateas a 5;* no.74, *Unus ex duobus discipulis a 5* [secunda pars *Cum pervenisset beatus Andreas*]; no.75, *Sancte Paule Apostole a 5;* no.82, *Sancta et immaculata virginitas a 6* [secunda pars *Benedicta tua*]; no.89, *Fuit homo missus a Deo a 5;* no.97, *Puer qui natus a 5;* no.104, *Tu es Petrus a 7;* no.105, *Tu es Petrus a 6* [secunda pars *Quodcumque ligaveris*]; no.111, *Beatae Mariae Magdalenae a 5;* no.118, *Venit Michael Archangelus a 5;* no.123, *Corona aurea a 5* [secunda pars *Domine praevenisti eum*]; no.124, *Tradent eum vos in conciliis a 5;* no.125, *Omnipotens sempiterne Deus a 5.*

B0014 Berlin. Staatsbibliothek zu Berlin. Sammlung Bohn Mus.ms.5 [formerly Breslau, Stadtbibliothek. MS Mus. 5]. Six partbooks. Late 16th century. Provenance Breslau, copied for local evangelical church use.

Contains motets no.20, *Alleluia tulerunt Dominum a 5;* no.21, *Ascendit Dominus a 5;* no.26, *Haec dies a 6;* no.70, *Alleluia tulerunt Dominum a 5;* no.101, *Viri Galilaei a 6* [secunda pars *Ascendit Deus in iubilatione*]; no.112, *Ascendo ad Patrem a 5*; no.120, *Veni sancte spiritus a 8;* no.127, *Dum complerentur a 6;* no.166, *O beata et benedicta a 5* [secunda pars *O vera summa*]; no.184, *Fuit homo missus a Deo a 5;* no.190, *Tu es Petrus a 6* [secunda pars *Quodcumque ligaveris*]; no.197, *Beatae Mariae Magdalenae a 5*; no.204, *O lux et decus Hispaniae a 5* [secunda pars *O singulare orna mentum*]; no.206, *Omnipotens sempiterne Deus a 5;* no.213, *Venit Michael Archangelus a 5.*

B0015 Berlin. Staatsbibliothek zu Berlin. Sammlung Bohn Mus.ms.6 [formerly Breslau, Stadtbibliothek. MS Mus. 6]. Volume of intabulated scores. Dated 1567.

Contains motets no.41, *Hodie Christus natus est a 8;* No.42, *O magnum mysterium a 6* [secunda pars *Quem vidistis pastores*]; no.43, *Surge illuminare a 8;* no.50, *Nunc dimittis a 6* [Silla Pierluigi]; no.55, *Senex puerum portabat a 5* [secunda pars *Hodie beata virgo*]; no.58, *O admirabile commercium a 5;* no.59, *Stella quam viderant Magi a 5.*

B0016 Berlin. Staatsbibliothek zu Berlin. Sammlung Bohn Mus.ms.11 [formerly Breslau, Stadtbibliothek. MS Mus. 11]. Six partbooks. Dated 1583 on covers. Provenance Breslau, copied for local evangelical church use.

Contains motets no.2, *Unus ex duobus a 5* [secunda pars *Cum pervenisset beatus Andreas*]; no.27, *Veni Domine et noli tardare a 6* [secunda pars *Excita Domine*]; no.28, *Hierusalem cito veniet a 6* [secunda pars *Ego enim sum Dominus*]; no.29, *Canite tuba in Sion a 5* [secunda pars *Rorate coeli desuper*]; no.44, *Hodie Christus natus est a 8;* no.45, *Surge illuminare a 8;* no.92, *O admirabile commercium a 5;* no.101, *Stella quam viderant Magi a 5;* no.108, *Sancte Paule Apostole a 5;* no.110, *Nunc dimittis a 6* [Silla Pierluigi]; no.113, *Senex puerum portabat a 5* [secunda pars *Hodie beata virgo*]; no.122, *Sancta et immaculata virginitas a 6* [secunda pars *Benedicta tu*]; no.123, *Suscipe verbum Virgo Maria a 5* [secunda pars *Paries quidem filium*]; no.128, *O Domine Jesu Christe a 6;* no.140, *Lauda Sion salvatorem a 8;* no.142, *Vidi turbam magnam a 6* [secunda pars *Et omnes angeli stabant*]; no.147, *Corona aurea a 5* [secunda pars *Domine praevenisti eum*]; no.149, *Tradent eum vos a 5.*

B0017 Berlin. Staatsbibliothek zu Berlin. Sammlung Bohn Mus.ms.12 [formerly Breslau, Stadtbibliothek. MS Mus. 12]. Six partbooks. Early 17th century. Provenance Breslau, copied for local evangelical church use.

Contains motet no.11, *Tu es Petrus a 6* [secunda pars *Quodcumque ligaveris*].

B0018 Berlin. Staatsbibliothek zu Berlin. Sammlung Bohn Mus.ms.15 [formerly Breslau, Stadtbibliothek. MS Mus. 15]. Five partbooks (of an original 8 or more). Late 16th century (date 1587 in MS). Provenance Breslau, copied for local evangelical church use.

Contains motets no.57, *O Domine Jesu a 6;* no.69, *Hodie Christus natus est a 8;* no.150, *Alleluia tulerunt Dominum a 5;* no.175, *Tu es Petrus a 6* [secunda pars *Quodcumque ligaveris*]; no.296, *Haec dies a 6;* no.303, *Confitebor tibi Domine a 8* [secunda pars *Notas facite*].

B0019 Berlin. Staatsbibliothek zu Berlin. Sammlung Bohn Mus.ms.16 [formerly Breslau, Stadtbibliothek. MS Mus. 16]. Two partbooks (of an original six or more). Late 16th century. Provenance Breslau, copied for local evangelical church use.

Contains motet no.9, *Vidi turbam magnam a 6* [secunda pars *Et omnes angeli stabant*].

B0020 Berlin. Staatsbibliothek zu Berlin. Sammlung Bohn Mus.ms.18 [formerly Breslau, Stadtbibliothek. MS Mus. 18]. Volume of intabulated scores. Dated 1580.

Contains motets no.24, *Hodie Christus natus est a 8;* no.25, *Surge illuminare a 8;* no.72, *O Domine Jesu a 6;* no.135, *Viri Galilei a 6* [secunda pars *Ascendit Deus in iubilatione*]; no.160, *Dum complerentur a 6* [secunda pars *Dum ergo essent*].

B0021 Berlin. Staatsbibliothek zu Berlin. Sammlung Bohn Mus.ms.20 [formerly Breslau, Stadtbibliothek. MS Mus. 20]. Volume in folio of intabulated scores. Dated ca.1600.

Contains no.34, *Hodie Christus natus est a 8.*

B0022 Berlin. Staatsbibliothek zu Berlin. Sammlung Bohn Mus.ms.22 [formerly Breslau, Stadtbibliothek. MS Mus. 22]. Eight partbooks. Early 17th century (date 1614 in MS).

Contains no.19, *Hodie Christus natus est a 8.*

B0023 Berlin. Staatsbibliothek zu Berlin. Sammlung Bohn Mus.ms.23 [formerly Breslau, Stadtbibliothek. MS Mus. 23]. Six partbooks of an original eight. First half of 17th century. Various hands [parts for compositions intabulated in Wroclaw MSS 20 and 21].

Contains no.78, *Hodie Christus natus est a 8.*

B0024 Berlin. Staatsbibliothek zu Berlin. Sammlung Bohn Mus.ms.28 [formerly Breslau, Stadtbibliothek. MS Mus. 28]. Three partbooks of an original five. Early 17th century (dates 1613 and 1616 in MS). Various hands.

Contains no.6, *O Domine Jesu a 6.*

B0025 Berlin. Staatsbibliothek zu Berlin. Sammlung Bohn Mus.ms.31 [formerly Breslau, Stadtbibliothek. MS Mus. 31]. Seven partbooks of an original nine. 17th century. Various hands.

Contains no.4, *Hodie Christus natus est a 8.*

B0026 Berlin. Staatsbibliothek zu Berlin. Sammlung Bohn Mus.ms.32 [formerly Breslau, Stadtbibliothek. MS Mus. 32]. One partbook (basso continuo). Early 17th century.

Contains no.1, *Hodie Christus natus est a 8.*

B0027 Berlin. Staatsbibliothek zu Berlin (Staatsbibliothek Preussischer Kulturbesitz). Sammling Bohn. Mus.ms. 357. Section I: six partbooks, dated to 1580–1600; section II: German organ tablature.

Section I contains motets no.18, *O admirabile commercium a 5;* no.30, *Viri Galilei a 6* [secunda pars *Ascendit Deus in iubilatione*]; no.32, *Dum complerentur a 6* [secunda pars *Dum ergo essent*]; no.267, *O Domine Jesu*

Christe a 6; no.268, *Nunc dimittis a 6* [Silla Pierluigi]; no.274, *Cantabo Domino in vita mea a 6* [secunda pars *Deficiant peccatores*].

Section II contains no.25, *O admirabile commercium a 5;* no.42, *Viri Galilei a 6* [transposed a fourth; secunda pars *Ascendit Deus in iubilatione*]; no.44, *Dum complerentur a 6* [transposed a fourth; secunda pars *Dum ergo essent*]; no.271, *O Domine Jesu Christe a 6* [transposed a fourth]; no.272, *Nunc dimittis a 6* [Silla Pierluigi; transposed a fourth]; no.279, *Cantabo Domino in vita mea a 6* [transposed a fourth; secunda pars *Deficiant peccatores*].

B0028 Berlin. Staatsbibliothek zu Berlin (Staatsbibliothek Preussischer Kulturbesitz). Ms. Mus. 40039 [olim 239]. Twelve partbooks. Dates 1570 and 1628 in MS. Copied by various hands.

Contains no.54, *Laudate Dominum in sanctis eius a 8* (f.52); no.77, *Heiliger Geist du Tröster mein a 8* [=*Veni sancte Spiritus*] (f.68v).

B0029 Berlin. Staatsbibliothek zu Berlin (Staatsbibliothek Preussischer Kulturbesitz). Ms. Mus. 40073. One partbook. First quarter of 17th century. Provenance Poland. 162ff.

Contains no.9, Mass, C-Ionian, number of voices uncertain (f.23).

B0030 Berlin. Former Preussische Staatsbibliothek. Ms. Mus. 40192. Dated 1581 [MS missing since 1945].

Reported to contain one work by Palestrina.

B0031 Berlin. Staatsbibliothek zu Berlin (Staatsbibliothek Preussischer Kulturbesitz). Ms. Mus. 40209 [olim 40257]. Five partbooks. First quarter of 17th century. Provenance Saxony.

Contains motets no.7, *Stellam quam viderant magi a 5* (f.7v); no.17, *Senex puerum portabat a 5* [with secunda pars *Hodie beata virgo Maria*] (f.21).

B0032 Berlin. Staatsbibliothek zu Berlin (Staatsbibliothek Preussischer Kulturbesitz). Ms. Mus. 40212. Partbook. Dated after 1582. Provenance Germany.

Contains motet, no.93, *Alleluia! tulerunt Dominum a 5*; madrigals no.5, *Il tempo vola e se non fuggon a 5* [with seconda parte *Ivi vedrai la gloria*]; no.10, *Vestiva i colli a 5* [with seconda parte *Così le chiome mie*]; no.11, *Io son ferito ahi lasso a 5.*

B0033 Berlin. Staatsbibliothek zu Berlin (Staatsbibliothek Preussischer Kulturbesitz). Ms. Mus. 40299. Partbook. Dated circa 1615. Provenance Eastern Germany. 20ff.

Contains motet no.5, *O Domine Jesu Christe adoro te a 6.*

B0034 Bologna. Archivio di San Petronio. Choirbook (partitura) Lib. P.12–II. 17th–18th century.

Contains masses *Missa Ecce sacerdos a 4* [with organ part]; *Missa Salvum me fac a 5* [with organ part]; motet *Caro mea a 4.*

B0035 Bologna. Civico Museo Bibliografico Musicale. MS C.33. Treatise *Il dolcimelo d'Aurelio Virgiliano dove si contengono variati pasaggi, e diminutioni cosi per voci, come per tutte sorte d'instrumenti musicali; con loro accordi, e modi di sonare.* Dated circa 1600.

Contains madrigal f.35v, *Vestiva i colli* with diminuitions.

B0036 Bologna. Civico Museo Bibliografico Musicale. MS F.888. Score. Undated but probably early 18th century. Copied by Antonio Maria Pacchioni.

Contains mass *Missa Ecce sacerdos magnus a 4*; motets *Sicut cervus a 4; Lauda Sion a 4; Veni sancte Spiritus a 8; Ave Regina coelorum a 8; In diebus illis a 4; Quae est ista a 4; Nativitas tua a 4; Nos autem gloriari a 4; Dum aurora a 4; Doctor bonus a 4; Regem cui omnia a 5; Miserere a 5; Stabat Mater a 4 et 8.*

B0037 Bologna. Civico Museo Bibliografico Musicale. MS F.889. Score. Undated but probably early 18th century. Copied by Antonio Maria Pacchioni.

Contains *Missa L'homme armé a 5* [labelled in source "Missa vulgo dell'Uomo Armato"].

B0038 Bologna. Civico Museo Bibliografico Musicale. MS F.891. Score. Undated but probably early 18th century. Copied by Antonio Maria Pacchioni.

Contains motets *Hic est vere; Gaudent in coelis; Ego sum panis; Caro mea vere est; Salvator mundi; Coenantibus illis; Congratulamini mihi; Q quantus luctus; Cantabitur organis* [Cantantibus organis]*; Biduanis; Angelus Domini; Et introeuntes; Inclytae sanctae; Fuit homo; Erat Joannes; O lux et decus; O singulare praesidium; Tradent enim vos; Significavit Dominus; O quoniam metuendus; Pax vobis; Cum ortus fuerit; Rex pacificus; Haec dies quam fecit Dominus; Virgo singularis; Sit laus* [marked *Canon* in Gaspari]; hymns *Lucis creator optime; Ne meus; Praesta Pater; O lux beata Trinitas; Deo Patri; Ad preces nostras; Crimina lata; Christe lux vera; Tu nobis dona; Gloria Deo* [marked *Canon* in Gaspari]; *Ad coenam agni; Protecti Pasche; O vere digna Hostia; Quaesumus auctor; Jesu nostra redemptio; Inferni claustra; Tu esto* [marked *Canon* in Gaspari]; *Quodcumque vinctis; Doctor egregie; Vexilla regis; Impleta sunt; Beata cuius; O crux; Te fons.*

B0039 Bologna. Civico Museo Bibliografico Musicale. MS Q.22. Four partbooks. 16th to 17th century.

Contains *Missa Sine nomine a 4* [Cas. v.19] [anon. in source].

B0040 Bologna. Civico Museo Bibliografico Musicale. MS Q.31. Choirbook. Dated 1580 in MS. Provenance Rome.

Contains hymns f.54v, *Lauda mater ecclesia a 4* [not in Haberl]; f.56v, *Quicumque Christum quaeritis* (strophes 2, 4); f.58v, *Quicumque Christum quaeritis a 4* [not in Haberl]; f.70v, *Vox primae Christi a 4* [=*Salvete flores martyrum*] (strophe 2).

B0041 Bologna. Civico Museo Bibliografico Musicale. MS Q.34. Score. Dated

1613. Copied by Joannes Amigonus Mantuanus.

Contains motets f.46v, *Corona aurea a 5;* f.50, *Introduxit me rex a 5*; f.51v, *Pulchra es amica mea a 5*; madrigals f.27, *Vestiva i colli a 5;* f.31, *Io son ferito a 5.*

B0042 Bologna. Civico Museo Bibliografico Musicale. MS Q.35. Dated 1603. Provenance Brescia.

Contains f.73, *Stabat Mater a 4 et 8* [two choirs].

B0043 Bologna. Civico Museo Bibliografico Musicale. MS Q.40. Score. 17th century.

Contains p.1, *Stabat Mater a 8.*

B0044 Bologna. Civico Museo Bibliografico Musicale. MS Q.117. Large choirbook. Dated 1617.

Contains 4 *Magnificat a 4* [beginning *Anima mea* verse: f.1v, tone 1; f.7v, tone 2; f.13v, tone 3; f.19v, tone 4].

B0045 Bologna. Civico Museo Bibliografico Musicale. MS R.281. Score. First half of 19th century. Scoring by Fortunato Santini. [Contains two otherwise undocumented motets attributed to Palestrina.]

Contains motets *Ascendit Deus a 4*; *Panis angelicus a 4; Pater noster a 4* [*recte* Willaert]; p.12, *Lumen a 4 et 5;* p.20, *O bone Jesu o piissime a 4; Qui pacem a 4.*

B0046 Bologna. Civico Museo Bibliografico Musicale. MS S/9. Choirbook. Dated ca 1600. Copied by Teodore Clingher.

Contains hymns f.57, *Conditor alme siderum a 4;* f.59v, *Christe redemptor omnium a 4;* f.65, *A solis ortus cardine a 4;* f.66, *Salvete flos a 4;* f.68, *Hostes Herodes impie a 4;* f.71v, *Lucis creator optime a 4;* f.74, *O lux beata Trinitas a 4;* f.75, *Ad preces nostras a 4;* f.82, *Vexilla regis a 4* [Hab.VIII.35]; f.86v, *Ad coenam agni a 4;* f.90v, *Jesu nostra redemptio a 4.*

B0047 Bologna. Archivio Musicale della Fabbriceria di San Petronio. MS A.XXXIX. Dated 1552 [badly deteriorated].

Reported to contain music by Palestrina, although catalogue cites twenty-eight anonymous works in this source.

B0048 Breslau. Former Stadtbibliothek. MS Mus. 2 [presently lost; contents known from Bohn catalogue]. Score in intabulated notation. Dated 1573 [Palestrina motets are transposed to the lower fourth].

Contains motets no.45, *Haec dies a 6;* no.114, *Alleluia tulerunt Dominum a 5* [secunda pars no.115, *Angelus Domini a 5*]; no.155, *Viri Galilei a 6* [secunda pars *Ascendit Deus in iubilatione*]; no.166, *Ascendo ad Patrem a 5.*

B0049 Cambridge. Fitzwilliam Museum. Music MS 279 (AC) [olim 52 A 33–35]. Three partbooks of an original five. Copied late 16th to early 17th century.

Provenance English, Paston household.
Reported to contain three works by Palestrina.

B0050 Cambridge. King's College, Rowe Music Library. MS316. Partbook (contratenor). Dated ca. 1560 with late 16th-century additions [description in Iain Fenlon, *Cambridge Music Manuscripts 900–1700*, Cambridge 1982, pp.135–137].
Reported to contain two works by Palestrina.

B0051 Chicago. Newberry Library, Case MS 7A/2. Late 17th to early 18th century.
Contains two Aldrich-Palestrina recompositions, including *Be thou exalted.*

B0052 Città di Castello. Cattedrale di San Florido, Archivio Capitolare MS 2084 (olim VI C 11). Choirbook. Late 1550s.
Contains three hymns, including *Lauda mater ecclesia.*

B0053 Civitanova Marche. Biblioteca Comunale. MSS s.s. (1). Four partbooks. Dated ca. 1555–1560. Provenance Florence.
Reported to contain three works by Palestrina.

B0054 Coimbra. Biblioteca Geral da Universidade. MS 44. Choirbook. 17th century. Provenance Santa Cruz, Coimbra.
Contains no.27, *Missa Quartus tonus* [*Missa Gabriel Arcangelus*] *a 4*; no.28, *Missa brevis a 4*.

B0055 Dresden. Sächsische Landesbibliothek. Musikabteilung MS Mus 1/B/98. Score entitled "Collectaneorum musicorum libri quatuor" [four volumes]. Dated 1718.
Vol. 3 contains masses by Palestrina, four to six voices.

B0056 Dresden. Sächsische Landesbibliothek. MS Mus. 2/D/22 (olim B.266) Partbooks. Dated ca. 1590–1600. Probable central German provenance.
Contains motets no.9, *O admirabile commercium a 5*; no.12, *Stella quam viderant a 5* [secunda pars *Tribus miraculis*].

B0057 Dresden. Sächsische Landesbibliothek. MS Grimma 56 (1–5). Partbooks. Dated ca. 1568–1585. Provenance Meissen.
Contains motets no.8, *O admirabile commercium a 5*; no.21, *Dum complerentur a 6* [secunda pars *Dum ergo essent*]; no.22, *Viri Galilaei a 6* [secunda pars *Ascendit Deus*]; no.70, *O magnum mysterium a 6* [secunda pars *Quem vidistis pastores*].

B0058 Escorial. Real Monasterio de San Lorenzo del Escorial, Biblioteca y Archivio de Musica. MS 2 (=BeniCAM 4). Choirbook. Dated 1604 in inscription. Copied at Escorial.
Contains masses f.1v, *Missa Iste confessor a 4*; f.11v, *Missa Brevis a 4;* f.81v, *Missa Nasce la gioia mia a 6*; motets f.28v, *Domine quando veneris a*

4 [secunda pars *Comissa mea pavesco*]; f.32v, *Heu mihi Domine a 4* [secunda pars *Anima mea turbata est*]; f.36v, *Ad te levavi oculos meos a 4* [secunda pars *Miserere nostri Domine*]; f.40v, *Ad Dominum cum tribularer a 4* [secunda pars *Sagittae potentis*]; f.42v, *Sicut cervus a 4*; f.43v, *Super flumina a 4*; f.45v, *Quia vidisti me Thoma a 4*; f.46v, *Magnus sanctus Paulus a 4*; f.48v, *Veni sponsa Christi a 4*; f.49v, *Nativitas tua a 4*; f.50v, *Nativitas tua*; f.51v, *Exaudi Domine a 4*; f.52v, *Veni sponsa Christi a 4* [=f.48v]; f.53v, *Gaudent in coelis a 4*; f.54v, *Tollite jugum meum a 4*; f.55v, *Beatus vir qui suffert a 4*; f.56v, *Iste est qui ante Deum*; f.60v, *Jesus junxit se a 4*; f.62v, *Loquebantur in variis linguis a 4*; f.64v, *Ego sum panis vivus a 4*; f.66v, *Exaudi Domine a 4* [=f.51v].

B0059 Escorial. Real Monasterio de San Lorenzo del Escorial, Biblioteca y Archivio de Musica. MS 3 (=BeniCAM 3). Choirbook. Late 16th to early 17th century. Copied at Escorial.

Contains motets f.11v, *Alleluia! tulerunt Dominum a 5*; f.13v, *O vera summa sempiterna Trinitas a 5*; f.15v, *Ego sum panis vivus a 5*; f.17v, *Crucem sanctam a 5*; f.22v, *Tradent enim vos a 5*; f.24v, *Sanctificavit Dominus a 5*; f.26v, *O lux et decus hispaniae a 5*; f.28v, *Puer qui natus est a 5*; f.30v, *Venit Michael Arcangelus a 5*; f.37v, *Beatae Mariae Magdalenae a 5*; f.39v, *Haec dies a 6*; f.40v, *Vidi turbam magnam a 6*; f.42v, *Beatus Laurentius a 5*; f.43v, *Viri Galilaei a 6* [secunda pars *Ascendit Deus*]; f.45v, *O beatum virum a 5*; f.48v, *O Domine Jesu Christe a 6*; f.49v, *Solve juvente Deo a 6*; f.51v, *Dum complerentur a 6* [secunda pars *Dum ergo essent*]; f.56v, *Hodie beata virgo Maria a 5*; f.58v, *Suscipe verbum a 5*; f.60v, *Hodie nata est beata virgo a 5*; f.62v, *Quam pulchri sunt a 5*; f.69v, *Maria virgo coelos ascendit a 7*; f.74v, *Cum pervenisset beatus Andreas a 5.*

B0060 Escorial. Real Monasterio de San Lorenzo del Escorial, Biblioteca y Archivio de Musica. MS 4 (=BeniCAM 2). Choirbook. Early 17th century. Copied at Escorial. 86ff.

Contains masses no.22, *Missa de feria a 4* (f.57v); no.26, *Missa de feria a 4* [=no.22] (f.70v); motet no.5, *Pueri Hebraeorum a 4* [*"de voces iguales"*] (f.9v).

B0061 Escorial. Real Monasterio de San Lorenzo del Escorial, Biblioteca y Archivio de Musica. MS 5 (=BeniCAM 1). Choirbook. Early 17th century. Copied at Escorial. 75ff.

Contains motet, no.2, *Pueri Hebraeorum* (f.1v); mass, no.9, "*Misa cum 6 vocibus*" [CCATTB] (f.54v).

B0062 Escorial. Real Monasterio de San Lorenzo del Escorial, Biblioteca y Archivio de Musica. MS 6. Choirbook. Dated between 1689 and 1750.

Contains masses no.3, *Missa brevis* (f.9v); no.4, *Missa Iste confessor* (f.31v); no.5, *Missa sexti toni* (f.53v); no.6, *Missa Aeterna Christi munera* (f.74v); no.7, *Missa Emendemus in melius* (f.96v).

B0063 Escorial. Real Monasterio de San Lorenzo del Escorial, Biblioteca y

Archivio de Musica. MS 8. Score. Dated 1786. Provenance Spanish. ii + 187ff.

Contains offertory motets p.1, *Ad te levavi oculos meos a 5*; p.7, *Deus tu convertens a 5*; f.11, *Benedixisti Domine a 5*; p.17, *Ave Maria a 5*; p.23, *Bonum est confiteri a 5*; p.29, *Perfice gressus meos a 5*; p.35, *Benedictus es Domine a 5*; p.41, *Scapulis suis a 5*; f.p.47, *Meditabor in mandatis tuis a 5*; p.53, *Justitiae Domini a 5*; p.59, *Laudate Dominum a 5*; p.65, *Confitebor tibi Domine a 5*; p.71, *Improperium a 5*; p.77, *Custodi me Domine a 5*; p.83, *Domine exaudi orationem meam a 4*.

B0064 Escorial. Real Monasterio de San Lorenzo del Escorial, Biblioteca y Archivio de Musica. MS 9. Score. Dated 1786. Provenance Spanish. iv + 56ff.

Contains offertory motet no.18, *"Miércoles santo"* [*Domine exaudi orationem a 4*].

B0065 Escorial. Real Monasterio de San Lorenzo del Escorial, Biblioteca y Archivio de Musica. MS 1.247. Four partbooks. Copied 18th century.

Contains masses no.1, *Missa Brevis a 4*; no.2, *Missa Iste confessor a 4*; no.3, *Missa sexti toni a 4*.

B0066 Escorial. Real Monasterio de San Lorenzo del Escorial, Biblioteca y Archivio de Musica. MS 1.248. Four partbooks. Copied 18th century.

Contains masses *Missa Aeterna Christi munera a 4*; *Missa Emendemus in melius a 4*.

B0067 Ferrara. Biblioteca Comunale Ariostea. *Officium defunctorum*. 18th century.

Contains *Missa defunctorum a voci pari* (three tenors, one bass) [ascribed to Palestrina in MS; argued to be correct attribution in 1975 by Adriano Cavicchi, but status is unresolved].

B0068 Florence. Biblioteca nazionale centrale. Cod. Miscelli 89. Treatise *Lezioni di contrappunto fatte da Francesco Maria Bassani, con alcuni toccate e vari madrigali rotti (ossia passeggiati) da Orazio Bassani suo zio anno 1621, come sta stritto nel verso della seconda carta*. 1621.

Contains madrigals f.16v, *Io son ferito ahi lasso* [with diminutions]; f.19v, *Cosi le chiome mie* [seconda parte of *Vestiva i colli*, with diminutions].

B0069 Florence. Archivio del Duomo, Archivio musicale dell'Opera di Santa Maria del Fiore. Ms. Polifonico 18. Choirbook. 16th to 17th century.

Contains f.1v, *Missa Gabriel Arcangelus a 4*.

B0070 Florence. Archivio del Duomo, Archivio musicale dell'Opera di Santa Maria del Fiore. Ms. Polifonico 20. Choirbook. Dated ca. 1650.

Contains motet f.79v, *Tota pulchra es a 5*; hymn f.88v, *Pange lingua corporis mysterium a 4*.

B0071 Florence. Archivio del Duomo, Archivio musicale dell'Opera di Santa Maria

del Fiore. Ms. Polifonico 21. Three partbooks. Dated ca. 1700.
Contains p.52, *Missa Sine nomine a 4.*

B0072 Florence. Archivio del Duomo, Archivio musicale dell'Opera di Santa Maria del Fiore. Ms.Polifonico 25. Choirbook. Dated ca. 1600.
Contains motet f.91v, *Tribulationes civitatum a 5.*

B0073 Florence. Archivio del Duomo, Archivio musicale dell'Opera di Santa Maria del Fiore. Ms. Polifonico 33. Small choirbook. Dated ca. 1655.
Contains masses f.1v, *Missa Papae Marcelli a 6*; f.53v, *Missa Sine nomine a 4*; hymn f.160v, *Iste Confessor a 4.*

B0074 Gdansk (Danzig). Stadtbibliothek, MS 4005. Six partbooks. End of 16th century. Provenance S. Bartholomei, Danzig.
Contains mass no.4, *Missa Papae Marcelli a 6*; no.42, *Missa O magnum mysterium* [*Missa Tertia*] *a 5.*

B0075 Gdansk (Danzig). Stadtbibliothek, MS 4007. Three partbooks of an original eight. End of 16th century. Provenance S. Bartholomei, Danzig.
Contains mass f.92v, *Missa Prima* [*Missa Eripe me de inimicis*] *a 5.*

B0076 Guadalupe. Real Monasterio de Santa Maria, Archivio de Musica. MS s.s.(1) (olim I; A; 1). Choirbook. Dated between 1603 and ca. 1675. Possible provenance Jeronimite monastery at Guadalupe.
Contains mass *Missa Signe* [*sic*; recte *Sine*] *nomine a 4* [pub. 1567, but with an additional final *Kyrie* that is absent from published version].

B0077 Guadalupe. Real Monasterio de Santa Maria, Archivio de Musica. MS s.s.(2) (olim II; B; 2). Choirbook. Dated between 1603 and ca. 1675. Possible provenance Jeronimite monastery at Guadalupe.
Contains masses f.151v, *Missa Aspice Domine a 5/6*; f.187v, *Missa Papae Marcelli a 6*; f.219v, *Missa Ut re mi fa sol la a 6.*

B0078 Guatemala City. Catedral, Archivio Capitular. MS 1. Choirbook. Dated 1760s, recopied partially from a collection dated 1602. 193ff.
Contains mass f.31v, *Missa Sine nomine a 4* [=from Book II of masses].

B0079 Guatemala City. Catedral, Archivio Capitular. MS 2. Choirbook. Early 17th century. Provenance Cathedral in Guatemala City. 259ff.
Contains f.20v–32, *Magnificat primi toni cum 4 vocibus paribus* [odd-numbered verses beginning *Anima mea* f.20v–26; even-numbered verses beginning *Et exultavit* f.26v–32].

B0080 Guatemala City. Catedral, Archivio Capitular. MS 4. Choirbook. Dated ca. 1600–1602. Provenance Guatemala City [description in AIM, *Census-Catalogue of Manuscript Sources of Polyphonic Music*].
Reported to contain two works, one attribued to Palestrina, one attributed "Morales/Palestrina."

B0081 Krakow. Archiwum Panstwowym Miasta Krakowa i Wojewodztwa Krakowskiego (State Archives of the Town and Province of Krakow). MSS D32–35. Partbooks. Dated late 17th to early 18th century. Provenance Krakow.

Reported to contain three works by Palestrina.

B0082 Liegnitz (Legnica). Former Königliche Ritter-Akademie. Bibliotheca Rudolfina. MS 7 (Pfudel catalogue). Six partbooks. 16th to 17th century [note: after World War II, parts of the Rudolfina collection were dispersed to various Polish libraries in Liegnitz, Warsaw, Wroclaw [Breslau], and Lublin. The location of individual items has not been ascertained by the present author. Inventories derived from Pfudel catalogue].

Contains motet no.17, *Salve Regina misericordiae a 5.*

B0083 Liegnitz (Legnica). Former Königliche Ritter-Akademie. Bibliotheca Rudolfina. MS 16 (=Pfudel). Volume of German organ tablature. Early 17th century.

Contains motet no.191, *Lauda Sion salvatorem a 8.*

B0084 Liegnitz (Legnica). Former Königliche Ritter-Akademie. Bibliotheca Rudolfina. MS 20 (=Pfudel). Six partbooks. Dated first half of 17th century. Compiled in various hands.

Contains madrigal no.29, *Vestiva i colli a 5.*

B0085 Liegnitz (Legnica). Former Königliche Ritter-Akademie. Bibliotheca Rudolfina. MS 24 (=Pfudel). Eight partbooks. 17th century [compilation in four sections].

Section 3 contains madrigal no.60, *Vestiva i colli a 5.*

B0086 Liegnitz (Legnica). Former Königliche Ritter-Akademie. Bibliotheca Rudolfina. MS 26 (=Pfudel). Volume of German organ tablature. Early 17th century. 346ff.

Contains motets no.275, *O magnum mysterium a 6* [secunda pars *Quem vidistis pastores*]; no.276, *Beatus Laurentius a 5*; no.277, *Lapidabant Stephanum a 5* (incomplete); no.279, *Ascendo ad Patrem a 5*; no.280, *Homo quidam fecit a 5*; no.281, *Canite tuba in Sion a 5* (incomplete).

B0087 Liegnitz (Legnica). Former Königliche Ritter-Akademie. Bibliotheca Rudolfina. MS 31 (=Pfudel). Volume of German organ tablature. 17th century. [Compilation in fourteen sections.]

Section III contains motets from the printed Books 1, 2, and 3: no.7, *O Antoni eremita a 5;* no.8, *Alleluia tulerunt Dominum a 5*; no.9, *Crucem sanctam a 5*; no.10, *O beata et gloriosa Trinitas a 5* [prima et secunda pars]; no.11, *Ego sum panis a 5* [prima et secunda pars]; no.12, *Beatus Laurentius a 5*; no.13, *Hodie nata est beata virgo a 5*; no.14, *O beatum virum a 5*; no.15, *O beatum pontificem a 5*; no.16, *Deus qui dedisti a 5*; no.17, *Lapidabant Stephanum a 5*; no.18, *Hic est discipulus a 5*; no.19, *Sicut lilium a 5*; no.20, *Quam pulchri sunt a 5*; no.21, *Viri Galilaei a 5* [prima et secunda pars]; no.22, *Dum complerentur a 6* [prima et secunda pars]; no.23, *Pulchra es a 6*; no.24, *Vidi turbam magnam a 6* [prima et secunda pars]; no.25, *Virgo prudentissima a 6* [prima et secunda pars]; no.26, *O virgo simul et mater a 5*; no.27, *Memor esto verbi tui a 5*; no.28, *O sacrum convivium a 5*; no.29, *Coenantibus illis a 5*; no.30, *Derelinquat impius a 5*; [no.31, Angelo Pierluigi, *Circuire possum Domine a 5*, prima et secunda pars]; no.32, *Gaude Barbara beata a 5* [prima et secunda pars]; [no.33, Silla Pierluigi, *Domine Pater a 5*; no.34, Rodolfo Pierluigi, *Confitebor tibi a 5*]; no.35, *Peccantem me quotidie a 5*; no.36, *Jesus in qua nocte a 5*; no.37, *Tribularer si nescirem a 6* [prima et secunda pars]; no.38, *Confitebor tibi Domine a 8* [prima et secunda pars]; no.40, *Laudate pueri Dominum a 8;* no.41, [secunda pars] *Quis sicut Dominus a 8*; no.42, *Domine in virtute tua a 8* [prima et secunda pars]; no.43, *Laudate Dominum onmes gentes a 8*; no.44, *Pater noster a 5*; no.45, *Ave Maria a 5*; no.46, *Cantantibus organis Caecilia a 5* [prima et secunda pars]; no.47, *Caro mea a 5*; no.48, *Congrega Domine a 5* [prima et secunda pars]; no.49, *Inclytae sancte virginis a 5.*

Section IX contains no.155, *O Domine Jesu Christe a 6.*

Section XIV contains no.169, *Beate Marie Magdalene a 5.*

B0088 Liegnitz (Legnica). Former Königliche Ritter-Akademie. Bibliotheca Rudolfina. MS 49 (=Pfudel 18). Six partbooks. Dated ca. 1625. Provenance Liegnitz.

Section 4 contains no.31, *O Domine Jesu a 6.*

B0089 Lisbon. Palácio Ducal da Sereníssima Casa de Bragança de Vila Viçosa. MS 12. Choirbook. Dated 1735.

Contains motet f.2v, *Pueri Hebraeorum*; f.26v, mass *Missa de Beata Virgine* [*Credo* only]; motet f.103v, *Dominus Jesus in qua nocte.*

B0090 Ljubljana. Narodna in Univezitetna Knjiznica, Rokopisni Oddelek. MS 207. Partbook. Dated late 16th to early 17th century. Provenance Slovenian. 79ff.

Reported to contain two works by Palestrina.

B0091 London. British Library, Reference Division. Department of Manuscripts. MSS Additional 17840. Score. 18th century. 154ff. [Palestrina-Aldrich recompositions].

Contains no.29, “We have heard with our ears” (f.66); no.30, “Hold not thy tongue” (f.68).

B0092 London. British Library, Reference Division. Department of Manuscripts. MSS Additional 17842. Score. 18th century. Provenance Oxford. 145ff. [Palestrina-Aldrich recompositions].

Contains no.4, “We have heard with our ears” (f.14) [with annotation “adapted by Dr. Aldrich from Palastrini (sic) and Carissimi”]; no.9, “Why art thou so vexed” (f.37); no.10, “My heart is fixt” (f.40); no.11, “The eye of the Lord” (f.43); no.17, “O God the King of Glory” (f.64).

B0093 London. British Library, Reference Division. Department of Manuscripts.

MSS Additional 29372–29377 ("Tristitiae Remedium" of Thomas Muriell). Partbooks. Dated 1618. Provenance London.

Contains madrigal f.56v, *Sound out my voice a 5* [=*Vestiva i colli*] ["Gianetto Palaestina"].

B0094 London. British Library, Reference Division. Department of Manuscripts. MSS Additional 29388–29392. Partbooks. Early 17th century. English provenance.

Contains motet f.1, *Dum complerentur a 6* [secunda pars *Dum ergo essent*].

B0095 London. British Library, Reference Division. Department of Manuscripts. MSS Additional 31398. Score. Dated circa 1759.

Contains f.34v, "O God the King of Glory" a 4 [with annotation "Altered by Dr. Aldrich from the motet 'O Rex gloriae' "].

B0096 London. British Library, Reference Division. Department of Manuscripts. MSS Additional 31399. Score. 18th century.

Contains "O Lord God of our Salvation" [attributed to Aldrich-Palestrina].

B0097 London. British Library, Reference Division. Department of Manuscripts. MSS Additional 31404. Organ part. 18th century.

Contains no.7, "We have heard with our ears" (f.87v).

B0098 London. British Library, Reference Division. Department of Manuscripts. MSS Additional 41156–41158. Partbooks. Early 17th century. English provenance.

Reported to contain one work by Palestrina.

B0099 British Library, Reference Division. Department of Manuscripts. MSS Egerton 2009, 2011, 2012. Three partbooks of original five. Dated early 17th century. English provenance.

Reported to contain works by Palestrina.

B0100 London. British Library, Reference Division. Department of Manuscripts. MS Egerton 2010. Partbook. Early 17th century. English provenance.

Reported to contain works by Palestrina.

B0101 London. British Library, Reference Division. Department of Manuscripts. MS Egerton 3665 ("Tregian Manuscript"). Early 17th century.

Contains madrigal, f.199v.

B0102 London. British Library, Reference Division. Department of Manuscripts. MS Harley 7337–7342. Score [six volumes]. Late 17th to early 18th century. [Note volume 2, Harley 7338, 254 ff: the following works were "set to English words by ye Revd. Dr. Aldrich, Dean of Xt Church"].

Contains no.23, "We have heard with our ears" [*Doctor bonus*, f.154v];

no.24, "Why art thou so vexed, O my soul" [*Ave Maria*, f.156v]; no.25, "My heart is fixt, O God [*Nos autem gloriari*, f.158]; no.26, "The eye of ye Lord" [*Jesus junxit se*, f.159v]; no.27 "O God, ye King of Glory" [*O Rex gloriae*, f.161]; no.28., "Hold not thy tongue" [*Nativitas tua*, f.162v].

B0103 London. British Library, Reference Division. Music Library. MS Madrigal Society G.27. Partbook. Early 17th century. English provenance.
Reported to contain one work by Palestrina.

B0104 London. Royal College of Music. MS 2041. Partbook (of original 8?). Early 17th century. English provenance. [Missing since 1960s].
Reported to contain one work by Palestrina.

B0105 Loreto. Biblioteca della Santa Casa. MS 35. Choirbook. 17th century.
Contains f.1v, *Missa Già fu che m'ebbe cara a 4;* f.15v, *Missa In illo tempore a 4;* f.37v, *Missa Dum esset summus Pontifex a 4;* f.67v, *Missa Sine nomine (Je suis desheritée) a 4.*

B0106 Loreto. Biblioteca della Santa Casa. MS 37. Choirbook. Early 17th century. Possible provenance Loreto, Cappella Lauretana.
Contains motets f.145v, *Pulchra es amica mea a 5;* f.147v, *Quae est ista quae progreditur a 5;* f.149v, *Vulnerasti cor meum soror mea a 5;* f.151v, *Surge amica mea a 5;* f.155v, *Dilectus meus descendit a 5*; f.166v, *Veni dilecti mi a 5;* f.172v, *Isti sunt viri sancti a 4*; f.174v, *Tollite jugum meum a 4;* f.178v, *Veni sponsa Christi a 4;* f.180v, *Valde honorandus est a 4;* f.182v, *O admirabile commercium a 5.*

B0107 Loreto. Biblioteca della Santa Casa. MS 81. Choirbook. 16th to 17th century.
Contains masses [all anonymous in source] f.25v, *Missa Petra sancta a 5;* f.75v, *Missa Memor esto a 5;* f.141v, *Missa Papae Marcelli a 6.*

B0108 Lucca. Biblioteca del Seminario Arcivescovile. MS A 8 (or A VIII). Choirbook. Dated ca. 1576–1577. Provenance Rome.
Contains hymn f.47v, *Veni Sancte Spiritus a 4.*

B0109 Mexico City. Biblioteca Octaviano Valdés. Choirbook ("Valdés Codex"). Dated to ca. 1561–1571. Paper of Madrid provenance. 139ff.
Contains masses f.5v, *Missa Quem dicunt homines a 5;* f.18v, *Missa Già fu chi m'ebbe cara* [anonymous in source] f.56v, *Missa Aeterna Christi munera a 5;* f.86v, *Missa Ave regina coelorum a 4;* f.101v, *Missa Christus resurgens* [last is unicum source, either by Palestrina or Pierre Colin].

B0110 Mexico City. Metropolitan Cathedral of Mexico. Ms.5. Choirbook. Dated 16th to 17th century.
Reported to contain masses by Palestrina.

B0111 Milan. Biblioteca del Conservatorio di Musica Giuseppe Verdi, MS s.s.

("Tarasconi Codex," "Clerici Codex"). Dated last third of 16th century, completed 1585–1586. Provenance Parma.

Contains madrigals f.48v, *Piovommi amare lacrime* a 5 [seconda parte *Ma gli spiriti miei*] (attribution to Palestrina uncertain); f.49v, *Come in più negre tenebre*; f.49v, *Il gran splendor* [seconda parte *Io fui in poter*]; f.78v, *Vestiva i colli* [seconda parte *Così le chiome*]; f.79v, *Se fra quest'erb'e fiori*; f.80v, *Io son ferito*; f.92v, *Il tempo vola* [seconda parte *Ivi vedrai la gloria*]; f.128v, *Dolor non fu né fia;* f.193v, *In dubio di mio stato* [seconda parte *Or fia giammai*] (attribution to Palestrina uncertain).

B0112 Milan. Biblioteca del Conservatorio di Musica Giuseppe Verdi, Ms. Fondo Santa Barbara MS 14. Five partbooks. Last third of 16th century.

Contains p.1, *Missa In duplicibus (minoribus I) a 5;* p.9, *Missa De beata Marie (Virginis III) a 5*; p.17, *Missa Festis Apostolor(um I) a 5;* p.25, [*Missa*] *in D*[*omi*]*nicis diebus a 4*; p.33, *Missa In semiduplicibus (majoribus II) a 5.*

B0113 Milan. Biblioteca del Conservatorio di Musica Giuseppe Verdi, Ms. Fondo Santa Barbara MS 109. Four partbooks. Dated late 16th century.

Contains *Missa Sine nomine a 4.*

B0114 Milan. Biblioteca del Conservatorio di Musica Giuseppe Verdi, Ms. Fondo Santa Barbara. MS 164. Choirbook. Dated 1587, copied by Franceso Sforza. [Alternatim polyphony format].

Contains f.1v, *Missa In duplicibus (minoribus I) a 5;* f.23v, *Missa In duplicibus (minoribus II) a 5;* f.44v, *Missa De beata Marie (Virginis I) a 5;* f.66v, *Missa De beata Marie (Virginis II) a 5;* f.84v, *Missa De beata Marie (Virginis III) a 5.*

B0115 Milan. Biblioteca del Conservatorio di Musica Giuseppe Verdi, Ms. Fondo Santa Barbara. MS166. Choirbook. 1592, copied by Francesco Sforza.

Contains f.23v, *Missa Festis Apostolor(um I) a 5;* f.44v, *Missa Festis Apostolor(um II) a 5;* f.85v, *Missa In semidupl(icibus) major(ibus I) a 5;* f.103v, *Missa In semiduplicibus (majoribus II) a 5.*

B0116 Modena. Duomo, Biblioteca e Archivio Capitolare. MS Mus. VI. Partbook (cantus or tenor). Dated ca. 1560–1570. Provenance Modena.

Contains f.11v, *"Missa Pilastrina"* [attribution doubtful]; f.24v, *Missa Ut, re, mi, fa, sol, la a 6.*

B0117 Modena. Duomo, Biblioteca e Archivio Capitolare. MS Mus. XII. Choirbook. Dated 16th century, in several layers. Provenance Modena.

Contains f.32v, *Missa Papae Marcelli a 6.*

B0118 Modena. Biblioteca Estense. Ms.mus. D.303. Three partbooks. Dated 17th to 18th century [attribution doubtful, but considered authentic by Jeppesen].

Contains *Missa Sine nomine a 4* [without *Gloria* or *Credo,* with organ and violone parts added].

B0119 Modena. Biblioteca Estense. Ms.mus. D.305. Partbooks. Dated 17th to 18th century.

Contains *Missa Emendemus a 5* [with organ or violone part; lacks *Gloria* in organ part].

B0120 Modena. Biblioteca Estense. Ms.mus. F.888. Score. Dated to beginning of 18th century. Possibly copied by Antonio Maria Pacchioni.

Contains sequence p.41, *Stabat Mater a 4 et 8* (incomplete); motet p.83, *Miserere mei a 5.*

B0121 Modena. Biblioteca Estense. Ms.mus. F.889. Score. Dated to beginning of 18th century. "From the hand of the celebrated Don Antonio Maria Pacchioni."

Contains *Missa L'homme armé a 5.*

B0122 Montserrat. Biblioteca del Monestir. MS 767. Dated 1586. Provenance Madrid.

Reported to contain one work by Palestrina.

B0123 Munich. Bayerische Staatsbibliothek, Musiksammlung. Mus. Ms 46 (olim Maier 18). Choirbook. Dated ca. 1565. Provenance Munich.

Contains *Missa Benedicta es coelorum Regina a 6* ["Gianetto"].

B0124 Munich. Bayerische Staatsbibliothek, Musiksammlung. Mus. MS 64 (olim Maier 23). Choirbook. Dated ca. 1570. Provenance Benedictine Cloister, Tegernsee. 231ff.

Contains f.2, *Missa Octo vocum a 8 VII. toni* [copied by F. Flori, ca. 1565–1588]; f.59, *Missa Escoutes tous gentilz a 8* [parody mass based on Jannequin model; copied by J. Pollet, ca. 1555–1570] ["Janetto Palestrino"; attributions doubtful].

B0125 Munich. Bayerische Staatsbibliothek. Musiksammlung Anh. Mus. Ms 259 (olim Maier 218). Score. Dated 1628. Made by Wilhelm Krumper, organist of the Augustinian cloister in Polling, based on the print *Hortus Musicus (1606).* 178ff.

Contains no.23, *Succurite ahi lasso vos sancti Dei* [contrafactum=*Io son ferito ahi lasso a 5*]; no.25, *Festiva dies agitur a 5* [contrafactum=*Vestiva i colli a 5*].

B0126 Munich. Bayerische Staatsbibliothek. Musiksammlung Mus. Ms 511 (olim Maier 53). Choirbook. Dated 1596–1597. Provenance Benedictine cloister, Thierhaupten. 133ff.

Contains f.49v, *Missa Secunda (Veni Sancte Spiritus) a 5 (Et incarnatus est only)* [Hab. XXVIII.239].

B0127 Munich. Bayerische Staatsbibliothek. Musiksammlung Mus. Ms 668. Score. Dated 1834. In hand of F. M. Clos of Grafrath.

Contains p.203, *Miserere mei a 5.*

B0128 Munich. Bayerishce Staatsbibliothek, Musiksammlung. Musica Ms 1536 (olim Lat.16527b; Maier 132). Five partbooks (of original 8). Dated 1583. Provenance south Bavaria.

Contains motets no.106, *Surge illuminare a 6;* 107, *Hodie Christus natus est a 8;* no.108, *Veni sancte spiritus a 8;* no.109, *Lauda Sion a 8;* no.110, *Ave regina coelorum a 8*; no.111, *Jubilate Deo omnis terra a 8.*

B0129 Munich. Bayerishce Staatsbibliothek, Musiksammlung. Mus. Ms 1641 (olim Maier 257). Volume of German organ tablature. End of 16th century. Provenance Augustinian cloister in Au am Inn. 221ff.

Contains motets no.31, *Fuit homo missus a Deo a 5* [secunda pars *Erat Johannes in deserto*]; no.56, *Susanna ab improbis senibus a 6* [secunda pars *Postquam autem falso*]; no.62, *Haec dies quam fecit Dominus a 6;* no.121, *Fuit homo missus a Deo a 5* [secunda pars *Erat Johannes in deserto*; this item transposed one tone higher than no.31].

B0130 Munich. Bayerische Staatsbibliothek, Musiksammlung. Mus. Ms 6483 (no Maier number). Two partbooks of original eight. Dated 1596. Provenance Bavarian Augustinian cloister.

Contains motets Part I, no.9, *Surge illuminare a 8*; Part II, no.15, *Deus qui ecclesiam tuam a 6* [secunda pars *Tribue nobis*].

B0131 Munich. Metropolitankirche zu Unserer Lieben Frau. Mf. Chb.11. Choirbook. Dated 1741, copied by Sebastian Pattinger. Palestrina material copied from RISM 1646[1].

Contains f.27, *Missa Iste Confessor a 4.*

B0132 Münster. Bibliothek Fortunato Santini. MS 872. Score. First half of 19th century, in hand of Fortunato Santini.

Contains motets f.10v, *Da pacem Domine a 6.*

B0133 Münster. Bibliothek Fortunato Santini. MS 1208. Score. First half of 19th century, in hand of Fortunato Santini.

Contains motet p.5, *Lauda Sion salvatorem a 6* [with note "ex Corsiniana e ne esiste altra copia nella Barberiana"]; p.28, *Christus resurgens a 5.*

B0134 Münster. Bibliothek Fortunato Santini. MS 1236. Score. First half of 19th century, in hand of Fortunato Santini.

Contains motet p.16, *Cum invocarem a 6;* p.26, *Ecce nunc benedicite a 6;* p.34, *Nunc dimittis a 6;* p.37, *Ave regina coelorum a 4* [attribution questioned]; hymns p.31, *Te lucis ante terminum a 4;* p.39, *Fortem virili pectore a 4* [=*Lauda mater ecclesia*].

B0135 Münster. Bibliothek Fortunato Santini. MS 1244. Score. First half of 19th century, in hand of Fortunato Santini.

Contains motet p.50, *Christus factus est a 4.*

B0136 Münster. Bibliothek Fortunato Santini. MS 2332. Score. First half of 19th

century, in hand of Fortunato Santini.
Contains p.8, *Nunc dimittis a 4.*

B0137 Münster. Bibliothek Fortunato Santini. MS 2762. Four partbooks. 18th century.
Contains motet p.17, *Vidi acquam a 4.*

B0138 Münster. Bibliothek Fortunato Santini. MS 2932. Score. First half of 19th century, in hand of Fortunato Santini.
Contains motets f.1v, *Cantabant sancti a 4*; f.4, *Domine secundum actum a 4;* f.6, *Deus qui animae a 4;* f.8, *Ecce nunc benedicite a 4*; f.10v, *Gaude Barbara a 4*; f.13, *Innocentes pro Christe a 4;* f.15, *Princeps gloriosissime a 4;* f.16v, *Veni sancte Spiritus a 8;* f.21, *Haec dies a 8.*

B0139 Münster. Bibliothek Fortunato Santini. MS 4283. Score. First half of 19th century, in hand of Fortunato Santini.
Contains motets f.47v, *O salutaris Hostia a 4;* f.77, *Inter vestibulum a 4;* f.114v, *Ascendens Christus a 4;* f.126v, *Vidi acquam a 4*; hymns f.49v, *Gloria laus a 4* [Hab. XXXI]; f.166v, *Tantum ergo a 4.*

B0140 New Haven. Yale University, Music Library. Miscellaneous MS 170, Filmer 1/a–e (olim Beinecke Library for Rare Books and Manuscripts, MA21/F48/A11) ("Filmer Partbooks"). Five partbooks. Dated ca. 1588–1603. Copied in England.
Contains one work by Palestrina.

B0141 New York. The Hispanic Society Library. MS **HC 392/278. Choirbook. Early 17th century. Copied at the Escorial.
Contains motet f.3, *Pueri Hebraeorum a 4.*

B0142 New York. The Hispanic Society Library. MS **HC380/861. Choirbook. Early 17th century. Copied at the Escorial.
Contains masses f.51, *Missa Iste confessor a* 4; f.66, *Missa Ut re mi fa sol la a* 6; f.85, *"Missa Pasce la giona mia"* [*sic*; recte *Missa Nasce la gioia mia a 6*].

B0143 New York. The Hispanic Society Library. MS **HC380/871. Choirbook. Early 17th century. Copied at the Escorial.
Contains f.1, *Missa Ut re mi fa sol la a 6.*

B0144 New York. Public Library, Music Division. MSS Mus. Res. Drexel 4180–4185. Six partbooks. First half of 17th century. Probably western England provenance.
Contains madrigals: *Vergine bella* à 5, *Vergine saggia* à 5, *Vergine pura* à 5, *Vergine santa* à 5, *Vergine sol'al monio* à 5, *Vergine chiara* à 5, *Vergine quanti* [*lagrime*] à 5.

B0145 Oporto. Biblioteca Publica Municipale. MS Musical 40 [olim 1609]. Choir-

book. Second half of 16th century. Provenance Portugal. 358ff.
Reported to contain one work by Palestrina.

B0146 Oxford. Bodleian Library. MSS Tenbury 340. Volume of lute tablature. Dated circa 1600.
Contains motet no.4, *Dum complerentur a 6* (f.6v).

B0147 Oxford. Bodleian Library. MSS Tenbury 349–353. Five partbooks. Early 17th century. English provenance.
Reported to contain three works by Palestrina; titles ascribed but not authors.

B0148 Oxford. Bodleian Library. MSS Tenbury 359–363. Five partbooks. Early 17th century. English provenance.
Reported to contain two works by Palestrina, of which one is no.52, *Pacem relinquo* (f.47v).

B0149 Oxford. Bodleian Library. MSS Tenbury 374–378. Five partbooks. Early 17th century. English provenance.
Reported to contain six works by Palestrina, of which one is *Pacem relinquo* (f.16v).

B0150 Oxford. Bodleian Library. MSS Tenbury Tenbury 385–388. Four partbooks of an original five. Late 16th century.
Contains f.26v, *Sancta et immaculata*; f.27v, *O beata et benedicta*; f.28v [secunda pars], *O vera summa.*

B0151 Oxford. Christ Church Library. MS 8. Score. 17th century.
Contains *Madrigali spirituali a 5* (1594) in score; first work is texted, the rest are without text.

B0152 Oxford. Christ Church Library. MSS Mus.10. Score. Late 17th century, in hands of William Husbands and Henry Aldrich.
Contains *Liber quintus motettum* (complete, in Husbands's hand).

B0153 Oxford. Christ Church Library. MSS Mus. 16. Score. Dated to 1670s, in hand of Henry Aldrich [contains Aldrich reworkings/recompositions based on Palestrina].
Contains no.22, "Hold not thy tongue" [*Nativitas tua*] (p.103); no.24, "O God the king of glory" [*O rex gloriae*] (p.107); no.25, "Hold not thy tongue" [second version based on *Nativitas tua*] (p.109); no.26, "We have heard with our ears" [*Doctor bonus*] (p.112); no.27, "Why art thou so vexed" [*Ave Maria*] (p.115); no.28, "The eye of the Lord" [*Jesus junxit se*] (p.118); no.29, "My heart is fixed" [*Nos autem gloriari*] (p.121); no.30, "The eye of the Lord" [second version based on *Jesus junxit se*] (p.123).

B0154 Oxford. Christ Church Library. MSS Mus. 48. Score. Late 17th century [Aldrich-Palestrina attributions].

Contains "O Lord God of our salvation" [attributed to Palestrina in London, British Library, MS Add. 31399]; "Be thou exalted" [attributed to Palestrina by John Gostling in Newberry Library Case MS 7A/2].

B0155 Oxford. Christ Church Library. MSS Mus. 521–524. Partbooks, late 17th century.

Contains motets *Liber primus motettum* (complete); "O God the King of Glory" [Palestrina-Aldrich, based on *O rex gloriae a 4*]; "Why art thou so vexed" [Palestrina-Aldrich, based on *Ave Maria a 4*].

B0156 Oxford. Christ Church Library. MS Mus.1142B. Guardbook of miscellaneous items. Late 17th century.

Contains f.59, "Hold not thy tongue" [short score of second version based on *Nativitas tua*].

B0157 Oxford. Christ Church Library. MSS 1220–1224. Five partbooks. Dated 1643–1644, with later additions. Provenance Oxford [Palestrina-Aldrich recompositions].

Contains "O God the King of Glory" [*O rex gloriae a 4*]; "Why art thou so vexed" [*Ave Maria a 4*].

B0158 Oxford. Christ Church Library. MS Mus. 1230. Book of organ music. Dated probably ca. 1710–1718, in hand of Richard Goodson senior [Palestrina-Aldrich recompositions].

Contains "Hold not thy tongue" [*Nativitas tua a 4*]; "Behold now praise the Lord" [*a 5,* uncertain attribution or source]; "My heart is fixed" [*Nos autem gloriari a 4*]; "O Lord God of my salvation" [uncertain source]; "The eye of the Lord" [*Jesus junxit se a 4*]; "We have heard with our ears" [*Doctor bonus a 4*]; "Why art thou so vexed" [*Ave Maria a 4*].

B0159 Paris. Bibliothèque nationale. Département de la Musique. Fonds du Conservatoire. MS Res. Vma. 851 ("Bourdeney Manuscript"). Dated to late 16th century. Copied in Parma or Ravenna. i + 290 + i ff. [motets probably copied from *Motecta festorum, Liber I, Liber III*; Masses from *Liber I* and *III*].

Contains masses *Missa Virtute magna a 4; Missa Ecce sacerdos magnus a 4; Missa O regem coeli a 4; Missa Gabriel Archangelus a 4; Missa Ad cenam Agni providi a 4; Missa Spem in alium a 4; Missa Primi toni [super Io son giovenetta] a 4; Missa Brevis a 4; Missa De feria a 4; Missa L'homme armé a 5; Missa Repleatur os meum a 5; Missa De beata Virgine a 6; Missa Ut re mi fa sol la a 6*; motets *Dies sanctificatus a 4; Lapidabant Stephanum a 4; Valde honorandus est a 4; Magnum haereditatis a 4; Tribus miraculis a 4; Hodie beata Virgo a 4; Ave Maria gratia a 4; Jesus iunxit se discipulis a 4; O rex gloriae a 4; Loquebantur variis linguis a 4; Benedicta sit sancta Trinitas a 4; Lauda Sion a 4; Fuit homo missus a 4; Tu es pastor ovium a 4; Magnus Sanctus Paulus a 4; Surge propera amica a 4; In diebus illis a 4; Beatus Laurentius a 4; Quae est ista a 4; Misso Herodes a 4; Nativitas tua a 4; Nos autem gloriari a 4; Salvator mundi a 4; O quantus luctus a 4; Congratulamini a 4; Dum aurora finem daret a 4; Doctor bonus a 4; Quam pul-*

chri sunt a 4; Isti sunt viri a 4; Hic est vere martir a 4; Tollite iugum meum a 4; Gaudent in celis a 4; Iste est qui ante Deum a 4; Beatus vir qui suffert a 4; Veni sponsa Christi a 4; Exaudi Domine a 4; Pater noster a 5; Ave Maria a 5; Tribularer si nescirem a 6; Accepit Jesus calicem a 6; Sicut lilium a 5; Introduxit me rex a 5 [incomplete]; madrigals *Io son ferito ahi lasso a 5; Vestiva i colli a 5* [seconda parte *Così le chiome mie*]; *Io felice sarei a 5*; *O bella Ninfa mia a 5.*

B0160 Pelplin. Biblioteka Seminarium. MSS 304–308, 308a [or 382–386, 386a]. Volumes (six in all) in "new" German organ tabulature. Dated ca. 1620–1630.

Contains no.314, *Quanti mercenarii a 5*; no.396, *Domine in virtute tua a 5.*

B0161 Pistoia. Archivio Capitolare. Ms.mus. B.21, N.6. Partbooks (incomplete). Dated 16th to 17th century.

Contains (no.6) incomplete part material for a mass *Sine nomine* in sixteen parts/four choirs "del Palestina." Attribution doubtful.

B0162 Plasencia. Archivio del Cathedrale. MS 3. Choirbook. 17th century.

Contains motets no.1, *Asperges me a 4;* no.2, *Vidi acquam a 4;* masses no.3, *Missa Brevis a 4;* no.4, *Missa Iste Confessor a 4;* no.5, *Missa Sexti toni a 4;* no.6, *Missa Aeterna Christi munera a 4*; no.7, *Missa Emendemus in melius a 4.*

B0163 Puebla (Mexico). Archivo de Musica Sacra de la Catedral. MS I. Choirbook. Second half of 17th century. Provenance Puebla.124 ff.

Reported to contain one work by Palestrina (liturgical music).

B0164 Puebla (Mexico). Archivo de Musica Sacra de la Catedral. MS10. Choirbook. Early 17th century.

Contains masses f.10, *Missa brevis a 4*; f.32v, *Missa Iste Confessor a 4*; f.75v, *Missa Aeterna Christi munera a 4*; f.97v, *Missa Emendemus a 4*; motet f.1v, *Aspersorium per annum a 4.*

B0165 Puebla (Mexico). Archivo de Musica Sacra de la Catedral. MS13. Choirbook. Early 17th century.

Contains masses f.2v, *Missa Sine nomine a 6*; f.20v, *Missa Nasce la gioia mia a 6*; f.37v, *Missa Nigra sum a 5*; f.55v, *Missa Sicut lilium inter spinas a 5*; f.72v, *Missa Aeterna Christi munera a 4*; f.82v, *Missa Iste Confessor a 4*; f.92v, *Missa Jam Christus astra ascenderat a 4*; f.106v, *Missa Panis quem ego dabo a 4.*

B0166 Puebla (Mexico). Archivo de Musica Sacra de la Catedral. MS20. Choirbook. Early 17th century.

Contains masses f.10v, *Missa Quem dicunt homines a 4*; f.28, *Missa Dum esset Summus Pontifex a 4*; f.41v, *Missa O admirabile commercium a 5*; f.60v, *Missa Memor esto a 5*; f.79v, *Missa Dum complerentur a 6*; f.106v, *Missa Sacerdotes Domini a 6.*

B0167 Regensburg. Bischöfliche Zentralbibliothek. MS A.R. 728–732. Five partbooks. First quarter of 17th century. Provenance German.
Contains motet no.119, *Justorum animae a 5.*

B0168 Regensburg. Bischöfliche Zentralbibliothek. MS A.R. 775–777. Six partbooks. Dated 1579. Provenance South German or Austrian.
Contains motet no.98, *Laudate Dominum in sanctis eius a 8* [attribution questioned].

B0169 Regensburg. Bischöfliche Zentralbibliothek. MS A.R. 942–946. Six partbooks. Dated 1609–1610. Provenance Regensburg.
Contains motet no.78, *O admirabile commercium a 5.*

B0170 Regensburg. Bischöfliche Zentralbibliothek. MS A.R. 985–986. Two partbooks of an original six. Dated ca. 1602. Provenance Regensburg [possibly transcribed from RISM 1585^1 (ed. Lindner)].
Contains motets no.14, *O magnum mysterium a 6* [secunda pars *Quem vidistis pastores*]; no.21, *O admirabile commercium a 5.*

B0171 Regensburg. Bischöfliche Zentralbibliothek. MS A.R. 1011–1017. Seven partbooks of an original eight. Dated ca. 1610. Provenance possibly Neuburg or Augsburg.
Contains motets no.18, *Justorum animae a 5;* no.29, *Haec dies quam fecit Dominus a 6;* no.32. *Hodie Christus natus est a 8;* no.125, *O admirabile commercium a 5.*

B0172 Regensburg. Bischöfliche Zentralbibliothek, MS B. 205–210. Five partbooks of an original eight. Beginning of 17th century. Provenance Augsburg.
Contains motets no.48, *Hodie Christus natus est a 8;* no.55, *Surge illuminare Hierusalem a 8;* no.59, *Jubilate Deo omnis terra a 8.*

B0173 Regensburg. Bischöfliche Zentralbibliothek, MS B. 268–270. Two partbooks of an original eight. Beginning of 17th century. Provenance Augsburg.
Contains motets no.25, *Surge illuminare a 8;* no.62, *Veni sancte spiritus a 8.*

B0174 Regensburg. Bischöfliche Zentralbibliothek, MS B. 271–274. Three partbooks of an original six. Beginning of 17th century. Provenance Augsburg.
Contains motets no.90, *Exultate Deo a 5;* no.91, *Exi cito in plateas a 5;* no.92, *Justorum animae a 5;* no.95, *Ad te levavi animam meam a 5.*

B0175 Regensburg. Bischöfliche Zentralbibliothek, MS B.H. 6002 (olim C. II). Choirbook. 16th to 17th century. Provenance Church of San Spirito in Sassia, Rome.
Contains f.2v, *Veni Domine a 6;* f.31v, *Missa Emendemus in melius a 4;* f.55v, *Missa In illo tempore a 4;* f.71v, *Missa Già fu chi m'ebbe cara a 4;* f.84v, *Missa Sanctorum meritis a 4*; f.100v, *Missa Veni sponsa Christi a 4;* f.112v, *Thomas unus a 4;* f.116v, *O magnum mysterium a 6;* f.118v, *Missa Ut re mi fa sol la a 6*; f.158v, *Lauda Sion a 4.*

B0176 Regensburg. Bischöfliche Zentralbibliothek, MS B.H. 6004 (olim C. IV). Choirbook. Dated ca. 1700. Provenance Church of San Spirito in Sassia, Rome.

Contains motets p.90, *Sicut lilium a 5* [secunda pars *Quam pulchri sunt*]; p.134, *Hic est discipulus ille a 5.*

B0177 Regensburg. Bischöfliche Zentralbibliothek, MS B.H. 6005 (olim C.V.) Choirbook. End of 17th century. Provenance Church of San Spirito in Sassia, Rome.

Contains motet p.20, *Victimae paschali a 4 et 8.*

B0178 Regensburg. Bischöfliche Zentralbibliothek. MS B.H. 6007 (olim C.VII). Choirbook. Dated 1625, copied by Paolo Troiano. Provenance Church of San Spirito in Sassia, Rome.

Contains offertory motets f.2v, *Deus tu conversus a 5;* f.4v, *Benedixisti Domine a 5;* f.6v, *Ave Maria a 5; Ad te levavi a 5;* f.8v, *Tui sunt coeli a 5;* f.10v, *Elegerunt Apostoli a 5;* f.12v, *Justus ut palma a 5;* f.14v, *Anima nostra a 5;* f.17v, *Posuisti Domine a 5;* f.18v, *Deus enim firmavit a 5;* f.20v, *Inveni David a 5;* f.22v, *Reges Tharsis a 5;* f.24v, *Jubilate Deo omnis terra a 5;* f.26v, *Jubilate Deo universa a 5;* f.28v, *Dextera Domini a 5;* f.30v, *Bonum est confiteri a 5;* f.32v, *Perfice gressus a 5;* f.34v, *Benedictus es a 5*; f.36v, *Scapulis suis a 5;* f.38v, *Meditabor in mandatis a 5;* f.40v, *Justitiae Domini rectae a 5;* f.42v, *Laudate Dominum quia a 5;* f.44v, *Confitebor tibi Domine a 5;* f.46v, *Improperium exspectavit a 5;* f.48v, *Terra tremuit a 5*

B0179 Regensburg. Bischöfliche Zentralbibliothek. MS B.H. 6008 (olim C.VIII). n.d.

Contains motet f.20v, *Lauda Sion salvatorem a 4;* f.47v, *Peccantem me quotidie a 5*

B0180 Regensburg. Bischöfliche Zentralbibliothek. MS C. 119. Volume of organ tablature. Dated 1590–1593. Provenance possibly Gmunden. 188ff.

Contains motet no.98, *Susanna ab improbis senibus a 6* [secunda pars *Postquam autem*].

B0181 Regensburg. Bischöfliche Zentralbibliothek. MS AN 1. Five partbooks of an original six. Dated 1607. Provenance possibly Regensburg.

Contains motets no.6, *O magnum mysterium a 6;* no.43, *O admirabilis commercium a 5.*

B0182 Rome. Archivio della Congregazione dell'Oratorio dei Padri Filippini. Ms. I, II, III. Probably early 17th century.

Contains *Missa Papae Marcelli a 12* [arranged probably by Stefano Nascimbeni].

B0183 Rome. Archivio del Pio Sodalizio dei Piceni. Miscellaneous items, no shelf number known. Provenance S. Maria di Loreto di Marchegiani, Rome. n.d.

Contains motet *Domine quando veneris a 4* [see Lepanto de Angelis *NdA* 1939, item E0171].

B0184 Rome. Biblioteca Casanatense, MS 2564 (olim O. II.184). Score. Early 19th century, partially transcribed by Giuseppe Baini.

Contains motets in section 17, *Lumen ad revelationem gentium a 4 et 5.*

B0185 Rome. Biblioteca Casanatense. MS 2748 (olim O. III.48). Score. End of 17th century. Provenance Bernardo Pasquini, later Giuseppe Baini.

Contains masses no.1, *Missa De beata Virgine a 4;* no.2, *Missa Ad fugam a 4;* no.3, *Missa Ad coenam Agni providi a 5;* no.4, *Missa Papae Marcelli a 6.*

B0186 Rome. Biblioteca Casanatense. MS 2760 (olim O. IV.174). Score. First half of 19th century [formerly belonging to Giuseppe Baini, containing in part otherwise unknown or dubiously attributed works].

Contains motets p.12, *Stabat Mater a 8;* p.70, *Veni sancte Spiritus a 4;* p.97, *Magnus sanctus Paulus a 4;* p.99, *Gaudent in coelis a 4;* p.101, *Valde honorandus est a 4;* p.103, *Nos autem gloriari oportet a 4;* p.111, *O Domine Jesu a 4;* p.113, *Adoramus te Christe a 4;* p.119, *Popule meus a 4* [two choirs]; p.134, *Asperges me a 4*; magnificat p.122 *Magnificat a 8* [tone 1].

B0187 Rome. Biblioteca Casanatense 2852 (olim O. II.196). Score in quarto notebook. Early 19th century [formerly belonging to Giuseppe Baini, made with reference to sources apparently derived in part from the archive of the Cappella Giulia and which, though known to Haberl, are now thought to be lost].

Contains *Missa Papae Marcelli a 6* [*Agnus Dei II* only]; motets *Alma redemptoris mater a 8; Ave regina coelorum a 8; Fratres ego enim accepi a 8; Haec dies a 8; Hic est panis a 8; Jesus junxit se a 8; Lauda Sion salvatorem a 8; Miserere mei a 12; Regina coeli a 4; Stabat Mater a 8; Sub tuum praesidium a 8; Tria sunt munera a 8; Tu es pastor ovium a 5; Veni sancte Spiritus a 8; Venite exultemus a 8; Victimae paschali a 8;* hymns *O gloriosa Domina a 4 et 12.*

B0188 Rome. Biblioteca Corsiniana. Ms. M 14 (olim 2490). Score. Dated ca. 1600.

Contains 8 *Ricercari* [questionable attribution although usually accepted in practice as by Palestrina].

B0189 Rome. Biblioteca Musicale Governativa del Conservatorio di Musica Santa Cecilia. MS G.389. Score. Copied 1617. Provenance Rome [once owned by Alexander Nison, organist of Santa Maria sopra Minerva, Rome].

Contains motets f.1, *Congratulamini mihi a 6* [unicum]; f.33v, *Surgam et circuibo a 5;* f.37, *Vulnerasti cor meum soror mea a 5;* f.46, *Ego rogabo patrem a 5*; f.49v, *Homo quidam fecit a 5.*

B0190 Rome. Biblioteca Musicale Governativa del Conservatorio di Musica Santa Cecilia, MSS G.792–795 [formerly Riserva B. I. I] [read in conjunction with Biblioteca Nazionale mss 117–121, cited below]. Four partbooks of original twelve. Dated ca. 1590–1620, copied probably in Rome. Provenance Chiesa Nuova, Rome.

Contains motets no.2, *Assumpta est Maria a 6*; no.6, *Sacerdotes Domini a 5;* no.13, *O admirabile commercium a 5;* no.14, *Crucem sanctam a 5;* no.43, *Derelinquat impius a 6;* no.44, *O bone Jesu a 6;* no.45, *O bone Jesu a*

6; no.47, *Vidi turbam magnam a 6* [ascribed to Vincenzo Ruffo]; no.49, *Salve regina mater misericordiae a 6;* no.71, *O pretiosum et admirabile convivium a 8;* no.75, *Magna est gloria a 8;* no.77, *Surge illuminare a 8;* no.78, *Ave regina coelorum a 8;* no.82, *Laudate Dominum omnes gentes a 8;* no.88, *O admirabile commercium a 8;* no.89, *Videntes stellam Magi a 8;* no.98, *O Domine Jesu a 8;* no.103, *Laudate Dominum in tympanis a 12;* no.104, *Ecce nunc benedicite a 12;* no.115, *Stabat Mater a 12* [ascribed to F. Anerio]; no.116, *Nunc dimittis a 12.*

B0191 Rome. Biblioteca Musicale Governativa del Conservatorio di Musica Santa Cecilia MSS 796–805 (olim 761–770). Ten partbooks (two exemplars of each voice part). Dated ca. 1580. Provenance Church of San Spirito in Sassia, Rome.

Contains motets p.1, *Coenantibus illis a 5;* p.7, *Misit me vivens Pater a 5;* p.12, *Ascendo ad Patrem a 5*; p.14, *Confirma hoc a 5;* p.15, *Benedicite gentes a 5*; p.16, *Tu es Petrus a 5;* p.17, *Domine Pater a 5* [Silla Pierluigi]; p.18, *O sapientia a 5;* p.20, *Confitebuntur coeli a 5*; p.26, *Corona aurea a 5.*

B0192 Rome. Biblioteca Musicale Governativa del Conservatorio di Musica Santa Cecilia. MS 1147. Choirbook. Late 17th century. Provenance possibly San Giovanni in Laterano.

Contains mass p.185, *Missa Già fu chi m'ebbe cara a 4*; magnificat p.211, *Magnificat a 4* [tone 6, Hab. XXVII.26]; p.225, *Magnificat a 4* [tone 4, Hab. XXVII.15].

B0193 Rome. Biblioteca Musicale Governativa del Conservatorio di Musica Santa Cecilia. Riserva B. I. I. Single-sheet parts on leaves. Provenance unknown [believed to be in Palestrina's autograph]. Late 16th century.

Contains motets *Beata es a 8; Omnis pulchritudo Domine a 8.*

B0194 Rome. Biblioteca Nazionale Centrale Vittorio Emanuele II. MSS Musicali 77–88. Twelve partbooks. Copied 16th and 17th centuries in various hands. Provenance Chiesa Nuova, Rome.

Contains motets p.3v, *Laudate Dominum omnes gentes a 8;* p.8, *Beati omnes a 12*; p.9v, *O Domine Jesu a 6;* p.10, *O bone Jesu a 6;* p.17, *Ad te levavi a 12;* p.22v, *Salve Regina a 4/8/12;* f.25v, *Regina coeli a 4.*

B0195 Rome. Biblioteca Nazionale Centrale Vittorio Emanuele II. MSS Musicali 117–121 Five partbooks of original twelve. Dated ca. 1590–1620. Provenance probably Rome [the Rome Santa Cecilia mss 792–795 are four more from the same original set; the B1, Q, S books have been missing since 1958. A transcription of the entire set was made by Fortunato Santini in 1821 and is preserved in Münster].

Contains motets no.2, *Assumpta est Maria a 6*; no.6, *Sacerdotes Domini a 5;* no.13, *O admirabile commercium a 5;* no.14, *Crucem sanctam a 5;* no.43, *Derelinquat impius a 6;* no.44, *O bone Jesu a 6;* no.45, *O bone Jesu a 6;* no.47, *Vidi turbam magnam a 6* [ascribed to Vincenzo Ruffo]; no.49, *Salve regina mater misericordiae a 6;* no.71, *O pretiosum et admirabile con-*

vivium a 8; no.75, *Magna est gloria a 8;* no.77, *Surge illuminare a 8;* no.78, *Ave regina coelorum a 8;* no.82, *Laudate Dominum omnes gentes a 8;* no.88, *O admirabile commercium a 8;* no.89, *Videntes stellam Magi a 8;* no.98, *O Domine Jesu a 8;* no.103, *Laudate Dominum in tympanis a 12;* no.104, *Ecce nunc benedicite a 12;* no.115, *Stabat Mater a 12* [ascribed to F. Anerio]; no.116, *Nunc dimittis a 12.*

B0196 Rome. San Giovanni in Laterano. Archivio Musicale. MS 48. Choirbook. Late 16th century.

Contains *Missa Sacerdotes et pontifex a 5.*

B0197 Rome. San Giovanni in Laterano. Archivio Musicale MS 55. Choirbook. Dated 1607.

Contains *Missa Assumpta est Maria a 6.*

B0198 Rome. San Giovanni in Laterano. Archivio Musicale. MS 56. Choirbook. 16th century.

Contains 8 *Magnificat* [beginning with even-numbered *Et exultavit* verse: no.1, tone 1 *a 5*; no.2, tone 2 *a 5*; no.3, tone 3 *a 6*; no.4, tone 4 *a 6*; no.5, tone 5 *a 5*; no.6, tone 6 *a 6*; no.7, tone 7 *a 5*; no.8, tone 8 *a 6*].

B0199 Rome. San Giovanni in Laterano. Archivio Musicale. MS 58. Choirbook. 16th century.

Contains Lamentations f.45v, *Aleph. Quomodo obscuratum a 4*; f.54v, *Recordare a 6*; f.62, *Jod. Manum suam a 6*; f.67, *Heth. Peccatum peccavit a 5.* [Works attributed to Francesco Soriano in MS but, according to Jeppesen, undoubtedly by Palestrina].

B0200 Rome. San Giovanni in Laterano. Archivio Musicale MS 59. Small choirbook. Second half of 16th century [Contains material in Palestrina's autograph.]

Contains motets f.1, *Miserere mei a 5;* f.26v, *Ecce nunc benedicite a 4 et 5;* f.27v, *Nunc dimittis a 4 et 5;* f.59v, *Lucis creator optime a 4;* f.65v, *Coeli Deus sanctissime a 4;* f.67v, *Magnae Deus a 4;* f.71v, *O lux beata Trinitas a 4;* f.90v, *Hodie Christus natus est a 4;* f.89v, *Popule meus a 4* [two choirs]; f.92v, *Libera me a 3 et 4*; f.94v, *Benedictus Dominus a 4*; hymns f.6v, *Aurea luce et decore a 4;* f.7v, *Lauda mater ecclesia a 4;* f.8v, *Petrus beatus a 4;* f.8v, *Quicumque Christum quaeritis a 4;* f.9v, *Tibi Christe splendor a 4* [strophes 1 and 3]; f.10v, *Christe redemptor omnium a 4;* f.11v, *Exultet coelum a 4* [Hab.VIII]; f.13v, *Deus tuorum militum a 4;* f.14v, *Sanctorum meritis a 4;* f.15v, *Iste Confessor a 4;* f.16v, *Jesu corona virginum a 4* [Hab.VIII.123]; f.17v, *Huius obtentu a 4;* f.17v, *Urbs beata Jerusalem a 4;* f.19v, *Rex gloriose martyrum a 4;* f.20v, *Jesu corona virginum a 4* [Hab.VIII.127]; f.21v, *Vexilla regis a 4* [Hab.VIII.70]; f.22v, *Tibi Christe splendor a 4;* f.45v, *Creator alme siderum a 4;* f.46v, *Conditor alme siderum a 4* [strophes 2, 4]; f.49v, *Christe redemptor omnium a 4* [strophe 2, *a 4;* strophe 4, *a 3;* strophe 6, *a 5*]; f.53v, *A solis ortus cardine a 4;* f.55v, *Salvete flos a 4;* f.56v, *Hostes Herodes impie a 4* [strophes 2 and 4, Casimiri, *Codice*

59, 21]; f.61v, *Immense coeli conditor a 4;* f.62v, *Tristes erant Apostoli a 4;* f.63v, *Telluris ingens a 4;* f.68v, *Deus tuorum militum a 4;* f.69v, *Plasmator hominis a 4;* f.72v, *Audi benigne a 4;* f.73v, *Ad preces nostras a 4;* f.75v, *Vexilla regis a 4* [Hab.VIII.35]; f.80v, *Ad coenam agni a 4;* f.82v, *Jesu nostra redemptio a 4;* f.84v, *Veni creator a 4* [Hab.VIII]; f.86v, *Pange lingua a 4* [Hab.VIII]; f.87v, *Doctor egregie a 4;* f.87v, *Quodcunque vinclis a 4;* f.91v, *Ut queant laxis a 4;* f.97v, *Ave maris stella a 4*; magnificat f.77v, *Magnificat* [tone 4 *a 4*, Hab. XXVII.244]; lamentations f.1, *Heth. Misericordiae a 4*; f.1v, *Aleph. Quomodo sedet a 4*; f.2v, *Heth. Peccatum peccavit a 4*; f.3v, *Heth. Cogitavit a 4*; f.5v, *Heth. Misericordiae a 4*; f.5v, *Pars mea a 4*; f.23v, *Recordare a 6*; f.28v, *Aleph. Quomodo sedet a 4*; f.29v, *Vau. Et egressus a 4*; f.31v, *Jod. Manum suam a 5*; f.33v, *Lamed. Matribus a 4*; f.34v, *Heth. Cogitavit a 4*; f.34v, *Theth a 4*; f.37v, *Aleph. Ego vir a 5*; f.39v, *Aleph. Quomodo obscuratum a 5*; f.42v, *Recordare a 6.*

B0201 Rome. San Giovanni in Laterano. Archivio Musicale. MS 61. Choirbook. Dated 1575. Provenance Rome, possibly copied by Annibale Stabile for use at S. Giovanni Laterano. i + 158ff.

Contains hymns f.136v, *Veni Creator a 4* [Hab. XXX]; f.140v, *Pange lingua a 4*; f.143v, *Tristes erant Apostoli a 5* [Hab. XXXI].

B0202 Rome. San Giovanni in Laterano. Archivio Musicale. MS 87. Choirbook. Dated ca. 1600 and early 17th century. Provenance San Giovanni in Laterano, Rome. 78ff.

Contains Lamentations [attributed to Dragoni in MS but identical to those in Spoleto 9 attributed to Palestrina]. *Feria V. in coena Domini*; *Feria VI. In Parasceve*.

B0203 Rome. San Giovanni in Laterano. Archivio Musicale. MS A52–54. Three volumes. Late 16th to early 17th century.

Contains *Missa Cantantibus organis Caecilia a 12.* [Palestrina=*Et in terra pax*].

B0204 Rome. San Giovanni in Laterano. Archivio Musicale. MS Mazzo IV. Six volumes. End of 16th century.

Contains motets no.7, *Ingrediente Domino a 4* [unique attribution]; no.9, *O bone Jesu miserere a 4*; no.10, *O Redemptor a 4;* no.11, *Salve Regina misericordiae a 4*; hymn no.5, *Gloria laus a 4* [Hab. XXXI].

B0205 Saragossa. Iglesia Metropolitana de la Virgen del Pilar. Archivo Musical. Armario B-2, MS 34. Partbook. Dated last third of 16th century (date 1570 on f.29). Provenance presumably Saragossa.

Reported to contain three works by Palestrina.

B0206 Segovia. Archivo Capitular de la Catedral. MS 1. Choirbook. Early 17th century. Provenance Segovia, copied for use by cathedral choir.

Reported to contain one work by Palestrina.

B0207 Segovia. Archivo Capitular de la Catedral. MS 2. Choirbook. Early 17th century, with additions in 1759. Provenance Segovia, copied for cathedral choir use. i + 161ff.

Reported to contain four works by Palestrina.

B0208 Spoleto. Archivio Capitolare, Cod. 9. Small choirbook. Probably compiled ca. 1564. 102ff.

Contains Lamentations *a 4* f.1v–4, 11v–15, 15v–19 [identical to those in Lateran 87 attributed to Dragoni]: f.1v, *Aleph. Quomodo sedet a 4*; f.4v, *Vau. Et egressus a 4*; f.7v, *Jod. Manum suam a 4*; f.11v, *Heth. Cogitavit a 4*; f.15v, *Lamed. Matribus a 4*; f.19v, *Aleph. Ego vir a 4*; f.23v, *Theth. Misericordiae a 4*; f.26v, *Aleph. Quomodo obscuratum a 4*; f.30v, *Recordare a 4.*

B0209 Stockholm. Kungliga Musikaliska Akademiens Biblioteket. MS Tyska Kyrkans Samling 32. Four partbooks of original six. Late 16th century (date 1595 in tenor book). Provenance, possibly copied in Stockholm.

Reported to contain one work by Palestrina.

B0210 Tarazona. Archivo Capitular de la Catedral. MS 1. Choirbook, 16th century.

Contains motets f.35v, *Dies sanctificatus a 4;* f.36v, *Lapidabant Stephanum a 4;* f.38v, *Valde honorandus est a 4;* f.40v, *Magnum haereditatis a 4;* f.42v, *Tribus miraculis a 4;* f.45v, *Hodie beata virgo a 5;* f.47v, *Ave Maria a 4*; f.49v, *Jesus junxit se a 4;* f.51v, *O rex gloriae a 4;* f.53v, *Loquebantur in variis linguis a 4;* f.56v, *Benedicta sit a 4*; f.59v, *Lauda Sion Salvatorem a 4;* f.61v, *Tu es pastor ovium a 4;* f.64v, *Magnus sanctus Paulus a 4;* f.67v, *Surge propera amica mea et veni a 4;* f.70v, *Quae est ista quae processit a 4;* f.72v, *Misso Herodes spiculatore a 4;* f.74v, *Nativitas tua Dei genetrix a 4;* f.76v, *Nos autem gloriari oportet a 4;* f.78v, *Salvator mundi a 4;* f.80v, *O quantus luctus hominum a 4;* f.82v, *Congratulamini mihi a 4*; f.84v, *Dum aurora a 4;* f.86v, *Doctor bonus et amicus Dei a 4*; f.89v, *Quam pulchri sunt a 4.*

B0211 Tarazona. Archivo Capitular de la Catedral. MS 4. Choirbook. Late 16th century. Provenance Tarazona, copied for use by cathedral choir. 151ff.

Contains mass f.118v, *Missa sine nomine a 4*; motets (all *a 4*): f.35v, *Dies sanctificatus a 4;* f.37v, *Lapidabant Stephanum a 4;* f.39v, *Valde honorandus est a 4;* f.41v, *Magnum haereditatis a 4;* f.43v, *Tribus miraculis a 4;* f.46v, *Hodie beata Virgo a 4;* f.48v, *Ave Maria a 4;* f.50v, *Jesus iunxit se a 4;* f.52v, *Rex gloriae a 4;* f.54v, *Loquebantur a 4;* f.57v, *Benedicta sit a 4;* f.60v, *Lauda Sion a 4;* f.62v, *Tu es Pastor a 4;* f.65v, *Magne Sancte Paule a 4;* f.68v, *Surge propera a 4;* f.71v, *Quae est ista a 4;* f.73v, *Misso Herodes a 4;* f.75v, *Nativitas tua a 4;* f.77v, *Nos autem gloriari a 4;* f.79v, *Salvator mundi a 4;* f.81v, *Quantum luctum a 4* [O quantus luctus]; f.83v, *Congratulamini a 4;* f.85v, *Dum aurora a 4;* f.87v, *Doctor bone a 4* [Doctor bonus];f.90v, *Quam pulchri a 4*.

B0212 Tarazona. Archivo Capitular de la Catedral. MS 7. Choirbook. Second half of 16th century. Provenance Tarazona, probably copied for use by cathedral choir. 100ff (originally 111+).

Contains hymn f.76v, *O lux et decus Hispaniae a 5.*

B0213 Tarazona, Archivo Capitular de la Catedral. MS10. Choirbook (paper). Dated 16th century. 89ff.

Contains magnificat, f.1v–41, *Magnificat a 4* [a set through the eight tones, odd-numbered verse settings only]; f.41v–89, *Magnificat a 4* [a set through the eight tones, even-numbered verse settings only].

B0214 Tarazona, Archivo Capitular de la Catedral. MS11. Choirbook (paper). 17th to 18th century. 17ff total.

Contains motet *Pulchra es amica mea a 4.*

B0215 Tarazona, Archivo Capitular de la Catedral. MS16. One partbook (cantus) of a probable original eight. Early 17th century. Provenance Tarazona, possibly copied in Tarazona by a Spanish copyist.

Contains motet *Petre amas me* [attribution to Palestrina, *unicum*, argued as genuine]; magnificat *Magnificat sexti toni* [doubtful attribution].

B0216 Trento. Collection L. Feininger. Volume of organ intabulations. Dated 17th century. Italian provenance. 97ff. [cit. Willi Apel, *Keyboard Music*, 805; identification R. Shindle].

Contains *Missa O magnum mysterium a 5* [*Kirie a 5* and *Benedictus a 3* only].

B0217 Treviso. Biblioteca Capitolare del Duomo. MS 29. Five partbooks of original six. Dated ca. 1570–1575 in Treviso for use of cathedral choir [destroyed 1944 but contents known from catalogue made by archivist Giovanni d' Alessi].

Contains motets no.27, *Tu es Petrus a 6* [secunda pars: *Quodcumque ligaveris*]; no.38, *Beatus Dei famulus a 5* [secunda pars: *Gaude tarvisina civitas*]; no.74, *O sancte praesul Nicolae a 5* [secunda pars: *Gaude praesul optime*]; no.76, *Columna es a 6*; no.82, *In medio eccelsiae a 5* [secunda pars: *Jucunditatem*]; no.84, *Silvester beatissimus a 5*; no.100, *Tradent enim vos a 5*; no.104, *Corona aurea a 5* [secunda pars: *Domine prevenisti*]; no.107, *Filiae Jerusalem a 5* [secunda pars: *Quoniam confortavit*]; no.111, *Haec est vera fraternitas a 5* [secunda pars: *Ecce quam bonus*]; no.126, *Sanctificavit Dominus a 5*; no.127, *O quam metuendus a 5*; no.128, *Inclitae sanctae virginis a 5*; no.129, *Fuit homo missus a 5* [secunda pars: *Erat Joannes*]; no.130, *O lux et decus Hispaniae a 5* [secunda pars: *O singulare praesidium*]; no.131, *Praeceptor bonum est a 5* [secunda pars: *Non enim*]; no.132, *Omnipotens sempiternae Deus a 5;* second series, no.32, *O virgo simul et mater a 5*; no.33, *Sancta et immaculata a 6* [secunda pars: *Benedicta tu*]; also contains Angelo Pierluigi, *Circuire possum a 5* [secunda pars: *In hac cruce*].

B0218 Turin. Biblioteca Nazionale Universitaria. MS Riserva musicale IV.45 (olim Regia Biblioteca dell' Università, qm VI.86). Six partbooks now bound together. Late 16th century. Provenance probably Turin, copied for use of court chapel of Carlo Emanuele I (1562–1630) of Savoy.

Reported to contain five works by Palestrina.

B0219 Valencia. Colegio y Seminario del Corpus Christi del Patriarca, Archivo. MS20. Eight partbooks. Early 17th century. Provenance Valencia.

Contains motet p.55, *Surge propera amica mea et veni a 4;* p.56, *Veni veni dilecti mi a 5.*

B0220 Valladolid. Catedral Metropolitana, Archivo de Musica. MS 17. Partbook. Dated to last third of 16th century. Provenance probably Valladolid. 136ff. of original 200.

Contains motet f.181v, *O bone Jesu a 6*; two other works.

B0221 Vatican City. Biblioteca Apostolica Vaticana. MS Barberini lat. 4184 (formerly XLVII.55). Score. 17th century. Provenance possible Spanish. 206ff.

Contains masses f.1, *Missa Laudate Dominum a 8;* f.23, *Missa Hodie Christus natus est a 8;* f.42v, *Missa Fratres ego enim accepi a 8*; f.63, *Missa Confitebor tibi Domine a 8*; motets f.106, *Pater noster a 8;* f.108, *Ave Maria a 8;* f.110, *Fratres ego enim accepi a 8;* f.113, *Expurgate vetus fermentum a 8;* f.116v, *Apparuit gratia a 8* [anonymous in source]; f.119v, *Sub tuum praesidium a 8;* f.121v, *Caro mea a 8;* [anonymous in source]; f.126v, *Ave mundi spes a 8;* f.131v, *Dies sanctificatus a 8;* f.134v, *Haec est dies praeclara a 8;* f.136v, *Disciplinam et sapientiam a 8;* f.139v, *Congratulamini mihi a 8* [anonymous in source]*;* f.141v, *Magnus sanctus Paulus a 8;* f.146v, *O quam suavis a 8;* f.148v, *Nunc dimittis a 8;* f.151v, *Omnes gentes plaudite a 8;* f.156v, *Surge illuminare Jerusalem a 8;* f.158v, *Lauda Sion a 8;* f.161, *Veni sancte Spiritus a 8;* f.164v, *Hodie Christus natus est a 8;* f.171, *Victimae paschali a 8;* f.173v, *Alma redemptoris mater a 8* [anonymous in source]; f.176, *Ave regina coelorum a 8;* f.178v, *Regina coeli a 8;* f.181v, *Salve regina a 8;* f.184v, *Confitebor tibi Domine a 8;* f.194v, *Laudate pueri a 8;* f.197v, *Domine in virtute a 8*; f.204, *Laudate Dominum omnes gentes a 8*; litanies f.87, *Litaniae sacrae eucharistiae a 8* [Hab. XXVI.125]; f.90v, *Litaniae Domini a 8* [Hab. XXVI.119]; f.94, *Litaniae Beatae Mariae Virginis a 8* [Hab. XXVI.78]; f.103, *Litaniae Beatae Mariae Virginis a 8* [Hab. XXVI.95].

B0222 Vatican City. Biblioteca Apostolica Vaticana. MS Cappella Giulia VIII.39 (olim Cod.47). Choirbook. Second half of 16th century. Provenance Rome, copied for use by Cappella Giulia. 220ff.

Contains motets f.190v, *Sancta Dei genetrix a 4*; f.191v, *Petrus apostolus a 4*; f.192v, *Da pacem Domine a 4*; magnificat f.214, *Magnificat* [tone 6 *a 4*, Hab. XXVII.251].

Note: Palestrina also added *si placet* parts to two *Magnificat* by Cristobal de Morales in this source.

B0223 Vatican City. Biblioteca Apostolica Vaticana. MS Cappella Giulia XII.6 (olim Cod.50). Choirbook. Dated 1540–1541, with additions in 1587. Provenance Rome, copied for use by Cappella Giulia. 142ff.

Contains hymns f.63v, *Monstra te esse a 4* [=*Ave maris stella a 3* by Costanzo Festa, to which Palestrina added the fourth *Si placet* part]; f.94v, *Deus tuorum militum a 4* [Hab. XXX]; f.97v, *Exultet coelis a 4 et 5* [Hab. XXX].

B0224 Vatican City. Biblioteca Apostolica Vaticana. MS Cappella Giulia XIII.16. Choir part material (with basso continuo). Dated to 17th to 18th century. 56ff.

Contains f.37, *Missa sine nomine a 4* [with basso continuo].

B0225 Vatican City. Biblioteca Apostolica Vaticana. MS Cappella Giulia XIII.17. Choir part material (with basso continuo). Dated to early 18th century.

Contains hymns no.1, *Placare Christe a 4* [=*Christe redemptor omnium a 4*]; no.2, *Veni Creator a 4* [Hab. XXX]; no.3, *Aurea luce et decore a 4;* no.4, *Tantum ergo a 4* [unicum].

B0226 Vatican City. Biblioteca Apostolica Vaticana. MS Cappella Giulia XIII.18. Scored music and parts. Dated 17th and 18th to early 19th century [apparently gatherings of Palestrina material in various hands, some of which is in autographs of Giuseppe Ottavio Pitoni and Giuseppe Baini]. 554pp.

Contains motets f.1, *Confitebor tibi Domine a 8* [secunda pars *Notas facite*]; f.49, *Accepit Jesus calicem a 6*; f.73, *Tu es Petrus a 6* [with basso continuo]; f.223, *Tu es Petrus a 6* [with basso continuo]; f.269, *Domine Jesus in qua nocte a 5*; f.291, *Caro mea vere a 5*; f.312, *Ego sum panis vivus a 5* [secunda pars *Panis quem ego dabo*]; f.357, *O sacrum convivium a 5*; f.279, *Sicut cervus a 4*; f.398, *Coenantibus illis a 5*; f.422, *Domine quando veneris a 4* [with basso continuo]; f.465, *Peccavimus a 5*; f.487, *Fratres ego enim accepi a 8*; f.497, *Fratres ego enim a 8* [=f.487; this layer contains scorings of several motets by Baini].

B0227 Vatican City. Biblioteca Apostolica Vaticana. MS Cappella Giulia XIII.19. Twenty-one parts including some copies. 17th to early 18th century. 128ff. [Cantus III is headed "Palestrina."]

Contains *Missa Tu es Petrus a 18* [eighteen parts in three choirs, with basso continuo].

B0228 Vatican City. Biblioteca Apostolica Vaticana. MS Cappella Giulia XIII.20. Scored music and parts. Dated 17th to 18th century. Provenance Rome [much of this material is in the autograph of Giuseppe Ottavio Pitoni]. 158ff.

Contains offertory motets f.1, *Justus ut palma a 5*; f.7, *Confessio et pulchritudo a 5*; f.13, *Hodie beata virgo Maria a 4*; f.35, *Confitebor tibi Domine a 5*; f.47, *Improperium expectavit a 5*; f.59, *Dextera Domine a 5*; f.78, *Constitues eos a 5* [with basso continuo]; f.90, *Inveni David a 5* [with basso continuo]; f.99, *O angelorum principes a 6*; f.107, *Justus ut palma a 5* [with basso continuo]; f.114, *Posuisti Domine a 5*; f.120, *Veritas mea a 5* [with basso continuo]; f.140, *Stetit angelus a 5* [with basso continuo]; f.147, *Tui sunt coeli a 5*; f.153, *Lauda Sion salvatorem a 8*.

B0229 Vatican City. Biblioteca Apostolica Vaticana. MS Cappella Giulia XIII.21. Sixteen partbooks bound in parchment. Dated 1708–1718. Copied by Corradini. 28ff.

Contains motets f.3v, *Pueri Hebraeorum a 4;* f.4, *Gloria laus a 4* [Hab. XXX]; f.8r–v, *O Redemptor a 4;* f.8r–v, *Sicut cervus a 4* [secunda pars *Sitivit anima mea*]; hymns f.5–5v, *Vexilla regis a 4* [Hab. XXX]; f.5v–7, *Pange lingua a 4* [Hab. XXX]; f.9–10v, *Veni creator spiritus a 4* [Hab. XXX].

B0230 Vatican City. Biblioteca Apostolica Vaticana. MS Cappella Giulia XIII.24 (olim Cod. 60). Eight partbooks. Second half of 16th century.

Contains motets f.3–3v, *Regina coeli a 4 in 2 cori* [secunda pars *Resurrexit a 8 in 2 cori*]; f.4–4v, *Salve regina a 8 in 2 cori;* f.4v, *Ave regina coelorum a 8;* f.5v, *Alma redemptoris mater a 8;* f.7v, *Ave mundi spes a 8;* f.8–8v, *Beata es a 8* [secunda pars *Ave Maria*]; f.9, *O quam suavis a 8;* f.9v–10, *Disciplinam et sapientiam a 8;* f.10v, *Domine quis habitabit a 12 in 3 cori;* f.11, *Laudate Dominum omnes gentes a 8;* f.12, *Tantum ergo a 4;* f.14v, *O bone Jesu a 8;* f.15, *O Domine Jesu Christe a 8;* f.17, *Nunc dimittis a 8;* f.17v, *Omnes gentes plaudite a 8;* f.18v, *Fratres ego enim accepi a 8;* f.19–19v, *Expurgate vetus fermentum a 8;* f.24, *Laudate Dominum de coelis a 8;* f.25, *Sub tuum praesidium a 8;* p.46, *Beata es a 8* [attribution in source: Ruggiero Giovanelli]; f.26v, *Pater noster a 8;* f.35–35v, *Salve regina a 4/8/12 in 3 cori;* f.36v, *Jubilate Deo omnes terra a 12* [secunda pars *Laudate nomen eius*]; f.39, *Ave Maria a 8;* f.43v, *O gloriosa Domina a 12 in 3 cori;* f.44, *O quantum bonus a 12 in 3 cori;* f.46, *Ad te levavi a 12;* f.46v, *Beati omnes qui timent a 12*; litanies f.16–16v, *Litaniae Beatae Mariae Virginis a 6* [Hab. XXVI.71]; f.21v–22, *Litaniae Domini a 4 et 8* [Hab. XXVI.102]; f.26–26v, *Litaniae Domini a 8* [Hab. XXVI.113]; f.29–29v, *Litaniae Beatae Mariae Virginis a 8* [Hab. XXVI.78]; f.38v–39, *Litaniae Beatae Mariae Virginis a 8* [Hab. XXVI.95]; f.39v–40, *Litaniae Domini a 8* [Hab. XXVI.119]; f.40r–v, *Litaniae sacrae eucharistiae a 8* [Hab. XXVI.125]; f.41v, *Litaniae sacrae eucharistiae a 8* [Hab. XXVI.133].

B0231 Vatican City. Biblioteca Apostolica Vaticana. MS Cappella Giulia XIII.25. Four partbooks. 17th century.

Contains p.49, *Magnificat a 8* [tone 1, Hab. XXVII.235].

B0232 Vatican City. Biblioteca Apostolica Vaticana. MS Cappella Giulia XIII.26. Choirbook. Late 16th century, with additions dated 1675. Provenance Vatican. 16ff.

Contains motets f.7, *Pueri Hebraeorum a 4*; f.8, *Sicut cervus a 4* [secunda pars *Sitivit anima mea*]; f.10v, *O redemptor sume carnem a 4*; hymns f.5, *Vexilla regis prodeunt a 4*; f.5v, *Veni creator spiritus a 4*; f.7v, *Gloria laus a 4*; f.11v, *Pange lingua a 4.*

B0233 Vatican City. Biblioteca Apostolica Vaticana. MS Cappella Giulia XV.15 (olim Cod.13) [exemplar of print of *Liber primus missarum* with manuscript appendix].

Appendix contains mass f.1v, *Missa pro defunctis a 5*; motet f.15v, *Libera me a 5.*

B0234 Vatican City. Biblioteca Apostolica Vaticana. MS Cappella Giulia XV.19 (olim Cod.15) Choirbook, inscribed on cover "Inni del Palestrina." Dated late 16th and early 17th centuries.

Contains hymns f.1v, *Conditor alme siderum a 4;* f.7v, *Christe redemp-*

tor omnium a 4; f.13v, *A solis ortus cardine a 4;* f.18v, *Salvete flos martyrum a 4;* f.20v, *Hostes Herodes impie a 4;* f.24v, *Lucis creator optime a 4;* f.278v, *Immense coeli conditor a 4;* f.31v, *Telluris ingens a 4;* f.34v, *Coeli Deus a 4;* f.37v, *Magnae Deus a 4;* f.40v, *Plasmator hominis a 4;* f.43v, *O lux beata Trinitas a 4;* f.46v, *Audi benigne a 4;* f.49v, *Ad preces nostras a 4;* f.54v, *Vexilla regis a 4* [Hab.VIII.35]; f.60v, *Ad coenam agni a 4;* f.65v, *Jesu nostra redemptio a 4;* f.69v, *Veni creator a 4* [Hab.VIII]; f.75v, *Pange lingua a 4* [Hab.VIII]; f.80v, *Quodcunque vinclis a 4;* f.82v, *Doctor egregie a 4;* f.84v, *Ave maris stella a 4;* f.89v, *Ut queant laxis a 4;* f.94v, *Aurea luce et decore a 4;* f.98v, *Lauda mater ecclesia a 4;* f.101v, *Petrus beatus a 4;* f.103v, *Quicumque Christum quaeritis a 4;* f.107v, *Tibi Christe splendor a 4;* f.111v, *Christe redemptor omnium a 4;* f.117v, *Exultet coelum a 4* [Hab.VIII]; f.122v, *Tristes erant Apostoli a 4;* f.125v, *Vexilla regis a 4* [Hab.VIII.70]; f.128v, *Deus tuorum militum a 4* [Hab.VIII.110]; f.131v, *Rex gloriose martyrum a 4;* f.133v, *Jesu corona virginum a 4* [Hab.VIII.127]; f.137v, *Deus tuorum militum a 4* [Hab.VIII.105]; f.142v, *Sanctorum meritis a 4;* f.145v, *Iste confessor a 4;* f.149v, *Jesu corona virginum a 4* [Hab.VIII.123]; f.152v, *Huius obtentu a 4;* f.153v, *Urbs beata Jerusalem a 4;* f.159v, *Deus tuorum militum a 4* [Hab. XXX]; f.166v, *Exultet coelis a 4 et 5* [Hab. XXX]; f.174v, *Forte virili pectore a 4* [=*Lauda mater ecclesia*]; f.178v, *Pater superni luminis a 4* [=*Lauda mater ecclesia*]; f.184v, *Laus et perennis gloria a 5* [=*Gloria tibi Domine* (Hab.VIII)].

B0235 Vatican City. Biblioteca Apostolica Vaticana. MS Cappella Giulia XV.21 (olim Cod.10). Choirbook, inscribed "Libro con le lamentatione della settimana santa del Palestrina." Second half of 16th century. 57ff.

Contains lamentations f.1v, Feria V: *Incipit lamentatio a 5*; f.7v, *Vau. Et egressus a 5;* f.14v, *Jod. Manum suam a 6;* Feria VI: f.20v, *Heth. Cogitavit a 5*; f.26v, *Lamed. Matribus suis a 5;* f.33v, *Aleph. Ego vir a 6*; Sabbato sancto f.38v, *Heth. Misericordiae a 5;* f.44v, *Aleph. Quomodo obscuratum a 5*; f.51v, *Recordare a 6.*

B0236 Vatican City. Biblioteca Apostolica Vaticana. MS Cappella Giulia XV.22 (olim Cod.16). Choirbook, entitled "Palestina con 16 Magnificat dentro." Late 16th century. 129ff.

Contains sixteen *Magnificat* [beginning even-numbered *Et exultavit* verse; f.2v, tone 1 *a 5*; f.10v, tone 2 *a 5*; f.17v, tone 3 *a 6*; f.26v, tone 4 *a 6*; f.37v, tone 5 *a 5*; f.45v, tone 6 *a 6*; f.55v, tone 7 *a 5*; f.64v, tone 8 *a 6*. Beginning odd-numbered *Anima mea* verse: f.74v, tone 1 *a 4*; f.82v, tone 2 *a 4*; f.89v, tone 3 *a 4*; f.95v, tone 4 *a 4*; f.102v, tone 5 *a 4*; f.109v, tone 6 *a 4*; f.116v, tone 7 *a 4*; f.123v, tone 8 *a 4*].

B0237 Vatican City. Biblioteca Apostolica Vaticana. MS Cappella Giulia XV.62. Nine partbooks. 17th century. 68pp [page numbers from cantus 1 partbook].

Contains motets p.62, *Ave Maria a 8;* p.65, *Sub tuum praesidium a 8*; litany p.18, *Litaniae Beatae Mariae Viriginis a 8* [Hab. XXVI.95].

B0238 Vatican City. Biblioteca Apostolica Vaticana. MS Cappella Giulia XV.66. Eight partbooks. 17th to 18th century.

Contains motets f.8, *Domine quando veneris a 4*; f.9, *Heu mihi Domine a 4.*

B0239 Vatican City. Biblioteca Apostolica Vaticana. MS Cappella Giulia XVI.15. Choirbook. Dated 1602. Provenance Rome, copied by G.A. Fanensis.

Contains f.1v, *Missa Tu es pastor ovium a 5;* f.23v, *Missa Vestiva i colli a 5;* f.50v, *Missa O admirabile commercium a 5*; f.73v, *Missa Sine nomine a 5;* f.102v, *Missa Sacerdotes Domini a 6;* f.131v, *Missa Assumpta est Maria a 6.*

B0240 Vatican City. Biblioteca Apostolica Vaticana. MS Ottoboniani lat. 3386. Choirbook. Dated 1607. Provenance Altaemps library.

Contains no.1, *Missa Assumpta est Maria a 6*; no.2, *Missa Tu es Petrus a 6;* no.3, *Missa Te Deum laudamus a 6.*

B0241 Vatican City. Biblioteca Apostolica Vaticana. MS Ottoboniani lat. 3387. Choirbook. Dated ca. 1600. Provenance Altaemps library.

Contains motet *Popule meus a 4* [two choirs]; Lamentations: no.1, *Aleph. Quomodo sedet a 5*; no.2, *Vau. Et egressus a 5*; no.3, *Jod. Manum suam a 5*; no.4, *Heth. Cogitavit a 5*; no.5, *Lamed. Matribus a 6*; no.6, *Aleph. Ego vir a 6*; no.7, *Heth. Misericordiae a 5*; no.8, *Aleph. Quomodo obscuratum a 5*; no.9, *Recordare a 6.*

B0242 Vatican City. Biblioteca Apostolica Vaticana. MS Ottoboniani lat. 3389. Choirbook. Dated ca. 1600. Provenance Altaemps library.

Contains masses no.6, *Missa Sanctorum meritis a 4;* no.8, *Missa In majorius duplicibus a 4;* no.9, *Missa In minoribus duplicibus a 4*; hymns no.1, *Immense coeli conditor a 4;* no.2, *Telluris ingens a 4;* no.3, *Coeli Deus sanctissime a 4;* no.4, *Magnae Deus a 4;* no.5, *Plasmator hominis a 4.*

B0243 Vatican City. Biblioteca Apostolica Vaticana. MS Ottoboniani lat. 3391. Choirbook. Dated ca. 1600. Provenance Altaemps library, copied by Luca Orpheo Fano.

Contains *Missa Assumpta est Maria a 6.*

B0244 Vatican City. Biblioteca Apostolica Vaticana. MS Cappella Sistina 22. Choirbook. Dated ca. 1565 and 1568. Provenance Rome, copied for use by Cappella Sistina. 144ff.

Contains f.42v, *Missa Benedicta es coelorum Regina a 6*; f.71v, *Missa Papae Marcelli a 6*; f.94v, *Missa Illumina oculos meos*.

B0245 Vatican City. Biblioteca Apostolica Vaticana. MS Cappella Sistina 29. Choirbook. Dated ca. 1590. Provenance Rome, copied for use by Cappella Sistina. i + 197ff.

Contains motets f.15v, *Ierusalem cito veniet a 6* [secunda pars *Ego enim sum Dominus*]; f.29v, *Cum autem esset Stephanus a 6* [secunda pars *Possitis autem genibus*]; f.36v, *Hic est beatissimus Evangelista a 6* [secunda pars *Hic est discipulus ille*]; f.43v, *Surge illuminare Jerusalem a 8* [secunda pars *Et ambulabunt gentes*]; f.50v, *Responsum accepit Simeon a 6* [secunda pars *Cum inducerent puerum Jesum*]; f.84v, *Surrexit pastor bonus a 8* [two choirs: secunda pars *Et enim Pascha nostrum*]; f.89v, *Iesus iunxit se discipulis a 8* [two choirs: secunda pars *Et increpavit eos*]; f.94v, *Spiritus sanctus replevit a 8;* f.98v, *Hodie gloriosa semper Virgo a 8* [secunda pars *Regina mundi*]; f.111v, *Tradent enim vos a 6*; sequence f.76v, *Stabat mater a 8*; magnificat f.165v, *Magnificat a 8* [tone 1].

B0246 Vatican City. Biblioteca Apostolica Vaticana. MS Cappella Sistina 30. Choirbook. Dated 1594. Provenance Rome. 161ff.

Contains masses f.25v, *Missa Salve Regina a 5*; f.100v, *Missa O sacrum convivium a 4*; f.135v, *Missa Ecce ego Iohannes a 6.*

B0247 Vatican City. Biblioteca Apostolica Vaticana. MS Cappella Sistina 32. Choirbook. Dated 1585. Provenance Rome. 148ff.

Contains masses f.26v, *Missa Viri Galilei a 6*; f.56v, *Missa Dum complerentur a 6*; f.88v, *Missa Aspice Domine a 5*; f.123v, *Missa Te Deum laudamus a 6.*

B0248 Vatican City. Biblioteca Apostolica Vaticana. MS Cappella Sistina 33. Choirbook. Dated 1610. Provenance Rome, copied by Orazio Griffio. 112ff.

Contains motets f.2v, *Viri Galilei a 6* [secunda pars *Ascendit Deus*]; f.11v, *Dum complerentur a 6* [secunda pars *Dum ergo essent*]; f.20v, *Veni Domine e noli tardare a 6* [secunda pars *Excita Domine*]; f.33v, *O magnum mysterium a 6* [secunda pars *Quem vidistis pastores*].

B0249 Vatican City. Biblioteca Apostolica Vaticana. MS Capppella Sistina 38. Choirbook. Dated 1563. Provenance Rome, copied by Johannes Parvus. 163ff.

Contains motets f.79v, *Beatus Laurentius a 5*; f.155v, *Estote fortes in bello a 6.*

B0250 Vatican City. Biblioteca Apostolica Vaticana. MS Cappella Sistina 39. Choirbook. Dated 1563. Provenance Rome, copied by Johannes Parvus. 131ff.

Contains mass f.59v, *Missa Ut re mi fa sol la a 6.*

B0251 Vatican City. Biblioteca Apostolica Vaticana. MS Cappella Sistina 43. Choirbook. Dated 1619. Provenance Rome, copied by Nicola de Fantis. i, ii + 161ff.

Contains offertory motets (all a 5): f.3v, *Iubilate Deo omnis terra;* f.7v, *Dextera Domini fecit virtutem;* f.11v, *Bonum est confiteri Domino;* f.15v, *Angelus Domini descendit de coelo;* f.19v, *Deus meus ad te de luce vigilio;* f.23v, *Lauda anima mea Dominum;* f.27v, *Iubilate Deo universa terra;* f.31v, *Benedicite gentes Dominum;* f.36v, *Ascendit Deus in iubilatione;* f.40v, *Confirma hoc Deus;* f.44v, *Sacerdotes Domini incensum;* f.49v, *Domine convertere;* f.53v, *Sperent in te omnes;* f.58v, *Illumina oculos meos;* f.62v, *Benedicam Dominum qui tribuit mihi;* f.66v, *Perfice gressus meos;* f.70v, *Sicut in holocaustus arietum;* f.74v, *Populem humilem;* f.78v, *Iustitiae Domini rectae;* f.82v, *Ad te levavi animam meam;* f.86v, *Exaltabo te Domine;* f.90v, *Praeca-*

tus est Moises; f.94v, *In te speravi Domine;* f.98v, *Immittit Angelus Domini;* f.102v, *Expectans expectavi Dominum;* f.106v, *Domine in auxilium meum respice;* f.110v, *Oravi ad Dominum; f.114v, Sanctificavit Moises altare Domino;* f.118v, *Si ambulavero in medio tribulationis;* f.122v, *Super flumina Babilonis;* f.126v, *Vir erat in terra Hus;* f.130v, *Recordare mei Domine;* f.134v, *De profundis clamavi;* f.139v, *Tradent enim vos in conciliis;* f.144v, *Corona aurea super caput eius;* f.148v, *Iustorum animae in manu Dei sunt;* f.152v, *Veritas mea et misericordia mea;* f.156v, *Afferentur Regi virgines.*

B0252 Vatican City. Biblioteca Apostolica Vaticana. MS Cappella Sistina 47. Choirbook. Dated 1616 [some material recopied 1704; manscript restored 1724]. Provenance Rome, copied by Domenico Brancadore. 165ff.

Contains masses f.4v, *Missa* [*sine nomine*] *a 4* (doubtful attribution?); f.26v, *Missa Lauda Sion salvatorem a 4;* f.46v, *Missa O admirabile commercium a 5*; f.80v, *Missa Memor esto a 5* [recopied in 1708]; f.107v, *Missa O virgo simul et mater a 5* [recopied 1708]; f.134v, *Missa Octavi toni a 6* [*lacks Agnus Dei II*].

B0253 Vatican City. Biblioteca Apostolica Vaticana. MS Cappella Sistina 52. Choirbook. Dated 1612 and 1613. Provenance Rome, copied by Ippolito Fersini. i + 99ff.

Contains masses f.1v, *Missa Sacerdos et pontifex a 5;* f.37v, *Missa Ascendo ad Patrem a 5*; f.67v, *Missa Tu es Petrus a 6.*

B0254 Vatican City. Biblioteca Apostolica Vaticana. MS Cappella Sistina 54. Choirbook conflated from various fascicles. 16th and 17th centuries. Provenance Rome, some materials apparently copied by Johannes Parvus. 151ff.

Contains motets f.111v, *Viri Galilaei 6* [secunda pars *Ascendit Deus in iubilatione*]; f.121v, *Per lignum a 5* [ascribed to Palestrina in Haberl edition; work is probably by Divitis]; f.127v, *Tu es Petrus a 6* [secunda pars *Quodcumque ligaveris*]; f.133v, *Ego sum panis vivus qui a 5* [secunda pars *Panis quem ego dabo*]; f.139v, *Ascendo a Patrem meum a 5* [secunda pars *Ego rogabo patrem*]; f.147v, *O beata et benedicta et gloriosa Trinitas a 5* [secunda pars *O vere summa sempiterna Trinitas*].

B0255 Vatican City. Biblioteca Apostolica Vaticana. MS Cappella Sistina 57. Choirbook, conflated from various fascicles. Mid-16th century. Provenance Rome, in various hands, some material in hand of Johannes Parvus. 139ff.

Contains masses f.3v, *Missa O magnum mysterium (Missa Tertia) a 5*; f.24v, *Missa Veni creator spiritus a 6.*

B0256 Vatican City. Biblioteca Apostolica Vaticana. MS Cappella Sistina 66. Choirbook. Dated 1671. Provenance Rome. 33ff.

Contains mass f.2v, *Missa Beatus Laurentius a 5.*

B0257 Vatican City. Biblioteca Apostolica Vaticana. MS Cappella Sistina 68. Choirbook. Dated 1618. Provenance Rome, copied by Domenico Brancadore. 114ff.

Contains masses f.3v, *Missa Pater noster a 4;* f.31v, *Missa Veni Sponsa Christi a 4;* f.57v, *Missa Iesu nostra redemptio (Missa Tertia) a 4*; f.81v, *Missa Pietra santa a 5.*

B0258 Vatican City. Biblioteca Apostolica Vaticana. MS Cappella Sistina 70. Choirbook. Dated 1666. Provenance Rome, in hand of Bartolomeo Belleschi. 50ff.

Contains mass f.2v, *Missa Nativitas tua Dei genetrix a 5* [anonymous in source; attributed to Palestrina by Bernhard Janz in 1997].

B0259 Vatican City. Biblioteca Apostolica Vaticana. MS Cappella Sistina 71. Choirbook. Dated 1631. Provenance Rome, copied by Orazio Felice and Giuseppe Dosi. 61ff.

Contains antiphon motet f.1v, *Lumen ad revelationem gentium a 4 et 5,* with canticle *Nunc dimittis.*

B0260 Vatican City. Biblioteca Apostolica Vaticana. MS Cappella Sistina 72. Choirbook, a conflation of several fascicles. 16th century [restoration work done in 1721]. i + 103ff.

Contains motets: f.3v, *Salvatorem expectamus Dominum a 6* [secunda pars *Sobrie e juste*] [questioned attribution]; f.19v, *O Rex gloriae a 4*; f.25v, *Suscipe verbum virgo Maria a 5* [secunda pars *Paries quidem filium*]; f.47v, *Salvum me fac a 5* [questioned attribution; possibly by Jachet?]; f.53v, *Angelus Domini descendit de coelo a 5* [secunda pars *Et introeuntes*] a 5; f.87v, *Fuit homo missus a Deo a 5* [secunda pars *Erat Joannes in deserto*].

B0261 Vatican City. Biblioteca Apostolica Vaticana. MS Cappella Sistina 73. Choirbook, conflation of several fascicles. Dated 1659. Provenance Rome, in various hands. 49ff.

Contains motets f.3v, *Salvator mundi a 4*; f.11v, *Confessio et pulchritudo a 5*; f.36v, *Derelinquat impius a 5.*

B0262 Vatican City. Biblioteca Apostolica Vaticana. MS Cappella Sistina 76. Choirbook, conflation of several fascicles. Dated 1599. Provenance Rome, in various hands. 191ff.

Contains masses f.4v, *Missa Assumpta est Maria a 6*; f.26v, *Missa Beatus Laurentius a 5*; f.50v, *Missa Dilexi quoniam a 5*; f.80v, *Missa Vestiva i colli a 5*; motet f.177v, *Tu es Petrus a 6.*

B0263 Vatican City. Biblioteca Apostolica Vaticana. MS Cappella Sistina 78. Choirbook. 16th century. Provenance Rome. i + 29ff.

Contains f.2v, *Missa Tu es pastor ovium a 5*; f.24v, motet, *Tu es pastor ovium a 5.*

B0264 Vatican City. Biblioteca Apostolica Vaticana. MS Cappella Sistina 88. Choirbook. 17th century. Provenance Rome, copied by Orazio Felice. 53ff.

Contains motets f.1v, *Pulchra es amica mea a 5*; f.7v, *O Antoni eremita a 5*; f.13v, *O quantus luctus a 4*; f.20v, *Cantantibus organis Cecilia* a 5; f.25v, *Misit Rex incredulus a 4*; f.29v, *O doctor optime* a 4; f.35v, *Dexteram meam et collum meum* a 5; f.41v, *Cum descendisset Iesus de monte a 4*; f.47v, *Quem dicunt homines a 5*.

B0265 Vatican City. Biblioteca Apostolica Vaticana. MS Cappella Sistina 91. Choirbook, conflation of various fascicles. Dated 1620, 1622. Provenance Rome, in hand of Giuseppe Dosi. 35ff.

Contains motet f.31v, *Beatus Laurentius orabat a 4*.

B0266 Vatican City. Biblioteca Apostolica Vaticana. MS Cappella Sistina 96. Choirbook. Dated 1630. Provenance Rome, copied for the use of the Sistine Chapel. i, ii + 52ff.

Contains motets f.18v, *Quam pulchri sunt a 4*; f.24, *Congratulamini mihi a 4*; f.28v, *Hodie nata est beata Virgo Maria a 5*; f.34, *Surge propera amica mea a 4*; f.40v, *Tempus est ut revertar a 5* [secunda pars *Nisi ego abiero*].

B0267 Vatican City. Biblioteca Apostolica Vaticana. MS Cappella Sistina 97. Choirbook. Dated 1687. Provenance Rome. i + 22ff.

Contains motets f.3v, *Surrexit pastor bonus a 8* [secunda pars *Etenim Pascha nostrum*]; f.11v, *Iesus iunxit se a 8* [secunda pars *Et increpavit eos*].

B0268 Vatican City. Biblioteca Apostolica Vaticana. MS Cappella Sistina 100. Choirbook, conflation of several fascicles. Dated 1659. Provenance Rome, in various hands. 33ff.

Contains motets f.9v, *Lauda Sion a 4*; f.25v, *Veni sponsa Christi a 4*; f.29v, *Valde honorandus est a 4*.

B0269 Vatican City. Biblioteca Apostolica Vaticana. MS Cappella Sistina 101. Choirbook. Dated 1638. Provenance Rome, in hand of Orazio Felice. 37ff.

Contains motets f.14v, *O beata et benedicta et gloriosa Trinitas a 5* [secunda pars *O vera summa*]; f.24v, *Vidi turbam magnam a 5* [secunda pars *Et omnes angeli*].

B0270 Vatican City. Biblioteca Apostolica Vaticana. MS Cappella Sistina 104. Choirbook. Dated 1709. Provenance Rome. i, ii + 28ff.

Contains motets f.2v, *Viri Galilei quid statis a 6* [secunda pars *Ascendit Deus*]; f.12v, *Dum complerentur dies Pentecostes a 6* [secunda pars *Dum ergo essent*].

B0271 Vatican City. Biblioteca Apostolica Vaticana. MS Cappella Sistina 105. Choirbook, conflation of several sources. 17th century; the Palestrina work was apparently copied in 1627. Provenance Rome. 57ff.

Contains motet f.52v, *Rex Melchior a 5*.

B0272 Vatican City. Biblioteca Apostolica Vaticana. MS Cappella Sistina 108. Choirbook. Dated 1697. Provenance Rome, copied by Jacopo Tartani. i + 40ff.

Contains motet f.10v, *Corona aurea a 5* [secunda pars f.16v, *Domine praevenisti eum*].

B0273 Vatican City. Biblioteca Apostolica Vaticana. MS Cappella Sistina 113. Choirbook. Dated 1709. Provenance Rome, copied by Jacopo Tartani. i + 46ff.

Contains mass f.1v, *Missa Virgo simul et matera 5.*

B0274 Vatican City. Biblioteca Apostolica Vaticana. MS Cappella Sistina 117. Choirbook. Dated 1662. Provenance Rome, copied by Bartolomeo Belleschi. 25ff.

Contains motets f.3v, *Fratres ego enim accepia 8*; f.10v, *Salvum me fac Dominea 5* [questioned attribution; possibly by Jachet?].

B0275 Vatican City. Biblioteca Apostolica Vaticana. MS Cappella Sistina 120. Choirbook. Dated 1791. Provenance Rome, copied by Enrico Giorgi. 20ff.

Contains mass f.2v, *Missa Nigra sum a 5.*

B0276 Vatican City. Biblioteca Apostolica Vaticana. MS Cappella Sistina 125. Choirbook. Dated 1760. Provenance Rome, copied by Francesco Biondini. i + 27ff.

Contains motet f.7v, *Princeps apostolorum a 6* [secunda pars *Quodcumque ligaveris*] [contrafactum text; music=*Solve jubente*].

B0277 Vatican City. Biblioteca Apostolica Vaticana. MS Cappella Sistina 126. Choirbook. Dated 1762. Provenance Rome, copied by Francesco Biondini. 31ff.

Contains motets f.2v, *Virtute magna reddebanta 5* [secunda pars *Repleti quidem spiritus*][contrafactum text; music=*Ascendo ad Patrem/Ego rogabo Patrem*]; f.10v, *Inveni David servum meum a 5* [contrafactum text; music=*Exi cito in plateas a 5*].

B0278 Vatican City. Biblioteca Apostolica Vaticana. MS Cappella Sistina 127. Choirbook. Dated 1786. Provenance Rome, copied by Bernardino Sebastiani. i + 33ff.

Contains mass f.2v, *Missa Assumpta est Maria a 6.*

B0279 Vatican City. Biblioteca Apostolica Vaticana. MS Cappella Sistina 129. Choirbook. Dated 1710. Provenance Rome, copied by Tommaso Altavilla. i + 47ff.

Contains mass f.2v, *Missa Memor esto a 5.*

B0280 Vatican City. Biblioteca Apostolica Vaticana. MS Cappella Sistina 131. Choirbook. Dated 1714. Provenance Rome, copied by Jacopo Tartano. i + 42ff.

Contains mass f.3v, *Missa Viri Galilaei a 6* [lacks *Agnus Dei II*].

B0281 Vatican City. Biblioteca Apostolica Vaticana. MS Cappella Sistina 132. Choirbook. 17th century. Provenance Rome, MS restoration with recopying 1753. 39ff.

Contains masses f.3v, *Missa Dilexi quoniam a 5*; f.21v, *Missa Nigra sum a 5.*

B0282 Vatican City. Biblioteca Apostolica Vaticana. MS Cappella Sistina 133. Choirbook. Dated 1709. Provenance Rome, copied by Tommaso Altavilla. i + 53ff.
Contains mass f.2v, *Missa O admirabile commercium a 5.*

B0283 Vatican City. Biblioteca Apostolica Vaticana. MS Cappella Sistina 134. Choirbook. Dated 1621. Provenance Rome, MS restoration 1721. i + 33ff.
Contains motets f.14v, *Osculetur me osculo oris sui a 5*; f.17v, *Trahe me post te a 5*; f.21v, *Vulnerasti cor meum a 5*; f.24v, *Sicut lilium inter spinas a 5*; f.28v, *Surge, propera amica mea formosa a 5.*

B0284 Vatican City. Biblioteca Apostolica Vaticana. MS Cappella Sistina 135. Choirbook. Dated 1703. Provenance Rome, copied by Jacopo Tartani. 47ff.
Contains mass f.1v, *Missa Tu es pastor ovium a 5* [lacks *Agnus Dei II*]; motet f.38v, *Tu es pastor ovium a 5.*

B0285 Vatican City. Biblioteca Apostolica Vaticana. MS Cappella Sistina 137. Choirbook. Dated 1668. Provenance Rome, copied by Bernardino Sebastiani. i + 34ff.
Contains mass f.3v, *Missa Assumpta est Maria a 6* [lacks *Agnus Dei II*].

B0286 Vatican City. Biblioteca Apostolica Vaticana. MS Cappella Sistina 140. Choirbook. Dated 1676. Provenance Rome, copied by Bartolomeo Belleschi. i + 34ff.
Contains mass f.3v, *Missa Papae Marcelli a 6* [lacks *Agnus Dei II* and *III*].

B0287 Vatican City. Biblioteca Apostolica Vaticana. MS Cappella Sistina 141. Choirbook. Dated 1660. Provenance Rome, copied by Bartolomeo Belleschi. i + 40ff.
Contains mass f.3v, *Missa Sine nomine (Cantabo Domino,* or *Beata Dei genetrix) a 6* [lacks *Agnus Dei II*].

B0288 Vatican City. Biblioteca Apostolica Vaticana. MS Cappella Sistina 143. Choirbook. 18th century. Provenance Rome. 29ff.
Contains mass f.1v, *Missa Beatus Laurentius a 5* [lacks *Agnus Dei II*].

B0289 Vatican City. Biblioteca Apostolica Vaticana. MS Cappella Sistina 144. Choirbook. Dated 1768. Provenance Rome. i + 21ff.
Contains mass f.2v, *Missa Papae Marcelli a 6* [lacks *Credo*, *Agnus Dei II* and *III*].

B0290 Vatican City. Biblioteca Apostolica Vaticana. MS Cappella Sistina 146. Choirbook. Dated 1747. Provenance Rome, copied by Biondini. i + 29ff.
Contains motets f.3v, *Loquebantur variis linguis a 4*; f.9v, *Sanctificavit Dominus a 5*; f.15v, *Cum pervenisset Beatus Andreas a 5.*

B0291 Vatican City. Biblioteca Apostolica Vaticana. MS Cappella Sistina 147. Choirbook, from different fascicles combined into a single volume. Dated 1785. Provenance Rome. i + 58ff.

Contains masses f.1v, *Missa Alma Redemptoris mater a 6* [lacks *Christe, Credô Benedictus, Agnus Dei II*]; f.26v, *Missa [Quinti toni] a 5* [lacks *Christe, Benedictus* and *Agnus Dei II*].

B0292 Vatican City. Biblioteca Apostolica Vaticana. MS Cappella Sistina 149. Choirbook. Mid-16th century. Provenance Rome, in hand of Johannes Parvus. i + 28ff.

Contains f.1v, *Missa Confitebor tibi Domine a 8.*

B0293 Vatican City. Biblioteca Apostolica Vaticana. MS Cappella Sistina 153. Choirbook. 16th century. Provenance Rome, copied by Luca Orpheus. 30ff.

Contains mass f.1v, *Missa Panem nostrum a 5* [lacks *Agnus Dei II*]; motet f.21v, *Ecce sacerdos magnus a 6* [secunda pars *Ideo iureiurando*].

B0294 Vatican City. Biblioteca Apostolica Vaticana. MS Cappella Sistina 171. Choirbook. 17th century. Provenance Rome, formerly owned by Girolamo Chiti. 48ff.

Contains f.19v, *Missa Laudate Dominum omnes gentes a 8*, chorus I [lacks *Agnus Dei II*].

B0295 Vatican City. Biblioteca Apostolica Vaticana. MS Cappella Sistina 172. Choirbook, 17th century. Provenance Rome, formerly owned by Girolamo Chiti, paired with MS 171. 41ff.

Contains f.19v, *Missa Laudate Dominum omnes gentes a 8*, chorus II [lacks *Agnus Dei II*].

B0296 Vatican City. Biblioteca Apostolica Vaticana. MS Cappella Sistina 182. Choirbook. Dated 1726. Provenance Rome. i + 11ff.

Contains improperia f.1v, *Popule meus a 8*, chorus I *a 4*.

B0297 Vatican City. Biblioteca Apostolica Vaticana. MS Cappella Sistina 183. Choirbook, dated 1726. Provenance Rome, paired with MS 182. i + 9ff.

Contains improperia f.1v [*Popule meus a 8*], *Quia eduxi te*, chorus II *a 4*.

B0298 Vatican City. Biblioteca Apostolica Vaticana. MS Cappella Sistina 194. Choirbook. 17th century. Provenance Rome, copied by Bartolomeo Belleschi. 37ff.

Contains mass f.1v, *Missa Lauda Sion salvatorem a 4* [lacks *Agnus Dei II*].

B0299 Vatican City. Biblioteca Apostolica Vaticana. MS Cappella Sistina 198. Choirbook, conflation of various fascicles. 17th century, restored 1724. i + 92ff.

Contains lamentation f.22v, *Feria VI Lectio II Lamentatio Ieremiae Prophetae: Matribus cui comparabo* and *Ierusalem a 4*; f.26, *Aleph. Quomodo sedet a 5*; f.31v, *Heth. Cogitavit a 5* [anonymous in source].

B0300 Vatican City. Biblioteca Apostolica Vaticana. MS Cappella Sistina 205.

Choirbook, conflation of various fascicles. 17th century. 58ff.

Contains improperia f.2v, *Popule meus a 8*, chorus I; f.42v, Psalm 50, *Miserere mei Deus a 9*, chorus I; f.44v, improperia *Popule meus a 8*, chorus I.

B0301 Vatican City. Biblioteca Apostolica Vaticana. MS Cappella Sistina 206. Choirbook, conflation of various fascicles. 17th century. Paired with MS 205. 61ff.

Contains improperia f.2v [*Popule meus a 8*], *Quia eduxi te*, chorus II; f.39v, Psalm 50, *Miserere mei Deus* a 9, chorus II; f.44v, improperia [*Popule meus a 8*] *Quia eduxi te*, chorus II.

B0302 Vatican City. Biblioteca Apostolica Vaticana. MS Cappella Sistina 215.25, 215.27–33. Partbooks. Dated 1721. Provenance Rome.

Contains motets f.26v, *Fratres ego enim accepi a Domino a 8*; f.28, *Iubilate Deo omnis terra a 8* [from *cantus primi chori*].

B0303 Vatican City. Biblioteca Apostolica Vaticana. MS Cappella Sistina 219. Choirbook. Mid-18th century. Provenance Rome, copied by singer Giovanni Celio for use in the Sistine Chapel. 36ff.

Contains mass f.1v, *Missa pro defunctis a 5* [*Kyrie, Offertorium, Sanctus, Benedictus, Agnus Dei*]; f.25v, responsory *Libera me a 3 et 4.*

B0304 Vatican City. Biblioteca Apostolica Vaticana. MS Cappella Sistina 221. Choirbook. Dated 1688. Provenance Rome, copied by Niccolo Porta. i + 189ff.

Contains motet f.34v, *Derelinquat impius a 5;* hymn f.110 [anonymous], *Crudelis Herodes a 4* [=*Hostes Herodes impie*].

B0305 Vatican City. Biblioteca Apostolica Vaticana. MS Cappella Sistina 267. Score. Dated 1792. 5ff.

Contains scoring of canon *Cantabimus canticum novum a 4* [not in Haberl or Casimiri]. This canon was said to have been incised in stone on the funeral monument to the papal singers situated until 1640 in Santa Maria in Vallicella (Chiesa Nuova), where it was ascribed to Palestrina. The 1792 transcription was written out by Leander Piazza [Llorens, *Capellae Sixtinae Codices,* p.304]. The canon was more likely to have been composed by Gregorio Allegri; see item E0198.

B0306 Vatican City. Biblioteca Apostolica Vaticana. MS Cappella Sistina 273. Choirbook. Dated 1753. Provenance Rome, copied by Francesco Biondini. i + 38ff.

Contains mass f.2v, *Missa Gabriel Archangelus a 4* [lacks *Benedictus, Agnus Dei II* and *III*].

B0307 Vatican City. Biblioteca Apostolica Vaticana. MS Cappella Sistina 276. Choirbook. Dated 1724. Provenance Rome, copied by Giovanni Domenico Biondini. 28ff.

Contains mass f.1v, *Missa sine nomine a 4* [lacks *Agnus Dei II* and *III*].

B0308 Vatican City. Biblioteca Apostolica Vaticana. MS Cappella Sistina 280. Choirbook. Dated 1724. Provenance Rome, copied by Piero Fiori. i + 72ff.

Contains masses f.1v, *Missa brevis a 4* [lacks *Agnus Dei II*]; f.37v, *Missa Aeterna Christi munera a 4* [lacks *Agnus Dei II*].

B0309 Vatican City. Biblioteca Apostolica Vaticana. MS Cappella Sistina 281. Choirbook. Dated 1734. Provenance Rome, copied by Giovanni Domenico Biondini. i + 30ff.

Contains mass f.2v, *Missa Iste Confessor a 4* [lacks *Agnus Dei II*].

B0310 Vatican City. Biblioteca Apostolica Vaticana. MS Cappella Sistina 285. Choirbook. Dated 1795. Provenance Rome, copied by Leonardo Testa. i + 61ff.

Containts masses f.19v, *Missa Iste Confessor a 4* [*Credo* only]; f.28v, *Missa Aeterna Christi munera a 4* [*Credo* only].

B0311 Vatican City. Biblioteca Apostolica Vaticana. MS Cappella Sistina 286. Choirbook. Dated 1791. Provenance Rome, restored 1850. i + 40ff.

Contains masses f.2v, *Missa Dilexi quoniam a 5* [lacks *Credo*, *Benedictus*, *Agnus Dei II* and *III*]; f.21v, *Missa Nigra sum a 5* [lacks *Benedictus* and *Agnus Dei III*].

B0312 Vatican City. Biblioteca Apostolica Vaticana. MS Cappella Sistina 287. Choirbook. Dated 1750. Provenance Rome, copied by Giovanni Domenico Biondini. 44ff.

Contains mass f.3v, *Missa Repleti sunt omnes a 4* [lacks *Agnus II* and *III*].

B0313 Vatican City. Biblioteca Apostolica Vaticana. MS Cappella Sistina 288. Choirbook. Dated 1707. Provenance Rome, copied by Tommaso Altavilla, restored 1768. 54ff.

Contains masses f.3v, *Missa Pietra sancta a 4* [lacks *Credo* and *Agnus Dei II* and *III*]; f.33v, *Missa Vestiva i colli a 5* [lacks *Credo*, *Benedictus*, and *Agnus Dei II* and *III*].

B0314 Vatican City. Biblioteca Apostolica Vaticana. MS Cappella Sistina 289. Choirbook. Dated 1796. Provenance Rome. 21ff.

Contains mass f.2v, *Missa Papae Marcelli a 6* [lacking *Credo* and *Agnus Dei II* and *III*].

B0315 Vatican City. Biblioteca Apostolica Vaticana. MS Cappella Sistina 291. Choirbook. Dated 1739. Provenance Rome, copied by Giovanni Domenico Biondini for use in the Sistine Chapel. i + 33ff.

Contains mass f.2v, *Missa pro defunctis a 5*; f.24v, responsory *Libera me a 3 et 4.*

B0316 Vatican City. Biblioteca Apostolica Vaticana. MS Cappella Sistina 292. Choirbook. Dated 1749. Provenance Rome, copied by Giovanni Domenico Biondini. i + 37ff.

Contains motets f.3v, *O magnum mysterium a 5* [secunda pars *Natum vidimus*]; f.11v, *Surge illuminare a 8* [secunda pars *Et ambulabunt gentes*]; f.23v, *Responsum accepit Simeon a 6* [secunda pars *Cum inducerent puerum*]; f.31v, *Derelinquat impius a 5*.

B0317 Vatican City. Biblioteca Apostolica Vaticana. MS Cappella Sistina 293. Choirbook. Dated 1748. Provenance Rome, copied by Giovanni Domenico Biondini. i + 55ff.

Contains motets f.31v, *Plangant eum a 6* [contrafactum text; music=*Deus qui ecclesiam tuam a 6*]; f.42v, *Stabat mater* a 8 [secunda pars *Eja mater*].

B0318 Vatican City. Biblioteca Apostolica Vaticana. MS Cappella Sistina 294. Choirbook. Dated 1748. Provenance Rome, copied by Francesco Biondini. 55ff.

Contains motets f.13v, *Iesus iunxit se a 8*; f.27v, *Angelus Domini a 8*; f.37v, *Viri Galilaei a 6*; f.45v, *Dum complerentur dies Pentecostes a 6* [secunda pars *Dum ergo essent*].

B0319 Vatican City. Biblioteca Apostolica Vaticana. MS Cappella Sistina 295. Choirbook. Dated 1749. Provenance Rome, copied by Francesco Biondini. 51ff.

Contains motets f.3v, *O beata et gloriosa Trinitas a 5* [secunda pars *O vere summa*]; f.13v, *Vidi turbam magnam* [secunda pars *Et omnes Angeli stabant*]; f.23v, *Salvatorem exspectamus a 6* [secunda pars *Sobrie et juste*]; f.33v, *Ierusalem cito veniet a 6* [secunda pars *Ego enim*]; f.42v, *Canite tuba a 5* [secunda pars *Rorate coeli*].

B0320 Vatican City. Biblioteca Apostolica Vaticana. MS Cappella Sistina 296. Choirbook. Dated 1749. Provenance Rome, copied by Giovanni Domenico Biondini. i + 47ff.

Contains motets f.3v, *Veni Domine et noli tardare a 6* [secunda pars *Excita Domine*]; f.30v, *Cum autem esset Stephanus a 6* [secunda pars *Positis autem genibus*]; f.38v, *Hic est beatissimus Evangelista a 6* [secunda pars *Hic est discipulus*].

B0321 Vatican City. Biblioteca Apostolica Vaticana. MS Cappella Sistina 297. Choirbook. Dated 1749 and 1777. Provenance Rome, copied by Giovanni Domenico Biondini. i + 62ff.

Contains motets f.19v, *Ne timeas Maria a 6* [secunda pars *Et dabit illi Dominus*]; f.53v, *Fuit homo missus a Deo a 5* [secunda pars *Erat Johannes in deserto*].

B0322 Vatican City. Biblioteca Apostolica Vaticana. MS Cappella Sistina 298. Choirbook. 18th century. Provenance Rome, copied by Giovanni Domenico Biondini. i + 63ff.

Contains motets f.5v, *Sancte Paule Apostole a 5*; f.13v, *Tu es pastor ovium a 4*; f.18v, *Solve iubente Deo a 6* [secunda pars *Quodcumque ligaveris*]; f.29v, *Surge Petre a 5*; f.54v, *Tu es Petrus a 6* [secunda pars *Quodcumque ligaveris*].

B0323 Vatican City. Biblioteca Apostolica Vaticana. MS Cappella Sistina 299. Dated 1743. Provenance Rome, copied by Giovanni Domenico Biondini. i + 40ff.

Contains motet f.15v, *Corona aurea a 5*; f.30v, *Tu es Petrus a 6* [secunda pars *Quodcumque ligaveris*].

B0324 Vatican City. Biblioteca Apostolica Vaticana. MS Cappella Sistina 300. Choirbook. Dated 1749. Provenance Rome, copied by Giovanni Domenico Biondini. i + 38ff.

Contains motet f.25v, *Sancta et immaculata virginitas a 6* [secunda pars *Benedicta tu*].

B0325 Vatican City. Biblioteca Apostolica Vaticana. MS Cappella Sistina 301. Choirbook. Dated 1743. Provenance Rome, copied by Giovanni Domenico Biondini. i + 34ff.

Contains motet f.4v, *Memor esto verbi tui a 5.*

B0326 Vatican City. Biblioteca Apostolica Vaticana. MS Cappella Sistina 302. Choirbook. Dated 1742. Provenance Rome, copied by Giovanni Domenico Biondini. i + 44ff.

Contains motet f.14v, *Veni sponsa Christi a 4*; f.21v, *Iste est qui ante Deum a 4*; f.29v, *Nos autem gloriari a* 4; f.36v, *Hic est vere martyr a 4.*

B0327 Vatican City. Biblioteca Apostolica Vaticana. MS Cappella Sistina 306. Choirbook, conflated from several fascicles. 18th century. Provenance Rome, copied by Giuseppe Lorenzini. i + 50ff.

Contains motet f.1v, *Haec dies a 6.*

B0328 Vatican City. Biblioteca Apostolica Vaticana. MS Cappella Sistina 308. Choirbook in two parts. Dated 1752 and 1798. Provenance Rome, copied by Francesco Grimaldi. i + 39ff.

Contains motet f.2v, *Fratres ego enim accepi a 8.*

B0329 Vatican City. Biblioteca Apostolica Vaticana. MS Cappella Sistina 309. Choirbook. 18th century. i + 17 ff.

Contains motet [sequence] f.9v, *Lauda Sion salvatorem a 5* [strophes 1, 2, 23].

B0330 Vatican City. Biblioteca Apostolica Vaticana. MS Cappella Sistina 310. Choirbook. Dated 1795. Provenance Rome, copied by Leonardo Testa. 26ff.

Contains motet f.3v, *Mirificat Dominus a 5* [contrafactum text; music=*Deus qui dedisti legem a 5*].

B0331 Vatican City. Biblioteca Apostolica Vaticana. MS Cappella Sistina 311. Choirbook. Dated 1761 and 1760. Provenance Rome, copied by Giuseppe Lorenzini. i + 35 ff.

Contains motets f.3v, *Descendit lux magna a 8* [secunda pars *Dies sanctificatus*] [contrafactum text; music=*Laudate pueri Dominum*]; f.16v, *Psallite Deo nostro a 8* [contrafactum text; music=*Domine in virtute a 8*]; f.26v,

Germinavit radix Iesse a 5 [secunda pars *Hodie beata virgo*] [contrafactum text; music=*Senex puerum portabat*].

B0332 Vatican City. Biblioteca Apostolica Vaticana. MS Cappella Sistina 314. Choirbook. Dated 1761. Provenance Rome, copied by Francesco Biondini. i + 21 ff.

Contains motet f.3v, *Advenit ignis a 6* [contrafactum text; music=*Responsum accepit Simeon a 6*].

B0333 Vatican City. Biblioteca Apostolica Vaticana. MS Cappella Sistina 315. Choirbook. Dated 1767. Provenance Rome, copied by Francesco Biondini. 40ff.

Contains motets f.3v, *Exultate Deo adjutori nostro a 8* [contrafactum text; music=*Magna est gloria*]; f.16v, *Coronas aureas a 5.*

B0334 Vatican City. Biblioteca Apostolica Vaticana. MS Cappella Sistina 320. Choirbook. Dated 1780. Provenance Rome, copied by Giuseppe Lorenzini. i + 33 ff.

Contains mass f.1v, *Missa Papae Marcelli a 4* [Anerio's reduced version of the original mass *a 6*].

B0335 Vatican City. Biblioteca Apostolica Vaticana. MS Cappella Sistina 321. Choirbook. Dated 1830. i + 25ff.

Contains motets f.2v, *Salvator mundi a 4*; f.6v, *Dies sanctificatus a 4*; f.10v, *O rex gloriae a 4*; f.14v, *Loquebantur variis linguis a 4*; f.18v, *Benedicta sit sancta Trinitas a 4*; f.22v, *Sicut cervus a 4.*

B0336 Vatican City. Biblioteca Apostolica Vaticana. MS Cappella Sistina 331. Choirbook, conflated from three fascicles. 18th century. Provenance Rome, in various hands. 57ff.

Contains hymn f.8v, *Salutis humnae sator a 4* [=*Jesu nostra redemptio*] [verses 1, 3, 5 in polyphony; other verses in plainchant].

B0337 Vatican City. Biblioteca Apostolica Vaticana. MS Cappella Sistina 340. Choirbook. Dated 1748 and 1777. Provenance Rome, hands of Giovanni Domenico Biondini and Giuseppe Lorenzini. 35ff.

Contains f.17v, *Improperia a 4* [second chorus] [see also B0338].

B0338 Vatican City. Biblioteca Apostolica Vaticana. MS Cappella Sistina 341. Choirbook. Dated 1748 and 1777. Provenance Rome, hands of Giovanni Domenico Biondini and Giuseppe Lorenzini. 37ff.

Contains f.19v, *Improperia* a 4 [first chorus] [see also B0337].

B0339 Vatican City. Biblioteca Apostolica Vaticana. MS Cappella Sistina 342. Choirbook, "Liber Lamentationum." Dated 1733. Provenance Rome, copied by Giovanni Domenico Biondini. i + 31 ff.

Contains Lamentation f.16v, *Feria VI in Parasceve Lamentatio Jeremiae prophetae Lectio I* [three sections].

B0340 Vatican City. Biblioteca Apostolica Vaticana. MS Cappella Sistina 354. Choirbook, conflated from numerous fascicles. Late 18th to early 19th century. In several hands. 458ff.

Contains f.164, *Missa [Sine nomine] a 8;* f.195, *Missa Veni sponsa Christi a 4*; motets f.220, *Coronas aureas a 5;* f.228, *Descendit lux magna a 8* [contrafactum text; music=*Laudate pueri a 8*]; f.244, *Exultate Deo a 8* [contrafactum text; music=*Magna est gloria*]; f.258, *Germinavit radix Jesse a 5* [contrafactum text; music=*Senex puerum portabat*]; f.266, *Mirificavit Dominus a 5* [contrafactum text; music=*Deus qui dedisti legem a 5*]; f.270v, *Princeps apostolorum a 6* [contrafactum text; music=*Solve jubente*]; f.282, *Princeps apostolorum a 6* [*sic*, as with f.270v]; f.290, *Tanquam sponsum a 7* [contrafactum text; music=*Tu es Petrus a 7*]; f.298, *Virtute magna a 5;* f.407, *Psallite Domino nostro a 8.*

B0341 Vatican City. Biblioteca Apostolica Vaticana. MS Cappella Sistina 355. Score, inscribed as containing unpublished compositions by Palestrina. Dated 19th century. Material copied from Ottoboniani sources MSS 2923 and 2928, formerly owned by Giuseppe Baini. 522ff.

Contains masses f.22, *Missa Tu es Petrus a 6*; f.53, *Missa in maioribus duplicibus a 4*; f.80, *Missa in minoribus duplicibus a 4*; f.104, *Missa Papae Marcelli a 4* [cantus only]; f.108, *Missa Iste Confessor a 4* [cantus only]; f.111, *Missa Sine nomine* [cantus only]; hymn f.120, *Immense coeli conditor a 4.*

B0342 Vatican City. Biblioteca Apostolica Vaticana. MS Cappella Sistina 452. Score. 19th century. Provenance Giuseppe Baini. 133 ff.

Contains f.11, *Improperia a 8*; f.27, motets *Pueri Hebraeorum, Gloria laus et Ingrediente Domino a 4;* f.91, *Lamentationes Ieremiae prophetae a 4.*

B0343 Vatican City. Biblioteca Apostolica Vaticana. MS Cappella Sistina 453. Score. 19th century. Provenance Giuseppe Baini. 118 ff.

Contains masses f.1, *Missa Brevis a 4*; f.24, *Missa Papae Marcelli a 6*; f. 56, *Missa Quem dicunt homines a 4*; f.79, *Missa Ut re mi fa sol la a 6* [some voices missing in each item].

[Vatican City. Biblioteca Apostolica Vaticana. MS Cappella Sistina 456–472. Scores. 19th century.

A series of scorings in the hand of Giuseppe Baini of primary source prints of Palestrina's music in several genres.]

B0344 Vatican City. Biblioteca Apostolica Vaticana. MS Cappella Sistine 473. Scores. Early 19th century. In the hand of Giuseppe Baini, described as works "found in various manuscripts with the name of Gio. Pierluigi da Palestrina," including material formerly located by Girolamo Chiti in Roman archives. Baini notes that authorship of several works was uncertain. i–vi + 40 ff.

Contains hymns fasc I: f.1, *Audi benigne Conditor a 4;* f.3, *Te lucis ante terminum a 4;* f.5, *Immense coeli conditor a 4;* f.5v, *Telluris ingens conditor a 4;* f.6v, *Coeli Deus sanctissime a 4;* f.8, *Magnae Deus potentiae a 4*; fasc III: responsories f.3v, *In manus tuas* and *Nunc dimittis a 4;* f.15, *In monte*

Oliveti a 5; f.16, *Ecce vidimus a 5;* f.17, *Amicus meus a 5;* f.18, *Judas mercator a 5;* f.18v, *Unus ex discipulus a 5;* f.19v, *Erat quasi agnus a 5;* f.20v, *Una hora a 5;* f.21v, *Seniores populi a 5;* f.22v, *In monte Oliveti a 5;* f.23v, *Judas mercator;* f.24, *Unus ex discipulus a 4;* f.24v, *Erat quasi agnus a 4;* f.25, *Una hora a 4;* f.26, *Seniores populi*; fasc V: motets f.27, *Ave verum a 5;* f.28, *Exaudi Domine a 5;* f.29v, *Illumina oculos meos a 5;* f.31, *Qui manducat meam carnem a 5;* f.32, *Ne reminiscaris Domine a 5;* f.35v, *Venite exultemus a 5;* f.38, *Tu es pastor ovium a 5* [secunda pars *Quodcumque ligaveris*].

[Vatican City. Biblioteca Apostolica Vaticana. MS Cappella Sistina 474–478, 480. Scores. 19th century.

A series of scorings in the hand of Giuseppe Baini of primary source prints of books of Palestrina's motets.]

B0345 Vatican City. Biblioteca Apostolica Vaticana. MS Cappella Sistina 479. Score. 19th century. Partly in hand of Giuseppe Baini [certain works in this score, printed in Haberl, are based on sources located by Girolamo Chiti but are now believed lost]. i–iv + 69 ff.

Contains Lamentations f.25, *Incipit Lamentatio* et seq.; motets f.50, *Stabat mater a 8*; f.55v, *Sub tuum praesidium a 8;* f.57, *Fratres ego enim a 8*; f.59v, *Caro mea vere est cibus a 8*; f.61v, *Hic est panis a 8*; f.63v, *Tria sunt munera a 8*; f.66, *Fili non te frangunt a 8*; f.68, *Ecce veniet dies illa a 8.*

[Vatican City. Biblioteca Apostolica Vaticana. MS Cappella Sistina 481. Scores. 19th century.

Scorings in the hand of Giuseppe Baini of masses by Palestrina.]

B0346 Vatican City. Biblioteca Apostolica Vaticana. MS Cappella Sistina 484–489. Six partbooks. Mid-18th century, circa 1751. Provenance Rome, in hand of Giovanni Celi [foliation from cantus part].

Contains motets f.8, *Qui manducat meam carnem a 5*; f.8v–9, *Ne reminiscaris Domine a 5*; f.9v, *Ave verum a 5*; f.10v, *Caro mea vere est cibus a 4*; f.12, *Exaudi Domine preces a 5*; f.15, *Salvatorem exspectamus a 6*; f.18, *Ecce sacerdos magnus a 6* [anonymous in source]; f.19, *Responsum accepit Simeon a 6*; f.19v, *Cum autem esset Stephanus a 6* [secunda pars *Positis autem genibus*]; f.20v, *Hic est beatissimus Evangelista a 6* [secunda pars *Hic est discipulus*]; f.23v, *Assumpta est Maria a 6* [secunda pars *Quae est ista a 6*]; f.25, *O beata et benedicta et gloriosa Trinitas a 5* [secunda pars *O vera summa et sempiterna Trinitas a 6*]; f.26, *Ne timeas Maria a 6* [secunda pars *Et dabit illi Dominus*] [contrafactum text; music=*Dum complerentur a 6*]; f.35v, *O magnum misterium a 6* [secunda pars *Quem vidistis pastores*]; f.37v, *De profundis clamavi a 4*; f.48v, *Laudate coeli a 5*; f.50v, *O vos omnes a 4*; f.48r–v, *Litaniae beatae Mariae virginis* a 5; motets f.48v, *Laudate coeli a 5*; f.52v, *Lumen ad revelationem gentium a 4 et 5*; f.54v, *Alma redemptoris Mater a 8*; f.55, *Regina coeli a 8*; f.55v, *Salve Regina a 8.*

B0347 Vatican City. Biblioteca Apostolica Vaticana. MS Cappella Sistina 527–530.

Partbooks. Dated 1746. Provenance Rome, in hand of Giovanni Celi. 42 ff [foliation from cantus].

Contains masses f.3, *Missa Io mi son giovinetta a 4*; f.9, *Missa Brevis a 4*; f.13, *Missa De Feria a 4*; f.15, *Missa Sine nomine pulcherrima a 4*; f.18, *Missa Prima* [Quarti Libri] *a 4*; f.22, *Missa Secunda* [Quarti Libri] *a 4*; f.26, *Missa Tertia* [Quarti Libri] *a 4*; f.30, *Missa Quarta* [Quarti Libri] *a 4*; f.34, *Missa Ave regina coelorum a 4*; f.38v, *Missa Pater noster a 4.*

B0348 Vatican City. Biblioteca Apostolica Vaticana. MS Cappella Sistina 531–534. Partbooks. Dated 1748. Provenance Rome, in hand of Giovanni Celi. 39 ff [foliation from cantus].

Contains masses f.3, *Missa Inviolata a 4*; f.7, *Missa Spem in alium a 4*; f.11, *Missa Veni sponsa Christi a 4*; f.15, *Missa Già fu chi m'ebbe cara a 4*; f.18, *Missa Repleti sunt omnes a 4*; f.22, *Missa Regina coeli a 4*; f.27, *Missa O rex gloriae a 4*; f.31, *Missa ad fugam a 4*; f.34, *Missa de beata virgine a 4.*

B0349 Vatican City. Biblioteca Apostolica Vaticana. MS Cappella Sistina 535–539. Partbooks. Mid-18th century. Provenance Rome, in hand of Giovanni Celi and others. 37 ff [foliation from cantus].

Contains masses f.3, *Missa Repleatur os meum a 5*; f.9, *Missa Vestiva i colli a 5*; f.16v, *Missa O virgo simul et mater a 5*; f.21v, *Missa Sine nomine a 5*; f.27, *Missa Petra sancta a 5*; f.31, *Missa Beatus Laurentius a 5.*

B0350 Vatican City. Biblioteca Apostolica Vaticana. MS Cappella Sistina 604. Score. 19th century. Provenance Rome. 122 ff.

Contains motet [sequence] f.21, *Veni sancte spiritus a 8.*

B0351 Vatican City. Biblioteca Apostolica Vaticana. MS Santa Maria Maggiore [Jeppesen says MS 11 (olim 27)]. Choirbook. Second half of 16th century. 100ff [MS reported to be in poor condition; present state unknown].

Contains hymns f.2v, *Deus tuorum militum a 4* [Hab. XXX]; f.8v, *Exultet coelum a 4 et 5* [Hab. XXX]; f.11v, *Immense coeli conditor a 4;* f.14v, *Telluris ingens a 4;* f.17v, *Coeli Deus sanctissime a 4;* f.20v, *Magnae Deus a 4;* f.23v, *Plasmator hominis a 4;* f.26v, *Audi benigne a 4*; Lamentations f.55v, *Aleph. Quomodo sedet a 5*; f.59v, *Vau. Et egressus a 5*; f.64v, *Jod. Manum suam a 6*; f.70v., *Heth. Cogitavit a 5*; f.74v, *Lamed. Matribus a 5*; f.79v, *Aleph. Ego vir a 6*; f.84v, *Heth. Misericordiae a 5*; f.89v, *Aleph. Quomodo obscuratum a 5*; f.93v, *Recordare a 6.*

B0352 Vatican City. Biblioteca Apostolica Vaticana. MS Santa Maria Maggiore 29 [olim J.J. III.7]. Choirbook. Dated circa 1580. Provenance Rome, copied by Johannes Parvus. 139 ff [all items anonymous in source].

Contains f.1v, *Missa Papae Marcelli a 6*; f.22v, *Missa Sine titulo (Io mi son giovinetta) a 6;* f.53v, *Missa Benedicta es coelorum Regina a 6*; f.89v, *Missa Ut re mi fa sol la a 6;* f.112v, *Missa De beata Virgine a 6*; motet f.82v, *Beata es a 6.*

B0353 Vatican City. Biblioteca Apostolica Vaticana. MS Santa Maria Maggiore 32 [olim J.J.III.10]. Choirbook. Second half of 16th century. Provenance Rome, copied partly by Johannes Parvus, partly by another hand. 153 ff.

Contains f.134v, *Magnificat* [beginning *Et exultavit* verse: tone 6 *a 4*, Hab. XXVII.251].

B0354 Vatican City. Biblioteca Apostolica Vaticana. MS Vaticani Latini 10776. Second half of 16th century. Provenance presumably Rome. 59 ff [believed once owned by Palestrina, contains autograph material].

Contains f.55v, *Dixit Dominus a 4* [this work has been identified as by Palestrina; there are fourteen anonymous works in the MS].

B0355 Vienna. Österreichische Nationalbibliothek Musiksammlung. MS Mus. 15507. Choirbook. Dated 1637. Copied by Georg Moser.

Contains hymns p.41, *O solis ortus cardine a 4;* p.69, *Deus tuorum militum a 4* [Hab. XXX]; p.363, *Quicumque Christum quaeritis a 4.*

B0356 Vienna. Österreichische Nationalbibliothek, Musiksammlung, MS Mus. 15807. "Partidura." Dated 1601.

Contains masses f.67v, *Missa Jesu nostra redemptio (Missa Tertia) a 4;* f.75v, *Missa Iam Christus astra a 4;* f.82v, *Missa Aeterna Christi munera a 4;* f.87, *Missa Sanctorum meritis a 4;* f.94v, *Missa Iste Confessor a 4;* f.99, *Missa Ecce sacerdos magnus a 4;* f.109v, *Missa O Regem coeli a 4;* f.118, *Missa Virtute magna a 4;* f.125v, *Missa De beata Virgine a 4;* f.132v, *Missa Inviolata a 4;* f.140v, *Missa Spem in alium a 4;* f.149v, *Missa Primi toni (Io mi son giovinetta) a 4;* f.162v, *Missa Sine nomine (Je suis desheritée) a 4*; hymns f.1, *Conditor alme siderum a 4*; f.3v, *Christe redemptor omnium a 4*; f.5v, *A solis ortus cardine a* 4; f.8, *Hostes Herodes impie a 4;* f.8v, *Lucis creator optime a 4;* f.9v, *O lux beata Trinitas a 4;* f.10v, *Ad preces nostras a 4;* f.13, *Vexilla regis a 4* [Hab.VIII.35]; f.14v, *Ad coenam agni a 4;* f.16v, *Jesu nostra redemptio a 4;* f.20, *Veni creator a 4* [Hab.VIII]; f.22, *Pange lingua a 4* [Hab.VIII]; f.23v, *Quodcunque vinclis a 4*; f.24, *Doctor egregie a 4;* f.26v, *Ave maris stella a 4;* f.26v, *Vexilla regis a 4* [Hab.VIII.70]; f.27v, *Ut queant laxis a 4;* f.29v, *Aurea luce et decore a 4;* f.31v, *Lauda mater ecclesia a 4;* f.32v, *Petrus beatus a 4;* f.33v, *Quicumque Christum quaeritis a 4;* f.34, *Tibi Christe splendor a 4;* f.36, *Placare Christe a 4* [=*Christe redemptor omnium a 4*]; f.37v, *Exultet coelum a 4* [Hab.VIII]; f.39v, *Tristes erant Apostoli a 4;* f.41, *Deus tuorum militum a 4;* f.42, *Deus tuorum militum a 4*; f.42v, *Sanctorum meritis a 4;* f.43v, *Rex gloriose martyrum a 4;* f.45, *Iste confessor a 4;* f.46v, *Jesu corona virginum a 4* [Hab.VIII.123]; f.48, *Jesu corona virginum a 4* [Hab.VIII.127]; f.48v, *Huius obtentu a 4;* f.49v, *Urbs beata Jerusalem a 4;* f.51v, *Magne Pater Augustine a 4;* f.54, *Laudibus summis a 4;* f.55v, *En gratulemur a 4*; f.56v, *Proles de coelo a 4;* f.58v, *Decus morum a 4;* f.59v, *Christe qui lux est a 4;* f.61v, *Prima lux surgens a 4;* f.63v, *Nunc juvat celsi a 4;* f.65, *Mensis Augusti a 4;* f.66v, *Hymnus canoris a 4.*

B0357 Vienna. Österreichische Nationalbibliothek. Musiksammlung. MS Mus. 15942. Choirbook. 17th century. Copied by Georg Moser.

Contains hymn f.161v, *Vexilla regis prodeunt a 4* [Hab.VIII.35].

B0358 Vienna. Österreichische Nationalbibliothek. Musiksammlung. MS Mus. 15943 (olim A.N.43.E.21). Choirbook. Mid-17th century. Provenance Vienna, copied for use of court chapel of Emperor Ferdinand III. 270 + i ff.

Contains f.96, *Benedictus a 4*; f.161v, *Magnificat a 4* [odd verses, tone 1].

B0359 Vienna. Österreichische Nationalbibliothek. Musiksammlung. MS Mus. 15944. Choirbook. Mid-17th century.

Contains masses f.1, *Missa Lauda Sion salvatorem a 4;* f.29, *Missa Jesu nostra redemptio (Missa Tertia) a 4;* f.60, *Missa L'homme armé (Missa Quarta) a 4;* f.91, *Missa Secunda (primi toni) a 4;* f.122, *Missa Ad fugam;* f.143, *Missa Sine nomine a 4;* f.166, *Missa Brevis a 4;* f.198, *Missa Papae Marcelli a 4* [*4vv version*].

B0360 Vienna. Österreichische Nationalbibliothek. Musiksammlung. MS Mus. 15945. Choirbook. 17th century. Copied by Georg Moser. i + 259ff.

Contains masses f.1, *Missa Primi toni (Io mi son giovinetta) a 4;* f.44, *Missa Gabriel Arcangelus a 4;* f.83, *Missa Spem in alium a 4;* f.127, *Missa Virtute magna a 4;* f.172, *Missa O Regem coeli a 4;* f.214, *Missa Ecce sacerdos magnus a 4.*

B0361 Vienna. Österreichische Nationalbibliothek. Musiksammlung. MS Mus. 16199. Choirbook. Dated 1646. Copied by Georg Moser. v + 194ff.

Contains hymns f.1v, *Creator alme siderum a 4* [=*Conditor alme siderum a 4*]; f.6v, *Jesu redemptor a 4* [=*Christe redemptor omnium a 4*]; f.12v, *Deus tuorum militum a 4* [Hab. XXX]; f.14v, *Exultet orbis a 4* [=*Salvete flos*]; f.16v, *Salvete flos a 4;* f.20v, *Crudelis Herodes a 4* [=*Hostes Herodes impie*]; f.26v, *Lucis creator optime a 4;* f.31v, *Jam sol recedit a 4* [=*O lux beata Trinitas*]; f.36v, *Audi benigne a 4;* f.40v, *Vexilla regis prodeunt a 4* [Hab.VIII.35]; f.45v, *Ad coenam agni a 4* [text=*Ad regias agni*]; f.50v, *Salutis humanae sator a 4* [=*Jesu nostra redemptio*]; f.56v, *Veni creator a 4* [Hab.VIII]; f.61v, *Pange lingua a 4* [Hab.VIII]; f.64v, *Rex gloriose martyrum a 4;* f.68v, *Quodcumque in orbe a 4* [=*Quodcunque vinclis*]; f.74v, *Egregie Doctor a 4* [=*Doctor egregie*]; f.80v, *Ave maris stella a 4;* f.84v, *Tristes erant Apostoli a 4* [=*Vexilla regis*]; f.91v, *Ut queant laxis a 4;* f.96v, *Aurea luce et decore a 4*; f.102v, *Pater superni luminis a 4* [=*Lauda mater ecclesia*]; f.111v, *Quicumque Christum quaeritis a 4;* f.115v, *Te splendor et virtus a 4* [=*Tibi Christe splendor*]; f.119v, *Custodes hominum a 4* [=*Sanctorum meritis*]; f.125v, *Proles de coelo a 4;* f.129v, *Decus morum a 4;* f.133v, *Placare Christe a 4* [=*Christe redemptor omnium a 4*]; f.139v, *Exultet orbis gaudiis a 4* [=*Exultet coelum a 4*] [Hab.VIII]; f.144v, *Tristes erant Apostoli a 4;* f.149v, *Deus tuorum militum a 4* [Hab.VIII.105]; f.154v, *Deus tuorum militum a 4;* f.158v, *Sanctorum meritis a 4;* f.167v, *Iste confessor a 4*; f.169, *Iste confessor a 4*; f.174v, *Fortem virili pectore a 4* [=*Jesu corona virginum*] [Hab.VIII.123]; f.178v, *Jesu corona virginum a 4* [Hab.VIII.127]; f.183v, *Fortem virili pectore a 4* [=*Jesu corona virginum*] [Hab.VIII.123]; f.187v, *Coelestis urbs Jerusalem a 4* [=*Urbs beata Jerusalem*].

B0362 Vienna. Österreichische Nationalbibliothek. Musiksammlung. MS Mus.

16200. Choirbook. Early 17th century.

Contains mass f.31r, *Missa Ave regina coelorum a 4*.

B0363 Vienna. Österreichische Nationalbibliothek. Musiksammlung. MS Mus. 16704 (olim A.N.62.G.3). Choirbook. Early 17th century. Provenance Graz, copied for use of court of Ferdinand, Archduke of Styria (1578–1637, Emperor Ferdinand II from 1619). 309ff.

Contains motets f.15v, *Unus ex duobus a 5* [secunda pars *Beatus Andreas*]; f.24v, *Canite tuba a 5* [secunda pars *Rorate coeli*]; f.28v, *Suscipe verbum virgo Maria a 5;* f.32v, *Veni Domine a 6* [secunda pars *Excita Domine potentiam*]; f.39v, *O sancte praesul Nicolae a 5* [secunda pars *Gaude praesul optime*]; f.48v, *Suscipe verbum virgo Maria a 5* [secunda pars *Paries quidem filium*]; f.58v, *Columna es a 6;* f.62v, *Quia vidisti me Thoma a 4;* f.114v, *Lapidabant Stephanum a 5;* f.118v, *Hic est discipulus ille a 5;* f.132v, *O bone Jesu exaudi me a 6;* f.139v, *Stella quam viderant a 5;* 151v, *Senex puerum portabat a 5* [secunda pars *Hodie beata Virgo Maria*]; f.165v, *Surge Petre a 5;* f.263v, *Crucem sanctam dubiit a 5;* f.267v, *Angelus Domini a 5* [secunda pars *Et introeuntes*]; f.279v, *Haec dies a 6;* f.302v, *Viri Galilei a 6* [secunda pars *Ascendit Deus in iubilatione*].

B0364 Vienna. Österreichische Nationalbibliothek. Musiksammlung. MS Mus. 16705. Choirbook. 16th century. 309ff.

Contains motets f.10v, *Dum complerentur a 5* [secunda pars *Cum ergo essent*]; f.21v, *Salve Regina a 5* [secunda pars *Eia ergo advocata*]; f.33v, *O beata et benedicta et gloriosa a 5* [secunda pars *O vere summa*]; f.42v, *Lauda Sion salvatorem a 4;* f.48v, *Coenantibus illis a 5;* f.52v, *Fuit homo missus a Deo a 5* [secunda pars *Erat Joannes in deserto*]; f.60v, *Tu es Petrus a 6* [secunda pars *Quodcumque ligaveris*]; f.68v, *Sancte Paule Apostole a 5;* f.72v, *Beatae Mariae Magdalenae a 5;* f.76v, *O lux et decus Hispaniae* [secunda pars *O singulare praesidium*]; f.84v, *Beatus Laurentius a 5;* f.92v, *Omnipotens sempiterne Deus a 5;* f.96v, *Hodie nata est beata Virgo Maria a 5;* f.104v, *Venit Michael a 5;* f.117v, *O beatum pontificem a 5;* f.122v, *Cantantibus organis Caecilia a 5* [secunda pars *Biduanis*]; f.130v, *Inclyta sanctae virginis Catharinae a 5;* f.134v, *Gaude Barbara a 5* [secunda pars *Gaude quia meruisti*]; f.145v, *Sanctificavit Dominus a 5* [secunda pars *O quam metuendus est*]; f.156v, *Domine Deus qui conteris a 5* [secunda pars *Tu Domine, cui humilium*]; f.181v, *Ave Maria a 5*; f.203v, *Quam pulchri sunt a 5;* f.208v, *Sancta et immaculata a 6* [secunda pars *Benedicta tu in mulieribus*]; f.235v, *Tradent enim vos a 5;* f.240, *Corona aurea super caput a 5* [secunda pars *Domine praevenisti*].

B0365 Vienna. Österreichische Nationalbibliothek. Musiksammlung. MS Mus. 16709 [MS source for motet *Ave regina coelorum a 8\4*, doubtful?; *Alma redemptoris mater a 4*, not in Haberl or Casimiri].

Contains motets f.58v, *Columna es a 6;* f.213v, *Salve Regina misericordiae a 4;* f.216v, *Alma redemptoris mater a 4;* f.219v, *Ave regina coelorum a 4;* f.221v, *Regina coeli;* f.263v, *Crucem sanctam a 5*; hymns f.4v, *Creator alme siderum a 4* [=*Conditor alme siderum a 4*]; f.10v, *Christe redemptor omnium a 4;* f.17v, *Salvete flos a 4;* f.19v, *Hostes Herodes impie a 4;* f.23v, *Ave maris stella a 4;* f.29v, *O lux beata Trinitas a 4;* f.33v, *Lucis creator optime a 4;* f.38v, *Quodcunque vinclis a 4;* f.41v, *Doctor egregie a 4;* f.43v, *Ad preces nostras a 4;* f.51v, *Vexilla regis a 4* [Hab.VIII.35]; f.60, *Ad coenam agni providi a 4;* f.68v, *Tristes erant Apostoli a 4;* f.73v, *Deus tuorum militum a 4* [Hab.VIII.110]; f.76v, *Rex gloriose martyrum a 4;* f.79v, *Jesu corona virginum a 4* [Hab.VIII.127]; f.85v, *Vexilla regis a 4* [Hab.VIII.70]; f.89v, *Te fons salutis a 4* [=*O crux ave* from *Vexilla regis*]; f.90v, *Jesu nostra redemptio a 4;* f.96v, *Veni creator a 4* [Hab.VIII]; f.104v, *Tantum ergo a 4;* f.106v, *Pange lingua a 4* [Hab.VIII]; f.112v, *Congratulemur hodie a 4* [=*En gratulemur*]; f.118v, *Ut queant laxis a 4;* f.124v, *Aurea luce et decore a 4;* f.129v, *Lauda mater ecclesia a 4;* f.133v, *Hymnus canoris a 4;* f.136v, *Petrus beatus a 4;* f.138v, *Quicumque Christum quaeritis a 4;* f.142v, *Magne Pater Augustine a 4;* f.148v, *Laudibus summis a 4;* f.154v, *Tibi Christe splendor a 4;* f.158v, *Proles de coelo a 4;* f.164v, *Decus morum a 4;* f.169v, *Christe redemptor omnium a 4;* f.175v, *Exultet coelis a 4;* f.180v, *Deus tuorum militum a 4* [Hab.VIII.105]; f.185v, *Sanctorum meritis a 4;* f.190v, *Iste confessor a 4;* f.196v, *Jesu corona virginum a 4;* [Hab.VIII.123]; f.201v, *Huius obtentu a 4;* f.203v, *Urbs beata Jerusalem a 4;* f.207v, *Magne Pater Augustine a 4;* f.210v, *Audi benigne a 4.*

[Vienna, Österreichische Nationalbibliothek. Musiksammlung. MS Mus. 17473–17523 inclusive.

A series of 18th-century copies of individual works, with one or two Palestrina works per MS.]

B0366 Vienna, Österreichische Nationalbibliothek. Musiksammlung. MS Mus. 19426 (olim A.N.43.E.13). iv + 324 + i paper folios. Dated 1630 (dated index), probably copied in Vienna for use of court chapel of Emperor Ferdinand II.

Contains mass f.151v, *Missa Dies sanctificatus a 4* [*Kyrie*, *Sanctus*, *Benedictus*, *Agnus Dei* only]; hymn f.85v, *Vexilla regis prodeunt a 4* [Hab.VIII.35]; canticles f.212v, *Benedicite Dominus Deus a 4;* f.254, *Magnificat a 4* [odd verses, tone 1].

B0367 Vienna, Österreichische Nationalbibliothek. Musiksammlung. MS Mus. 19428. Choirbook. 17th century. 86ff.

Contains f.58v, *Sicut cervus a 4* [secunda pars *Sitivit anima mea*].

B0368 Washington, DC. Catholic University of America. Mullen Library. Biblioteca Albani Urbinas F V.8 [MS 201]. Choirbook. Dated 1726. Provenance Rome, Sistine Chapel, copied by Giovanni Domenico Biondini. i + 147ff.

Contains motets f.2v, *O magnum mysterium a 5*; f.10v, *Surge illuminare Jerusalem a 8*; f.23v, *Responsum acceppit Simeon a 6*; f.31v, *Derelinquat impius a 5*; f.78v, *Stabat Mater dolorosa a 8*; f.91v, *Fratres ego enim accepi a 8*; f.108v, *Jesus junxit se a 8*; f.118v, *Surrexit pastor bonus a 8*; f.138v, *Ne timeas Maria a 6.*

B0369 Washington, DC. Catholic University of America. Mullen Library. Biblioteca Albani Urbinas F V.9 [MS 202]. Choirbook. Dated 1727. Provenance

Rome, Sistine Chapel, copied by Giovanni Domenico Biondini. i + 155ff.

Contains motets f.10v, *Viri Galilaei a 6;* f.20v, *Dum complerentur dies Pentecostes a 6*; f.30v, *O beata et gloriosa Trinitas a 5*; f.40v, *Fuit homo missus a Deo a 5*; f.50v, *Tu es Petrus a 6*; f.70v, *Vidi turbam magnam a 6*; f.83v, *Salvatorem expectamus a 6*; f.91v, *Jerusalem cito veniet a 6*; f.100v, *Veni Domine a 6*; f.111v, *Canite tuba in Sion a 5*; f.139v, *Cum autem esset Stephanus a 6*; f.147v, *Hic est beatissimus evangelista a 6.*

B0370 Washington, DC. Catholic University of America. Mullen Library. Biblioteca Albani Urbinas F V.10 [MS 203]. Choirbook. Dated 1726. Provenance Rome, Sistine Chapel, copied by Giovanni Domenico Biondini. i + 57ff.

Contains motet f.40v, *Ave Maris stella a 4.*

B0371 Washington, DC. Catholic University of America. Mullen Library. Biblioteca Albani Urbinas F V.11 [MS 204]. Choirbook. Dated 1726. Provenance Rome, Sistine Chapel, copied by Giovanni Domenico Biondini. i + 45ff [contains plainsong propers as well as polyphony].

Contains mass f.2v, *Missa Assumpta est Maria a 6*; motet f.25v, *Assumpta est Maria a 6.*

B0372 Washington, DC. Folger Shakespeare Library. MSS V.a.405–407 (olim 460328). Three partbooks of original four. Early 17th century. Provenance English, household of Edward Paston.

Reported to contain one work by Palestrina.

B0373 Wroclaw [Breslau]. Biblioteka Uniwersytecka, Oddzial Zbiorow Muzycznych. MS Brieger Musiakaliensammlung K.34. Six partbooks. Dated circa 1600. Provenance Brzeg [Brieg], derived from prints published 1597–1599, copied in various hands.

Contains no.10, *Confitebor tibi Domine a 8* [secunda pars *Notas facite*] [ascribed to Clavius in this source; Berlin, Staatsbibliothek zu Berlin, Sammlung Bohn, Mus.ms.15 (formerly Breslau, Stadtbibliothek, MS Mus. 15) ascribes this to Palestrina as no.303].

B0374 Wroclaw [Breslau]. Biblioteka Uniwersytecka, Oddzial Zbiorow Muzycznych. MS Brieger Musiakaliensammlung K.36. Six partbooks. Dated 1592. Provenance Brzeg [Brieg], contains contents of RISM 1585/17, RISM L981, RISM S2300, with MS additions.

Contains no.29, *O Domine Jesu Christe a 6.*

B0375 Wroclaw [Breslau]. Biblioteka Uniwersytecka, Oddzial Zbiorow Muzycznych. MS Brieger Musiakaliensammlung K.40. One partbook. Last quarter of 16th century, some additions possibly extend into early 17th century. Provenance Brzeg [Brieg], contains contents of RISM L880, U125, L871, with MS additions at end.

Contains no.30, *O Domine Jesu Christe a 6.*

B0376 Wroclaw [Breslau]. Biblioteka Uniwersytecka, Oddzial Zbiorow Muzycznych. MS Brieger Musiakaliensammlung K.53. Three partbooks. Late 16th century. Contents derive from prints dated 1568 and 1586, in various hands.

Contains no.17, *Hodie Christus natus est a 8.*

B0377 Zwickau. Ratsschulbibliothek. MS XXXI, 32 (=Vollhardt MS 17). Five partbooks of original six. Last third of 16th century. Provenance Zwickau, copied by C. Freund for use at Church of St. Mary.

Contains motet no.79, *Dum complerentur dies Pentecostes a 6* [secunda pars *Dum ergo essent*]; no.17, *Viri Galilaei qui statis a 6* [secunda pars *Ascendit Deus*].

B0378 Zwickau. Ratsschulbibliothek. MS XXXIII, 34 (=Vollhardt MS 19). Five partbooks. Dated ca. 1580. Provenance Zwickau, copied by C. Freund for use at Church of St. Mary.

Reported to contain one work by Palestrina, unidentified [only anonymous titles listed].

B0379 Zwickau. Ratsschulbibliothek. MS LIII, 1 (=Vollhardt MS 627). Four partbooks of an original five.

Contains madrigal *Io son ferito ahi lasso a 5.*

B0380 Zwickau. Ratsschulbibliothek. MS LXXIV, 1 (=Vollhardt MS 11). Six partbooks. Late 16th century. Provenance Zwickau, copied by Johann Stoll for use at Church of St. Mary.

Contains motets no.76, *Viri Galilaei a 6* [secunda pars *Ascendit Deus*]; no.79, *Dum complerentur a 6* [secunda pars *Dum ergo essent*]; no.128, *O admirabile commercium a 5.*

B0381 Zwickau. Ratsschulbibliothek. MS XCVII, 2 (=Vollhardt MS 47). Two partbooks. Dated 1625. Provenance Zwickau, probably copied by Daniel Ferber.

Reported to contain two works by Palestrina, unidentified [only anonymous titles listed].

Chapter 4

Modern Editions of Palestrina's Music I: Comprehensive Editions

I. The "Haberl" Edition (1862–1907)

C0001 Giovanni Pierluigi da Palestrina. *Opera omnia,* ed. Franz Xaver Haberl et al. Leipzig Breitkopf & Härtel, 1862–1907. 33 vols.

This is described as the first critically supervised collected edition. Each volume of music is printed with the cleffings and notes values found in the primary sources. Each has a substantial preface with detailed information about the sources consulted for the works contained in it. Volumes 1–6, however, were not initially designated as part of this edition and were published separately. Although this *opera omnia* is popularly known as the "Haberl" edition, several editors contributed: Theodor de Witt edited vols. 1–3, Franz Espagne edited vols. 4–8, and Franz Commer edited vol. 9. Haberl himself was responsible for vols. 10–33.

Reprints of This Edition

C0002 Giovanni Pierluigi da Palestrina. *Works.* Farnborough: Gregg International Publishers, 1968. 33 vols [facsimile reprint].

C0003 Giovanni Pierluigi da Palestrina. *Opera omnia,* ed. Franz Xaver Haberl et al., 1862–1907. New York: University Music Editions, 1968 [facsimile reprint on microfiche].

Contents

[Volume 1] *Motetten von Pierluigi da Palestrina in Partitur gesetzt und redigirt von Theodor de Witt. Erster Band. Fünf- Sechs- und Siebenstimmige Motetten* [pub. 1862]. [Book I of motets (1569), for five, six, and seven parts]

Five-Part Works

1. *O admirabile commercium* (pp.3–5)
2. *Stella quam viderant Magi* (pp.6–9)
3. *O Antoni eremita* (pp.10–13)
4. *Senex puerum portabat* (pp.14–17)
   [secunda pars:] *Hodie beata Virgo Maria* (pp.18–21)
5. *Suscipe verbum Virgo Maria* (pp.22–25)
   [secunda pars:] *Paries quidem filium* (pp.26–29)
6. *Alleluja! tulerunt Dominum* (pp.30–33)
7. *Crucem sanctam subiit* (pp.34–36)
8. *O beata et gloriosa Trinitas* (pp.37–40)
   [secunda pars:] *O vera summa sempiterna Trinitas* (pp.40–43)

9. *Ego sum panis vivus* (pp.43–46)
   [secunda pars:] *Panis quem ego dabo* (pp.47–50)
10. *Puer qui natus est* (pp.50–53)
11. *Beatae Mariae Magdalenae* (pp.54–57)
12. *Sancte Paule apostole* (pp.57–60)
13. *Beatus Laurentius orabat* (pp.61–63)
14. *Hodie nata est beata Virgo* (pp.64–67)
15. *O beatum virum* (pp.67–70)
16. *Venit Michael archangelus* (pp.71–74)
17. *O beatum pontificem* (pp.74–78)
18. *Deus qui dedisti legem* (pp.79–82)
19. *Lapidabant Stephanum* (pp.83–86)
20. *Hic est discipulus ille* (pp.87–90)
21. *Sicut lilium inter spinas* (pp.90–94)
22. *Quam pulchri sunt gressus* (pp.94–97)
23. *Unus ex duobus* (pp.98–101)
24. *Cum pervenisset beatus Andreas* (pp.101–104)

Six-Part Works

25. *Viri Galilaei quid statis* (pp.105–107)
   [secunda pars:] *Ascendit Deus in jubilatione* (pp.108–110)
26. *Dum complerentur dies pentecostes* (pp.111–114)
   [secunda pars:] *Dum ergo essent in unum discipuli* (pp.115–117)
27. *Pulchra es, O Maria Virgo* (pp.118–122)
28. *Solve jubente Deo* (pp.123–125)
   [secunda pars:] *Quodcumque ligaveris* (pp.126–129)
29. *Vidi turbam magnam* (pp.129–133)
   [secunda pars:] *Et omnes angeli stabant* (pp.134–137)
30. *O magnum mysterium* (pp.137–140)
   [secunda pars:] *Quem vidistis pastores* (pp.141–144)
31. *O Domine Jesu Christe* (pp.144–145)

Seven-Part Works

32. *Tu es Petrus* (pp.146–151)
33. *Virgo prudentissima* (pp.152–157)
   [secunda pars:] *Maria Virgo* (pp.158–162)

[Volume 2] *Motetten von Pierluigi da Palestrina in Partitur gesetzt und redigirt von Theodor de Witt. Zweiter Band. Fünf- Sechs- und Achtstimmige Motetten* [pub. 1862]. [Book II of motets (1572) for five, six, and eight parts]

Five-Part Works

1. *O Virgo simul et mater* (pp.3–7)
2. *Memor esto verbi tui servo tuo* (pp.7–11)
3. *Corona aurea* (pp.12–15)
   [secunda pars:] *Domine praevenisti eum* (pp.15–18)
4. *In illo tempore egressus* (pp.18–22)
5. *O sacrum convivium* (pp.23–26)
6. *Coenantibus illis accepi Jesus* (pp.26–29)
7. *Derelinquat impius viam* (pp.29–33)
8. *Ascendo ad patrem meam* (pp.33–36)
   [secunda pars:] *Ego rogabo patrem* (pp.37–39)

9. *Homo quidam fuit* (pp.39–43)
10. *Canite tuba in Sion* (pp.43–46)
    [secunda pars:] *Rorate coeli* (pp.46–50)
11. *Exi cito in plateas* (pp.50–53)
12. *Circuire* [Angelo Pierluigi] (pp.53–56)
    [secunda pars:] *In hac cruce te invenit* (pp.57–59)
13. *Gaude Barbara beata* (pp.59–62)
    [secunda pars:] *Gaude quia meruisti* (pp.63–67)
14. *Domine Pater* [Silla Pierluigi] (pp.67–70)
15. *Confitebor tibi Domine* [Rodolfo Pierluigi] (pp.70–73)
16. *Peccantem me quotidie* (pp.73–76)
17. *Dominus Jesus in qua nocte* (pp.77–80)

Six-Part Works

18. *Tribularer si nescirem* (pp.81–84)
    [secunda pars:] *Secundum multitudinem dolorum* (pp.84–88)
19. *Veni Domine et non tardare* (pp.88–91)
    [secunda pars:] *Excita Domine* (pp.91–94)
20. *Hierusalem, cito veniet salus tua* (pp.94–97)
    [secunda pars:] *Ego enim sum Dominus* (pp.98–101)
21. *Beata Barbara* (pp.101–105)
    [secunda pars:] *Gloriosem mortem* (pp.105–109)
22. *Sancta et immaculata Virginitas* (pp.109–112)
    [secunda pars:] *Benedicta tu* (pp.112–115)
23. *Cantabo Domino in vita mea* (pp.115–118)
    [secunda pars:] *Deficiant peccatores* (pp.119–121)
24. *Tu es Petrus et super hanc petram* (pp.121–124)
    [secunda pars:] *Quodcumque ligaveris* (pp.121–127)
25. *Nunc dimittis servum tuum* [Silla Pierluigi] (pp.128–131)

Eight-Part Works

26. *Confitebor tibi Domine* (pp.132–137)
    [secunda pars:] *Notas facite in populis* (pp.138–142)
27. *Laudate pueri Dominum* (pp.142–147)
    [secunda pars:] *Quis sicut Dominus Deus* (pp.148–153)
28. *Domine in virtuta tua* (pp.153–158)
    [secunda pars:] *Magna est gloria ejus* (pp.159–163)
29. *Laudate Dominum omnes gentes* (pp.164–168)

[Volume 3] *Motetten von Pierluigi da Palestrina in Partitur gesetzt und redigirt von Theodor de Witt. Dritter Band. Fünf- Sechs- und Achtstimmige Motetten* [pub. 1862]. [Book III of motets (1575) for five, six, and eight parts]

Five-Part Works

1. *Pater noster* (pp.3–6)
2. *Ave Maria gratia plena* (pp.6–9)
3. *Cantantibus organis, Caecilia* (pp.9–12)
   [secunda pars:] *Biduanis ac triduanis* (pp.12–15)
4. *Caro mea vere est cibus* (pp.15–18)
5. *Angelus Domini descendit de coelo* (pp.18–23)
   [secunda pars:] *Et introeuntes in momentum* (pp.23–27)
6. *Congrega, Domine* (pp.28–31)

[secunda pars:] *Afflige opprimentes nos* (pp.32–35)
7. *Inclytae sanctae virginis Catherinae* (pp.36–38)
8. *Fuit homo missus a Deo* (pp.39–41)
[secunda pars:] *Erat Joannes in deserto* (pp.42–44)
9. *O lux et decus Hispaniae* (pp.45–47)
[secunda pars:] *O singulare praesidium* (pp.48–51)
10. *Quid habes Hester* (pp.51–54)
[secunda pars:] *Vidi te Domine* (pp.55–58)
11. *Tradent enim vos* (pp.59–62)
12. *Sanctificavit Dominus* (pp.62–65)
13. *O quam metuendus* (pp.66–69)
14. *Jubilate Deo omnes terra* (pp.69–72)
[secunda pars:] *Laudate nomen ejus* (pp.72–75)
15. *Omnipotens sempiterne Deus* (pp.75–78)
16. *O sancte praesul Nicolae* (pp.78–82)
[secunda pars:] *Gaude praesul optime* (pp.82–85)
17. *Domine Deus, qui conteris* (pp.85–88)
[secunda pars:] *Tu Domine cui humilium* (pp.89–91)
18. *Manifesto vobis veritatem* (pp.92–95)
[secunda pars:] *Pax vobis, noli timere* (pp.96–99)

Six-Part Works
19. *Susanna ab improbis* (pp.100–103)
[secunda pars:] *Postquam autem* (pp.103–107)
20. *Cum ortus fuerit* (pp.107–110)
21. *Rex pacificus* (pp.111–113)
22. *Haec dies, quam fecit Dominus* (pp.114–116)
23. *Columna es immobilis* (pp.116–119)
24. *Judica me Deus, et discerne* (pp.120–123)
25. *Accepit Jesus calicem* (pp.123–126)
26. *O bone Jesu exaudi me* (pp.127–129)
27. *Deus qui ecclesiam tuam* (pp.129–133)

Eight-Part Works
28. *Surge illuminare Hierusalem* (pp.134–138)
29. *Lauda Sion* (pp.138–143)
30. *Veni Sancte Spiritus* (pp.143–149)
31. *Ave Regina coelorum* (pp.150–154)
32. *Hodie Christus natus est* (pp.155–159)
33. *Jubilate Deo* (pp.160–166)

[Volume 4] *Motetten von Pierluigi da Palestrina in Partitur gesetzt von Theodor de Witt. Vierter Band. Fünfstimmige Motetten redigirt und herausgegeben con Franz Espagne* [pub. 1874]. [Book IV of motets (*Canticum canticorum*, 1583–1584); Book V of motets (1584), five-part motets]

Book IV
1. *Osculetur me osculo oris sui* (pp.3–5)
2. *Trahe me post te* (pp.5–8)
3. *Nigra sum, sed formosa* (pp.8–11)
4. *Vineam meam non custodivi* (pp.11–13)

5. *Si ignoras te, o pulchra inter mulieres* (pp.14–16)
6. *Pulchrae sunt genae tuae* (pp.17–19)
7. *Fasciculus myrrhae* (pp.20–22)
8. *Ecce tu pulcher es, dilecte mi* (pp.22–24)
9. *Tota pulchra es amina mea* (pp.25–27)
10. *Vulnerasti cor meum* (pp.27–30)
11. *Sicut lillium inter spinas* (pp.30–33)
12. *Introduxit me Rex in cellam* (pp.34–36)
13. *Laeva ejus sub capite meo* (pp.36–38)
14. *Vox dilecti mei* (pp.39–41)
15. *Surge, propera amica mea* (pp.41–44)
16. *Surge amica mea, speciosa mea* (pp.44–47)
17. *Dilectus meus mihi et ego illi* (pp.47–49)
18. *Surgem et circuibo civitatem* (pp.50–52)
19. *Adjuro vos, filiae Hierusalem* (pp.52–55)
20. *Caput ejus aurum optimum* (pp.55–58)
21. *Dilectus meus descendit in hortum suum* (pp.58–60)
22. *Pulchra es amica mea* (pp.61–63)
23. *Quae est ista* (pp.63–65)
24. *Descendi in hortum meum* (pp.66–68)
25. *Quam pulchri sunt gressus tui* (pp.68–71)
26. *Duo ubera tua* (pp.71–74)
27. *Quam pulchra es et quam decora* (pp.75–77)
28. *Guttur tuum sicut* (pp.78–80)
29. *Veni, veni dilecte mi* (pp.81–83)

Book V

1. *Laetus Hyperboream* (pp.91–93)
   [secunda pars:] *O patruo pariterque* (pp.93–96)
2. *Paucitas dierum meorum* (pp.96–98)
   [secunda pars:] *Manus tuae Domine* (pp.98–100)
3. *Tempus est, ut revertar* (pp.101–103)
   [secunda pars:] *Nisi ego abiero* (pp.104–106)
4. *Domine secundum actum meum* (pp.106–109)
5. *Ave Trinitatis sanctuarium* (pp.109–112)
6. *Parce mihi Domine* (pp.112–115)
   [secunda pars:] *Peccavi, peccavi* (pp.115–118)
7. *Orietur stella* (pp.118–121)
8. *Aegypte noli flere* (pp.121–124)
9. *Ardens est cor meum* (pp.124–127)
10. *Sic Deus dilexit mundum* (pp.128–130)
11. *Surge Petre* (pp.130–134)
12. *Apparuit caro suo* (pp.134–137)
13. *Ecce merces Sanctorum* (pp.137–140)
14. *Videns secundus* (pp.140–143)
15. *Rex Melchior* (pp.143–145)
16. *Ave Regina coelorum* (pp.146–148)
17. *Gaude gloriosa* (pp.149–151)
18. *Exultate Deo* (pp.151–154)

19. *Tribulationes civitatum* (pp.154–157)
    [secunda pars:] *Peccavimus* (pp.157–159)
20. *Surge sancte Dei* (pp.159–162)
    [secunda pars:] *Ambula sancte Dei* (pp.162–165)
21. *Salve Regina* (pp.165–167)
    [secunda pars:] *Eia ergo advocata* (pp.167–169)

[Volume 5] *Motetten von Pierluigi da Palestrina. Fünfter Band. Vierstimmige Motetten redigirt und herausgegeben von Franz Espagne* [pub. 1875]. [Four-part motets of the *Motecta Festorum totius anni* (first pub. 1564). Espagne edition facsimile title page from print of 1590)]

Book I

1. In Festo Nativitatis Domini. *Dies sanctificatus* (pp.3–5)
2. In Festo S. Stephani. *Lapidabant Stephanum* (pp.5–8)
3. In Festo S. Joannis Evangelistae. *Valde honorandus est* (pp.8–10)
4. In Die Circumcisionis Domini. *Magnus haereditatis mysterium* (pp.11–13)
5. In Epiphania Domini. *Tribus miraculis* (pp.14–17)
6. In Festo Purificationis B. Mariae. *Hodie beata Virgo Maria* (pp.17–20)
7. In Festo Annuntiationis B. Mariae. *Ave Maria gratia plena* (pp.20–22)
8. In Festo Resurrectionis Domini. *Jesus junxit se* (pp.23–26)
9. In Festo Ascensionis Domini. *O Rex gloriae* (pp.26–29)
10. In Die Pentecostes. *Loquebantur variis linguis* (pp.29–32)
11. In Festo Sanctae Trinitatis. *Benedicta sit Sancta Trinitas* (pp.33–35)
12. In Festo Corporis Christi. *Lauda Sion Salvatorem* (pp.36–38)
13. In Festo S. Joannis Baptistae. *Fuit homo missus a Deo* (pp.38–41)
14. In Festo S. Petri Apostoli. *Tu es pastor ovium* (pp.41–43)
15. In Die Sancti Pauli Apostoli. *Magnus Sanctus Paulus* (pp.44–46)
16. In Festo Visitationis Beatae Mariae. *Surge, propera amica mea* (pp.47–49)
17. In Die Sanctae Mariae Magdalenae. *In diebus illis* (pp.50–53)
18. In Festo Sancti Laurentii. *Beatus Laurentius* (pp.54–56)
19. In Assumptione Beatae Mariae. *Quae est ista* (pp.57–59)
20. In Decollatione Sancti Joannes Baptistae. *Misso Herodes spiculatore* (pp.60–62)
21. In Festo Nativitatis Beatae Mariae. *Nativitas tua* (pp.63–65)
22. In Festo Sanctae Crucis. *Nos autem gloriari* (pp.66–68)
23. In Festo Omnium Sanctorum. *Salvator mundi salva nos* (pp.69–71)
24. In Festo Sancti Martini Episcopi. *O quantus luctus* (pp.72–74)
25. In Festo Presentationis Beatae Mariae. *Congratulamini mihi omnes* (pp.74–76)
26. In Festo Sanctae Caeciliae. *Dum aurora finem daret* (pp.77–79)
27. In Festo Sancti Andreae. *Doctor bonus* (pp.80–83)
28. In Festo Conceptionis Beatae Mariae. *Quam pulchri sunt* (pp.83–86)

Common of Saints

29. In Festo Apostolorum. *Tollite jugum meum* (pp.87–89)
30. In Festo Evangelistorum. *Isti sunt viri sancti* (pp.89–92)
31. In Festo Unius Martyris. *Hic est vere martyr* (pp.92–95)

32. In Festo Plurimorum Martyrum. *Gaudent in coelis* (pp.96–98)
33. In Festo Confessorum Pontificum. *Iste est qui ante Deum* (pp.99–102)
34. In Festo Confessorum non Pontificum. *Beatus vir qui suffert* (pp.102–105)
35. In Festo Virginum. *Veni sponsa Christi* (pp.105–107)
36. In Dedicatione Templi. *Exaudi Domine* (pp.107–109)

Book II (pub. 1587; fascimile title page from edition of 1604)

1. *Domine quando veneris* (pp.117–118)
   [secunda pars:] *Commissa mea* (pp.119–120)
2. *Heu mihi Domine* (pp.121–123)
   [secunda pars:] *Anima mea turbata* (pp.123–125)
3. *Super flumina Babylonis* (pp.125–127)
4. *Ecce nunc benedicite Dominum* (pp.128–130)
5. *Ad te levavi oculos meos* (pp.130–132)
   [secunda pars:] *Miserere nostri Domine* (pp.133–134)
6. *Ad Dominum cum tribularer* (pp.135–136)
   [secunda pars:] *Sagittae potentis* (pp.137–138)
7. *Fundamenta ejus* (pp.139–141)
   [secunda pars:] *Numquid Sion dicet* (pp.141–143)
8. *Quid vidisti me Thoma* (pp.144–145)
9. *Ego sum panis vivus* (pp.146–148)
10. *Sicut cervus desiderat* (pp.148–150)
    [secunda pars:] *Sitivit anima mea* (pp.150–152)
11. *Ave Regina coelorum*. Paribus Vocibus (pp.152–154)
    [secunda pars:] *Gaude gloriosa* (pp.154–156)
12. *Alma redemptoris mater*. Paribus Vocibus (pp.156–158)
    [secunda pars:] *Tu quae genuisti natura mirante* (pp.158–160)
13. *Salve Regina* (pp.160–162)
    [secunda pars:] *Eja ergo advocata nostra* (pp.162–164)
14. *Ave Maria gratia plena*. Paribus Vocibus (pp.164–167)
15. *Haec dies quam fecit* (pp.167–169)
16. *Confitemini Domino*. Paribus Vocibus (pp.170–171)
17. *Pueri Hebraeorum*. Paribus Vocibus (pp.172–173)
18. *Sub tuum praesidium*. Paribus Vocibus (pp.173–175)
19. *Adoramus te Christe*. Paribus Vocibus (pp.176–177)
20. *Surrexit pastor bonus* (pp.177–179)
21. *Gloriosi principes* (pp.180–181)

[Volume 6] *Werke von Pierluigi da Palestrina. Sechster Band. Fünf- sechs- und achtstimmige Motetten aus dem Nachlass. Herausgegeben von Franz Espagne* [pub. 1876]. [Five-, six-, and eight-part motets]

Eight-Part Works [pub. 1614]

1. *Sub tuum praesidium* (pp.1–4)
2. *Fratres ego enim accepi* (pp.4–9)
3. *Caro mea vere est cibus* (pp.10–14)
4. [secunda pars:] *Hic est panis* (pp.14–18)

"From the archive of the papal chapel"

Five-Part Works

5. *Tu es pastor ovium* (pp.21–24)

6. [secunda pars:] *Quodcumque ligaveris* (pp.24–27)

Six-Part Works

7. In Assumptione Beatae Mariae Virginis. *Assumpta est Maria* (pp.28–31)
8. [secunda pars:] *Quae est ista* (pp.31–35)
9. In Festo S. Stephani Protomartyris. *Cum autem esset Stephanus* (pp.36–38)
10. [secunda pars:] *Positis autem genibus* (pp.39–41)
11. In Festo S. Joannis Apostoli et Evangelistae. *Hic est beatissimus* (pp.41–44)
12. [secunda pars:] *Hic est discipulis ille* (pp.45–47)
13. In Festo Purificationis Beatae Mariae Virginis. *Responsum accepit* (pp.48–50)
14. [secunda pars:] *Cum inducerent puerum Jesum* (pp.50–53)
15. *Tradent enim vos in conciliis* (pp.53–56)

Eight-Part Works

16. *Surrexit pastor bonus* (pp.57–61)
17. [secunda pars:] *Et enim pascha nostrum* (pp.61–65)
18. *Jesus junxit se discipulis* (pp.66–71)
19. [secunda pars:] *Et increpavit eos dicens* (pp.71–75)
20. *Spiritus sanctus replevit* (pp.76–82)
21. In Assumptione Beatae Mariae Virginis. *Hodie gloriosa semper Virgo* (pp.82–86)
22. [secunda pars:] *Regina mundum hodie* (pp.86–89)
23. *Et ambulabunt gentes in lumine* [Secunda pars of the motet "Surge, illuminare Jerusalem" (see vol.3 p.134)] (pp.90–95)
24. *Stabat Mater dolorosa* (pp.96–108)

"From the archive of the Capella Giulia in the Vatican"

Eight-Part Works

25. *Ave mundi spes, Maria* (pp.111–118)
26. *Beata es, Virgo Maria* (pp.118–121)
27. *Ave Maria, gratia plena* (pp.121–124)
28. *O quam suavis est, Domine, spiritus tuus* (pp.125–129)
29. *Disciplinam et sapientiam docuit eos* (pp.129–134)
30. *O bone Jesu, exaudi me* (pp.135–139)
31. *O Domine Jesu Christe* (pp.140–143)
32. *Expurgate vetus fermentum* (pp.144–149)
33. *Pater noster, qui es in coelis* (pp.150–153)
34. *Salve Regina, mater misericordiae* (pp.153–158)
35. *Alma redemptoris Mater* (pp.159–164)
36. *Regina coeli, laetare* (pp.165–170)

[Volume 7] *Motetten von Pierluigi da Palestrina. Siebenter band. Vier- sechs- acht- und zwölfstimmige Motetten aus dem Nachlass. Herausgegeben von Franz Espagne* [pub. 1874]. [Four-, six-, eight-, and twelve-part motets, plus an alphabetical index (by text incipit) of vols.1–7 (pp.201–206)]

Six-Part Works

1. *Salve Regina, mater misericordiae* (pp.3–6)
2. [secunda pars:] *Eja ergo, advocata nostra* (pp.6–9)

Eight-Part Works
3. *O pretiosum et admirandum convivium* (pp.10–14)
4. *O admirabile commercium* (pp.14–19)
5. *Videntes stellam Magi* (pp.19–24)
Twelve-Part Works
6. *Laudate Dominum in tympanis* (pp.25–34)
7. *Ecce nunc benedicite Dominum* (pp.35–43)
8. *Nunc dimittis servum tuum, Domine* (pp.44–52)
"From the library of the Roman College"
Four-Part Works
9. In Ascensione Domini. *Ascendens Christus in altum* (pp.55–57)
10. *Domine secundum actum meum* (pp.57–59)
11. In Missis defunctorum. *Ne recorderis peccata mea* (pp.60–62)
12. *Ecce nunc benedicite Dominum* (pp.62–64)
13. In Festo S. Gregorii Papae. *Deus, qui animae famuli tui Gregorii* (pp.64–66)
14. *Innocentes pro Christo infantes* (pp.66–68)
15. In Festo S. Michaelis Archangeli. *Princeps gloriosissime* (pp.68–70)
16. In Festo S. Barbarae Virginis. *Gaude, Barbara beata* (pp.70–72)
Eight-Part Works
17. *Alma redemptoris Mater* (pp.73–75)
18. *Tria sunt munera pretiosa* (pp.76–80)
19. *Fili, non te frangant labores* (pp.80–83)
20. [secunda pars:] *Ecce veniet dies illa* (pp.84–87)
21. *Haec dies, quam fecit Dominus* (pp.88–91)
22. *Lauda Sion Salvatorem* (pp.91–105)
23. *Victimae paschali laudes* (pp.105–111)
24. *Victimae paschali laudes* (pp.112–117)
25. *Veni Sancte Spiritus* (pp.117–123)
26. *Ave Regina coelorum* (pp.124–129)
Twelve-Part Works
27. *Stabat Mater dolorosa* (pp.130–150)
"From the library of the Barberini Palace"
Eight-Part Works
28. *Apparuit gratia Dei* (pp.153–157)
29. *Dies sanctificatus* (pp.158–162)
30. *Haec est dies praeclara* (pp.163–167)
31. *Congratulamini mihi omnes* (pp.167–171)
32. *Magnus sanctus Paulus* (pp.171–175)
33. [secunda pars:] *Sancte Paule Apostole* (pp.176–180)
34. *Nunc dimittis servum tuum* (pp.181–186)
35. *Omnes gentes plaudite manibus* (pp.187–194)
36. *Victimae paschali laudes* (pp.194–199)

[Volume 8] *Hymnen von Pierluigi da Palestrina. Herausgegeben von Franz Espagne* [pub. 1878]. [Hymns, based on publication of 1589]
1. In Adventu Domini. *Conditor alme siderum* (pp.1–6)
2. In Nativitate et Circumcisione Domini. *Christe redemptor omnium* (pp.6–12)

3. In Nativitate. Ad Laudes. *A solis ortus cardine* (pp.12–17)
4. In Festo Sanctorum Innocentium. *Salvete flores martyrum* (pp.17–19)
5. In Epiphania Domini. *Hostes Herodes impie* (pp.19–22)
6. In Dominicis per Annum. *Lucis creator optime* (pp.23–26)
7. In Sabbatis. *O lux beata, Trinitas* (pp.27–29)
8. In Dominicis Quadragesimae. *Ad preces nostras* (pp.29–35)
9. In Dominica Passionis et Exaltatione S.Crucis. *Vexilla regis prodeunt* (pp.35–41)
10. In Dominicis Tempore Paschali. *Ad coenam Agni providi* (pp.42–46)
11. In Ascensione Domini. *Jesu, nostra redemptio* (pp.47–51)
12. In Festo Pentecostes. *Veni creator Spiritus* (pp.51–56)
13. In Festo Corporis Christi. *Pange lingua gloriosi* (pp.57–61)
14. In Festo Cathedrae S. Petri. *Quodcumque vinclis* (pp.62–63)
15. In Conversione et Commemoratione S.Pauli. *Doctor egregie* (pp.63–65)
16. In Festo Beatae Virginis. *Ave maris stella* (pp.65–69)
17. In Inventione S. Crucis. *Vexilla regis prodeunt* (pp.70–73)
18. In Festo S.Joannis Baptistae. *Ut queant laxis* (pp.73–77)
19. In Festo Apostolorum Petri et Pauli. *Aurea luce* (pp.78–81)
20. In Festo S. Mariae Magdalenae. *Lauda mater ecclesia* (pp. 82–84)
21. In Festo S.Petri ad Vincula. *Petrus beatus* (pp.85–86)
22. In Festo Transfigurationis Domini. *Quicumque Christum quaeritis* (pp.86–89)
23. In Festo S. Michaelis Archangeli. *Tibi Christe, splendor Patris* (pp.90–92)
24. In Festo Omnium Sanctorum. *Christe redemptor omnium* (pp.93–98)
25. In Communi Apostolorum et Evangelistarum. *Exultet coelum laudibus* (pp.98–101)
26. In Festo Apostolorum et Evangelistarum. Tempore Paschali. *Tristes erant Apostoli* (pp.102–105)
27. In Communi Unius Martyrus. *Deus tuorum militum* (pp. 105–109)
28. In Festo Unius Martyrus. Tempore Paschali. *Deus tuorum militum* (pp.110–112)
29. In Commune Plurimorum Martyrum. *Sanctorum meritis* (pp. 113–116)
30. In Festo Plurimorum Martyrum. Tempore Paschali. *Rex gloriose martyrum* (pp.117–119)
31. In Natali Confessorum. *Iste confessor* (pp.119–123)
32. In Natalitiis Virginum et Martyrum. *Jesu corona virginum* (pp. 123–126)
33. In Festo Virginum et Martyrum. Tempore Paschali. *Jesu corona virginum* (pp.127–131)
34. In Festo Sanctarum Mulierum. *Hujus obtentu* (pp.131–132)
35. In Festo Dedicationis Ecclesiae. *Urbs beata Jerusalem* (pp.132–138)
36. In Festo S. Augustini. *Magne pater Augustine* (pp.138–142)
37. In Festo S. Nicolai de Tolentino. *Laudibus summis* (pp.142–147)

38. In Festo S. Antonii de Padua. *En gratulemur hodie* (pp. 147–151)
39. In Festo S. Francisci. In Primis Vesperis. *Proles de coelo prodiit* (pp.152–157)
40. In Festo S. Francisci in Secundis Vesperis. *Decus morum, dux minorum* (pp.157–161)
41. In Quadragesima ad Completorium. *Christe, qui lux es et dies* (pp.161–165)
42. In Festo S. Elisaei. *Prima lux surgens* (pp.165–169)
43. In Festo S. Eliae. *Nunc juvat celsi* (pp.169–173)
44. In Festo S. Alberti. *Mensis Augusti* (pp.173–177)
45. In Festo S. Jacobi. *Hymnus canoris personet* (pp.177–179)

[Volume 9] *Offertorien von Pierluigi da Palestrina. Herausgegeben von Franz Commer* [pub. 1881]. [Offertories, all for five voices, based on 1593 publication]

First Part

1. Dominica prima Adventus. *Ad te levavi animam meam* (pp.3–6)
2. Dominica secunda Adventus. *Deus tu convertens* (pp.6–9)
3. Dominica tertia Adventus. *Benedixisti Domini terram tuam* (pp. 10–12)
4. Dominica quarta Adventus. *Ave Maria gratia plena* (pp.13–15)
5. In Nativitate Domini ad tertiam Missam, et in Circumcisione. *Tui sunt coeli* (pp.16–18)
6. In Festo Sancti Stephani protomartyris. *Elegerunt Apostoli Stephanum levitam* (pp.18–21)
7. In Festo S. Joannis Apostoli. *Justus ut palma* (pp.21–24)
8. In Festo Sanctorum Innocentium. *Anima nostra sicut passer* (pp.24–26)
9. In Festo Sancti Thomae Archiepiscopi et martyris. *Posuiste Domine in capite eius* (pp.27–29)
10. Dominica infra oct. Nativitatis Domini. *Deus enim firmavit orbem terrae* (pp.29–32)
11. In Festo Sancti Silvestri, Papae et conf. *Inveni David servum meum* (pp.32–34)
12. In Epiphania Domini. *Reges Tarsis et insulae* (pp.35–37)
13. Dominica infra octavum Epiphaniae. *Iubilate Deo omnes terra* (pp.37–40)
14. Dominica secunda post Epiphaniam. *Iubilate Deo universa terra* (pp.40–43)
15. Dominica tertia, quarta et V. post Epipha. *Dextera Domini fecit virtutem* (pp.43–45)
16. Dominica in Septuagesima. *Bonum est confiteri* (pp.46–48)
17. Dominica in Sexagesima. *Perfice gressus meos* (pp.48–51)
18. Dominica in Quinquagesima. *Benedictus domine doce me* (pp.51–54)
19. Dominica prima Quadragesimae. *Scapulis suis obumbrabit* (pp.54–57)

20. Dominica secunda Quadragesimae. *Meditabor in mandatis tuis* (pp.57–60)
21. Dominica tertia Quadragesimae. *Iustitiae Domini rectae* (pp.60–63)
22. Dominica quarta Quadragesimae. *Laudate Dominum quia benignus est* (pp.63–66)
23. Dominica de Passione. *Confitebor tibi Domine* (pp.66–69)
24. Dominica Palmarum. *Improperium exspectavit cor meum* (pp.69–72)
25. Dominica Resurrectionis Domini. *Terra tremuit et quievit* (pp.72–75)
26. Dominica in Albis, in octava Paschae. *Angelus Domini descendit* (pp.75–78)
27. Dominica secunda post Pascha. *Deus Deus meus ad te* (pp.78–81)
28. Dominica tertia post Pascha. *Lauda anima mea Dominum* (pp.81–83)
29. Dominica quinta post Pascha. *Benedicite gentes Dominum* (pp.84–87)
30. In Die Ascensione Domini. *Ascendit Deus in iubilatione* (pp.87–89)
31. In Dominica Pentecostes. *Confirma hoc Deus* (pp.90–92)
32. In Festo S.S.Trinitatis. *Benedictus sit Deus Pater* (pp.93–95)
33. In Solemnitate Corporis Christi. *Sacerdotes Domini* (pp.96–98)
34. Dominica secunda post Pentecosten. *Domine convertere* (pp.99–101)
35. Dominica tertia post Pentecosten. *Sperent in te omnes* (pp.102–105)
36. Dominica quarta post Pentecosten. *Illumina oculos neos* (pp.105–108)
37. Dominica quinta post Pentecosten. *Benedicam Dominum* (pp.108–111)
38. Dominica septima post Pentecosten. *Sicut in holocaustis* (pp.111–114)
39. Dominica octava post Pentecosten. *Populum humilem salvum* (pp.114–117)
40. Dominica nona post Pentecosten. *Iustitiae Domini rectae* (pp.117–120)

Second Part

41. Dominica XI post Pentecosten. *Exaltabo te Domine* (pp.125–127)
42. Dominica XII post Pentecosten. *Precatus est Moyses* (pp.128–130)
43. Dominica XIII post Pentecosten. *In te speravi Domine* (pp.131–133)
44. Dominica XIV post Pentecosten. *Immittet Angelus Domini* (pp.134–136)
45. Dominica XV post Pentecosten. *Expectans expectavi Dominum* (pp.137–139)
46. Dominica XVI post Pentecosten. *Domine in auxilium meum* (pp.140–142)
47. Dominica XVII post Pentecosten. *Oravi ad Dominum Deum meum* (pp.143–145)
48. Dominica XVIII post Pentecosten. *Sanctificavit Moyses* (pp.146–148)
49. Dominica XIX post Pentecosten. *Si ambulavero in medio* (pp.149–152)

50. Dominica XX post Pentecosten. *Super flumina Babylonis* (pp.152–154)
51. Dominica XXI post Pentecosten. *Vir erat in terra Hus* (pp.155–157)
52. Dominica XXII post Pentecosten. *Recordare mei Domine* (pp.158–160)
53. Dominica XXIII et XXIV post Pentecosten. *De profundis clamavi* (pp.161–163)
54. In Nativitate S. Joan. Baptistae. *Justus ut palma* (pp.164–166)
55. In Die S. Jacobi Apostoli. *Mihi autem nimis* (pp.167–169)
56. In Festo S. Laurentii Martyris. *Confessio et pulchritudo* (pp.170–172)
57. In Assumptione Beatae Mariae Virginis. *Assumpta est Maria* (pp.173–175)
58. In Festo Dedicationis S. Michaelis, Archang. *Stetit angelus juxta aram* (pp.176–178)
59. In die Commemorationis omnium Sanctorum. *Constitues eos principes* (pp.179–181)
60. In Festo SS. Apost. Philippi et Jacobi. *Confitebuntur coeli* (pp.182–184)
61. In Festo SS. Apost. Simonis et Judae. *In omnem terram exivit* (pp.185–187)
62. In Die S. Matthiae Apostoli. *Justorum animae in manu Dei* (pp.187–190)
63. Commune Sanctorum. *Veritas mea et misericordia* (pp.190–192)
64. Commune plurimum Martyrum. *Laetamini in Domino* (pp.193–195)
65. Commune Virginum. *Afferentur regi virgines* (pp.195–197)
66. In Festo Dedicationis Ecclesiae. *Domine Deus in simplicitate* (pp.198–200)
67. In Festo Purificationis B. Mariae Virginis. *Diffusa est gratia* (pp.200–203)
68. In Festo Cathedrae sancti Petri. *Tu es Petrus* (pp.203–206)

[Volume 10] *Erstes Buch der Messen von Pierluigi da Palestrina. Herausgegeben von Franz Xaver Haberl* [pub. 1880]. [Masses, Book I (1554), based on edition of 1591]

For Four Voices

1. *Missa Ecce sacerdos magnus* (pp.3–31)
2. *Missa O regem coeli* (pp.32–54)
3. *Missa Virtute magna* (pp.55–79)
4. *Missa Gabriel Archangelus* (pp.80–104)

For Five Voices

5. *Missa Ad cenam agni providi* (pp.105–137)
6. *Missa Pro defunctis* (pp.138–152)

For Six Voices

7. *Missa Sine nomine* (pp.153–174)

[Volume 11] *Zweites Buch der Messen von Pierluigi da Palestrina. Herausgegeben von Franz Xaver Haberl* [pub. 1881]. [Masses, Book II (1567)]

For Four Voices
1. *Missa de Beata Virgine* (pp.1–20)
2. *Missa Inviolata* (pp.21–40)
3. *Missa Sine nomine* (pp.41–56)
4. *Missa Ad fugam* (pp.57–70)
For Five Voices
5. *Missa Aspice Domine* (pp.71–96)
6. *Missa Salvum me fac* (pp.97–128)
For Six Voices
7. *Missa Papae Marcelli* (pp.128–155)

[Volume 12] *Drittes Buch der Messen von Pierluigi da Palestrina. Herausgegeben von Franz Xaver Haberl* [pub. 1881]. [Masses, Book III (1570)]
For Four Voices
1. *Missa Spem in alium* (pp.3–25)
2. *Missa Primi toni* (pp.26–49)
3. *Missa Brevis* (pp.50–65)
4. *Missa De Feria* (pp.66–74)
For Five Voices
5. *Missa L'homme arme* [*sic*] (pp.75–104)
6. *Missa Repleatur os meum* (pp.105–134)
For Six Voices
7. *Missa De beata Virgine vel Dominicalis* (pp.135–164)
8. *Missa Ut re mi fa sol la* (pp.165–193)

[Volume 13] *Viertes Buch der Messen von Pierluigi da Palestrina. Herausgegeben von Franz Xaver Haberl* [pub. 1882]. [Masses, Book IV (1582)]
For Four Voices
1. *Missa Prima (Lauda Sion)* (pp.1–14)
2. *Missa Secunda (Primi Toni)* (pp.15–28)
3. *Missa Tertia (Jesu, nostra redemptio)* (pp.29–44)
4. *Missa Quarta* (pp.45–58)
For Five Voices
5. *Missa Prima (Eripe me de inimicis meis)* (pp.59–84)
6. *Missa Secunda* (pp.85–109)
7. *Missa Tertia (O magnum mysterium)* (pp.110–139)

[Volume 14] *Fünftes Buch der Messen von Pierluigi da Palestrina. Herausgegeben von Franz Xaver Haberl* [pub. 1882]. [Masses, Book V (1590)]
For Four Voices
1. *Missa Aeterna Christi munera* (pp.1–14)
2. *Missa Jam Christus astra ascenderat* (pp.15–33)
3. *Missa Panis quem ego dabo* (pp.34–53)
4. *Missa Iste Confessor* (pp.54–65)
For Five Voices
5. *Missa Nigra sum* (pp.66–94)
6. *Missa Sicut lilium inter spinas* (pp.95–117)

For Six Voices
7. *Missa Nasce la gioia mia* (pp.118–139)
8. *Missa Sine nomine* [see Book I, vol.10, p.153]

[Volume 15] *Sechstes Buch der Messen von Pierluigi da Palestrina. Herausgegeben von Franz Xaver Haberl* [pub. 1883]. [Mass, Book VI (1594), based on 1596 Gardano print]
For Four Voices
1. *Missa Dies sanctificatus* (pp.1–21)
2. *Missa In te Domine speravi* (pp.22–43)
3. *Missa Sine nomine* (pp.44–59)
4. *Missa Quam pulchra es* (pp.60–83)
For Five Voices
5. *Missa Dilexi quoniam* (pp.84–112)
For Six Voices
6. *Missa Ave Maria* (pp.113–151)

[Volume 16] *Ioannis Petraloysii Praenestini. Opera Omnia. Tom.XVI. Missarum librum septimum curavit Franciscus Haberl* [pub. 1884]. [Masses, Book VII (1594)]
For Four Voices
1. *Missa Ave Maria* (pp.1–21)
2. *Missa Sanctorum meritis* (pp.22–43)
3. *Missa Emendemus* (pp.44–59)
For Five Voices
4. *Missa Sacerdos et pontifex* (pp.60–84)
5. *Missa Tu es pastor ovium* (pp.85–108)

[Volume 17] *Achtes Buch der Messen von Pierluigi da Palestrina. Herausgegeben von Franz Xaver Haberl* [pub. 1885]. [Masses, Book VIII (1599)]
For Four Voices
1. *Missa Quem dicunt homines* (pp.1–22)
2. *Missa Dum esset Summus Pontifex* (pp.23–37)
For Five Voices
3. *Missa O admirabile commercium* (pp.38–62)
4. *Missa Memor esto* (pp.63–84)
For Six Voices
5. *Missa Dum complerentur* (pp.85–112)
6. *Missa Sacerdotes Domini* (pp.113–140)

[Volume 18] *Neuntes Buch der Messen von Pierluigi da Palestrina. Herausgegeben von Franz Xaver Haberl* [pub. 1886]. [Masses, Book IX (1599)]
For Four Voices
1. *Missa Ave Regina coelorum* (pp.1–20)
2. *Missa Veni sponsa Christi* (pp.21–37)
For Five Voices
3. *Missa Vestiva i colli* (pp.38–63)
4. *Missa Sine nomine* (pp.64–90)

For Six Voices
5. *Missa In te Domine speravi* (pp.91–118)
6. *Missa Te Deum laudamus* (pp.119–143)

[Volume 19] *Zehntes Buch der Messen von Pierluigi da Palestrina. Herausgegeben von Franz Xaver Haberl* [pub. 1888]. [Masses, Book X (1600)]
For Four Voices
1. *Missa In illo tempore* (pp.1–21)
2. *Missa Già fù chi m'ebbe cara* (pp.22–36)
For Five Voices
3. *Missa Petra sancta* (pp.37–62)
4. *Missa O Virgo simul et mater* (pp.63–84)
For Six Voices
5. *Missa Quinti toni* (pp.85–108)
6. *Missa Illumina oculos meos* (pp.109–140)

[Volume 20] *Elftes Buch der Messen von Pierluigi da Palestrina. Herausgegeben von Franz Xaver Haberl* [pub. 1889]. [Masses, Book XI (1600)]
For Four Voices
1. *Missa Descendit angelus Domini* (pp.1–21)
For Five Voices
2. *Missa Regina coeli* (pp.22–49)
3. *Missa Quando lieta sperai* (pp.50–79)
For Six Voices
4. *Missa Octavi toni* (pp.80–105)
5. *Missa Alma redemptoris* (pp.106–132)

[Volume 21] *Zwölftes Buch der Messen von Pierluigi da Palestrina. Herausgegeben von Franz Xaver Haberl* [pub. 1889]. [Masses, Book XII (1601)]
For Four Voices
1. *Missa Regina coeli* (pp.1–21)
2. *Missa O rex gloriae* (pp.22–37)
For Five Voices
3. *Missa Ascendo ad Patrem* (pp.38–61)
4. *Missa Qual è il più grand'Amor* (pp.62–85)
For Six Voices
5. *Missa Tu es Petrus* (pp.86–110)
6. *Missa Viri Galilaei* (pp.111–136)

[Volume 22] *Dreizehntes Buch der Messen von Pierluigi da Palestrina. Herausgegeben von Franz Xaver Haberl* [pub. 1890]. [Masses, Book XIII (1601), four masses in eight parts]
For Eight Voices
1. *Missa Laudate Dominum omnes gentes* (pp.1–39)
2. *Missa Hodie Christus natus est* (pp.40–73)
3. *Missa Fratres ego enim accepi* (pp.74–109)
4. *Missa Confitebor tibi Domine* (pp.110–154)

[Volume 23] *Vierzehntes Buch der Messen von Pierluigi da Palestrina. Nach romis-*

chen Handschriften herausgegeben von Franz Xaver Haberl [pub. 1888]. [Masses, Book XIV, based on Roman manuscripts]
For Four Voices
1. *Missa In majoribus duplicibus* (pp.1–25)
2. *Missa Inminoribus duplicibus* (pp.26–47)
For Five Voices
3. *Missa Beatus Laurentius* (pp.48–70)
4. *Missa O sacrum convivium* (pp.71–96)
For Six Voices
5. *Missa Assumpta est Maria* (pp.97–121)
6. *Missa Veni Creator Spiritus* (pp.122–150)
Appendix:
Alternate Christe, *Missa Assumpta est Maria* (pp.151–152)

[Volume 24] *Fünfzehntes Buch der Messen von Pierluigi da Palestrina. Herausgegeben von Franz Xaver Haberl* [pub. 1887]. [Masses, Book XV, based on manuscript sources]
For Four Voices
1. *Missa Pater noster* (pp.1–19)
For Five Voices
2. *Missa Panem nostrum* (pp.20–45)
3. *Missa Salve Regina* (pp.46–71)
For Six Voices
4. *Missa Sine titulo* (pp.72–104)
5. *Missa Tu es Petrus* (pp.105–128)
6. *Missa Ecce ego Joannes* (pp.129–154)

[Volume 25] *Lamentationen. Herausgegeben von Franz Xaver Haberl* [pub. 1888]. [Principal primary sources: Book I from print of 1583; Book II on MS Lateran 59; Book III on MS Cappella Giulia XV.21; Book IV on MS Ottoboni 2928/3387]
Liber Primus [Book I]
Feria V. In coena Domini
Lectio I [*Incipit Lamentatio . . . Aleph. Quomodo sedet*] (pp.1–4)
Lectio II [*Vau. Et egreesus est*] (pp.4–7)
Lectio III [*Jod. Manum suam*] (pp.8–12)
Feria VI. In Parasceve
Lectio I [*De Lamentatione . . . Cogitavit*] (pp.12–16)
Lectio II [*Lamed. Matribus suis*] (pp.16–19)
Lectio III [*Aleph. Ego vir videns*] (pp.20–23)
Sabbato Sancto
Lectio I [*De Lamentatione . . . Heth. Misericordiae Domini*] (pp.24–28)
Lectio II [*Aleph. Quomodo obscuratum est*] (pp.28–31)
Lectio III [*Incipit oratio . . . Recordare Domine*] (pp.32–35)
Liber Secundus [Book II]
Feria V. In coena Domini
Lectio I [*Incipit Lamentatio . . . Aleph. Quomodo sedet*] (pp.39–42)

Lectio II [*Vau. Et egressus est*] (pp.43–48)
Lectio III [[*Jod. Manum suam*] (pp.49–53)
Feria VI. In Parasceve
Lectio I [*De Lamentatione . . . Cogitavit*] (pp.54–59)
Lectio II [*Lamed. Matribus suis*] (pp.60–65)
Lectio III [*Aleph. Ego vir videns*] (pp.65–69)
Sabbato Sancto.
Lectio I [*De Lamentatione . . . Heth. Misericordiae Domini*] (pp.70–74)
Lectio II [*Aleph. Quomodo obscuratum est*] (pp.74–79)
Lectio III [*Incipit oratio . . . Recordare Domine*] (pp.80–87)
Liber Tertius [Book III]
Feria V. In coena Domini
Lectio I [*Incipit Lamentatio . . . Aleph. Quomodo sedet*] (pp.91–96)
Lectio II [*Vau. Et egressus est*] (pp.97–104)
Lectio III [*Jod. Manum suam*] (pp.104–110)
Feria VI. in Parasceve
Lectio I [*De Lamentatione . . . Heth. Cogitavit*] (pp.111–116)
Lectio II [*Lamed. Matribus suis*] (pp.116–123)
Lectio III [*Aleph. Ego vir videns*] (pp.124–129)
Sabbato Sancto
Lectio I [*De Lamentatione . . . Heth. Misericordiae Domini*] (pp.130–137)
Lectio II [*Aleph. Quomodo obscuratum est*] (pp.137–143)
Lectio III [*Incipit oratio . . . Recordare Domine*] (pp.144–151)
Liber Quartus [Book IV]
Feria V. In coena Domini
Lectio I [*Incipit Lamentatio . . . Aleph. Quomodo sedet*] (pp.155–159)
Lectio II [*Vau. Et egressus est*] (pp.160–166)
Lectio III [*Jod. Manum suam*] (pp.166–173)
Feria VI. In Parasceve
Lectio I [*De Lamentatione . . . Cogitavit*] (pp.173–180)
Lectio II [*Lamed. Matribus suis*] (pp.180–187)
Lectio III [*Aleph. Ego vir videns*] (pp.187–192)
Sabbato Sancto
Lectio I [*De Lamentatione . . . Heth. Misericordiae Domini*] (pp.193–199)
Lectio II [*Aleph. Quomodo obscuratum est*] (pp.200–204)
Lectio III [*Incipit oratio . . . Recordare Domine*] (pp.204–209)

[Volume 26] *Drei Bucher Litaneien, Motetten und Psalmen* [pub. 1886]. *Herausgegeben von Franz Xaver Haberl.* [Three books of litanies, motets, and psalms]
Book I
Litaniae deiparae virginis a 4 (pp.1–29)
Book II
Litaniae deiparae virginis a 4 (pp.33–64)

Book III

1. *Litaniae de Beata Virgine Maria a 5* (pp.67–70)
2. *Litaniae de Beata Virgine Maria a 6* (pp.71–77)
3. *Litaniae de Beata Virgine Maria a 8* (pp.78–94)
4. *Litaniae de Beata Virgine Maria a 8* (pp.95–101)
5. *Litaniae Domini a 8* (pp.102–112)
6. *Litaniae Domini a 8* (pp.113–118)
7. *Litaniae Domini a 8* (pp.119–124)
8. *Litaniae Sacrosanctae Eucharistiae a 8* (pp.125–132)
9. *Litaniae Sacrosanctae Eucharistiae a 8* (pp.133–138)

Appendix

1. *Ad te levavi oculos meos a 12* [original chorus III parts missing; parts in this edition composed by Michael Haller] (pp.139–152)
2. *Beati omnes a 12* [original chorus III parts missing; parts in this edition composed by Michael Haller] (pp.153–165)
3. *Dominus, quis habitabit a 12* [chorus III missing, these parts composed by Michael Haller] (pp.166–177)
4. *Jubilate Deo omnis terra a 12* [secunda pars: *Laudate nomen ejus*; original chorus III parts missing; these parts composed by Michael Haller for the present edition] (pp.178–196)
5. *O quam bonus et suavis a 12* [chorus III missing; these parts composed by Michael Haller for the present edition] (pp.197–210)
6. Antiphona: *Salve Regina a 12* [chorus III missing; these parts composed by Michael Haller for the present edition] (pp.211–220)

[Volume 27] *35 Magnificat (Lobgesang Mariens). Herausgegeben von Franz Xaver Haberl* [pub. 1885]

Liber Primus

[four voices, odd-numbered verse settings]

Primi toni (pp.1–5)
Secundi toni (pp.6–10)
Tertii toni (pp.11–15)
Quarti toni (pp.15–20)
Quinti toni (pp.20–25)
Sexti toni (pp.26–30)
Septimi toni (pp.30–35)
Octavi toni (pp.35–40)

[Even-numbered verse settings]

Primi toni (pp.40–45)
Secundi toni (pp.45–49)
Tertii toni (pp.49–53)
Quarti toni (pp.54–58)
Quinti toni (pp.58–62)
Sexti toni (pp.63–67)
Septimi toni (pp.67–72)
Octavi toni (pp.72–76)

Liber Secundus

[four to five voices, even-numbered verse settings]

Primi toni (pp.79–87)
Secundi toni (pp.88–96)
Tertii toni (pp.97–104)
Quarti toni (pp.105–112)
Quinti toni (pp.113–120)
Sexti toni (pp.121–127)
Septimi toni (pp.128–135)
Octavi toni (pp.136–143)

Liber Tertius
[five to seven voices, odd-numbered verse settings]
Primi toni (pp.147–157)
Secundi toni (pp.158–167)
Tertii toni (pp.168–178)
Quarti toni (pp.178–191)
Quinti toni (pp.191–202)
Sexti toni (pp.202–214)
Septimi toni (pp.214–224)
Octavi toni (pp.225–234)

Appendix
Primi toni octonis vocibus [from Vatican Library, Cappella Sistina MS 29, all verses] (pp.235–243)
Quarti toni cum quatuor vocibus paribus [from Rome, San Giovanni in Laterano, MS59, even-numbered verses] (pp.244–250)
Sexti toni [from Vatican Library, Cappella Giulia MS47, even-numbered verses, four to five voices] (pp.251–258)

[Volume 28] *Vierstimmige Madrigale (1. und 2. Buch). Drei- bis sechstimmige Madrigale (3. Buch). Herausgegeben von Franz Xaver Haberl* [pub. 1884]. [Four-part madrigals, books 1 and 2. Three- to six-part madrigals, Book 3, based on publications in anthologies. Madrigal texts pp.xi–xxi]

Book I for Four Voices
1. *Deh or foss'io col vago* (pp.1–2)
2. *S'i'l dissi mai ch'i venga in odio* (pp.3–4)
3. *Queste saranno ben lagrime* (pp.5–7)
4. *Che non fia che giammai dal cor* (pp.7–9)
5. *Rime, dai sospir miei nati e dal pianto* (pp.10–12)
6. *Lontan dalla mia diva* (pp.12–14)
7. *Nessun visse giammai più* (pp.15–16)
8. *La ver l'aurora, che si dolce l'aura* (pp.17–18)
9. *Chiara, si chiaro e de'vostr'occhi* (pp.19–20)
10. *Che estinguerà il mio foco* (pp.21–23)
11. *Donna, vostra mercede ogni pietade eccede* (pp.24–26)
12. *Già fu chi m'ebbe cara* (pp.26–28)
13. *Ovver de'sensi è priva* (pp.29–30)
14. *Amor, Fortuna, e la mia mente* (pp.31–33)
    [seconda parte:] *Ne spero i dolci di tornino* (pp.33–34)
15. *Che debbo far, che mi consigli, Amore?* (pp.34–36)
16. *Gitene liete rime, ov'er si siede* (pp.37–39)
17. *Mentr a le dolci e le purpuree labbia* (pp.39–41)

18. *Amor, che meco in quest'ombre ti stava* (pp.42–43)
19. *Ecc'ove giunse prima* (pp.43–45)
20. *Vaghi pensier, che così passo* (pp.45–47)
21. *Mentre ch'al mar discenderanno* (pp.47–49)
22. *Quai rime fur si chiare* (pp.50–52)
23. *Ecc'oscurati i raggi al sole* (pp.52–54)
    [seconda parte:] *Rara beltà non mai più vista* (pp.54–56)
    [terza parte:] *Questo doglioso stil* (pp.57–58)
    [quarta parte:] *Mai fu più cruda* (pp.59–60)
    [quinta parte:] *Privo di fede oltra l'usato* (pp.61–62)
    [ultima parte:] *Ma voi, fioriti ed onorati* (pp.63–66)

Book II of Madrigals for Four Voices

1. *Così la fama scriva in sempiterni marmi* [dedication "All' illustrissi. ed eccellentissi. Sign. Giulio Cesare Colonna principe di Palestina"] (pp.71–72)
2. *S'un squardo un fa beato* (pp.73–75)
3. *Amor, ben puoi tu ormai* (pp.75–77)
4. *Partomi Donna, e teco lascio il core* (pp.77–80)
5. *Veramente inamore* (pp.80–82)
6. *Gioia m'abond'al cor* (pp.82–84)
7. *Donna gentil, quando talor degnate* (pp.85–87)
8. *Io dovea ben pensarmi* (pp.87–90)
9. *Se'l pensier che mi strugge* (pp.90–92)
10. *Che dunque fia, se voi donna* (pp.92–95)
11. *Mirate altrove, vita mia* (pp.95–97)
12. *Si è debile il filo a cui sattene* (pp.97–100)
13. *I vaghi fiori e l'amorose fronde* (pp.100–102)
14. *Mori quasi il mio core* (pp.103–105)
15. *Alla riva del Tebro* (pp.105–107)
16. *Amor, quando fioria mia speme* (pp.107–109)
17. *Beltà, se com'in ment'io* (pp.110–112)
18. *La cruda mia nemica* (pp.112–114)
19. *O che splendor de'luminosi rai* (pp.115–117)
20. *Io sento qui d'intorno* (pp.117–119)
21. *Deh! Fuss'or qui madonna* (pp.119–122)
22. *Se non fusse il pensier* (pp.122–124)
23. *Perche s'annida amore nelle luci* (pp.124–126)
24. *Ogni beltà, madonna, ch'io veggio* (pp.126–129)
25. *Ardo lungi e dappresso* (pp.129–131)

Book III of Madrigals for Three, Four, Five, and Six Voices:

1. *Ahi che quest'occhi miei a 3* (p.135)
2. *Da così dotta man sei stato a 3* (p.136)
3. *Pose un gran foco nel mio petto Amore a 4* (p.137)
4. *Vedrassi prima senza luce a 4* (pp.138–139)
5. *Ahi! letizia fugace a 5* [Ridolfo Pierluigi] (pp.140–143)
6. *Com'in più negre tenebre a 5* (pp.143–146)
7. *Dido, che giace entro quest'urna? a 5* (pp.146–148)
8. *Dolor non fu, ne fia a 5* (pp.149–153)
9. *Donna bell'e gentil a 5* (pp.153–156)

10. *Eran le vostre lagrime nel viso a 5* (pp.157–160)
11. *Febbre, ond'or per le vene a 5* (pp.160–163)
12. *Il dolce sonno in cui sepolto giace a 5* (pp.164–169)
13. *Il tempo vola, e se ne fuggon gli anni a 5* (pp.169–172)
    [seconda parte:] *Ivi vedrai la gloria* (pp.173–176)
14. *Io son felice sarei a 5* (pp.176–179)
15. *Io son ferito, ahi lasso a 5* (pp.179–183)
16. *Le selv'avea d' intorn'al lido Eusino a 5* (pp.183–186)
    [seconda parte:] *Quando fe'loro impallidir* (pp.186–189)
17. *Non son le vostre mani a 5* (pp.189–192)
18. *O bella Ninfa mia a 5* (pp.192–194)
19. *O felice ore, oh giorno fortunato a 5* (pp.195–198)
    [seconda parte:] *Per mostrar gioia* (pp.198–200)
20. *Ogni loco mi porge doglia e pianto a 5* (pp.201–204)
    [seconda parte:] *Poscia che per mio mal* (pp.204–206)
21. *Placide l'acqu'e placid'era il vento a 5* (pp.207–210)
22. *Saggio e santo Pastor a 5* (pp.210–213)
    [seconda parte:] *Onde seguendo l'onorata impresa* (pp.213–215)
23. *Se ben non veggon gl'occhi a 5* (pp.215–219)
24. *Se di pianti e di stridi a 5* (pp.219–222)
25. *Se fra quest'erb'e fiori a 5* (pp.222–226)
26. *Se lamentar augelli a 5* (pp.226–230)
27. *Soave fia il morir a 5* (pp.231–233)
28. *Struggomi, e mi disfaccio a 5* (pp.234–239)
29. *Vestiva i colli a 5* (pp.239–242)
    [seconda parte:] *Così le chiome mie* (pp.243–246)
30. *Quando dal terzo cielo a 6* (pp.246–249)

[Volume 29] *Fünfstimmige Madrigale (1. und 2. Buch). Herausgegeben von Franz Xaver Haberl* [pub. 1883]. [Five-part madrigals, books 1 and 2]
Book I of [Spiritual] Madrigals for Five Voices
[Madrigal texts (pp.xi–xiv)]

1. *Vergine bella, che di sol vestita* (pp.1–6)
2. *Vergine saggia, e del bel numer'una* (pp.7–11)
3. *Vergine pura d'ogni part' intera* (pp.11–15)
4. *Vergine santa, d'ogni grazia piena* (pp.16–20)
5. *Vergine sola al mondo* (pp.21–26)
6. *Vergine chiara e stabile in eterno* (pp.26–31)
7. *Vergine, quante lagrime ho già sparte* (pp.32–37)
8. *Vergine, tale è terra* (pp.37–42)
9. *Spirito santo, Amore* (pp.42–45)
10. *O Sol' incoronato* (pp.45–48)
11. *O cibo di dolcezza* (pp.49–51)
12. *O refrigerio acceso* (pp.52–54)
13. *Tu sei soave fiume* (pp.55–57)
14. *Paraclito amoroso, quando t'avrò io?* (pp.58–60)
15. *Amor, senza il tuo dono* (pp.60–62)
16. *Dunque divin Spiracolo* (63–65)
17. *O Manna saporito* (pp.65–67)

18. *Signor, dammi scienza* (pp.67–69)
19. *O Jesu dolce, o infinito amore* (pp.70–73)
20. *Giammai non resti a mille dolci modi* (pp.74–76)
21. *Quando più t'offend'io* (pp.76–78)
22. *Non basta ch'una volta tu portasti* (pp.79–81)
23. *S'io non ti conoscessi* (pp.82–84)
24. *Ma so ben, Signor mio* (pp.84–87)
25. *Et tu, anima mea, fatta da Dio* (pp.87–89)
26. *Per questo, Signor mio, non ti stancare* (pp.90–92)

Book II of [Spiritual] Madrigals for Five Voices

1. *Figlio immortal d'immortal padre* (pp.97–100)
2. *E se mai voci di quaggiù son grate* (pp.100–103)
3. *Or tu sol, che di vivi almi splendori* (pp.103–106)
4. *Dammi, scala del ciel e del ciel porta* (pp.107–109)
5. *E, se fur già de le mie mani* (pp.110–112)
6. *Dammi, vermiglia Rosa e bianco* (pp.113–116)
7. *E, se il pensier de la futura morte* (pp.116–119)
8. *Eletta Mirra, che soave odore* (pp.119–122)
9. *Cedro gentil dagli amorosi vermi* (pp.123–125)
10. *Fa, che con l'acque tue splendenti* (pp.126–128)
11. *Se amarissimo fiele e mortal tosco* (pp.129–131)
12. *Orto che sei si chiuso e si serrato* (pp.132–134)
13. *E se nel foco di lascivie ardendo* (pp.134–137)
14. *Vincitrice de l'empia idra infernale* (pp.137–140)
15. *Città di Dio, cui fan Tempi e Fortezze* (pp.141–144)
16. *Santo Altare, d'odor più veri e degni* (pp.144–147)
17. *Tu di fortezza torre* (pp.147–151)
18. *Specchio che fosti si polito* (pp.151–154)
19. *Vello di Gedeon, cui Dio si largo* (pp.154–157)
20. *Novella Aurora, che nascendo allegri* (pp.157–160)
21. *E questo spirto, de la propria sede* (pp.160–163)
22. *E dal letto di mille e mille colpe* (pp.163–166)
23. *Ed arda ognor sopra il lapideo altare* (pp.166–169)
24. *E tua mercè da così cieca e folta nebbia* (pp.169–172)
25. *E quella certa speme e quella fede* (pp.172–175)
26. *Anzi se foco e ferro e se veleno* (pp.176–179)
27. *E con i raggi tui splendenti e chiari* (pp.179–182)
28. *Regina delle Vergini e di tutte* (pp.182–186)
29. *Al fin, madre di Dio, che ne più bella cosa* (pp.186–190)
30. *E tu Signor, tu la tua grazia infondi* (pp.190–193)

[Volume 30] *Erster Nachtrag zur Gesammtausgabe der Werke von Pierluigi da Palestrina Herausgegeben von Franz Xaver Haberl* [pub. 1891]. [First supplement to the collected edition]

A. Ex Collectionibus Impressis Saeculi XVI et XVII

I. Cantiones Sacrae

1. *Jesu rex admirabilis a 3* [spiritual canzonetta] (p.3)
2. *Canon a 3 all'unisono* and *Resolutio* [doubtful attribution] (p.3)
3. *Tua Jesu dilectio a 3* [spiritual canzonetta] (p.4)

Intavulatura del cimbalo [of no.3] (p.4)
4. *Canon a 4 di quarta in quarta* and *Resolutio* [doubtful attribution] (pp.4–5)
5. *Jesu flos matris Virginis a 4* [spiritual canzonetta] (pp.5–6)
Intavolatura del cimbalo [of no.5] (p.6)
6. *O quam suavis est Domine a 4* [motet] (pp.7–9)
7. *Benedictus Dominus Deus Israel a 4* [canticle, odd-numbered verses] (pp.10–13)
8. *Miserere mei Dominus* [falsobordone] (p.14)
9. *Missa Papae Marcelli* [anonymous arrangement for four voices, pub. 1590] (pp.15–27)
10. *Missa Dominicales*, altus and bassus parts [pub. 1592] (pp.28–34)
11. *Laudate Dominum in sanctis ejus a 8* [motet, pub. 1607] [Haberl considered doubtful; presently accepted as genuine] (pp.35–41)
12. *Vos amici mei estis a 8* [motet, pub. 1591] (pp.42–46)

II. Cantiones Profanae
1. *Amor, se pur sei Dio* [cantus and bassus only] (pp.47–48)
2. *Chiare, fresche e dolci acque a 4* [canzone] (pp.48–50)
[seconda parte] *S'egli e pur mio destino* (pp.50–52)
[terza parte] *Tempo verra ancor forse* (pp.53–55)
[quarta parte] *Da'be'rami scendea* (pp.55–57)
[quinta parte] *Quante volte diss'io* (pp.58–60)
3. *Da fuoco così bel a 4* [canzone] (pp.61–63)
[II. stanza] *Rapace ingorda* (pp.63–65)
[III. stanza] *Amo, e non nacque del mio amor* (pp.65–67)
[IV. stanza] *Da l'empia gelosia* (pp.67–69)
[V. stanza] *Si mi vince talor* (pp.69–71)
[VI. stanza] *O effetto rio* (pp.72–74)
[VII. stanza] *Amore, non volendo io* (pp.74–76)
[VIII. stanza] *Non mi sferra il crudel* (pp.76–78)
[IX. stanza] *Poi che la vista* (pp.78–81)
[X. stanza] *Io ho non lingua* (pp.81–83)
[XI. stanza] *L'alta cagion* (pp.83–85)
[XII. stanza] *Misero stato degli amanti* (pp.85–87)
[XIII. stanza] *Fuggir dovriasi* (pp.87–90)
[XIV. et ultima stanza] *Sazio di tormentarmi* (pp.90–92)
4. *Con dolce, altiero ed amoroso cenno a 4* [madrigal] (pp.93–95)
5. *Se dai soavi accenti a 4* [madrigal] (pp.96–98)
6. *Voi me poneste in foco a 4* [canzona] (pp.99–100)
[II. parte] *Però che da'l ardore* (pp.101–102)
[III. parte] *Che se tant'a voi piace* (pp.102–104)
[IV. parte] *E di voi non mi doglio* (pp.104–106)
7. *Donna, presso al cui viso a 5* [madrigal, cantus and tenor lacking] (pp.107–109)
8. *Non fu già suon di trombe a 5* [madrigal, cantus and tenor lacking] (pp.110–112)
9. *Il caro è morto a 5* [madrigal, tenor lacking here] (pp.113–115)
[II. parte] *Or che la nobil lingua fredda* (pp.116–118)

10. *Anima, dove sei a 5* [madrigal; tenor, quinto, basso parts lacking here] (pp.119–121)
11. *Quand'ecco, donna, il vostro braccio a 5* [canzona, fifth stanza only by Palestrina, tenor I and basso lacking here] (pp.122–125)
12. *Dunque perfido Amante a 5* [madrigal] (pp.126–128)

B. Ex Archivo Capellae Juliae ad S. Petrum

1. Hymnus: In Sancti Stephani Protom [four to six voices, from I-Rvat CG50, CG15] (pp.129–132)
2. Hymnus: In Festo S. Joannis Apostoli et Evang [four to five voices, from I-Rvat CG50, CG15] (pp.133–137)
3. Hymnus: *Gloria, laus a 4* [questioned attribution] (p.138)
4. Ex hymno: *Ave maris stella a 4* [verse *Monstra te* only; cantus I] (p.139)
5. Hymnus: *O Redemptor a 4* [questioned attribution] (pp.140–141)
6. Hymnus: *Pange lingua a 4* (pp.142–149)
7. Antiphona: *Pueri Hebraeorum a 4* (pp.150–152)
8. Ex hymno: *Pange lingua [Tantum ergo] a 4* (pp.153–154)
9. Hymnus: *Veni Creator Spiritus a 4* (pp.155–160)
10. Hymnus: *Vexilla Regis prodeunt a 4* [questioned attribution] (pp.160–161)
11. Responsorium: *Beata es Virgo* cum II. parte *Ave Maria a 8* (pp.162–169)
12. *Laudate Dominum de coelis a 8* (pp.170–174)
13. Antiphona: *Regina coeli, laetare a 8* (pp.175–180)
14. Hymnus: *O gloriosa Domina a 12* (pp.181–188)

[Volume 31] *Zweiter Nachtrag zur Gesamtausgabe der Werke. Herausgegeben von Fraz Xaver Haberl* [pub. 1892]. [Second supplement to the collected edition, containing unpublished sources from the Sistine Chapel, the Vatican Library and the archive of St. John Lateran]

C. Ex Archivo Capellae Pontificiae

1. *Cum descendisset a 4* [doubtful attribution, from I-Rvat CS80] (pp.1–3)
2. *Lectio I. Feria VI. in Parasceve* ["Palestrina-Biordi," four to five voices] (pp.4–10)
3. In die Pentecostes. *Dum complerentur a 4* [doubtful attribution] (pp.11–13)
   [secunda pars:] *Et repleti sunt omnes* (pp.13–14)
4. *Gloria Patri a 4* [from I-Rvat CS76] (p.15)
5. *Lectio II. Feriae VI. In Parasceve a 4* (pp.16–18)
6. Responsorium: *Libera* [three to four voices, alternate choruses, from I-Rvat CS219] (pp.19–24)
7. *Miserere mei Deus* [falsobordoni, four and five voices] (pp.24–27)
8. *Miserere mei Deus in duplici choro 4 et 5 vocum* (pp.28–34)
9. *Misit rex a 4* [from I-Rvat CS88] (pp.35–36)
10. *O Doctor optime a 4* [from I-Rvat CS88] (pp.37–38)
11. *Dexteram meam a 5* [from I-Rvat CS88] (pp.39–40)
12. *Laudate coeli a 5* [doubtful attribution] (pp.41–43)

13. *Ne reminiscaris a 5* [doubtful attribution] (pp.44–47)
14. *Per lignum a 5* [doubtful attribution, from I-Rvat 54] (pp.48–51)
15. *Quem dicunt homines a 5* [from I-Rvat CS89] (pp.52–54)
16. *Qui manducat a 5* [doubtful attribution] (pp.55–57)
17. *Salvum me fac a 5* [doubtful attribution, from I-Rvat CS72 and 117] (pp.58–62)
18. *Tu es pastor ovium a 5* (pp.63–66)
    [secunda pars:] *Quodcumque ligaveris* (pp.66–69)
19. *Ecce sacerdos magnus a 6* [questioned attribution, from I-Rvat CS153] (pp.70–72)
    [secunda pars:] *Ideo jure jurando* (pp.72–74)
20. *Estote fortes in bello a 6* (pp.75–78)
21. *Salvatorem exspectamus a 6* (pp.79–81)
    [secunda pars:] *Sobrie et juste* (pp.82–84)

D. Ex Bibliotheca Vaticana
(5) Hymni Feriales ad Vesperas
1.Feriae II. *Immense coeli conditor a 4* (pp.85–87)
2.Feriae III. *Telluris ingens conditor a 4* (pp.87–89)
3. Feriae IV. *Coeli Deus sanctissime a 4* (pp.90–93)
4. Feriae V. *Magnae deus potentiae a 4* (pp.93–95)
5. Feriae VI. *Plasmator hominis Deus a 4* (pp.96–98)

XI exercizi sopra la scala [doubtful attribution]
6. I (pp.99–100)
7. II (pp.100–101)
8. III (pp.101–102)
9. IV (pp.102–103)
10. V (pp.103–104)
11. VI (pp.104–105)
12. VII (pp.105–106)
13. VIII (p.107)
14. IX (pp.108–109)
15. X (pp.109–110)
16. XI (pp.110–111)
17. Canticum: *Benedictus Dominus Deus Israel a 5* [odd-numbered verses in plainchant; even-numbered verses in polyphony] (pp.112–118)

E. Ex Archivo Basilicae S. Joannis ad Lateranum
1. *Sabbata Quadragesimae.* [*Audi benigne Conditor*] *Nostras preces* [hymn, four to five voices, odd-numbered verses in polyphony] (pp.119–122)
2. *In Adventu Domini.* [*Creator alme siderum*] *Aeterna lux credentium a 4* [hymn] (pp.123–124)
3. *Lectio I. Feriae VI. In Parasceve 4 et 5 vocum* (pp.125–129)
4. Fragmenta diversa:
    a. *Ex lectione II. Feriae V. In Coena Domini a 4* (pp.130–132)
    b. (pp.132–133)
5. *Gloria laus a 4* (p.134)
6. *Hodie Christus natus est a 4* (pp.135–137)

7. *Ingrediente Domino a 4* [doubtful attribution] (pp.137–139)
8. Respons. *Libera me, Domine a 4* (pp.140–144)
9. *O bone Jesu a 4* (p.145)
10. *O Redemptor a 4* (p.146)
11. *Salve Regina a 4* (pp.147–149)
    [secunda pars:] *Et Jesum, benedictum* (pp.150–151)
12. Hymnus de Communi Apostolorum temp. pasch. [*Tristes erant Apostoli*] *Sermone blando* [even-numbered verses] (pp.152–155)
13. *Ecce nunc benedicite a 4 et 5 vocum* [even-numbered verses in polyphony; baritone voice supplied by Michael Haller] (pp.156–157)
14. Canticum: *Nunc dimittis a 4 et 5 vocum* [even-numbered verses in polyphony] (pp.158–159)
15. *Miserere mei Deus* [falsobordone] (p.160)
16. *Lectio III. Sabbati sancti* [six to eight voices] (pp.161–168)
17. *Canticum Zachariae a 4* (pp.169–170)
18. a. *Improperia secundum autographum Praenestini* (pp.171–172)
    b. *Improperia Jo. Petri Aloysii Praenestini juxta Cod.205 et 206 Cap. Pontificiae* (pp.175–180)

[Volume 32] *Drittes Nachtrag zur Gesammtausgabe der Werke. Herausgegeben von Franz Xaver Haberl* [pub. 1892]. [Third supplement to the collected edition, containing unpublished sources from the archives of Santa Maria Maggiore, Biblioteca Altempsiana, and various libraries]

Note: The responsories marked as **, already considered doubtful attributions by Haberl, have since been firmly established as composed by Marc'Antonio Ingegneri.

F. Ex Archivo Basilicae Liberianae ad S. Mariam Majorem

1. *Beata es a 6* (pp.1–5)
   [secunda pars:] *Ave Maria gratia plena* (pp.5–9)
2. *Missa sine titulo a 6* [from I-Rsm 29] (pp.10–42)

G. Ex Bibliotheca olim Collegii Romani

1. Hymnus: *Tempore Quadragesimae.* [*Audi benigne conditor*] *Nostras preces a 4* [odd-numbered verses in polyphony] (pp.43–46)
2. Hymnus: *Te lucis ante terminum a 4* [verses 1, 3] (pp.47–48)
3. Resp. breve: *In manus a 4* (p.49)
4. Canticum Simeonis: *Nunc dimittis. Salva nos a 4* (pp.49–50)
5. *Regina coeli a 4* (pp.51–52)
6. *Venite exsultemus Domino a 5* (pp.53–58)
7. *Benedictus pro Hebdomada sancta a 9* (pp.59–67)
8. *Miserere mei Deus 12 vocum in 3 choris* (pp.68–79)

H. Ex diversis bibliothecis et archivis

VIII Ricercari a 4 vocum

1. I. tono (pp.80–81)
2. II. tono (pp.81–83)
3. III. tono (pp.83–84)
4. IV. tono (pp.84–86)
5. V. tono (pp.86–87)

6. VI. tono (pp.88–89)
7. VII. tono (pp.89–91)
8. VIII. tono (pp.91–92)

XXVII Responsoria Tridui Sacri** [4 vocum]

In Coena Domini ad Matutinum in Primo Nocturno

9. I. Responsorium. *In monte oliveti* (p.93–94)
10. II. Responsorium. *Tristis est anima mea* (pp.94–95)
11. III. Responsorium. *Ecce vidimus eum* (pp.96–97)

In Secundo Nocturno

12. IV. Responsorium. *Amicus meus osculi me tradidit* (pp.98–99)
13. V. Responsorium. *Judas mercator pessimus* (pp.99–100)
14. VI. Responsorium. *Unus ex discipulis* (pp.100–101)

In Tertio Nocturno

15. VII. Responsorium. *Eram quasi agnus innocens* (pp.101–102)
16. VIII. Responsorium. *Una hora non potui* (pp.102–103)
17. IX. Responsorium. *Seniores populi* (p.104)

In Parasceve ad Matutinum. In Primo Nocturno

18. I. Responsorium. *Omnes amici mei* (pp.105–106)
19. II. Responsorium. *Velum templum scissum est* (pp.106–107)
20. III. Responsorium. *Vinea mea electa* (pp.107–108)

In Secundo Nocturno

21. IV. Responsorium. *Tanquam ad latronem* (pp.109–110)
22. V. Responsorium. *Tenebrae factae sunt* (pp.110–111)
23. VI. Responsorium. *Animam meam dilectam* (pp.112–113)

In Tertio Nocturno

24. VII. Responsorium. *Tradiderunt me* (pp.114–115)
25. VIII. Responsorium. *Jesum tradidit impius summis* (pp.115–116)
26. IX. Responsorium. *Caligaverunt oculi* (pp.116–117)

Sabbato Sancto. In Primo Nocturno

27. I Responsorium. *Sicut ovis ad occisum* (p.118)
28. II. Responsorium. *Jerusalem surge* (p.119)
29. III. Responsorium. *Plange quasi virgo* (p.120)

In Secundo Nocturno

30. IV. Responsorium. *Recessit pastor noster* (pp.121–122)
31. V. Responsorium. *O vos omnes* (pp.122–123)
32. VI. Responsorium. *Ecce quomodo moritur* (pp.123–125)

In Tertio Nocturno

33. VII. Responsorium. *Astiterunt reges terrae* (p.125)
34. VIII. Responsorium. *Aestimatus sum* (pp.126–127)
35. IX. Responsorium. *Sepulto Domino signatum est* (pp.127–128)
36. *Et erexit a 4* [doubtful attribution] (p.128)
37. Ant. *Asperges me a 4* (pp.129–130)
38. *O bone Jesu a 4* (pp.131–132)
39. *O Domine Jesu Christe a 4* (p.133)
40. In festo sancti Thomae Apostoli. *Thomas unus ex duodecim a 4* (pp.134–136)
41. Sequentia in Festo Pentecostes. *Veni Sancte Spiritus* [four to six voices] (pp.137–142)

42. Antiph. in distributione candelarum. *Lumen ad revelationem* [four and five voices] (pp.143–154)
43. Respons: *Libera me Domine a 5* (pp.155–160)
44. *Miserere mei Deus* [falsibordone a 5] (p.161)
45. *Miserere a 6* (p.162)
46. *Lectio I. Feria V. In Coena Domini a 8* (pp.163–168)
47. *Lectio II. Feria V.* (pp.168–171)
48. *Lectio III.* (Fragmenta.) (p.172)
49. *Stabat Mater* [four and eight voices] (pp.173–179)
50. Sequentia: *Victimae paschali laudes* [two choruses; one lacking and composed here by Michael Haller] (pp.180–182)

[Volume 33] *Viertes Nachtrag zur Gesammtausgabe. Herausgegeben von Franz Xaver Haberl* [pub. 1907]. [Fourth supplement to the collected edition, with miscellaneous works and indexes]

1. *Missa Dominicalis a 5* [contains alternatim setting of *Gloria* and *Credo*] (pp.1–33)
2. *Opem nobis a 5* (pp.34–36)
3. *Surge propera a 5* (pp.37–39)
   [secunda pars:] *Veni dilecti mi* (pp.39–41)
4. *Quanti mercenarii a 5* (pp.41–44)
5. *Benedicta sit sancta Trinitas* (Diminuito) (pp.45–48)
6. *Ave Maria* (Diminuito) (pp.48–49)
7. *Hodie beata Virgo* (Diminuito) (pp.49–50)
8. *Fuit homo missus* (Diminuito) (p.51)
9. *Tota pulchra es* (Diminuito) (pp.52–53)
10. *Introduxit me Rex* (Diminuito) (pp.54–55)
11. *Pulchra es* (Diminuito) (pp.56–57)
12. *Veni, veni dilecti mi* (Diminuito) (pp.58–59)
13. *Vestiva i colli* (Diminuito) (pp.60–61)
14. *Io son ferito* (Diminuito) (p.62)
15. *Io son ferito* and *Ave verum corpus* (Diminuito) (pp.63–66)
16. *Donna, presso al cui a 5* (pp.67–69)
17. *Vestiva i colli* [embellished cantus part, including seconda parte *Così le chiome mie*, from dalla Casa II, p.36] (pp.70–71)
18. *Vestiva i colli* [lute intabulation, includes seconda parte *Così le chiome mie*, from Galilei 1584, p.26] (pp.71–73)
19. *Se tra quest'erbe e fiore* [lute intabulation, from Galilei 1584, p.53] (pp.73–74)
20. *Io son ferito ahi lasso* [lute intabulation, from Galilei 1584, p.121] (pp.74–75)
21. *Il dolce sonno in cui sepolto giace* [lute intabulation, from Galilei 1584, p.122] (p.75)
22. *Da poi ch'io viddi vostra falsa fede* [cantus and alto lacking here] (p.76)
23. *Perch'al viso d'amor* [cantus and alto lacking here] (pp.77–78)
24. *Qual più crudel martire* [cantus and alto lacking here] (pp.78–79)
25. *Misit me vivens Pater a 5* (pp.80–83)

Index alphabeticus verborum, a quibus modui operum Praenestini initium faciunt. (pp.84–96). Works, listed by text incipit or title.

Index musicus omnium operum Joannis Petraloysii Praenestini. (pp.97–129). Thematic index of works, listed by genre and musical incipit.

II. The "Casimiri" Edition (1939–1987)
Current editor: Lino Bianchi

C0004 Palestrina, Giovanni Pierluigi da. *Le opere complete.* Rome: Fratelli Scalera, 1939–1951 (vols.1–18); Rome: Istituto Italiano per la Storia della Musica, 1953 to date (vols.19–34). Thirty-four volumes to date; the most recent volume was published in 1987, and at least one further volume is forthcoming.

In 1934, Raffaele Casimiri (1883–1943) announced a new "national edition" of Palestrina's works, which in his view aimed to rework, modify, and correct the Haberl edition in light of the rules of historical criticism and the latest discoveries of musicological research. The actual editorship consisted of Casimiri for volumes 1–15, Lavinio Virgili for volumes 16–17, Knud Jeppesen for volumes 18–19, and Lino Bianchi for volumes 20–34. Each volume contains a critical report.

There are some significant differences between the contents of this and the Haberl edition. A number of items in "Haberl" do not appear in the present collection, but this edition also contains important newly recovered music, the most significant being the series of masses Palestrina wrote for Duke Guglielmo Gonzaga of Mantua that were located by Knud Jeppesen in Milan in the late 1940s. The scorings of this edition are characterized by the use of modern clefs and note values reduced by half. Sensitivity to issues of text underlay and to sixteenth-century Latin and Italian prosody is somewhat more evident here than in the Haberl edition. Casimiri retranscribed some passages of proportional notation in an interpretation different from Haberl's; his views on this admittedly difficult issue led to some strongly worded exchanges with other scholars, notably Antoine Auda. For a comparison of the critical and working methods evident in the Haberl and Casimiri editions, see Fischer 1997, item E0592.

Reprint of This Edition

C0005 New York: Edwin Kalmus, ca. 1965–1972. 74 volumes, paperbound.

The Kalmus reprint is incomplete. It divides volumes 1–17 and 20–31 of the Casimiri edition among seventy-four paperbound volumes. The Casimiri edition page numbers were retained in the Kalmus reprint even when the Kalmus volume number changed, so in the present listing the equivalent Kalmus reprints of Casimiri are indicated thus:

[Volume number and bibliographical citation for the Casimiri edition, followed by:
K1=pp.1–61; **K2**=pp.62–124; **K3**=pp.125–210, etc.]

For example, in locating *Missa Ad coenam Agni providi a 5*, the reader notes that it is printed in volume 1, pages 125–163 of the Casimiri edition. Beneath the bibliographical citation heading the list for that volume it will be noted that **K3** includes these pages; thus this mass would be found in the Kalmus edition, volume 3, pages 125–163.

Contents

[Volume 1] *Il libro primo delle messe a 4, 5 e 6 voci secondo la edizione originale del 1554 e la ristampa del 1591.* ed. Raffaele Casimiri. Rome: Fratelli Scalera, 1939

[**K1**=pp.1–61; **K2**=pp.62–124; **K3**=pp.125–210]

For Four Voices

1. *Missa Ecce sacerdos magnus* (pp.1–34)
2. *Missa O regem coeli* (pp.35–61)
3. *Missa Virtute magna* (pp.62–92)
4. *Missa Gabriel Archangelus* (pp.93–124)

For Five Voices

5. *Missa ad coenam agni providi* (pp.125–163)
6. *Missa Pro defunctis* [*Kyrie, Offertorium, Sanctus, Agnus Dei I–III*] (pp.164–181)

For Six Voices

7. *Missa Sine nomine* (pp.182–210)

[Volume 2] *Il libro primo di madrigali a 4 voci secondo la ristampa del 1596, con altri madrigali a 4 e 5 voci, pubblicati in raccolte dal 1554 e 1561.* ed. Raffaele Casimiri. Rome: Fratelli Scalera, 1939

[**K4**=pp.1–107; **K5**=pp.107–185]

Madrigals for Four Voices

1. *Deh or foss' io col vago de la Luna* (pp.1–3)
2. *S'i'l dissi mai ch'i'venga* (pp.3–5)
3. *Questa saranno ben lagrime* (pp.5–7)
4. *Che non fia che giammai* (pp.7–10)
5. *Rime, dai sospir miei nate e dal pianto* (pp.10–12)
6. *Lontan dalla mia diva* (pp.12–14)
7. *Nessun vissi giammai più di me lieto* (pp.15–16)
8. *La ver l'aurora che si dolce l'aura* (pp.16–18)
9. *Chiara, si chiaro e de'vostr'occhi il sole* (pp.18–20)
10. *Chi estinguerà il mio foco* (pp.20–23)
11. *Donna vostra mercede ogni pietade eccede* (pp.23–25)
12. *Già fu chi m'ebbe cara* (pp.25–27)
13. *Ovver de'sensi e priva* (pp.27–29)
14. *Amor, Fortuna e la mia mente* (pp.30–32)
15. [seconda parte:] *Ne spero i dolci di tornino* (pp.32–33)
16. *Che debbo far, che mi consigli, Amore?* (pp.33–35)
17. *Gitene liete rime, ov'or si siede* (pp.35–37)
18. *Mentre a le dolci e le purpuree* (pp.38–40)
19. *Amor, che meco in quest'ombre ti stavi* (pp.40–41)
20. *Vaghi pensier, che così passo passo* (pp.43–45)

21. *Mentre ch'al mar discenderanno* (pp.46–48)
22. *Quai rime fur si chiare* (pp.48–50)
23. *Ecc'oscurati i chiari raggi al sole* (pp.51–52)
    [seconda parte:] *Rara beltà non mai più vista* (pp.52–53)
    [terza parte:] *Questo doglioso stil colmo di pianto* (pp.54–56)
    [quarta parte:] *Mai fu più cruda o più spietata morte* (pp.56–58)
    [quinta parte:] *Privo di fede oltra l'usato* (pp.58–60)
    [ultima parte a 6:] *Ma voi, fioriti ed onorati colli* (pp.60–63)
24. *Con dolce, altiero ed amoroso cenno* (pp.64–66)
25. [prima stanza:] *Da fuoco così bel nasce il mio ardore* (pp.67–69)
    [seconda stanza:] *Rapace ingorda e venenosa* (pp.69–71)
    [terza stanza:] *Amo e non nacque del mio amor giammai* (pp.72–74)
    [quarta stanza:] *Da l'empia gelosia nasce il tormento* (pp.75–77)
    [quinta stanza:] *Si mi vince talor l'aspro martir* (pp.77–80)
    [sesta stanza:] *O effettorio che'l più felice stato* (pp.81–83)
    [settima stanza:] *Amore non volendo il che'l mio gioire* (pp.84–86)
    [ottava stanza:] *Non mi sferra il crudel* (pp.86–89)
    [nona stanza:] *Poi che la vista del mio caro sole* (pp.89–92)
    [decima stanza:] *Io non ho lingua e senza gli occhi* (pp.92–96)
    [decimauna stanza:] *L'alta cagion del mio fermo pensiero* (pp.96–98)
    [decimaseconda stanza:] *Misero stato degli amanti* (pp.99–101)
    [decimaterza stanza:] *Fuggir dovriasi se fuggir* (pp.101–104)
    [decimaquarta et ultima stanza:] *Sazio si tormentarmi* (pp.104–107)
26. [prima parte:] *Chiare, fresche et dolci acque* (pp.107–109)
    [seconda parte:] *S'egli e pur mio destino* (pp.110–112)
    [terza parte:] *Tempo verrà ancor forse* (pp.113–115)
    [quarta parte:] *Da'be'rami scendea* (pp.115–119)
    [quinta parte:] *Quante volte diss'io* (pp.119–122)
27. ["Anno 1558":] *Se da'soavi accenti* (pp.122–126)
28. ["Anno 1558." Canzona: prima parte:] *Voi me poneste in foco* (pp.127–129)
    [seconda parte:] *Però che da l'ardore* (pp.129–131)
    [terza parte:] *Che se tant'a voi piace* (pp.131–133)
    [quarta parte:] *E di voi non mi doglio* (pp.133–136)
29. ["Anno 1559" prima parte:] *Ogni loco mi porge doglia a 5* (pp.137–140)
    [seconda parte:] *Poscia che per mio mal a 5* (pp.141–143)
30. ["Anno 1560"] *Donna bell'e gentil a 5* (pp.144–148)
31. ["Anno 1561"] *Dolor non fu, ne fia a 5* (pp.148–153)
32. ["Anno 1561"] *Il dolce sonno in cui sepolto giace a 5* (pp.153–161)
33. ["Anno 1561"] *Io son ferito, ahi lasso a 5* (pp.161–165)
34. ["Anno 1561"] *Se ben non veggon gl'occhi a 5* (pp.165–169)
35. ["Anno 1561"] *Se fra quest'erb'e fiore a 5* (pp.170–175)
36. ["Anno 1561"] *Se lamentar augelli a 5* (pp.175–180)
37. ["Anno 1561"] *Struggomi, e mi disfaccio a 5* (pp.180–185)

[Volume 3] *Il libro primo dei mottetti a 4 voci secondo la ristampa del 1590.* ed. Raffaele Casimiri. Rome: Fratelli Scalera, 1939. [Edition of *Motecta festorum totius anni*, 1563]

[**K6**=pp.1–70; **K7**=pp.70–137]

1. In festo Nativitatis Domini. *Dies sanctificatus* (pp.1–4)
2. In festo S. Stephani. *Lapidabant Stephanum* (pp.4–8)
3. In festo S. Joannis Evangelistae. *Valde honorandus est* (pp.8–11)
4. In die Circumcisionis Domini. *Magnum haereditatis mysterium* (pp.11–15)
5. In Epiphania Domini. *Tribus miraculis* (pp.15–19)
6. In festo Purificationis Beatae Mariae. *Hodie beata Virgo* (pp.19–22)
7. In Annuntiatione Beatae Mariae. *Ave Maria* (pp.23–25)
8. In Resurrectione Domini. *Jesus junxit se* (pp.26–30)
9. In Ascensione Domini. *O Rex gloriae* (pp.30–34)
10. In die Pentecostes. *Loquebantur variis linguis* (pp.34–38)
11. In festo Sanctae Trinitatis. *Benedicta sit* (pp.38–42)
12. In festo Corporis Christi. *Lauda Sion* (pp.42–45)
13. In Nativitatis Joannis Baptistae. *Fuit homo* (pp.46–49)
14. In die Sancti Petri Apostoli. *Tu es pastor ovium* (pp.49–53)
15. In die Sancti Pauli Apostoli. *Magnus sanctus Paulus* (pp.53–57)
16. In Visitatione Beatae Mariae. *Surge propera* (pp.57–61)
17. In die Sanctae Mariae Magdalenae. *In diebus illis* (pp.61–66)
18. In festo Sancti Laurentij. *Beatus Laurentius* (pp.66–70)
18. In Assumptione Beatae Mariae. *Quae est ista* (pp.70–74)
19. In Decollatione Sancti Joannis Baptistae. *Misso Herodes spiculatore* (pp.74–78)
21. In festo Nativitatis Beatae Mariae. *Nativitas tua* (pp.78–82)
22. In festo Sanctae Crucis. *Nos autem gloriari* (pp.82–86)
23. In festo Omnium Sanctorum. *Salvator mundi* (pp.86–90)
24. In festo Sancti Martini Episcopi. *O quantus luctus* (pp.90–93)
25. In festo Praesentationis Beatae Mariae. *Congratulamini mihi* (pp.94–96)
26. In festo Sanctae Caeciliae. *Dum aurora* (pp.97–100)
27. In festo Sancti Andreae. *Doctor bonus* (pp.100–104)
28. In festoo Conceptionis Beatae Mariae. *Quam pulchri sunt* (pp.104–108)
29. In festo Apostolorum. *Tollite jugum meum* (pp.109–112)
30. In festo Evangelistarum. *Isti sunt viri sancti* (pp.113–116)
31. In festo unius Martyris. *Hic est vere Martyr* (pp.116–120)
32. In festo plurimorum Martyrum. *Gaudent in coelis* (pp.121–124)
33. In festo Confessorum pontificum. *Iste est* (pp.125–129)
34. In festo Confessorum non pontificum. *Beatus vir* (pp.129–132)
35. In festo Virginum. *Veni sponsa Christi* (pp.132–135)
36. In Dedicatione Templi. *Exaudi Domine* (pp.135–137)

[Volume 4] *Il libro secondo delle messe a 4, 5 e 6 voci secondo la stampa originale del 1567 e la ristampa del 1600.* ed. Raffaele Casimiri. Rome: Fratelli Scalera, 1939.

[**K8**=pp.1–73; **K9**=pp.74–166; **K10**=pp.167–201]

For Four Voices
1. *Missa De Beata Virgine* (pp.1–25)
2. *Missa Inviolata* (pp.26–52)
3. *Missa Sine nomine* (pp.53–73)
4. *Missa Ad fugam* (pp.74–90)
For Five Voices
5. *Missa Aspice Domine* (pp.91–125)
6. *Missa Salvum me fac* (pp.126–166)
For Six Voices
7. *Missa Papae Marcelli* (pp.167–201)
Appendix: *Gloria* ex missa *De Beata* [edition of 1600] (pp.i–iv)

[Volume 5] *Il libro primo dei mottetti a 5, 6 e 7 voci secondo la ristampa del 1600.* ed. Raffaele Casimiri. Rome: Fratelli Scalera, 1939. [Book I of motets] [**K11**=pp.1–78; **K12**=pp.79–149; **K13**=pp.149–218]
1. *O admirabile commercium a 5* (pp.1–4)
2. *Stella quam viderant Magi a 5* (pp.5–9)
3. *O Antoni eremita a 5* (pp.10–14)
4. *Senex puerum portabat a 5* (pp.15–19)
   [secunda pars:] *Hodie beata Virgo* (pp.20–24)
5. *Suscipe verbum Virgo Maria a 5* (pp.25–29)
   [secunda pars:] *Paries quidem filium* (pp.30–35)
6. *Alleluja: Tulerunt Dominum a 5* (pp.35–40)
7. *Crucem sanctam subiit a 5* (pp.41–44)
8. *O beata et gloriosa Trinitas a 5* (pp.45–49)
   [secunda pars:] *O vera summa sempiterna Trinitas* (pp.50–53)
9. *Ego sum panis vivus a 5* (pp.54–58)
   [secunda pars:] *Panis quem ego dabo* (pp.59–63)
10. *Puer qui natus est a 5* (pp.64–68)
11. *Beatae Mariae Magdalenae a 5* (pp.69–73)
12. *Sancte Paule apostole a 5* (pp.74–78)
13. *Beatus Laurentius a 5* (pp.79–83)
14. *Hodie nata est a 5* (pp.83–88)
15. *O beatum virum a 5* (pp.88–93)
16. *Venit Michael Archangelus a 5* (pp.94–98)
17. *O beatum Pontificem a 5* (pp.98–104)
18. *Deus, qui dedisti legem a 5* (pp.104–109)
19. *Lapidabant Stephanum a 5* (pp.110–115)
20. *Hic est discipulus ille a 5* (pp.116–120)
21. *Sicut lilium a 5* (pp.121–125)
22. *Quam pulchri sunt a 5* (pp.126–130)
23. *Unus ex duobus a 5* (pp.131–135)
24. *Cum pervenisset beatus Andreas a 5* (pp.135–140)
25. *Viri Galilaei a 6* (pp.141–144)
   [secunda pars:] *Ascendit Deus* (pp.145–149)
26. *Dum complerentur a 6* (pp.149–153)
   [secunda pars:] *Dum ergo essent* (pp.154–158)
27. *Pulchra es, o Maria a 6* (pp.158–164)

28. *Solve, jubente Deo a 6* (pp.165–168)
    [secunda pars:] *Quodcumque ligaveris* (pp.169–173)
29. *Vidi turbam magnam a 6* (pp.174–179)
    [secunda pars:] *Et omnes Angeli* (pp.179–183)
30. *O magnum mysterium a 6* (pp.184–188)
    [secunda pars:] *Quem vidistis pastores* (pp.188–192)
31. *O Domine Jesu Christe a 6* (pp.193–195)
32. *Tu es Petrus a 7* (pp.196–204)
33. *Virgo prudentissima a 7* (pp.204–211)
    [secunda pars:] *Maria Virgo* (pp.212–218)

[Volume 6] *Il libro terzo delle messe a 4, 5 e 6 voci secondo la edizione originale del 1570.* ed. Raffaele Casimiri. Rome: Fratelli Scalera, 1939. [Masses, Book III, 1570]

[**K14**=pp.1–61; **K15**=pp.62–135; **K16**=pp.136–253]

For Four Voices

1. *Missa Spem in alium* (pp.1–29)
2. *Missa Primi toni* (pp.30–61)
3. *Missa Brevis* (pp.62–83)
4. *Missa De feria* (pp.84–96)

For Five Voices

5. *Missa L'homme armé* (pp.97–135)
6. *Missa Repleatur os meum* (pp.136–174)

For Six Voices

7. *Missa De beata Virgine* (pp.175–215)
8. *Missa Ut re mi fa sol la* (pp.216–253)

[Volume 7] *Il libro secondo dei mottetti a 5, 6 ed 8 voci secondo la ristampa del 1573*. ed. Raffaele Casimiri. Rome: Fratelli Scalera, 1940. [Book II of motets]

[**K17**=pp.1–64; **K18**=pp.65–134; **K19**=pp.135–225]

1. *O virgo simul et mater a 5* (pp.1–6)
2. *Memor esto a 5* (pp.7–12)
3. *Corona aurea a 5* (pp.13–16)
    [secunda pars:] *Domine praevenisti eum* (pp.17–20)
4. *In illo tempore a 5* (pp.21–27)
5. *O sacrum convivium a 5* (pp.27–31)
6. *Coenantibus illis a 5* (pp.31–36)
7. *Derelinquat impius a 5* (pp.37–41)
8. *Ascendo ad Patrem a 5* (pp.42–46)
    [secunda pars:] *Ego rogabo Patrem* (pp.47–50)
9. *Homo quidam a 5* (pp.50–55)
10. *Canite tuba a 5* (pp.56–59)
    [secunda pars:] *Rorate coeli* (pp.60–64)
11. *Exi cito a 5* (pp.65–69)
12. *Circuire possum Domine a 5* [Angelo Pierluigi] (pp.70–74)
    [secunda pars:] *In hac cruce* (pp.75–77)
13. *Gaude Barbara a 5* (pp.78–82)

[secunda pars:] *Gaude, quia meruisti* (pp.83–88)
14. *Domine Pater a 5* [Silla Pierluigi] (pp.89–92)
15. *Confitebor tibi Domine a 5* [Rodolfo Pierluigi] (pp.93–97)
16. *Peccantem me quotidie a 5* (pp.98–101)
17. *Dominus Jesus a 5* (pp.102–106)
18. *Tribularer si nescirem a 6* (pp.107–111)
[secunda pars:] *Secundum multitudinem* (pp.112–116)
19. *Veni Domine a 6* (pp.117–120)
[secunda pars:] *Excita Domine* (pp.121–125)
20. *Hierusalem, cito veniet a 6* (pp.125–130)
[secunda pars:] *Ego enim sum Dominus* (pp.130–134)
21. *Beata Barbara a 6* (pp.135–140)
[secunda pars:] *Gloriosam mortem* (pp.140–145)
20. *Sancta et immaculata a 6* (pp.146–149)
[secunda pars:] *Benedicta tu* (pp.150–154)
21. *Cantabo Domine a 6* (pp.154–158)
[secunda pars:] *Deficiant peccatores a 6* (pp.158–161)
23. *Tu es Petrus a 6* (pp.162–166)
[secunda pars:] *Quodcumque ligaveris* (pp.166–170)
22. *Nunc dimittis a 6* [Silla Pierluigi] (pp.171–175)
24. *Confitebor tibi Domine a 8* (pp.176–184)
[secunda pars:] *Notas facite in populis* (pp.184–190)
25. *Laudate pueri a 8* (pp.190–197)
[secunda pars:] *Quis sicut Dominus* (pp.197–204)
26. *Domine in virtuta tua a 8* (pp.205–212)
[secunda pars:] *Magna est gloria ejus* (pp.212–219)
27. *Laudate Dominum omnes gentes a 8* (pp.219–225)

[Volume 8] *Il libro terzo dei mottetti a 5, 6 ed 8 voci secondo l' edizione originale del 1575.* ed. Raffaele Casimiri. Rome: Fratelli Scalera, 1940. [Book III of motets]

[**K20**=pp.1–84; **K21**=pp.85–150; **K22**=pp.151–216]
1. *Pater noster a 5* (pp.1–5)
2. *Ave Maria a 5* (pp.5–10)
3. *Cantantantibus organis a 5* (pp.10–14)
[secunda pars:] *Biduanis ac triduanis* (pp.14–18)
4. *Caro mea a 5* (pp.19–22)
5. *Angelus Domini descendit a 5* (pp.23–28)
[secunda pars:] *Et introeuntes in monumentum* (pp.29–34)
6. *Congrega Domine a 5* (pp.35–40)
[secunda pars:] *Afflige opprimentes nos* (pp.40–45)
7. *Inclytae sanctae virginis Catherinae a 5* (pp.45–49)
8. *Fuit homo missus a Deo a 5* (pp.49–53)
[secunda pars:] *Erat Joannes in deserto* (pp.53–57)
9. *O lux et decus Hispaniae a 5* (pp.57–61)
[secunda pars:] *O singulare praesidium* (pp.61–65)
10. *Quid habes Hester? a 5* (pp.66–70)
11. *Vidi te Domino a 5* (pp.70–75)

12. *Tradent enim vos a 5* (pp.75–80)
13. *Sanctificavit Dominus a 5* (pp.80–84)
14. *O quam metuendus est a 5* (pp.85–89)
15. *Jubilate Deo a 5* (pp.89–93)
    [secunda pars:] *Laudate nomen ejus* (pp.94–97)
16. *Omnipotens sempiterne Deus a 5* (pp.98–101)

16 bis. *O sancte praesul Nicolae* (pp.102–106)
    [secunda pars:] *Gaude praesul optime* (pp.107–110)

17. *Domine Deus qui conteris bella a 5* (pp.111–115)
    [secunda pars:] *Tu Domine cui humilium* (pp.115–119)
18. *Manifesto vobis veritatem a 5* (pp.120–124)
    [secunda pars:] *Pax vobis* (pp.125–129)
19. *Susanna ab improbis a 6* (pp.130–134)
    [secunda pars:] *Postquam autem* (pp.135–139)
20. *Cum ortus fuerit sol a 6* (pp.140–143)
21. *Rex pacificus a 6* (pp.144–147)
22. *Haec dies a 6* (pp.148–150)
23. *Columna es immobilis a 6* (pp.151–155)
24. *Judica me Deus a 6* (pp.155–159)
25. *Accepit Jesus calicem a 6* (pp.160–164)
26. *O bone Jesu a 6* (pp.165–167)
27. *Deus qui Ecclesiam tuam a 6* (pp.168–173)
28. *Surge illuminare Hierusalem a 8* (pp.174–179)
29. *Lauda Sion Salvatorem a 8* (pp.180–185)
30. *Veni Sancte Spiritus a 8* (pp.186–194)
31. *Ave Regina coelorum a 8* (pp.195–201)
32. *Hodie Christus natus est a 8* (pp.202–207)
33. *Jubilate Deo a 8* (pp.208–216)

[Volume 9] *Il libro primo dei madrigali (spirituali) a 5 voci secondo la stampa originale del 1581, con appendice di madrigali pubblicati in raccolte dal 1566 al 1576.* ed. Raffaele Casimiri. Rome: Fratelli Scalera, 1940. [Book I of spiritual madrigals; madrigals from anthologies 1566–1576.]

[**K23**=pp.1–80; **K24**=pp.81–165]

1. *Vergine bella, che di Sol vestita* (pp.1–8)
2. *Vergine saggia, e del bel numer'una* (pp.9–15)
3. *Vergine pura d'ogni parte intera* (pp.15–22)
4. *Vergine santa, d'ogni grazia piena* (pp.22–29)
5. *Vergine sola al mondo senzza esempio* (pp.29–37)
6. *Vergine chiara e stabile in eterno* (pp.38–44)
7. *Vergine, quante lagrime ho già sparte* (pp.45–51)
8. *Vergine, tale è terra e post'ha in doglia* (pp.52–58)
9. *Spirito santo, Amore, consolator* (pp.58–62)
10. *O Sol'incoronato di sette adorni lumi* (pp.63–66)
11. *O cibo di dolcezza* (pp.67–70)
12. *O refrigerio acceso d'un nutricante foco* (pp.70–74)
13. *Tu sei soave fiume de'bei parlar profondi* (pp.74–77)
14. *Paraclito amoroso, quando t'avro io?* (pp.78–80)

15. *Amor, senza il tuo dono* (pp.81–83)
16. *Dunque divin Spiracolo inspira il mio cor vano* (pp.84–86)
17. *O Manna saporito d'ogni dolcezza* (pp.86–89)
18. *Signor, dammi scienza* (pp.89–92)
19. *O Jesu dolce, o infinito amore* (pp.93–96)
20. *Giammai non resti a mille dolci modi* (pp.97–99)
21. *Quanto più t'offend'io* (pp.99–102)
22. *Non basta ch'una volta tu portasti* (pp.102–105)
23. *S'io non ti conoscessi in altre cose* (pp.106–108)
24. *Ma so ben, Signor mio* (pp.108–111)
25. *E tu, anima mia, fatta da Dio* (pp.111–113)
26. *Per questo, Signor mio, non ti stancare* (pp.114–116)

Appendix: [Secular] Madrigals for Five Voices

1. ["Anno 1566"] *Vestiva i colli a 5* (pp.117–121)
   [seconda parte:] *Così le chiome mie* (pp.122–125)
2. ["Anno 1568"] *Il tempo vola* (pp.126–129)
   [seconda parte:] *Ivi vedrai la gloria* (pp.129–132)
3. ["Anno 1574"] *Io felice sarei se gli occhi a 5* (pp.133–136)
4. ["Anno 1574"] *Ahi letizia fugace a 5* [Rodolfo Pierluigi] (pp.137–140)
5. ["Anno 1574"] *Le selv'avea d'intorn'al lido a 5* (pp.141–144)
   [seconda parte:] *Quando de'loro inpallidir a 5* (pp.144–148)
6. ["Anno 1574"] *Saggio e santo Pastor a 5* (pp.148–151)
   [seconda parte:] *Onde seguendo l'onorata impresa* (pp.152–154)
7. ["Anno 1574"] *Se di pianti e di stridi a 5* (pp.155–158)
8. ["Anno 1576"] *Placide l'acque e placid'era il vento a 5* (pp.158–161)
9. ["Anno 1576"] *Soave fia il morir a 5* (pp.162–165)

[Volume 10] *Il libro quarto delle messe a 4 e 5 voci secondo la stampa originale del 1582*. ed. Raffaele Casimiri. Rome: Fratelli Scalera, 1940. [Book IV of masses]

[**K25**=pp.1–78; **K26**=pp.79–188]

For Four Voices

1. *Missa prima. Lauda Sion* (pp.1–18)
2. *Missa secunda.* [*Primi toni*] (pp.19–37)
3. *Missa tertia. Jesu nostra redemptio* (pp.38–59)
4. *Missa quarta. L' homme armé* (pp.60–78)

For Five Voices

5. *Missa prima. Eripe me de inimicis meis* (pp.79–114)
6. *Missa secunda* (pp.115–149)
7. *Missa tertia. O magnum mysterium* (pp.150–188)

[Volume 11] *Il libro secondo dei mottetti a 4 voci secondo la ristampa del 1604. Il libro quarto dei mottetti a 5 voci [Cantico dei Cantici] secondo la ristampata del 1588*. ed. Raffaele Casimiri. Rome: Fratelli Scalera, 1941. [Book II of motets; Book IV of motets]

[**K27**=pp.3–62; **K28**=pp.63–138; **K29**=pp.139–200]

Mottetti a 4 Voci Dispari e Pari

1. *Domine quando veneris a 4* (pp.3–5)
   [secunda pars:] *Commissa mea pavesco* (pp.6–8)
2. *Heu mihi Domine a 4* (pp.8–11)
   [secunda pars:] *Anima mea turbata est* (pp.11–14)
3. *Super flumina Balylonis a 4* (pp.14–16)
4. *Ecce nunc benedicite Dominum a 4* (pp.17–19)
5. *Ad te levavi oculos meos a 4* (pp.20–22)
   [secunda pars:] *Miserere nostri Domine a 4* (pp.23–25)
6. *Ad Dominum cum tribularer a 4* (pp.26–28)
   [secunda pars:] *Sagittae potentis acutae* (pp.28–30)
7. *Fundamenta ejus a 4* (pp.30–33)
   [secunda pars:] *Numquid Sion dicet* (pp.33–36)
8. *Quia vidisti me Thoma a 4* (pp.36–39)
9. *Ego sum panis vivus a 4* (pp.39–42)
10. *Sicut cervus a 4* (pp.42–44)
    [secunda pars:] *Sitivit anima mea* (pp.44–47)
11. *Ave Regina coelorum a 4.* Paribus vocibus (pp.47–49)
    [secunda pars:] *Gaude, Virgo gloriosa* (pp.50–52)
12. *Alma Redemptoris Mater a 4.* Paribus vocibus (pp.52–54)
    [secunda pars:] *Tu quae genuisti* (pp.55–57)
13. *Salve Regina a 4.* Paribus vocibus (pp.57–60)
    [secunda pars:] *Eja ergo* (pp.60–62)
14. *Ave Maria a 4.* Paribus vocibus (pp.63–66)
15. *Haec dies a 4.* Paribus vocibus (pp.66–70)
16. *Confitemini Domino a 4.* Paribus vocibus (pp.70–72)
17. *Pueri Hebraeorum a 4.* Paribus vocibus (pp.72–74)
18. *Sub tuum praesidium a 4.* Paribus vocibus (pp.75–77)
19. *Adoramus te Christe a 4.* Paribus vocibus (pp.78–79)
20. *Surrexit pastor bonus a 4.* Paribus vocibus (pp.79–82)
21. *Gloriosi Principes terrae a 4.* Paribus vocibus (pp.83–85)

Il Libro Quarto dei Mottetti a 5 Voci [Cantico dei Cantici]

1. *Osculetur me* (pp.89–92)
2. *Trahe me post te* (pp.93–97)
3. *Nigra sum sed formosa* (pp.97–101)
4. *Vineam meam non custodivi* (pp.101–104)
5. *Si ignoras te* (pp.105–108)
6. *Pulchrae sunt genae tuae* (pp.109–112)
7. *Fasciculus myrrae* (pp.113–116)
8. *Ecce tu pulcher es* (pp.116–120)
9. *Tota pulchra es* (pp.120–123)
10. *Vulnerasti cor meum* (pp.124–127)
11. *Sicut lilium inter spinas* (pp.128–131)
12. *Introduxit me rex* (pp.132–135)
13. *Laeva ejus* (pp.135–138)
14. *Vox dilecti mei* (pp.139–142)
15. *Surge propera* (pp.142–146)
16. *Surge amica mea* (pp.146–150)
17. *Dilectus meus mihi* (pp.150–154)

18. *Surgam et circuibo civitatem* (pp.154–157)
19. *Adjuro vos filiae Jerusalem* (pp.157–162)
20. *Caput ejus* (pp.162–165)
21. *Dilectus meus descendit* (pp.166–169)
22. *Pulchra es* (pp.169–173)
23. *Quae est ista* (pp.173–176)
24. *Descendi in hortum meum* (pp.177–180)
25. *Quam pulchri sunt* (pp.181–184)
26. *Duo ubera tua* (pp.185–189)
27. *Quam pulchra es* (pp.189–192)
28. *Guttur tuum* (pp.193–196)
29. *Veni dilecte mi* (pp.197–200)

[Volume 12] *Il libro quinto dei mottetti a 5 voci secondo la ristampa del 1588.* ed. Raffaele Casimiri. Rome: Fratelli Scalera, 1941. [Book V of motets]
[**K30**=pp.1–53; **K31**=pp.54–113]

1. *Laetus Hyperboream* (pp.1–4)
   [secunda pars:] *O patruo* (pp.5–9)
2. *Paucitas dierum* (pp.9–12)
   [secunda pars:] *Manus tuae* (pp.12–15)
3. *Tempus est* (pp.16–19)
   [secunda pars:] *Nisi ego abiero* (pp.20–23)
4. *Domine secundum actum meum* (pp.23–27)
5. *Ave Trinitatus sacrarium* (pp.27–31)
6. *Parce mihi Domini* (pp.31–36)
7. *Peccavi quid faciam tibi* (pp.36–39)
8. *Orietur stella* (pp.40–44)
9. *Aegypte noli flere* (pp.45–49)
10. *Ardens est cor meum* (pp.49–53)
11. *Sic Deus dileit mundum* (pp.54–58)
12. *Surge Petre* (pp.58–63)
13. *Apparuit caro suo Joanni* (pp.64–67)
14. *Ecce merces Sanctorum* (pp.68–72)
15. *Videns Secundus* (pp.73–76)
16. *Rex Melchior* (pp.76–80)
17. *Ave Regina coelorum* (pp.80–84)
18. *Gaude [Virgo] gloriosa* (pp.84–87)
19. *Exsultate deo* (pp.88–92)
20. *Tribulationes civitatum* (pp.92–96)
    [secunda pars:] *Peccavimus* (pp.96–99)
21. *Surge sancte Dei* (pp.100–103)
    [secunda pars:] *Ambula sancte Dei* (pp.104–107)
22. *Salve Regina* (pp.108–110)
    [secunda pars:] *Eja ergo* (pp.111–113)

[Volume 13] *Le lamentazioni a 4, 5, 6 ed 8 voci seconda la stampa originale del 1589 e codici sincroni.* ed. Raffaele Casimiri. Rome: Fratella Scalera, 1941
[**K32**=pp.1–41; **K33**=pp.42–102; **K34**=pp.103–174;

K35=pp.175–270]
Liber Primus
Feria V. In Coena Domini
Lectio I. *Incipit Lamentatio . . . Aleph. Quomodo sedet* (pp.1–4)
Lectio II. *Vau. Et egressus est* (pp.5–9)
Lectio III. *Jod. Manum suam* (pp.9–13)
Feria VI. In Parasceve
Lectio I. *De lamentatione . . . Heth. Cogitavit* (pp.14–18)
Lectio II. *Lamed. Matribus suis* (pp.18–22)
Lectio III. *Aleph. Ego vir videns* (pp.22–26)
Sabbato Sancto
Lectio I. *De lamentatione . . . Heth. Misericordiae Domini* (pp.27–31)
Lectio II. *Aleph. Quodomo obscuratum* (pp.32–36)
Lectio III. *Incipit Oratio . . . Recordare* (pp.36–41)
Liber Secundus
Feria V. In Coena Domini
Lectio I. *Incipit Lamentatio . . . Aleph. Quomodo sedet* (pp.42–46)
Lectio II. *Vau. Et egressus est* (pp.47–53)
Lectio III. *Iod. Manum suam* (pp.54–60)
Feria VI. In Parasceve
Lectio I. *De Lamentatione . . . Heth. Cogitavit* (pp.61–67)
Lectio II. *Lamed. Matribus suis* (pp.68–74)
Lectio III. *Aleph. Ego vir videns* (pp.74–79)
Sabbato Sancto
Lectio I. *De Lamentatione . . . Heth. Misericordiae* (pp.80–86)
Lectio II. *Aleph. Quomodo obscuratum* (pp.86–92)
Lectio III. *Incipit Oratio . . . Recordare* (pp.94–102)
Liber Tertius
Feria V. In Coena Domini
Lectio I. *Incipit Lamentatio . . . Aleph. Quomodo sedet* (pp.103–109)
Lectio II. *Vau. Et egressus est* (pp.110–119)
Lectio III. *Iod. Manum suam* (pp.120–127)
Feria VI. In Parasceve
Lectio I. *De Lamentatione . . . Heth. Cogitavit* (pp.128–133)
Lectio II. *Lamed. Matribus suis* (pp.134–142)
Lectio III. *Aleph. Ego vir videns* (pp.142–149)
Sabbato Sancto
Lectio I. *De Lamentatione . . . Heth. Misericordiae* (pp.150–158)
Lectio II. *Aleph. Quomodo obscuratum est* (pp.158–165)
Lectio III. *Incipit Oratio . . . Recordare* (pp.166–174)
Liber Quartus, 5 et 6 Vocibus
Feria V. In Coena Domini
Lectio I. *Incipit Lamentatio . . . Aleph. Quomodo sedet* (pp.175–181)
Lectio II. *Vau. Et egressus est* (pp.181–189)
Lectio III. *Iod. Manum suam* (pp.190–197)
Feria VI. In Parasceve
Lectio I. *De Lamentatione . . . Cogitavit* (pp.198–206)
Lectio II. *Lamed. Matribus suis* (pp.206–215)

Lectio III. *Aleph. Ego vir videns* (pp.216–222)
Sabbato Sancto
Lectio I. *De Lamentatione . . . Heth. Misericordiae* (pp.223–231)
Lectio II. *Aleph. Quomodo obscuratum est* (pp.231–237)
Lectio III. *Incipit Oratio . . . Recordare* (pp.237–242)
Appendix
Lectio I. Feria VI. In Parasceve (pp.243–248)
Lectio II. Feria VI. In Parasceve (pp.249–252)
Lectio II. Sabbato Sancto (pp.252–257)
Lectio III. Sabbato Sancto (pp.258–267)
Lectio IV. Feria V. In Coena Domini [fragment] (pp.268–270)

[Volume 14] *Inni di tutto l' anno a 4, 5 e 6 voci secondo la stampa originale del 1589.* ed. Raffaele Casimiri. Rome: Fratelli Scalera, 1942. [Hymns]
K36=pp.1–73; **K37**=pp.74–155; **K38**=pp.155–237]

1. In Adventu Domini. *Conditor alme siderum* [odd strophes] (pp.1–70)
2. In Nativitate et Circumcisione Domini. *Christe redemptor omnium* [odd] (pp.8–14)
3. In Nativitate Domini. *A solis ortus cardine* [odd] (pp.15–20)
4. In festo Sanctorum Innocentium. *Salvete flos Martyrum* [odd] (pp.21–22)
5. In Epiphania Domini. *Hostis Herodes impie* [odd] (pp.23–27)
6. In Dominicis per Annum. *Lucis Creator optime* [odd] (pp.28–33)
7. In Sabbatis. *O lux beata Trinitas* [odd] (pp.33–37)
8. In Dominicis Quadragesimae. *Ad preces nostras* [odd] (pp.37–45)
9. In Dominica Passionis et Exaltationis S. Crucis. *Vexilla regis prodeunt* [odd] (pp.46–53)
10. In Dominicis, Tempore Paschali. *Ad coenam agni providi* [odd] (pp.54–60)
11. In Ascensione Domini. *Jesu nostra redemptio* [odd] (pp.60–66)
12. In festo Pentecostes. *Veni Creator Spiritus* [odd] (pp.67–73)
13. In festo Corporis Christi. *Pange lingua gloriosi* [odd] (pp.74–80)
14. In festo Cathedrae S. Petri. *Quodcumque ligaveris* [odd] (pp.80–83)
15. In Conversione et Commemoratione S. Pauli. *Doctor egregie* [odd] (pp.83–85)
16. In festis beatae Virginis. *Ave maris stella* [odd] (pp.85–91)
17. In Inventione S. Crucis. Tempore paschali. *Vexilla regis prodeunt* [even] (pp.91–96)
18. In festo S. Joannis Baptistae. *Ut queant laxis* [odd] (pp.96–103)
19. In festo apostolorum Petri et Pauli. *Aurea luce* [odd] (pp.103–108)
20. In festo S. Mariae Magdalenae. *Lauda mater Ecclesiae* [odd] (pp.109–112)
21. In festo S. Petri ad Vincula. *Petrus beatus* [odd] (pp.112–114)
22. In festo Transfigurationis Domini. *Quicumque Christum quaeritis* [odd] (pp.114–118)
23. In festo S. Michaelis Archangeli. *Tibi Christe splendor Patris* [odd] (pp.119–122)
24. In festo Omnium Sanctorum. *Christe Redemptor omnium* [odd] (pp.123–129)

25. In Communi Apostolorum et Evangelistarum. *Exsultet caelum laudibus* [odd] (pp.130–135)
26. In festo Apostolorum et Evangelistarum. Tempore paschali. *Tristis erant apostoli* [odd] (pp.136–140)
27. In Communi unius Martyris. *Deus tuorum militum* [odd] (pp.141–145)
28. In festo unius Martyris. Tempore paschali. *Deus tuorum militum* [odd] (pp.146–149)
29. In Communi plurimorum Martyrum. *Sanctorum meritis* [odd] (pp.150–155)
30. In festo plurimorum Martyrum. Tempore paschali. *Rex glorisose martyrum* [odd] (pp.155–158)
31. In Natali Confessorum. *Iste Confessor* [odd] (pp.158–164)
32. In Natalitiis Virginum et Martyrum. *Jesu corona Virginum* [odd] (pp.164–168)
33. In festo Virginum et Martyrum. Tempore paschali. *Jesu corona Virginum* [odd] (pp.169–175)
34. In festo Sanctarum Mulierum. *Hujus obtentu* [odd] (pp.175–176)
35. In festo Dedicationis Ecclesiae. *Urbs beata Jerusalem* [odd] (pp.177–183)
36. In festo S. Augustini. *Magnus pater Augustine* [odd] (pp.184–189)
37. In festo S. Nicolai de Tolentino. *Laudibus summis* [odd] (pp.190–195)
38. In festo S. Antonii de Padua. *En gratulemur hodie* [odd] (pp.196–201)
39. In festo S. Francisci. In primis Vesperis. *Proles de coelo prodiit* [odd] (pp.202–208)
40. In festo S. Francisci. In secundis Vesperis. *Decus morum dux minorum* [odd] (pp.208–214)
41. In Quadragesima. Ad Completorium. *Christe qui lux es et dies* [odd] (pp.215–219)
42. In festo S. Elisaei. *Prima lux surgens* [odd] (pp.220–224)
43. In festo S. Eliae. *Nunc juvat celsi* [odd] (pp.225–229)
44. In festo S. Alberti. *Mensis Augusti* [odd] (pp.230–234)
45. In festo S. Jacobi. *Hymnus canoris* [odd] (pp.235–237)

[Volume 15] *Il libro quinto delle messe a 4, 5 e 6 voci secondo la stampa originale del 1590.* ed. Raffaele Casimiri. Rome: Fratelli Scalera, 1941. [Book V of masses]

[**K39**=pp.1–88; **K40**=pp.89–190]

For Four Voices

1. *Missa Aeterna Christi munera* (pp.1–19)
2. *Missa Jam Christus astra ascenderat* (pp.20–44)
3. *Missa Panis quem ego dabo* (pp.45–71)
4. *Missa Iste Confessor* (pp.72–88)

For Five Voices

5. *Missa Nigra sum* (pp.89–129)
6. *Missa Sicut lilium inter spinas* (pp.130–160)

For Six Voices
7. *Missa Nasce la gioja mia* (pp.161–190)

[Volume 16] *I Magnificat a 4, 5, 6 ed 8 voci secondo la stampa originale del 1591 e i codici manoscritto dell'epoca.* ed. Lavinio Virgili. Rome: Fratelli Scalera, 1950. [*Magnificat*]
[**K41**=pp.1–97; **K42**=pp.98–189; **K43**=pp.190–302; **K44**=pp.303–334]
Liber Primus
Primi toni a 4 [odd-numbered verses] (pp.1–7)
Secundi toni a 4 [odd] (pp.7–13)
Tertii toni a 4 [odd] (pp.13–18)
Quarti toni a 4 [odd] (pp.19–25)
Quinti toni a 4 [odd] (pp.25–31)
Sexti toni a 4 [odd] (pp.23–37)
Septimi toni a 4 [odd] (pp.38–44)
Octavi toni a 4 [odd] (pp.44–49)
Primi toni a 4 [even-numbered verses] (pp.50–55)
Secundi toni a 4 [even] (pp.56–61)
Tertii toni a 4 [even] (pp.62–67)
Quarti toni a 4 [even] (pp.68–73)
Quinti toni a 4 [even] (pp.74–79)
Sexti toni a 4 [even] (pp.80–85)
Septimi toni a 4 [even] (pp.86–92)
Octavi toni a 4 [even] (pp.93–97)
Liber Secundus
Primi toni a 4 [even] (pp.98–111)
Secundi toni a 4 [even] (pp.111–124)
Tertii toni a 4 [even] (pp.124–135)
Quarti toni a 4 [even] (pp.136–146)
Quinti toni a 4 [even] (pp.147–157)
Sexti toni a 4 [even] (pp.157–167)
Septimi toni a 4 [even] (pp.168–179)
Octavi toni a 4 [even] (pp.179–189)
Liber Tertius 5et 6 Vocum
Primi toni a 5 [even] (pp.190–203)
Secundi toni a 5 [even] (pp.203–215)
Tertii toni a 6 [even] (pp.215–228)
Quarti toni a 6 [even] (pp.229–245)
Quinti toni a 5 [even] (pp.246–259)
Sexti toni a 6 [even] (pp.260–275)
Septimi toni a 5 [even] (pp.276–290)
Octavi toni a 6 [even] (pp.290–302)
Appendix
Quarti toni cum quatuor vocibus paribus [even] (pp.303–311)
Sexti toni [even] (pp.312–322)
Primi toni octonis vocibus [complete] (pp.323–334)

[Volume 17] *Offertori di tutto l' anno a 5 voci secondo la stampa originale del 1593.* ed. Lavinio Virgili. Rome: Fratelli Scalera, 1952. [Offertories]

[**K45**=pp.1–89; **K46**=pp.90–195; **K47**=pp.196–257]

1. Dominica prima Adventus. *Ad te levavi animam meam* (pp.1–5)
2. Dominica secunda Adventus. *Deus tu convertens* (pp.5–9)
3. Dominica tertia Adventus. *Benedixisti Domini* (pp.10–13)
4. Dominica quarta Adventus. *Ave Maria* (pp.14–17)
5. In Nativitate domini ad tertiam Missam, et in Circumcisione. *Tui sunt coeli* (pp.18–22)
6. In festo Sancti Stephani protomartyris. *Elegerunt Apostoli* (pp.22–26)
7. In festo S. Joannis Apostoli. *Justus ut palma* (pp.26–30)
8. In festo sanctorum Innocentium. *Anima nostra* (pp.30–34)
9. In festo sancti Thomae Archiepiscopi et martyris. *Posuisti Domine* (pp.34–37)
10. Dominica infra oct. Nativitatis Domini. *Deus enim firmavit* (pp.38–39)
11. In festo sancti Silvestri, Papae et conf. *Inveni David* (pp.41–45)
12. In Epiphania Domini. *Reges Tharsis* (pp.45–48)
13. Dominica infra oct. Epiphania. *Jubilate Deo omnis terra* (pp.49–52)
14. Dominica secunda post Epiphaniam. *Jubilate Deo universa terra* (pp.53–57)
15. Dominica tertia, quarta et V. post Epiphaniam. *Dextera Domini* (pp.57–60)
16. Dominica in Septuagesima. *Bonum est confiteri* (pp.61–64)
17. Dominica in Sexagesima. *Perfice gressus meos* (pp.64–68)
18. Dominica in Quinquagesima. *Benedictus es* (pp.69–73)
19. Dominica prima Quadragesimae. *Scapulis suis* (pp.73–77)
20. Dominica secunda Quadragesimae. *Meditabor* (pp.77–81)
21. Dominica tertia Quadragesimae. *Justitiae Domini* (pp.81–85)
22. Dominica quarta Quadragesimae. *Laudate Dominum quia benignus est* (pp.85–89)
23. Dominica de Passione. *Confitebor tibi* (pp.90–94)
24. Dominica Palmarum. *Improperium exspectavit* (pp.94–99)
25. Dominica Resurrectionis Domini. *Terra tremuit* (pp.99–103)
26. Dominica in Albis, in Octava Paschae. *Angelus Domini* (pp.103–107)
27. Dominica secunda post Pascha. *Deus Deus meus* (pp.107–110)
28. Dominica tertia post Pascha. *Lauda anima mea* (pp.111–114)
29. Dominica quinta post Pascha. *Benedicite gentes* (pp.115–119)
30. In die Ascensione Domini. *Ascendit Deus* (pp.120–123)
31. In Dominica Pentecostes. *Confirma hoc* (pp.123–127)
32. In festo SS. Trinitatis. *Benedictus sit Deus* (pp.128–132)
33. In Solemnitate Corporis Christi. *Sacerdotes Domini* (pp.132–136)
34. Dominica secunda post Pentecosten. *Domine convertere* (pp.136–140)
35. Dominica tertia post Pentecosten. *Sperent in te* (pp.141–145)
36. Dominica quarta post Pentecosten. *Illumina oculos meos* (pp.145–149)
37. Dominica quinta post Pentecosten. *Benedicam Dominum* (pp.150–153)
38. Dominica septima post Pentecosten. *Sicut in holocaustis* (pp.154–158)

39. Dominica octava post Pentecosten. *Populum humilem* (pp.158–162)
40. Dominica nona post Pentecosten. *Justitiae Domini* (pp.162–166)

Offertoria Secunda Pars

41. Dominica XI. post Pentecosten. *Exaltabo te* (pp.167–170)
42. Dominica XII. post Pentecosten. *Precatus est Moyses* (pp.171–175)
43. Dominica XIII. post Pentecosten. *In te speravi* (pp.175–179)
44. Dominica XIV. post Pentecosten. *Immittet Angelus* (pp.179–183)
45. Dominica XV. post Pentecosten. *Exspectans expectavi* (pp. 183–187)
46. Dominica XVI. post Pentecosten. *Domine in auxilium* (pp.187–191)
47. Dominica XVII. post Pentecosten. *Oravi ad Dominum* (pp.191–195)
48. Dominica XVIII. post Pentecosten. *Sanctificavit Moyses* (pp.196–200)
49. Dominica XIX. post Pentecosten. *Si ambulavero* (pp.200–204)
50. Dominica XX. post Pentecosten. *Super flumina* (pp.205–208)
51. Dominica XXI. post Pentecosten. *Vir erat in terra Hus* (pp.209–212)
52. Dominica XXII. post Pentecosten. *Recordare me* (pp.213–217)
53. Dominica XXIII. et XXIV. post Pentecosten. *De profundis* (pp.217–221)
54. In Nativitae S. Joan. Baptistae. *Justus ut palma* (pp.221–225)
55. In die S. Jacobi Apostoli. *Mihi autem nimis* (pp.225–229)
56. In festo S. Laurentii Martyris. *Confessio et pulchritudo* (pp.229–233)
57. In Assumptione Beatae Mariae Virginis. *Assumpta est Maria* (pp.233–237)
    [In festo S. Bartholomaei: vide *Mihi autem*, p.225]
58. In festo Dedicationis S. Michaelis Archang. *Stetit Angelus* (pp.237–241)
59. In die SS. Apostol. Petri et Pauli. *Constitues eos* (pp.241–246)
    [In Annuntiatione B. M.V. *Ave Maria*]
60. In festo SS. Apostol. Philippi et Jacobi. *Confitebuntur coeli* (pp.246–250)
61. In festo SS. Apostol. Simonis et Judae. *In omnem terram* (pp.250–254)
62. In die Commemorationis Omnium Sanctorum. *Justorum animae* (pp.254–257)
63. Commune Sanctorum. *Veritas mea* (pp.258–261)
64. Commune plurimorum Martyrum. *Laetamini in Domino* (pp.262–265)
65. Commune Virginum. *Afferentur Regi* (pp.266–268)
66. In festo Dedicatione Ecclesiae. *Domine Deus* (pp.269–272)
67. In festo Purificationis B. Mariae Virginis. *Diffusa est gratia* (pp.272–276)
68. In festo Cathedrae Sancti Petri. *Tu es Petrus* (pp.277–281)

[Volume 18] *Le messe di Mantova (1). Inedite dai manoscritti di Santa Barbara.* ed. Knud Jeppesen. Rome: Istituto Italiano per la Storia della Musica, 1954. [Pages ix–xxvi contain prefatory matter by Jeppesen on the recovery, sources, and construction of these masses]

For Five Voices
1. *Missa In duplicibus (minoribus I)* (pp.1–41; alternatim setting)
2. *Missa In duplicibus (minoribus II)* (pp.42–82; alternatim setting)
3. *Missa Beatae Mariae Virg(inis I)* (pp.83–125; alternatim setting)
4. *Missa Beatae Mariae Virg(inis II)* (pp.126–161; alternatim setting)
5. *Missa Beatae Mariae Virg(inis III)* (pp.162–201; alternatim setting)

[Volume 19] *Le messe di Mantova (2). Inediti dai manoscritti di Santa Barbara.* ed. Knud Jeppesen. Rome: Istituto Italiano per la Storia della Musica, 1954.
For Five Voices
1. *Missa In festis Apostolor(um I)* (pp.1–42; alternatim)
2. *Missa In festis Apostolor(um II)* (pp.43–86; alternatim)
3. *Missa In semidupl(icibus) maior(ibus I)* (pp.87–128; alternatim)
4. *Missa In semidupl(icibus) maior(ibus II)* (pp.129–167; alternatim)

For Four Voices
5. *Missa (Sine nomine)* [polyphony throughout] (pp.168–193)

[Volume 20] *Le litanie a 3, 4, 5, 6 e 8 voci secondo la ristampa del 1600 e i diversi codici manoscritti.* ed. Lino Bianchi. Rome: Istituto Italiano per la Storia della Musica, 1955. [Litanies]
[**K48**=pp.1–71; **K49**=pp.72–160]

Liber Primus

Litaniae Deiparae Virginis a 4:
Prima pars [*Kyrie eleison . . . Virgo Mater*] (pp.1–6); *Ave Maria* (pp.6–9); Secunda pars [*Kyrie eleison . . . Maria Mater gratiae*] (pp.10–15); Tertia pars [*Kyrie eleison . . . Virgo Maria*] (pp.15–20); Quarta pars [*Kyrie eleison . . . Ave de coelis*] (pp.21–26); Quinta pars [*Kyrie eleison . . . Ab omni malo*] (pp.27–35).

Litaniae Liber Secundus Ternis et Quaternis Vocibus Aequalibus si Relinquatur Superior Pars

Prima pars [*Kyrie eleison . . . Virgo Mater*] (pp.36–42); *Ave Maria* (pp.42–44); Secunda pars [*Kyrie eleison . . . Maria Mater gratiae*] (pp.45–51); Tertia pars [*Kyrie eleison . . . Virgo Maria*] (pp.51–58); Quarta pars [*Kyrie eleison . . . Ave de coelis*] (pp.58–65); Quinta pars [*Kyrie eleison . . . Ab omni malo*] (pp.65–71).

Appendix
1. *Litaniae de Beata Virgine Maria a 5* (pp.72–76)
2. *Litaniae de Beata Virgine Maria a 6* (pp.77–85)
3. *Litaniae de Beata Virgine Maria a 8* (pp.86–105)
4. *Litaniae de Beata Virgine Maria a 8* (pp.106–115)
5. *Litaniae Domini a 8* (pp.116–128)
6. *Litaniae Domini a 8* (pp.129–135)
7. *Litaniae Domini a 8* (pp.136–143)
8. *Litaniae Sacrosanctae Eucharistiae a 8* (pp.144–153)
9. *Litaniae Sacrosanctae Eucharistiae a 8* (pp.154–160)

[Volume 21] *Il libro sesto delle messe a 4, 5 e 6 voci secondo la stampa originale del 1594, la seconda edizione del 1596, e codici manoscritti.* ed. Lino Bianchi. Rome: Istituto Italiano per la Storia della Musica, 1956. [Book

VI of masses]
[**K50**=pp.1–104; **K51**=pp.105–187]

For Four Voices

1. *Missa Dies sanctificatus* (pp.1–25)
2. *Missa In te Domine speravi* (pp.26–51)
3. *Missa Sine nomine* (pp.52–72)
4. *Missa Quam pulchra es* (pp.73–104)

For Five Voices

5. *Missa Dilexi quoniam* (pp.105–141)

For Six Voices

6. *Missa Ave Maria* (pp.142–187)

[Volume 22] *Il libro secondo dei madrigali spirituali a 5 voci [Priego alla B. Vergine], secondo la stampa originale del 1594.* ed.Lino Bianchi. Rome: Istituto Italiano per la Storia della Musica, 1957. [Madrigal texts pages xiii–xv.] [Book II of spiritual madrigals]
[**K52**=pp.1–97]

1. *Figlio immortal d'immortal Padre* (pp.1–4)
2. *E se mai voci di qua giù son grate* (pp.4–7)
3. *Hor tu sol, che di vivi almi splendori* (pp.7–10)
4. *Dammi, scala del ciel e del ciel porta* (pp.10–13)
5. *E se fur già de le mie mani immonde* (pp.13–15)
6. *Dammi, vermiglia rosa e bianco e puro* (pp.16–19)
7. *E se'l pensier de la futura morte* (pp.19–22)
8. *Eletta Mirra, che soave odore* (pp.22–25)
9. *Cedro gentil, da gli amorosi vermi* (pp.25–28)
10. *Fa che con l'acque tue splendenti e vive* (pp.28–31)
11. *S'amarissimo fele e mortal tosco* (pp.31–34)
12. *Horto che sei si chiuso e si serrato* (pp.34–37)
13. *E se nel foco di lascivi ardendo* (pp.37–40)
14. *Vincitrice de l'empia hidra infernale* (pp.40–43)
15. *Città di Dio, cui fan tempi e fortezze* (pp.43–46)
16. *Santo Altare, d'odore più veri e degni* (pp.46–50)
17. *Tu di fortezza torre e torre eburna* (pp.50–53)
18. *Specchio che fosti si polito e terso* (pp.54–57)
19. *Vello di Gedeon, cui Dio si largo* (pp.57–60)
20. *Novella Aurora, che nascend'allegri* (pp.60–63)
21. *E questo spirito, de la propria sede* (pp.63–66)
22. *E dal letto di mille e mille colpe* (pp.66–69)
23. *Et arda ogn'hor sopra'l lapideo altare* (pp.70–72)
24. *E tua mercè da così cieca e folta* (pp.73–75)
25. *Et quella certa speme e quella fede* (pp.76–79)
26. *Anzi, se foco e ferro e se veleno* (pp.79–82)
27. *E con i raggi tuoi splendenti e chiari* (pp.82–86)
28. *Regina de le Vergini e di tutte* (pp.86–89)
29. *Al fin, Madre di Dio, che ne più bella* (pp.90–93)
30. *E tu Signor, tu la grazia infondi* (pp.94–97)

[Volume 23] *Il libro settimo delle messe a 4 e 5 voci secondo la stampa originale del 1594, le edizioni del 1605 e del 1609, e codici manoscritti.* ed. Lino Bianchi. Rome: Istituto Italiano per la Storia della Musica, 1957. [Book VII of masses]

[**K53**=pp.1–81; **K54**=pp.82–148; **K55**=pp.149–212]

For Four Voices

1. *Missa Ave Maria* (pp.1–29)
2. *Missa Sanctorum meritis* (pp.30–60)
3. *Missa Emendemus* (pp.61–81)

For Five Voices

4. *Missa Sacerdoes et pontifex* (pp.82–114)
5. *Missa Tu es pastor ovium* (pp.115–148)

Appendix: For Four Voices

6. *Missa In majoribus duplicibus* (pp.149–181)
7. *Missa In minoribus duplicibus* (pp.182–212)

[Volume 24] *Il libro ottavo delle messe a 4, 5 e 6 voci secondo la stampa originale del 1599, la seconda edizione del 1609, e codici manoscritti.* ed. Lino Bianchi. Rome: Istituto Italiano per la Storia della Musica, 1958. [Book VIII of masses]

[**K56**=pp.1–85; **K57**=pp.86–156; **K58**=157–263]

For Four Voices

1. *Missa Quem dicunt homines* (pp.1–31)
2. *Missa Dum esset summis pontifex* (pp.32–51)

For Five Voices

3. *Missa O admirabile commercium* (pp.52–85)
4. *Missa Memor esto* (pp.86–116)

For Six Voices

4. *Missa Dum complerentur* (pp.117–156)
5. *Missa Sacerdotes Domini* (pp.157–193)

Appendix: For Five Voices

6. *Missa Beatus Laurentius* (pp.194–226)
7. *Missa O sacrum convivium* (pp.227–263)

[Volume 25] *Il libro nono delle messe a 4, 5 e 6 voci. Secondo la stampa originale del 1599, la seconda edizione del 1608, e codici manoscritti.* ed. Lino Bianchi. Rome: Istituto Italiano per la Storia della Musica, 1958. [Book IX of masses]

[**K59**=pp.1–92; **K60**=pp.93–171; **K61**=pp.172–286]

For Four Voices

1. *Missa Ave Regina coelorum* (pp.1–29)
2. *Missa Veni sponsa Christi* (pp.30–53)

For Five Voices

3. *Missa Vestiva i colli* (pp.54–92)
4. *Missa Sine nomine* (pp.93–130)

For Six Voices

5. *Missa In te Domine speravi* (pp.131–171)

6. *Missa Te Deum laudamus* (pp.172–208)
Appendix: For Six Voices
7. *Missa Assumpta est Maria* (pp.209–245)
8. *Missa Veni Creator Spiritus* (pp.246–286)

[Volume 26] *Messa Tu es Petrus, a 18 voci, in tre cori. Prima stampa secondo il codici Manoscritto.* ed. Lino Bianchi. Rome: Istituto Italiano per la Storia della Musica, 1959.
[**K62**=pp.1–76]
1. *Kyrie* (pp.1–10)
2. *Gloria* (pp.11–32)
3. *Credo* (pp.33–61)
4. *Sanctus* (pp.62–70)
5. *Agnus Dei* (pp.71–76)

[Volume 27] *Il libro decimo delle messe a 4, 5 e 6 voci. Secondo la stampa originale del 1600, stampe del tempo, e codici manoscritti.* ed. Lino Bianchi. Rome: Istituto Italiano per la Storia della Musica, 1959. [Book X of masses]
[**K63**=pp.1–88; **K64**=pp.89–198; **K65**=pp.199–258]
For Four Voices
1. *Missa In illo tempore* (pp.1–29)
2. *Missa Già fu chi m'ebbe cara* (pp.30–51)
For Five Voices
3. *Missa Petra Sancta* (pp.52–88)
4. *Missa O Virgo simul et Mater* (pp.89–119)
For Six Voices
4. *Missa Quinti toni* (pp.120–154)
5. *Missa Illumina oculos meos vel ad beneplacitum* (pp.155–198)
Appendix: For Four Voices
6. *Missa Pater noster* (pp.199–225)
For Five Voices
7. *Missa Panem nostrum* (pp.226–258)

[Volume 28] *Il libro decimoprimo delle messe a 4, 5 e 6 voci. Secondo la stampa originale del 1600 e codici manoscritti.* ed. Lino Bianchi. Rome: Istituto Italiano per la Storia della Musica, 1960. [Book XI of masses]
[**K66**=pp.1–113; **K67**=pp.114–221; **K68**=pp.222–302]
For Four Voices
1. *Missa Descendit Angelus Domini* (pp.1–31)
For Five Voices
2. *Missa Regina coeli* (pp.32–70)
3. *Missa Quando lieta sperai* (pp.73–113)
For Six Voices
4. *Missa Octavi toni* (pp.114–147)
5. *Missa Alma redemptoris* (pp.148–184)
Appendix: For Five Voices
6. *Missa Salve Regina* (pp.185–221)

For Six Voices
7. *Missa Sine titulo* (pp.222–267)
8. *Missa Tu es Petrus* (pp.268–302)

[Volume 29] *Il libro decimosecondo delle messe a 4, 5 e 6 voci. Secondo la stampa originale del 1601 e codici manoscritti.* ed. Lino Bianchi. Rome: Istituto Italiano per la Storia della Musica, 1961. [Book XII of masses]
[**K69**=pp.1–87; **K70**=pp.88–158; **K71**=pp.159–234]
For Four Voices
1. *Missa Regina coeli* (pp.1–29)
2. *Missa O rex gloriae* (pp.30–53)
For Five Voices
3. *Missa Ascendo ad Patrem* (pp.54–87)
4. *Missa Qual'è il più grande amor* (pp.88–122)
For Six Voices
5. *Missa Tu es Petrus* (pp.123–158)
6. *Missa Viri Galilaei* (pp.159–196)
Appendix: For Five Voices
7. *Missa Ecco ego Joannes* (pp.197–234)

[Volume 30] *Le messe a 8 voci. Secondo le stampe originali del 1585 e del 1601 e codici manoscritti.* ed. Lino Bianchi. Rome: Istituto Italiano per la Storia della Musica, 1961. [Masses for eight voices]
[**K72**=pp.1–109; **K73**=pp.110–227]
1. *Missa Laudate Dominum omnes gentes* (pp.1–58)
2. *Missa Hodie Christus natus est* (pp.59–109)
3. *Missa Fratres ego enim accepi* (pp.110–162)
4. *Missa Confitebor tibi Domine* (pp.163–227)

[Volume 31] *Il libro secondo dei madrigali a 4 voci. Secondo la stampa originale del 1586.* ed. Lino Bianchi. Rome: Istituto Italiano per la Storia della Musica, 1965. [Book II of madrigals a 4]
[**K74**=pp.1–79]
1. *Così la fama scriva in sempiterni marmi* (pp.1–4)
2. *S'un sguardo un fa beato* (pp.4–7)
3. *Amor, ben puoi tu hormai* (pp.7–10)
4. *Partomi, donna, e teco* (pp.10–13)
5. *Veramente in amore* (pp.14–16)
6. *Gioia m'abond'al cor* (pp.17–20)
7. *Donna gentil* (pp.20–24)
8. *Io dovea ben pensarmi* (pp.24–28)
9. *Se'l pensier che mi strugge* (pp.28–30)
10. *Chi dunque fia* (pp.31–34)
11. *Mirate altrove* (pp.34–37)
12. *Si è debile il filo* (pp.37–41)
13. *I vaghi fiori* (pp.41–44)
14. *Mori quasi il mio core* (pp.44–47)
15. *Alla riva del Tebro* (pp.47–50)

16. *Amor, quando fioriva* (pp.50–53)
17. *Beltà se come in ment'io* (pp.54–56)
18. *La cruda mia nemica* (pp.57–59)
19. *O che splendor* (pp.60–62)
20. *Io sento qui d'intorno* (pp.62–65)
21. *Deh, fuss'hor qui madonna* (pp.65–68)
22. *Se non fusse il pensier* (pp.68–70)
23. *Perché s'annida amor* (pp.70–73)
24. *Ogni beltà, madonna* (pp.73–76)
25. *Ardo lungi e dapresso* (pp.77–79)

[Volume 32] *Le composizioni Latine a 12 voci.* ed. Lino Bianchi. Rome: Istituto Italiano per la Storia della Musica, 1972.

Five Motets
1. *Ecce, nunc benedicite Dominum* (pp.1–14)
2. *Servum verbum tuum* [*Nunc dimittis servum tuum Domine*] (pp.15–27)
3. *Laudate Dominum in tympanis* (pp.28–43)
4. *O gloriosa Domina* (pp.44–55)
5. *Miserere mei Deus* (pp.56–70)

Mass
6. *Missa Cantantibus organis Caecilia* [complete] (pp.71–173)
   Et in terra pax . . . filius Patris [*Gloria*] contributed by Palestrina (pp.84–95)

[Volume 33] *Composizioni Latine a 8 e 9 voci.* ed. Lino Bianchi. Rome: Istituto Italiano per la Storia della Musica, 1981.

1. *Surrexit pastor bonus a 8* (pp.15–21)
   [secunda pars:] *Etenim Pascha nostrum a 8* (pp.21–27)
2. *Iesus iunxit se discipulis a 8* (pp.28–35)
   [secunda pars:] *Et increpavit eos a 8* (pp.36–42)
3. *Stabat mater dolorosa a 8* (pp.43–49)
   [secunda pars:] *Eia mater fons amoris a 8* (pp.50–60)
4. *Hodie gloriosa a 8* (pp.61–66)
   [secunda pars:] *Regina mundi a 8* (pp.67–71)
5. *Spiritus sanctus replevit a 8* (pp.72–80)
6. *Et ambulabunt gentes a 8* (pp.81–89)
   [This is the secunda pars of *Surge illuminare Hierusalem*: see vol 8 pp.174–179]
7. *O pretiosum a 8* (pp.90–96)
8. *O admirabile commercium a 8* (pp.97–102)
9. *Videntes stellam Magi a 8* (pp.103–110)
10. *Miserere mei Deus* [*in duplici choro*] *4 et 5 vocum* (pp.111–117)
11. *Miserere mei Deus. In duplici choro 4 et 5 vocum* (pp.118–125)
12. *Qui statis in domo Domini (Ecce nunc benedicite)* [*In duplici choro*] *4 et 5 vocum* (pp.126–127)
13. *Quia viderunt oculi mei (Nunc dimittis)* [*In duplici choro*] *4 et 5 vocum* (pp.128–129)

14. *Benedictus pro Hebdomanda sancta a 9* (pp.130–145)

[Volume 34] *Le composizioni Latine a 8 voci*. ed. Lino Bianchi. Roma: Istituto Italiano per la Storia della Musica, 1987.

1. *Regina caeli* (pp.1–10)
2. *Regina caeli* (pp.11–19)
3. [*Alma*] *Redemptoris* (pp.20–28)
4. *Ave mundi spes, Maria* (pp.29–40)
5. *Beata es Virgo Maria* (pp.41–46)
   [secunda pars:] *Ave Maria* (pp.47–53)
6. *O quam suavis* (pp.54–60)
7. *Disciplinam et sapientiam* (pp.61–69)
8. *Nunc dimittis* (pp.70–78)
9. *Omnes gentes plaudite* (pp.79–89)
10. *Fratres ego enim accepi* (pp.90–97)
11. *Expurgate vetus fermentum* (pp.98–106)
12. *Laudate Dominum de caelis* (pp.107–114)
13. *Sub tuum praesidium confugimus* (pp.115–120)
14. *Pater noster* (pp.121–125)
15. *Apparuit gratia Dei* (pp.126–133)
16. *Caro mea vere est cibus* (pp.134–140)
    [secunda pars:] *Hic est panis* (pp.141–147)
17. *Dies sanctificatus* (pp.149–155)
18. *Hic est dies praeclarus* (pp.156–162)
19. *Congratulamini mihi omnes* (pp.163–168)
20. *Magnus Sanctus Paulus* (pp.169–177)
    [secunda pars:] *Sancte Paule Apostole* (pp.178–186)
21. *Victimae paschali* (pp.187–195)
22. *Benedictus Dominus* (p.196)
23. *Popule meus* (pp.197–198)
24. *Popule meus* (pp.199–205)
25. *Vos amici mei estis* (pp.206–212)
26. *Tria sunt munera pretiosa* (pp.213–219)
27. *Haec dies, quam fecit Dominus* (pp.220–225)
28. *Lauda Sion Salvatorem* (pp.226–250)
29. *Victimae paschali laudes* 251–260)
30. *Veni Sancte Spiritus* (pp.261–271)

[Volume 35] Miscellaneous compositions, not yet published

III. The Palestrina Foundation Series (1975–)

C0006 Giovanni Pierluigi da Palestrina. *Edizione anastatica delle fonti palestriniane*. ed. Lino Bianchi. Palestrina (Rome): Fondazione Giovanni Pierluigi da Palestrina, 1975ff.

The stated mission of the Fondazione Giovanni Pierluigi da Palestrina is to publish all surviving original sources for Palestrina's life and works. This edition is projected as a photoreproduction with critical apparatus of three series of important materials dealing with Palestrina's life and works. The projected series are: 1) *Opere a stampa* [printed music]; 2) *Opera manoscritte* [manuscript works]; 3) *Documenti* [documents, including letters, church records, iconographic material, etc.].

To date, the Palestrina Foundation has published the following:

[**Series 1, Volume 1**. Palestrina, Giovanni Pierluigi da] *Missarum liber primus.* ed. Giancarlo Rostirolla. Edizione anastatica delle fonte Palestriniani, Prima serie: Opere a stampa 1. Palestrina (Rome): Fondazione G.P. da Palestrina, 1975. 81pp. M3.1.P25.V62.1975.

Introduction by Giancarlo Rostirolla, pp.1–22, followed by facsimiles of the *First Book of Masses* as published by Dorico in 1554, reduced in size so as to fit four reproductions per page.

Contains *Missa Ecce sacerdos magnus a 4*; *Missa O Regem celi a 4*; *Missa Virtute magna a 4*; *Missa Gabriel archangelus a 4*; *Missa Ad cenam Agni providi a 5*.

[**Series 1, Volume 2**. Palestrina, Giovanni Pierluigi da] *Il primo libro dei madrigali a quattro voci*. ed. Giuliana Gialdroni. Edizione anastatica delle fonti Palestriniani, Prima serie: Opere a stampa 2. Palestrina (Rome): Fondazione Giovanni Pierluigi da Palestrina, 1989.

Introduction by Giuliana Gialdroni, pp.7–23; facsimiles, pp.25–213. Presentation of facsimiles of all known extant prints of the *First Book of Madrigals* issued by a variety of printers between 1555 and 1605. Nine editions are represented; each page of the facsimile edition presents one page of the original as found in each of the contemporary prints.

Two further volumes in this series are projected but not yet published. Volume 3 is planned as an edition of the *Hymni totius anni* (Rome: Tornieri e Donangelo, 1589). Further information regarding the contents of Volume 4 is not yet generally available.

[**Series 2, Volume 1**. Palestrina, Giovanni Pierluigi da] *Il codice 59 dell'Archivio musicale della Basilica di San Giovanni in Laterano: autografo di Giovanni Pierluigi da Palestrina.* ed. Giancarlo Rostirolla. Edizioni anastatica (Opere manoscritte 1). Palestrina: Fondazione Giovanni Pierluigi da Palestrina, 1996.

Reproduction and examination of the principal Palestrina musical autograph.

One further volume in this series is projected but not yet published.

[**Series 3, Volume 1**] Projected, but not yet published.

Chapter 5

Modern Editions of Palestrina's Music II: Collected and Individual Works

I. Selections in Anthologies, Collections, Sets, and Series

D0001 [No editor listed] *Musica sacra quae cantatur quotannis per Hebdomadam sanctam Romae in Sacello pontificio.* Lipsiae [Leipzig]: Sumptibus C.F. Peters, 1808. Contents listing on paper cover.

This edition is evidently based on Burney's 1771 publication, as layout and annotations follow the earlier print in most details. This is likely the edition referred to by Fétis in his *Biographie universelle* article on Palestrina, although he lists the publisher as Breitkopf und Härtel.

Contains *Stabat Mater a 8* (pp.2–12); *Fratres ego enim a 8* (pp.13–17); *Improperia* [from *Popule meus* to *miserere nobis*] *a 8* (pp.23–24). [Also contains Allegri's *Miserere* and Tommaso Bai's *Miserere.*]

D0002 [no editor listed] *Palestrina. 4 Misas. De Beata Virgine paráfrasis; L' homme armé tenor; Tu es Petrus parodia; Ad fugam libre.* Serie Musica callada 2. Madrid: Editorial Música mundana, n.d. [1990s].

Evidently items reprinted from the Casimiri edition [not named here], in miniature score.

Contains *Missa de Beata Virgine a 6* (pp.6–30); *Missa L' homme armé a 4* (pp.31–49); *Missa Tu es Petrus a 6* (pp.50–84); *Missa Ad fugam a 4* (pp.85–101).

Also contains an appendix including various Gregorian mass movements (pp.102–107), the *L'homme armé* melody (p.107), and the model for the *Missa Tu es Petrus*, the Palestrina motet *Tu es Petrus a 6* (together with its secunda pars, *Quodcumque ligaveris*) (pp.108–116).

D0003 [No editor listed] [Madrigals, four voices]. Dartmouth Collegium Musicum series 3, part 1. Hanover, NH: Dartmouth Publications, 1966.

SATB, English text taken from *Musica transalpina* [1589] translations, Italian text also given.

Contains madrigals *Joy so delights my heart* [*Gioia m'abond'al cor*]; *What meaneth love to nest him?* [*Perché s'annida Amore*].

D0004 Alfieri, Pietro, ed. *Excerpta ex celebrioribus de musica viris Jo. Petro Aloisio Praenestino, Thoma Ludovico a Victoria Abulensi et Gregorio Allegrio Romano: in usum cathedralium et collegialium ecclesiarum: concinenda in Dominica Palmarum et majori hebdomada. . . .* Roma: Petri Pitarelli et Socii, 1840.

Contains Sistine Holy Week repertory, including Palestrina items *Pueri Hebraeorum* (SSAT, pp.5–9); *Lamentatio I Feria V. In coena Domini* (SSAT, pp.29–39); *Feria VI in Parasceve ad Matutinum. Lectio I* (SSAT to SSATB, pp.39–58); *Ad Missum dum fit adoratio Crucis canuntur Improperia* (SATB SATB, pp.67–76).

D0005 Alfieri, Pietro, ed. *Raccolta di musica sacra in cui contengonsi i capi lavori de'più celebri compositori italiani consistente in messe, sequenze, offertori, mottetti, salmi, inni, responsori, ec.* Roma: P. Pittarelli e Comp., 1841–1846. Seven vols. M3.P13A4.

Although far from complete, this set constitutes an early and representative collected edition of Palestrina's sacred music, complete with catalogue in Volume 7.

Vol 1 contains masses: *Papae Marcelli* ["*di Papa Marcello*"]; *pro defunctis a 5* ["*per I Defonti*"]; *Missa Canonica a 4; O regem coeli a 4; Aeterna Christi munera a 4; Dies sanctificatus a 4; De feria a 4; Brevis* ["*Breve*"] *a 4; Ego enim accepi a 8.*

Vol 2 contains motets for five voices: *Adjuro vos; Ave Trinitatis sacrarium; Beatus Laurentius; Canite tuba in Sion; Caput ejus; Caro mea; Coenantibus illis; Crucem sanctam subiit; Derelinquat impius; Descendit in hortum meum; Dilectus meus descendit; Dilectus meus mihi; Domine secundum actum meum; Duo ubera tua; Ecce tu pulcher es; Exi cito in plateas; Exultate Deo adjutori nostro; Fasciculus myrrhae; Guttur tuum; Introduxit me Rex; Lapidabant Stephanum; Leva ejus; Manus tuas Domine; Nigra sum, sed formosa; O admirabile commercium; O beata, o benedicta; O sacrum convivium; O vera summa sempiterna; Osculetur me osculo; Parce mihi Domine; Pater noster; Paucitas dierum meorum; Peccantem me quotidie; Peccavi quid faciam tibi; Peccavimus cum patribus nostris; Pulchra es amica mea; Pulchrae sunt genuae tuae; Quae est ista; Quam pulchra es; Quam pulchri sunt; Rorate coeli; Salve Regina; Si ignoras te; Sicut lilium inter spinas; Surgam, et circuibo; Surge amica mea; Surge propera; Tota pulchra es; Trahe me post te; Tribulationes civitatum; Veni veni dilecte mi; Vineam meam; Vox dilecti mei; Vulnerasti cor meum.*

Vol 3 contains *Hymni totius anni* (pub. Rome, 1589) [complete].

Vol 4 contains "Lamentazioni di G.P. da Palestrina. Liber tre" [Books I, II, III; Feria VI. in Parasceve, Lectio I "as used in papal chapel 1587"].

Vol 5 contains *Offertoria totius anni . . . quinque vocibus concinenda* (Rome, 1593) "Offertorii a 5 voci di G.P. da Palestrina" [complete].

Vol 6 contains motets, antiphons, and sequences: *Jerusalem cito veniet a 6* [secunda pars *Ego enim*]; *Veni Domine a 6* [secunda pars *Excita Domine*]; *O magnum mysterium a 6* [secunda pars *Quem vidistis pastores*]; *Cum ortus fuerit sol a 6; Responsum accepit Simeon a 6; Cum inducerent a 6; Sancta et immaculata a 6* [secunda pars *Benedicta tu*]; *Haec dies a 6; Viri Galilei a 6* [secunda pars *Ascendit Deus*]; *Dum complerentur a 6*; *Tu es Petrus a 6* [secunda pars *Quodcumque ligaveris*]; *Solve jubente Deo a 6* [secunda pars *Quodcumque ligaveris*]; *Deus qui Ecclesiam tuam a 6; Vidi turbam magnam a 6* [secunda pars *Et omnes angeli*]; *Columna est immobilis a 6*; *Cantabo Domino a 6* [secunda pars *Deficiant peccatores*]; *Regina mater misericordiae a 6; Tu es Petrus a 7; Virgo prudentissima* [secunda pars *Maria Virgo*]; *Surge illuminare a 8* [secunda pars *Et ambulabunt*]; *Caro mea vere est cibus* [secunda pars *Hic est panis*]; *Laudate Dominum*; *Alma redemptoris mater a*

8; Ave regina coelorum a 8; *Jubilate Deo, psalm Laudate Dominumn a 8*; [secunda pars *Quis sicut Dominus*]; sequence *Victimae paschali a 8;* sequence *Veni Sancte spiritus a 8;* sequence *Stabat Mater a 8.*

Vol 7 contains hymn *O gloriosa virginum à 12*; sequence *Stabat Mater a 12*; *Absolutio in messa defunct. a 4: Libera me, Kyrie, etc*; motet *In messa defunct. a 4: Ne recorderis. Domine secundum actum meum*; motet *Innocentes pro Christo a 4;* motet *Valde honorandus a 4;* motet *Deus qui animae famuli Gregorii a 4;* motet *Ascendens Christus a 4;* motet *Princeps gloriossisime Michael;* hymn *Gaude Barbara a 4;* psalm *Venite a 5;* motet *Cantantibus organis Caecilia a 5* [secunda pars *Biduanis*]; motet *Assumpta est Maria a 6* [secunda pars *Quae est ista*]; motet *Cum autem esset Stephanus à 6* [secunda pars *Positis autem*]; motet *Hic est beatissimus Evangelista a 6* [secunda pars *Hic est discipulis*]; motet *Fratres ego enim a 8*; motet *Jesu junxit se a 8* [secunda pars *Et increpavit eos*]; motet *Spiritus sanctus*; magnificat *Primi toni a 8*; magnificat *Primi toni a 5 et 6*; magnificat *Secundi toni a 5 et 6*; magnificat *Tertii toni a 6*; magnificat *Octavi toni a 6*; magnificat *Octo tonorum a 4. Pars 1: 1,2,3,4,5,6,7,8. Altera pars: 1,2,3,4,5,6,7,8.* Catalogo de tutte le opere del Palestrina.

D0006 Alfieri, Pietro, ed. *Raccolta di musica sacra di Giovanni Pierluigi da Palestrina principe della musica opera publicata da Monsignor Pietro Alfieri Romano. Seconda edizione/vol. I/dedicato all'Eminentissimo Cardinale Costantino Patrizi Vicario di Nostro Signore Papa Pio IX.* Rome: Federico Chiapperini, 1876. Two vols.

Vol 1 contains *Missa Papae Marcelli a 6; Missa Per defonti a 5* [*Missa Pro defunctis*]; *Missa Canonica a 4* [*Missa Ad fugam*]; *Missa O regem coeli a 4; Missa Aeterna Christi munera a 4; Missa Dies sanctificatus a 4; Missa De feria a 4; Missa Brevis a 4; Missa Fratres ego enim accepi a 8.*

Vol 2 contains a selection of motets.

D0007 Anderson, Arthur Olaf, ed. *Selected Compositions of Palestrina.* Chicago: Hall & McCreary, 1940.

Score, 32pp. SATB, with piano accompaniment for rehearsal only.

Contains motets *O sacrum convivium a 4*; *O Domine Jesu Christe a 4*; *Dies sanctificatus a 4*. Masses: *Missa sine nomine a 4* [*Kyrie* only]; *Missa Aeterna Christi munera a 4* [*Sanctus* only]; *Missa Brevis a 4* [*Benedictus* only].

D0008 Arnold, Samuel, ed. *Cathedral Music: Being a Collection in Score of the Most Valuable and Useful Compositions for that Service, by the Several English Masters, of the Seventeenth & Eighteenth Centuries.* 1790; rev. ed. Edward F. Rimbault, London, 1843.

Vol 1 contains "We Have Heard with Our Ears" [Aldrich-Palestrina recomposition of *Doctor bonus*].

D0009 Bäuerle, Hermann, ed. *Pierluigi da Palestrina.* Leipzig: Breitkopf und Härtel, 1904+. Eight vols [seven + one unnumbered volume].

These items were also issued either individually or in small groups [*Hefte*] over a period of several years beginning in 1904. They were advertised as "altklassisiche Kirchenmusik in moderner Notation" [i.e. old classical church music in modern notation], that is, the polyphony was arranged in systems of two or three staves. Many were reissued individually in the 1950s and can still be found in libraries with that imprint. Introductions by Hermann Bäuerle.

Vol 1, *Vierstimmige Messen*, all designated SATB, contains no.1, *Missa Aeterna Christi munera;* no.2, *Missa Brevis;* no.3, *Missa Dies sanctificatus;* no.4, *Missa Emendemus;* no.5, *Missa Jesu nostra redemptio;* no.6, *Missa Iste Confessor;* no.7, *Missa Lauda Sion;* no.8, *Missa Sine nomine I (X. toni);* no.9, *Missa Sine nomine 2 (IV. toni);* no.10, *Missa Veni Sponsa Christi.*

Vol 2, *Vierstimmige Messen,* all designated SATB, contains no.1, *Missa De Feria;* no.2, *Missa Secunda;* no.3, *Missa Dum esset summus Pontifex;* no.4, *Missa Quarta;* no.5, *Missa Iam Christus astra ascenderat;* no.6, *Missa Pater noster;* no.7, *Missa Regina coeli;* no.8, *Missa De Beata Virgine;* no.9, *Missa Sanctorum meritis;* no.10, *Missa Ave regina coelorum.*

Vol 3, *Fünfstimmige Messen*, all designated SATTB, contains no.1, *Missa Ascendo ad Patrem;* no.2, *Missa Beatus Laurentius;* no.3, *Missa Dilexi quoniam;* no.4, *Missa O admirabile commercium;* no.5, *Missa O sacrum convivium;* no.6, *Missa Petra sancta;* no.7, *Missa Pro defunctis;* no.8, *Missa Regina coeli;* no.9, *Missa Sacerdos et Pontifex;* no.10, *Missa Sicut lilium.*

Vol 4, *30 Vierstimmige Motetten* (in twelve *Hefte)* include no.1, *Ave Maria; Benedicta sit*; no.2, *Salvator mundi; Exaudi Domine*; no.3, *Loquebantur variis linguis; O Rex gloriae;* no.4, *Dies sanctificatus; Nos autem gloriari;* no.5, *Lauda Sion; Ego sum panis vivus; Sicut cervus* [secunda pars *Sitivit anima mea*]; no.6, *Tu es pastor ovium; Magnus sanctus Paulus;* no.7, *Veni sponsa Christi; Gaudent in coelis;* no.8, *Lapidabant Stephanum; Quia vidisti me, Thoma;* no.9, *Dum aurora; Doctor bonus;* no.10, *Quae est ista; Nativitas tua;* no.11, *O quantus luctus; Fuit homo;* no.12, *Domine, quando veneris; Commissa mea pavesco; Heu mihi Domine; Anima mea turbata est; Super flumina Babylonis; Ecce nunc benedicite.*

Vol 5, *Achtstimmige Motetten,* includes no.1, *Stabat mater;* no.2, *Pater noster;* no.3, *Ave Maria;* no.4, *Jubilate Deo*; no.5, *Haec dies.*

Vol 6, *Fünfstimmige Offertorien,* (two *Hefte* in partitura) consists of *Heft I: Für die Adventzeit,* containing no.1, *Ad te levavi;* no.2, *Deus tu convertens*; no.3, *Benedixisti Domine;* no.4, *Ave Maria. Heft II: Für die Weihnachtzeit,* contains no.1, *Deus firmavit;* no.2, *Tui sunt coeli*; no.3, *Elegerunt Apostoli;* no.4, *Anima nostra.*

Vol 7, *Achtstimmige Messen* (in partitura) contains no.1 *Missa Confitebor tibi Domine;* no.2, *Missa Fratres ego enim accepi.*

Unnumbered volume, *19 Et incarnatus est,* "aus den übrigen vierstimmigen Messen."

D0010 Becker, Carl Ferdinand, ed. *Kirchengesänge berühmter Meister aus der 15.–17. Jahrhundert.* Five vols. Dresden: Wilhelm Paul, n.d. M2082.B395.

D0011 Bellermann, Heinrich, ed. *Palestrinas Werke. Herausgegeben von Heinrich Bellermann. Erster Theil. Vierstimmigen Motetten. Liber I.* (*Liber secundus*). Bergedorf: H. Weissenborn, 1869.

Second edition or reissue, Bergedorf, H. Weissenborn, 1871.

This item was originally intended as part of a six-volume *Denkmäler der Tonkunst* series under the general editorship of Friedrich Chrysander. It also exists in a version with an English title page, "The Works of Palestrina edited by H. Bellermann. Volume the First. 66 four part Motets" and on the outside bottom margin carries the statement "To be completed in 16 Volumes."

Contains the motets of the *Motecta festorum* and of Book II. Original note values observed; Latin text underlaid; several motets in transposition.

D0012 Böhme, Franz Magnus, ed. *Die hohen Feste in Liedern. 50 Weihnachtslieder, Neujahrs-, Passions- und Pfingstgesänge für eine Stimme mit Pianoforte Begleitung.* Dresden: W. Bock, n.d. [ca.1880].

Includes a version of part of *Stabat Mater a 8* [two strophes; the two canto/soprano voices are reduced to one, and the remaining voices are reduced to a piano accompaniment].

D0013 Bonnet, Joseph, ed. *Historical Organ-Recitals, in Six Volumes.* New York: G. Schirmer, 1917–1940.

Vol 1, ed. Joseph Bonnet, *Forerunners of Bach*, contains "Ricercare" [primo tuono, H xxxii,80] (pp.15–18). *Manualiter*, detailed registration directions.

D0014 Bordes, Charles, ed. *Anthologie des maîtres religieux primitifs des quinzième, seizième et dix-septième siècles.* Paris: Durand et Fils, 1893. Six vols. Reprint New York: Da Capo, 1981.

All items also issued separately in the series *Anthologie des maîtres religieux ancients pour chant et orgue, ser. 1. Répetoire des chanteurs de Saint-Gervais.* Edition populaire. Paris: Bureau d'Edition de la Schola Cantorum, c. 1893–1912. Each of the motets was published with a vocal reduction for keyboard (organ), and was extensively edited.

Vol 1, *Première année, Livre de messes,* contains *Missa Brevis a 4* (pp.1–22), *Missa Ascendo ad Patrem a 5* (pp.42–69), *Missa O regem coeli a 4* (pp.152–183).

Vol 2, *Première année, Livre de motets,* contains no.2, *Peccantem me quotidie* (pp.4–6); no.6, *Coenantibus illis a 5* (pp.21–24); no.7, *Trois repons* [*In monte Oliveti* (pp.25–27); *Tristis est anima mea* (pp.27–29); *Ecce vidimus eum* (pp.29–31)]; no.13, *Trois repons* [*Sicut oves ad occisum* (pp.58–60); *Jerusalem surge* (pp.60–62); *Plange quasi Virgo* (pp.62–63)]; no.21, *Trois repons* [*Omnes amici mei* (pp.98–100); *Velum templi* (pp.100–102); *Vinea mea electa* (pp.102–103)]; no.32, *Exultate Deo a 5* (pp.164–167); no.34, *Alma redemptoris mater a 4* (pp.174–176); no.40, *Veni sponsa Christi a 4* (pp.191–194).

Vol 3, *Deuxième année, Livre de messes,* contains the *Missa Papae Marcelli a 6* (pp.1–41).

Vol 4, *Deuxième année, Livre de motets*, contains no.44, *Trois repons* [*Recessit Pastor noster; O vos omnes; Ecce quomodo moritur justus* (pp.16–21)]; no.49, *Stabat Mater a 8* (SATB/SATB, interlinear-type French translation on a single empty stave, pp.40–53); no.50, *Dextera Domini a 5* (pp.54–56)]; no.51, *Ave Maria a 4* (pp.57–60); no.53, *Assumpta est Maria a 6* (SSATTB, untransposed, pp.63–67, with no.53a, *Quae est ista a 6,* pp.68–72); no.57, *Loquebantur in variis linguis a 4* (pp.85–89); no.64, *O admirabile commercium a 5* (SATTB, untransposed, pp.121–124); no.68, *Congratulamini mihi a 4* (pp.159–162); no.72, *Tantum ergo a 4* (pp.177–180).

Vol 5, *Troisieme année, Livre de messes,* contains *Missa Salve Regina à 5* (pp.69–99) and *Missa Sine nomine à 4* (pp.100–123).

Vol 6, *Troisième année, Livre de motets,* contains no.77, *Dum aurora finem daret a 4* (pp.4–8); no.81, *Ego sum panis vivus a 4* (pp.16–19); no.83, *Ave Maria à 4 voix égales* (SSSA, pp.32–35); no.85, *Ne recorderis peccata mea Domine* (SSSA or TTTB, pp.43–46); no.86, *Miserere mei Deus* (falsobordone) *a 4* (TTBB, p.48); no.87, *Adoramus te Christe à 4 voix égales* (TTTB or TTBarB, pp.51–52); no.91, *Sicut cervus a 4* [secunda pars *Sitivit anima mea*] (pp.60–65); no.92, *Tantum ergo sacramentum à 4 voix égales* (TTBarB, pp.66–67); no.94, *Vexilla regis prodeunt* (odd-numbered verses in square plainchant notation; even-numbered verses for various vocal ensembles from two choirs) (pp.70–73) , with no.94bis, *O crux ave a 4* (pp.74–75); no.103, *Tribulationes civitatum a 4* (with secunda pars, *Peccavimus,* pp.121–126); no.106, *Dies sanctificatus a 4* (pp.137–140); no.110, *Domine quando veneris a 4* (pp.151–153); no.112, *Exaudi Domine a 4* (pp.157–160); no.115, *Innocentes pro Christo à 4 voix égales* (pp.169–171); no.120, *O rex gloriae a 4* (pp.180–184); no.125, *Ad te levavi a 4* (pp.192–195); no.125bis, *Miserere nostri* (pp.196–199).

D0015 Brace, Geoffrey, ed. *Partsongs for Equal Voices.* Something to Sing 3. Cambridge: Cambridge University, 1966. 51 pp.

These are choral scores directed to younger performers. Latin text, with English adaptations by the editor. Contains motet *Jesu rex admirabilis* (SSA or TTB). Items also published separately (ref. 521 04299 2).

D0016 Brandt, William Edward, and Arthur Corra, William Christ, Richard Delone, and Allen Winold, eds. *The Comprehensive Study of Music. Vol. 1: Anthology of Music from Plainchant through Gabrieli.* New York: Harper's College Press, 1980.

Contains complete motet *O magnum mysterium a 6* (SSAATB, pp.185–189; secunda pars *Quem vidistis (*pp.190–194), and large excerpts from *Missa O magnum mysterium* (pp.195–221). A substantial part of each movement of the mass is printed; those sections which are omitted are identified by their text. Useful for study of parody/imitation technique if a complete score is not available. Text translation into English, p.15.

D0017 Burkhart, Charles, ed. *Anthology for Musical Analysis.* 3rd ed. New York: Holt, Rinehart and Winston, 1979.

Contains *Missa Aeterna Christi munera* [*Sanctus* and *Benedictus* only] (pp.33–28). The second edition (pub.1972) contains *Missa Aeterna Christi munera* [*Sanctus, Benedictus, Agnus Dei I, Agnus Dei II*] (pp.27–36).

D0018 Burney, Charles, ed. *La musica che si canta annualmente nelle funzioni della settimana santa nella Cappella Pontificia composta dal Palestrina,*

Allegri, e Bai: raccolta e pubblicata da Carlo Burney. London: Robert Bremner, 1771.

Preface by the editor, pp. i–iv, including a biographical notice of Palestrina. Contains *Stabat Mater a 8* (SATB SATB) "si canta nella Funzione delle Palme alla Messa" (pp.1–13); motet *Fratres ego enim accepi a 8* (SATB SATB) "si canta il Giovedi Santo alla Messa" (pp.14–23); Improperia *Popule meus* [to *miserere nobis*] (SATB SATB) "Improperia Petrus Aloysius Prenestinus/Si cantano nella Mattina del Venerdi Santo, all'Adorazione della Croce" (pp.31–34). There is another version of this publication with the imprint "Londra: Stampata per [blank] nella Strand" that also apparently dates from the early 1770s.

D0019 Busch, Hermann J., ed. *Two Settings of Palestrina's Missa Papae Marcelli.* Recent Researches in the Music of the Baroque Era 16. Madison, WI: A–R Editions, 1973.

Both versions of this mass are by younger contemporaries and associates of Palestrina and reflect changing perspectives on the *prima prattica* in the generation active ca.1590–1620. Preface (pp.5–9); facsimiles from two publications: Anerio's version (pp.13–14) and Soriano's (pp.55–56). Version 1 (pp.15–51), by Giovanni Francesco Anerio (1567–1630), is an arrangement for four voices (SATB) and basso continuo; Version 2 (pp.57–106) is by Francesco Soriano [Suriano] (1549–c.1621), arranged for eight voices in *cori spezzati* (SATB/SATB) with figured bass.

D0020 Calahorra Martinez, Pedro, ed. *Missae sex IV.V. et VI. Vocum . . . /Pedro Ruimonte.* Publicaciones de la Sociedad Española de Musicologia. Sección D. Ediciones de música antigua 3. Zaragoza: Sociedad Española de Musicologia, 1982.

Contains Palestrina motets *In diebus illis*; *Lapidabant Stephanum.* Ruimonte published these two motets and other music by Guerrero as models on which his imitation masses were based. Critical notes in Spanish.

———. Carver, Anthony F., ed. *Cori Spezzati: The Development of Sacred Polychoral Music to the Time of Schütz. Vol.2: An Anthology of Sacred Polychoral Music.* Cambridge: Cambridge University Press, 1988.

See E0192 for description of main text. Vol. 2 contains motet *Videntes stellam Magi* (pp.86–92), based on the Casimiri edition.

D0021 Casimiri, Raphael [Raffaele]. *Anthologia polyphonica auctorum saeculi XVI paribus vocibus.* Roma: Edizioni "Psalterium" [c.1924–1932]

Works in score.

———. Casimiri, Raffaele. *Il "Codice 59" dell'Archivio Musicale Lateranense. Autografo di Giov. Pierluigi da Palestrina.* Rome: Tipografia Poliglotta Vaticana, 1919. ML410.P15C26.

See item E0193 for bibliographical entry. Casimiri's meticulous examination of the most extensive Palestrina autograph contains an appendix of transcriptions of previously unpublished works, as well as eight fold-out pages of manuscript facsimiles (including Lateran 59, ff.9v, and 57v, which are among the material transcribed here). The appendix includes hymns pp.1–6, *Tibi Christe splendor Patris a 4* [from ff.9v–10]; pp.7–10, *Conditor alme siderum a 3 et 4* [from ff.46v–47]; pp.11–20, *Christe redemptor omnium a 3, 4 et 5* [from ff.49v–52]; pp.21–27, *Hostes Herodes impie* [from ff.56v–58]. Original clefs and note values are preserved, and hymn strophes are indicated.

Transcriptions of sections of other works appear throughout the text.

D0022 Casimiri, Raphael [Raffaele], ed. *Monumenta polyphoniae Italicae*. Rome: Pontificium Institutum Musicae Sacrae, 1930.

Vol 1: *Missa cantantibus organis, Caecilia: 12 vocibus*. ed. Raphael Casimiri.

Preface in Italian and Latin (pp.xi–xxi); two pages of facsimiles from primary source, Lateran cod.52. Palestrina contributed part of the *Gloria* [*Et in terra pax . . . filius patris*] (pp.11–19) to this work. The motet on which this mass was based, *Cantantibus organis a 5*, also by Palestrina, is printed here as well (pp.87–91).

D0023 Casimiri, Raphael [Raffaele], ed. *Societas Polyphonica Romanae . . . Repertorium; cura et studio Raph. Casimri.* Vols. 1–6. Rome: "Psalterium," 1925–1934.

Note values are halved, and the music is edited for dynamics and other performance indications. Listed on the inside covers of each volume are the Latin text and a short commentary for every selection.

Vol 1 (1925) contains no.1, offertory *Laudate Dominum a 5* (SATTB, pp.1–6); no.2, offertory *Vox dilecti mei a 5* (SATTB, pp.7–14); no.3, offertory *Improperium exspectavit a 5* (SATTB, pp.12–17); no.6, offertory *Ad te levavi a 5* (SATTB, pp.30–35); no.7, motet *O quantus luctus a 4* (SATB, pp.36–40); no.10, motet *Exultate Deo a 5* (STTBarB, pp.51–56).

Vol 2 (1925) contains no.1, offertory *Bonum est a 5* (SATTB, pp.1–5); no.5, motet *Alleluja, tulerunt Dominum a 5* (SATTB, pp.20–27); no.6, motet *Adjuro vos a 5* (STTBarB, pp.28–34); no.7, motet *Paucitas dierum meorum* [seconda pars *Manus tuae*] *a 5* (STTBarB, pp.35–43); no.8, mass movement *Missa Papae Marcelli* [*Credo* only] *a 6* (SATTBB, pp.44–57).

Vol 3 (1925) contains no.1, offertory *Exaltabo te a 5* (pp.1–3); no.2, motet *Nigra sum a 5* (SATTB, pp.6–11); no.3, motet *Tribulationes civitatum* [seconda pars *Peccavimus*] *a 5* (SATTB, pp.12–21); no.5, motet *Tota pulchra es a 5* (SATTB, pp.25–29); no.6, offertory *Dextera Domini a 5* (SATTB, pp.30–34); no.8, *Super flumina Babylonis a 4* (SATB, pp.39–42); no.9, motet *Introduxit me Rex a 5* (SATTB, pp.43–47); no.10, Improperium *Incipit Hieremiae a 6/8* (pp.48–59).

Vol 4 (1927) contains no.2, motet *Dilectus meus a 5* (SATTB, pp.6–10); no.6, *Sicut cervus a 4* (STTB, pp.19–21).

Vol 5 (1927) contains no.1, motet *Surge amica mea a 5* (SATTB, pp.1–6); no.3, motet *Hodie Christus a 4* (SSAT, pp.11–14); no.5, offertory *Confitebor a 5* (SATTB, pp.20–25).

Vol 6 contains no.1, motet *Peccantem me quotidie a 5* (STTBarB, pp.1–6); no.5, sequence *Stabat Mater a 8* (SATB SATB, pp.33–47).

———. Celler, Ludovic, ["L. Leclercq"], ed. *La Semaine sainte au Vatican: étude musicale et pittoresque: texte et musique.* Paris: Hachette et Cie., 1867. xii + 120pp.

See item E0477 for main bibliographical entry. The first part of this work is text describing events during Holy Week, including notes on performance practice of the Palestrina *Lamentations* and the history of the Sistine Chapel. The second part contains music by Palestrina, Victoria, Allegri, and others.

Palestrina, *Stabat Mater a 8* (printed on two staves, pp.1–14); Victoria, *Reponsiones populi* (pp.15–25); Allegri, *Miserere* (pp.26–31); Bai, *Miserere* (pp.32–41); Victoria, *Responsiones ad missam in passionem secundum Joannem* (pp.42–70); Palestrina, *Improperia* (after Burney, pp.49–70); Palestrina, motet *Christus factus est* (pp.71–72); Palestrina, *Missa Papae Marcelli* [*Kyrie* through *Agnus Dei I*] (pp.73–120).

D0024 Choron, Alexandre-Étienne, ed. *Collection des pièces de musique religieuse qui s'exécutent tous les ans à Rome, durant la Semaine Sainte, dans la Chapelle de souverain-pontife. Recuillies et publiées par M. Alexandre Choron, ancien chef de brigade à l'École Polytechnique. . . .* Paris: Chez l'Éditeur, au Pensionnat Royal de Chant [1810–1820].

Compilation derived from years of Choron's directorship, which included performance revivals of music by Palestrina and other sixteenth-century composers. See also Choron, *Raccolta generale delle opere classiche musicali* item D0026.

D0025 Choron, Alexandre-Étienne. *Principes de Composition des Ecoles d'Italie. Adoptés par le Gouvernement Français pour servir à l'instruction des Élèves des Maîtrises de Cathedrales.* 3 vols. Paris: Le Duc, 1808.

A massive treatise on composition, with examples included here rather than in Chapter 2 because of the post-1800 publication date. Book 6 represents a compendium of examples in church, chamber, and theatrical styles, in which both church and chamber music are represented by works by Palestrina.

Livre Sixième. Rhétorique Musicale contains the appendix *Modèles pour le sixième livre. Styles. Première section: Styles d'église*, including the following as examples written in the eight church modes.

Mode 1: pp.3–4, *Chori sanctorum a 4*; pp.4–5, *Sit laus Deo Patri summo Christo a 5*; pp.6–7, *Et exultavit a 5*.

Mode 2: pp.14–15, *Post fluxa carnis scandala a 5*; pp.15–16, *Sicut locutus est a 5*.

Mode 3: pp.26–27, *Quae vox quae poterit a 4*; pp.28–29, *Laus et perennis gloria a 5*; pp.29–30, *Sicut locutus est a 5*; pp.37, *Pleni sunt coeli a 3* [with note: "*Cet exemple est tiré de la Seconde Partie*"].

Mode 4: pp.39–40, *Hic ille Rex est gentium a 4*; pp.41–43, *O felix Roma a 5*; pp.44–46, *Sicut erat a 7* [with canons at diapente and diapason].

Mode 5: pp.50–51, *Legi prophetae gratiae a 4*; pp.51–52, *Praestet hoc nati genitor a 4*; pp.53–54, *Esurientes implevit bonis a 5*.

Mode 6: pp.65–67, *Gaudent in coelis a 4*.

Mode 7: pp.79–81, *Veni sponsa Christi a 4*; pp.84–86, *Sicut erat a 6*; pp.87–89, *Agnus Dei a 6*.

Mode 8: pp.91–92, *Hostem repellas longius a 4*; pp.93–95, *Beatus Laurentius a 5*; pp.100–101, *Quia fecit mihi magna a 6.*

Seconde Section: Style de Chambre. Première espèce: Madrigaux da Tavolino; pp.210–211, *Alla riva del Tebro a 4*; pp.228–230, *Tu di fortezza torre a 5.*

D0026 Choron, Alexandre-Étienne, ed. *Raccolta generale delle opere classiche musicali.* Paris: Auguste le Duc, ca. 1810.

These items, a by-product of Choron's association with the revival of early music and didactic activities, were apparently issued individually around 1810 and were subsequently reissued in different formats around 1825.

Includes no.2, *Missa ad fugam in perpetuo canone, in G, a quattro voci, da capella* (pub. ca. 1810), iii + 15pp; no.3, *Stabat Mater, motetto a otto voci reali, da cappella* (pub. ca. 1810), iii +14pp.

D0027 Cisilino, Siro, ed. *Sedici salmi a cinque voci di quattordici autori veneti cinquecenteschi dedicati a Giovanni Pierluigi da Palestrina.* Padova: G. Zanibon, 1978.

This is a modern edition of RISM 1592[3], a compilation of works by Asola and others, dedicated to Palestrina. Preface in Italian and English pp.iii–ix, providing notes on the preface, as well as biographies and publication histories of the various contributors. Two facsimiles on pp.x–xi. In addition to the publication contents, Cisilino has also published Palestrina's aptly titled response to this *Festschrift*, the motet *Vos amici mei estis a 8* (SATB SATB, pp.139–146).

D0028 Commer, Franz, ed. *Musica Sacra. Sammlung der besten Meisterwerke des 16. 17. und 18. Jahrhunderts. Gesammelt und herausgegeben von Franz Commer.* Berlin: Ed. Bote & G. Bock, 1838. 4 vols. New series beginning with vol 5, various editors, pub. ca. 1842–1846. Only volumes containing music by Palestrina listed here.

Vol 2, *Sammlung der besten Meisterwerke des 16. 17. und 18. Jahrhunderts für 2, 3, und 4 Männerstimmen* (German translation of texts by Wilhelm von Waldbrühl) contains "Quo cunque di Palestrina" ["Wohin du wallest Jungfrau"] (Latin and German texts both underlaid, pp.118–119).

Vol 3, *Sammlung der besten Meisterwerke des 16. 17. und 18. Jahrhunderts für 4 bis 8 Stimmen* [*gemischter Chor*], contains no.3, *Nos autem gloriari* (SATB, Latin text only underlaid, pp.12–14); no.10, *O crux ave* (SATTB, tranposed, Latin text only underlaid, pp.34–35)].

Vol 5, ed. A.H. Neidhardt, *Sammlung religiöser Gesänge älterer und neuester Zeit zum bestimmten Gebrauch für den Königlichen Berliner Domchor,* contains no.1, *Kyrie eleison* (SATB, pp.3–4); no.2, *Sanctus* ["*Heilig*"] (SATTBB, pp.5–9); no.3, Agnus Dei ["*O Lamm Gottes*"] (SATTBB, pp.10–14) [nos.1–3 are movements from the *Missa Papae Marcelli,* with Latin and German text underlay]; no.4, "*Wie der Hirsch schreit*" [*Sicut cervus*] (SATB, German text only underlaid); no.5, *Improperia* ["*Improperien,*" marked "*Der zweite Chor wird nur schwach, ein jeder Stimme von*

2.–3. besten Sängern besetzt"] (pp.18–19); no.6, "*Lasst uns mit Jesu ziehn*" [designated "*unterlegt unter den ersten Theil des Gesanges: Nos autem gloriari*" (SATB, pp.20–21); no.7, Hymnus *O crux ave* ["*O Jesu Christ dein theures Blut*," text by the poet Oleander] (SATTB).

Vol 6, ed. A. H. Neidhardt, J. Seyler, and C.J.A.H. Hoffmann, *Sammlung religiöser Gesänge älterer und neuester Zeit zum bestimmten Gebrauch für den Königlichen Berliner Domchor*, contains no.2a, *De lamentatione* (SSAT, with note "from 1587," pp.6–9); 2b, "*Jerusalem*" (SATB, with note "from 1587," pp.10–11); no.4, *Kyrie eleison* (SATB, Latin underlay, pp.16–17); no.5, *Benedictus qui venit* (SAT, Latin underlay, p.18); no.6, *Agnus Dei* (SATB, Latin underlay, pp.19–20); no.7, *Agnus Dei* (SAATB, Latin underlay, pp.21–22).

Vol 12, ed. A. H. Neidhardt, *Sammlung religiöser Gesänge älterer und neuester Zeit zum bestimmten Gebrauch für den Königlichen Berliner Domchor für Männestimmen,* contains no.1, *Adoramus te Christe* (TTBB, pp.3–4); no.2, *Crucifixus* (TTBB, pp.5–8); no.3, *Christus factus est* (TTBB, p.9); no.4, *Pueri Hebraeorum* (TTBB, pp.10–12); no.5, *Lamentation I* (TTBB, pp.13–17), no.6, *Lamentation II* (TTBB, pp.18–27). Latin underlay in each selection.

Vol 14, ed. R. von Hertzberg, *Sammlung religiöser Gesänge älterer und neuester Zeit zum bestimmten Gebrauch für den Königlichen Berliner Domchor,* contains no.2, *Responsorium "Velum templi scissum est"* (SATB, pp.7–8; Latin underlay with interlinear German translation).

Vol 15, ed. Albert E. A. Becker, *Sammlung religiöser Gesänge älterer Zeit zum bestimmten Gebrauch für den Königlichen Berliner Domchor*, contains no.1, *Quia vidisti me, Thoma* (SATB, pp.3–6); no.2, *Heu mihi Domine* (SATB, pp.7–10; secunda pars *Anima mea turbata est*, SATB, pp.11–14); no.3, *Ad te levavi oculos meos* (SATB, pp.15–19; secunda pars *Miserere nostri*, SATB, pp.20–23); no.4, *Super flumina Babylonis* (SATB, pp.24–27); no.5, *O sacrum convivium* (SATTB, pp.28–33); no.6, *Haec dies quam fecit Dominus* (SSATTB, pp.34–38); no.7, *Laudate Dominum omnes gentes* (SATB SATB, pp.39–47); no.8, *Agnus Dei a 7* (SSATTBB, with the second soprano and second tenor parts as resolved voices and the first bass part presenting the canon, pp.48–52). Latin underlay in all selections.

D0029 Crotch, William, ed. *Specimens of Various Styles of Music Referred to in a Course of Lectures Read at Oxford and London and Adapted to Keyed Instruments by William Crotch.* London: Robt. Birchall, ca. 1806–1808. MT6.5.C951.S7.

Vol 2 (pub. 1808) contains a *Deposuit potentes* adapted as "We have heard with our ears."

D0030 Cusma' Piccione, Cono. *Giovanni Pierluigi da Palestrina: Il quarto libro di Messe a quattro e cinque voci. Edizione critica.* Laureate thesis, Università degli Studi di Pavia, Scuola di Paleografia e Filologia Musicale, 1988–1989. 424pp.

Transcription, critical apparatus and commentary on the masses of Book

IV (1582). Includes *Missa Prima a 4*; *Missa Secunda a 4*; *Missa Tertia a 4*; *Missa Quarta a 4*; *Missa Prima a 5*; *Missa Secunda a 5*; *Missa Tertia a 5*.

D0031 Dakers, Lionel, ed. *The New Oxford Church Anthem Book.* Oxford and New York: Oxford University Press, 1992.

Contains preface. Latin underlay; note values halved, with some editorial indications for dynamics expression and liturgical uses.

Contains no.4, *Adoramus te, Christe a 4* (pp.14–17); no.77, *Salvator mundi a 4* (pp.404–412).

D0032 David, Hans Theodore, ed. *The Art of Polyphonic Song. Compositions of the 16th and 17th Centuries for Two to Eight Parts.* New York: G. Schirmer, 1940.

Includes an introduction (pp.6–37) containing discussions of polyphony, rhythm, melody, harmony, and dynamics as applied to this music. The introduction itself contains examples from various authors, including one of the disputed *Esercizi sopra la scala* (dated 1581, SSSA, keyboard accompaniment, pp.22–23). There are also notes on the motet *Alma Redemptoris Mater* (pp.32–33), as well as the complete music for this work, extensively edited (arr. SSSA, Latin and English texts both underlaid, pp.72–75, secunda pars *Tu quae genuisti,* pp.75–79).

D0033 David, Hans Theodore, ed. *Madrigals for Four Mixed Voices, by G.P. da Palestrina with Contemporary English Translations.* New York: Music Press, 1945.

Notes indicate that music is reprinted from vol 28 of the Haberl/Breitkopf & Härtel edition; English texts have been taken from the contemporary *Musica transalpina* (1589). Contains madrigals *a 4*, *Sweet Love when hope was flowring* [*Amor, quando floriva*] and *Joy so delights my heart* [*Gioia m'abond'al cor*]. Editing.

D0034 Davison, Archibald, and Willi Apel, eds. *Historical Anthology of Music. Volume I: Oriental, Medieval and Renaissance Music.* revised edition. Cambridge, MA: Harvard University Press, 1949.

Historical anthology popular in mid-twentieth century, with works arranged on short scores. Notes for each work provided at the back of the volume: Palestrina selections are annotated p.232.

Contains no.140, *Missa Papae Marcelli,* Agnus Dei I (six voices arranged on three staves, pp.152–153); no.141, *Sicut cervus* (motet *a 4* with secunda pars, *Sitivit anima mea*, four voices arranged on two staves, pp.153–154); no.142, *Alla riva del Tebro* (madrigal, four voices arranged on two staves, p.155).

———. Dehn, Siegfried. *Lehre von Contrapunkt, dem Canon und der Fugue. Nebst Analysen von Duetten, Terzetten, Fugen, etc. von Orlando di Lasso, Marcello, Palestrina u.a. Neu bearbeitet von Bernhard Scholz.* Berlin: W. Weber, 1882. 192pp. MT55.D31.1882. [Original edition 1859].

See item E0481 for main bibliographical entry. Contains a series of examples meant to be studied in conjunction with the text: pp.54–55, "*II. Terzett von Gio. Pier Luigi, genannt Palestrina*," with commentary on writing in the strict *a cappella* style, relates to example no.2, "*Terzetto di Palestrina*" [a *Benedictus*] (pp.147–149); pp.131–132, "*Achtstimmiger Satz*," dealing with writing for double choirs, refers to example no.12, *Sub tuum praesidium a 8* (pp.183–190), which is labelled as "*a cori battenti*."

D0035 Dixon, Graham, ed. *Masterworks from Rome.* Faber Motet Series. London: Faber & Faber, 1994.

Introduction by Dixon in English with German translation.

Contains motet *Jesus iunxit se* (pp.15–19). SATB with basso seguente organ part. Note values halved; transposed down a minor third.

D0036 Dixon, Jon, ed. *Alma Redemptoris. Dies sanctificatus.* Carshalton Beeches, Surrey: JOED Music, ca. 1994. 8pp. M2092.P25A46 1994.

SATB *da cappella.* Latin text, with English translations printed in captions. Transposed into modern clefs at a pitch suitable for SATB choirs. Edited from the Alfieri edition. Prefatory note indicates that the setting of *Alma redemptoris mater* "was not published in [Palestrina's] lifetime and it was first printed in the mid 19th century from a manuscript then in the possession of the Collegio Romano."

D0037 Dixon, Jon, ed. *Ave Regina. Alma Redemptoris. Salve Regina.* Carshalton Beeches, Surrey: JOED Music, 1994. 21pp. M2084.P35D5 1994.

SSSA *da cappella.* Latin text, with English translation printed in captions. Transposed into modern clefs at a pitch suitable for women's voices. Edited from the editions published in Venice by Gardane in 1596 and 1604. Prefatory note.

D0038 Dixon, Jon, ed. *Nunc dimittis. Ecce nunc benedicite. Stabat Mater.* Carshalton Beeches, Surrey: JOED Music, 1995. 28pp. M2082.P34D5 1995.

SATB SATB SATB *da cappella.* Latin text, with English translations printed in captions; transposed into modern clefs at a pitch suitable for SATB choirs. Edited from the Haberl edition. Prefatory note.

D0039 Dixon, Jon, ed. *Osculetur me. Quae est ista.* Carshalton Beeches, Surrey: JOED Music, 1995. 12pp.

Prefatory note to works edited from the edition published in Venice in 1613. SATTB and SSATB *da cappella*; Latin text, with English translations printed in captions; "transposed into modern clefs at a pitch suitable for SATB choirs."

D0040 Dixon, Jon, ed. *Surge propera. Veni dilecti me [mi].* Carshalton Beeches, Surrey: JOED Music, 1994. 12pp. M2092.P25M66 1994.

Prefatory note, indicating that works were edited from the Venice 1613 edition. SATTB *da cappella.* Latin text, with English translation printed in captions. Transposed into modern clefs at a pitch suitable for SATB choirs. Edited from the Venice, 1613 edition.

D0041 Druffel, Peter, ed. *Sechs ausgewählte Madrigale von Pierluigi da Palestrina. Zum praktischen Gebrauch für Freunde eines stylvollen mehrstimmigen Chorgesanges a capella* [*sic*]. Leipzig: Breitkopf und Härtel, 1887. Part.B.902; Ch.B.303.

Preface in German, with extensive introduction and analysis of selections; also contains a guide to pronunciation of Italian. German and Italian text both underlaid. Extensively edited.

Contains "*O Mutter voll Erbarmen*" [*Donna, vostra mercede*] (SATB, pp.19–23); "*Was soll ich nun auf Erden*" [*Che debbo far, che mi consigli*] (SATB, pp.24–27); "*O welch ein Glanz*" [*O che splendor*] (SATB, pp.28–32); "*Blick' ich umher, O Frau*" [*Ogni beltà, madonna*] (SATB, pp.33–38); "*Wie kannst du nur vergleichen*" [*Non son le vostre mani*] (SAATB, pp.39–45); "*O süsser Tod!*" [*Soave fia il morir*] (SAATB, pp.46–52).

D0042 Engel, Lehman, ed. *Renaissance to Baroque. Three Centuries of Choral Music.* vol. 2: *Italian Music.* Delaware Water Gap, PA: Harold Flammer, 1940.

Contains motet *Congratulamini mihi a 4* (SATB; piano part for rehearsal only, pp.49–57), editing. Preface (p.2) and English translation of Latin text (p.3); introductory remarks at head of work (p.49).

D0043 Erig, Richard, ed. and Veronika Gutmann, coll. *Italienische Diminutionen: Die zwischen 1553 und 1638 mehrmals bearbeiteten Sätze* [Italian diminutions: the pieces with more than one diminution from 1553 to 1638]. Prattica Musicale 1. Zürich: Amadeus, 1979.

Includes Palestrina works with more than one contemporaneous diminution, compiled in a comparative score format. The original work is printed out in score on the upper part of the page, and the variants are laid on staves beneath the original, one under the other.

Includes no.14, *Io son ferito ahi lasso*, with diminutions by Bassano, Bovicelli (2 versions, including Bovicelli's contrafactum *Ave verum corpus*), Rognoni (2 versions), and Bassani (pp.252–268); no.22, *Vestiva i colli*, together with its seconda parte, *Così le chiome mie*, with diminutions by dalla Casa, Bassano, Rognoni (2 versions), Terzi, Bartolomeo de Selma (2 versions), and Virgiliano (pp.347–376 and 377–388); no.23, *Pulchra es amica mea*, with diminutions by Bassano (2 versions) and Rognoni (2 versions) (pp.389–399).

D0044 Fellerer, Karl Gustav, ed. *Drei Motetten.* Heidelberg: Süddeutscher Musikverlag, Willy Müller, n.d. SM936.

Contains motets *Ave Maria; Benedicta sit sancta Trinitatis; Pulchra es amica mea*. SATB, *a cappella.*

D0045 Fellerer, Karl Gustav, ed. *Pre-Classic Polyphony.* Anthology of Music 28. Köln: Arno Volk, 1965.

Historical introduction, pp.5–14, in English translation by Robert Kolben.

Contains no.8, *Praestet hoc nati genitor a 5* (hymn strophe from *En gratulemur hodie*, pp.33–34). Note values halved; *Mensurstrich.*

D0046 Fellerer, Karl Gustav, ed. *Ricercari sopra li tuoni, a quattro. Vierstimmige Ricercare in den acht Kirchentonarten für ein Tasteninstrument oder beliebige Einzelinstrument.* Antiqua, eine Sammlung alter Musik. Mainz: B. Schotts Söhne; New York: Associated Music Publishers, 1933. 27pp.

For four unspecified instruments SATB in open score, together with an "intavolatura," here a keyboard reduction.

Contains no.1, *Ricercar del primo tuono* (pp.3–5); no.2, *Ricercar del secondo tuono* (pp.6–8); no.3, *Ricercar del tertio tuono* (pp.9–11); no.4, *Ricercar del quarto tuono* (pp.12–14); no.5, *Ricercar del quinto tuono* (pp.15–17); no.6, *Ricercar del sesto tuono* (pp.18–20); no.7, *Ricercar del settimo tuono* (pp.21–24); no.8, *Ricercar del ottavo tuono* (pp.25–27).

D0047 Guilmant, Alexandre, ed. *Concert historique d'orgue. Morceaux d'Autuers célèbres de differentes écoles du XVIe au XIXe siècle. Historical organ concert. Pieces by celebrated composers of different schools from the XVIth to the XIXth centuries.* Mainz: B. Schotts Söhne/London: Schott & Co. Ltd, n.d.

Contains a *Ricercare.*

D0048 Haas, Robert. *Aufführungspraxis der Musik.* Handbuch der Musikwissenschaft. Wildpark-Potsdam: Akademische Verlagsgesellschaft Athenaion, 1931.

Modern edition of diminutions of Palestrina works published by Giovanni Bassano in 1591: motet *Benedicta sit sancta Trinitas a 4* (2 versions, both p.115); madrigal *Vestiva i colli a 5 with seconda parte*, *Così le chiome mie* (p.117).

D0049 Haberl, Franx Xaver, ed. *Ad finem Laudum Tridui Sacri. Canticum "Benedictus" quatuor et quinque vocum auctore J. Petraloysis Praenestino, Antiph. "Christus factus est" quatuor et quinque voc. Auctore Joanne Franc. Anerio, quae ex codicibus originalibus redegit F. X. Haberl.* Regensburg: Friedrich Pustet, 1886.

Contains motet *Benedictus Dominus Deus Israel a 4 et 5.*

D0050 Hamburger, Povl, ed. *Four Motets.* Egtved [Denmark]: Musikhojskolens Forlag, n.d.

No.2 in *Orbis chori* series. Preface and commentary in German.

Contains *a cappella* motets *Ad te levavi oculos meos* [secunda pars *Miserere nostri Domine*] (SATB); *Ave regina coelorum* [secunda pars *Gaude virgo gloriosa*] (SSSA); *Isti sunt* (SATB); *Quae est ista* (SSATB).

D0051 Harman, Alec, ed. *Ten Four-Part Motets for the Church's Year.* London: Oxford University Press, 1964.

Preface by Alec Harman; Latin texts with English translations, both underlaid; optional keyboard accompaniment.

Contains *Ave Maria* (Advent, pp.1–9); *Dies sanctificatus* (Christmas, pp.10–18); *Tribus miraculis* (Epiphany, pp.19–31); *Ad te levavi oculos meos* (pars prima only, Lent, pp.31–40); *Nos autem gloriari oportet* (Passiontide, pp.41–51); *Haec dies quam fecit Dominus* (Easter, pp.52–60); *O Rex gloriae* (Ascension, pp.61–71); *Loquebantur variis linguis* (Pentecost/Whitsun, pp.72–83); *Benedicta sit sancta Trinitas* (Trinity, pp.84–95); *Salvator mundi* (All Saints, pp.84–95).

D0052 Hawke, H. William, ed. *Italian Keyboard Music.* Indianapolis: Ernest White Editions, 1970. 6 vols.

Vol 3 contains *Ricercar on the fifth tone* (pp.45–47); *Ricercar on the sixth tone* (pp.48–50), both arranged for two manuals and pedal. Collections prefaced by historical notes and notes on the performance of each work.

D0053 Hennefeld, Norman, ed. *The Liturgical Music Press, Inc. Masterpieces of Organ Music. Selected Compositions of the Old Masters.* New York: Liturgical Music Press, Inc., 1944–.

Folio 22 contains *Ricercar on the second tone; Ricercar on the fourth tone; Ricercar on the fifth tone; Ricercar on the sixth tone* (16pp).

Folio 55 contains *Ricercar on the seventh tone; Ricercar on the eighth tone.*

D0054 Hohn, Wilhelm. *Notenbeispiele zu Der Kontrapunkt. Palestrina und seinen Zeitgenossen.* Regensburg: Friedrich Pustet, 1918. MT55.H75

Examples intended to complement Bellermann's counterpoint text.

D0055 Hübsch, Hanns, ed. *Laudate Dominum.* Heidelberg: Süddeutscher Musikverlag Willy Müller, 1949 *et seq.*

This series was designed to provide suitable musical materials for various seasons of the liturgical year. Items issued separately. Latin text, score format. Heft 1 [SM1507] contains hymn *Creator alme siderum* (SATB to SATT to SATTB); Heft 2 [SM1516, pub.1953] contains motet *Hodie Christus natus est* (SSAT); *Gloria tibi Domine* (SSATTB); *Hunc coelum* (SATB); Heft 3 [SM1509, pub.1960] contains motet *Ad Dominum cum tribularer* (SATB); *Manus tuae Domine* (SATTB); *Paucitas dierum meum* (SATTB); Heft 4 [SM1517] contains *Cui comparabo te* (SATB); Heft 5 [SM1511, pub.1949] contains *Haec dies* (SSATTB); *Exsultate Deo* (SATTB); *Surrexit pastor bonus* (SATB).

D0056 Hüschen, Hans, ed. *The Motet.* Anthology of Music 47. General ed. Karl Gustav Fellerer. Köln: Arno Volk, 1975.

Historical introduction to the motet genre, pp.5–23.

Contains motet *Rex pacificus a 6* (pp.55–57). Note values halved; *Mensurstrich.*

D0057 Imrie, Martyn, ed. *Hodie Christus Natus Est! An Anthology of Motets for Advent and Christmas.* London: Vanderbeck & Imrie, 1986.

Preface containing biographical material and description of the motet selection (p.2). English translation at head of music; Latin text underlay.

Note values halved; transposed down 1 tone.

Contains *Canite tuba in Sion* [secunda pars *Rorate coeli desuper*] (pp.9–17).

D0058 Imrie, Martyn, ed. *Mapa Mundi. Renaissance Performing Scores.* Mapa Mundi, 1981.

Series E, *Italian Church Music*, contains no.9E, *Ascendo ad Patrem: For 5 Voices* [pub. 1981; motet SATTB, Latin text]; no.10, *Missa Ascendo ad Patrem for 5 Voices* [pub.1981; mass SATTB, Latin text]. Issued separately.

D0059 Jancsovics, Antal, ed. *Canticum canticorum: 29 motetta.* Musicotheca classica 5. Budapest: Editio Musica, 1976.

Contains the 29 motets of Book IV (1584) in one volume. Each motet was also issued separately, in series numbered 312–42000–312–42028, listed in brackets following the incipit below.

Contains *Osculetur me* [312–42000] (SATTB, pp.9–11); *Trahe me post te* [312–42001] (SATTB, pp.11–15); *Nigra sum, sed formosa* [312–42002] (SATTB, pp.15–19); *Vineam meam* [312–42003] (SATTB, pp.19–22); *Si ignoras te* [312–42004] (SATTB, pp.23–27); *Pulchrae sunt genuae tuae* [312–42005] (SATTB, pp.27–31); *Fasciculus myrrhae* [312–42006] (SATTB, pp.31–34); *Ecce tu pulcher es* [312–42007] (SATTB, pp.34–37); *Tota pulchra es* [312–42008] (SATTB, pp.38–41); *Vulnerasti cor meum* [312–42009] (SATTB, pp. 41–45); *Sicut lilium inter spinas* [312–42010] (SATTB, pp.45–49); *Introduxit me Rex* [312–42011] (SATTB, pp.49–52); *Laeva ejus* [312–42012] (SATTB, pp.53–56); *Vox dilecti mei* [312–42013] (SATTB, pp.56–60); *Surge propera amica mea* [312–42014] (SATTB, pp.60–63); *Surge, amica mea* [312–42015] (SATTB, pp.64–67); *Dilectus meus mihi* [312–42016] (SATTB, pp.68–71); *Surgam et circuibo* [312–42017] (SATTB, pp.71–74); *Adjuro vos, filiae* [312–42018] (SATTB, pp.75–79); *Caput ejus* [312–42019] (AATTB, pp.79–83); *Dilectus meus descendit* [312–42020] (AATTB, pp.83–87); *Pulchra es amica mea* [312–42021] (AATTB, pp.87–90); *Quae est ista* [312–42022] (AATTB, pp.90–94); *Descendi in hortum meum* [312–42023] (AATTB, pp.94–98); *Quam pulchri sunt* [312–42024] (SSATB, pp.98–102); *Duo ubera tua* [312–42025] (SSATB, pp.102–106); *Quam pulchra es et quam decora* [312–42026] (SAATB, pp.107–111); *Guttur tuum sicut* [312–42027] (SAATB, pp.111–115); *Veni veni dilecte mi* [312–42028] (SATTB, pp.115–119).

D0060 Jeppesen, Knud, ed. *Italia Sacra Musica. Musiche corali italiane sconosciute della prima metà del cinquecento.* Copenhagen: Wilhelm Hansen, 1962. 3 vols.

Vol 3, *Unknown Italian Cathedral Music of the Early 16th Century*, contains remarks on the publication, a list of manuscript and print sources, and notes on the various composers represented in the volume. Includes Palestrina: hymn *Quicumque Christum quaeritis* (pp.163–168, SATB, alternatim [even-numbered strophes in polyphony] with plainchant verses also printed); hymn *Salvete flos martyrum* (pp. 169–171, SATB, alternatim

[even] with plainchant verses also printed); *Lamentationes* (pp.172–191, SATB to SATTB: *Feria V. In coena Domini, Lectio I,* pp.172–177; *Feria VI. In Parasceve, Lectio I,* pp.178–184; *Lectio II* pp.185–191). *Mensurstrich.*

D0061 *Die junge Kantorei*. Stuttgart: Hänssler, 19—.

This series is divided into a number of subseries containing works by Palestrina, including: vol 5 (the first of a subseries of three volumes [5, 9, 10]), ed. Diethard Hellmann, *Introiten und Motetten zum Kirchenjahr*; vol 33 (the first of a subseries of two volumes [33, 38]), *Introiten und Psalmen*; vol 39, *Chorgesänge zum gottesdienstlichen Gebrauch*; vol 57, *100 Jahre Verband Evangelischer Kirchenchöre in Württemberg.*

D0062 Klein, Maynard, ed. *Eleven Motets for Treble Voices*. Chicago: G.I.A. Publications, 1978.

A collection of motet and mass excerpts for three and four voices, geared to younger performers. Provides Latin text with English translation. Bears edition number 2143; items also issued individually, but also under the same edition number, 2143. Contains *Adoramus te Jesu Christe* (SSAA); *Confitemini Domino* (SSAA); *Jesu rex admirabilis* (SSA); *Missa Lauda Sion* (*Benedictus* only, SSA); *Missa Sacerdotes Domini* (*Pleni sunt coeli* only, SSA); *Sicut cervus* (SATB).

D0063 *Königliche Akademie der Künste. Berlin. Musikalische Section. Auswahl vorzüglicher Musik-Werke in gebundener Schreibart von Meister alter und neuer Zeit . . . zur Beförderung des höhern Studiums der Musik.* No.1–48. 1–16 Lief. Berlin: T. Trautwein, 1835–1841.

No.28 contains motet *Tu es Petrus a 6.*

D0064 Köthe, Bernard, ed. *Musica Sacra. Sammlung von Hymnen und Motetten für Männerstimmen.* Leipzig: F.E.C. Leuckart, n.d.

D0065 Kraus, Eberhard, ed. *Cantantibus organis. Sammlung von Orgelstücken alter Meister.* Regensburg: Friedrich Pustet, 1958.

Contains editions of intabulations for organ of Palestrina motets made by Jacob Paix (1556–1623), from Paix's *Ein schön Nutz- und Gebräuchlich Orgel Tabular* (RISM 1583[22]).

Vol 1, *Die Orgel im Kirchenjahr: Advent/Weihnachten* (1958), contains Palestrina/Paix: no.10, *Hodie Christus natus est* (pp.25–28); no.15, *Lapidabant Stephanum* (pp.45–49); no.20, *Senex puerum* (pp.58–61).

Vol 6, *Orgelmusik an europäischen Kathedralen II: St. Peter in Rom* (1961), contains Palestrina/Paix: no.9, *Cantantibus organis* (pp.18–24).

———. Kuhn, Max. *Die Verzierungs-Kunst in der Gesangs-Musik des 16.–17. Jahrhunderts (1535–1650).* Beihefte der Internationalen Musikgesellschaft 7. Leipzig: Breitkopf und Härtel, 1902. KL1403.K96.

See item E0278 for main bibliographical entry. On pp.100–109 is printed Bassano's diminutions on Palestrina's *Benedicta sit sancta Trinitas* in a composite score drawn from pp.1 *et seq.* and p.9 of Bassano's text, with the soprano diminution on the top staff and the bass diminution on the lowest staff. On pp.122–125 Bovicelli's diminutions on *Io son ferito* [p.38 of his text] are printed in a system of two staffs, containing the embellished and unembellished lines respectively.

D0066 La Fage, Adrien de [Juste-Adrien-Lenoir de], ed. *Cinq messes tirées du répetoire de la chapelle sixtine à Rome.* Paris: Mme. Ve. Launer, n.d. [1840s]

Introductory notes discussing Palestrina's life and works [see item E0518]. Contains masses: *Papae Marcelli a 6* (pp. 1–52); *Per i deffonti [pro defunctis: Kyrie, Offertorium, Sanctus, Agnus Dei] a 5* (pp.53–76); *Canonica a 4* (pp.77–112); *O regem coeli a 4* (pp.113–156); *Aeterna Christi munera a 4* (pp.157–184).

D0067 La Fage, Adrien de [Juste-Adrien-Lenoir de], ed. *Vingt motets tirées du répetoire de la chapelle sixtine à Rome composés par Jean Pierluigi de Palestrina. Edition revue et corrigée avec le plus grand soin.* Paris: Mme. Ve. Launer, n.d. [1840s]

Contents all for five voices and derived from motet prints of 1569–1584. Includes introductory notes [see item E0515] 1. *Coenantibus illis accepit* (pp.1–6); 2. *Tribulationes civitatum* (pp.6–10; secunda pars *Peccavimus cum patribus* pp.10–14); 3. *Salve Regina* (pp.14–20); 4. *Exultate Deo* (pp.21–26); 5. *Pater noster* (pp.26–31); 6. *Parce mihi Domine* (pp.32–36; secunda pars *Peccavi* pp.37–40); 7. *Beatus Laurentius* (pp.41–45); 8. *Lapidabant Stephanum* (pp.46–52); 9. *Peccantem me quotidie* (pp.53–57); 10. *Caro me a vere est cibus* (pp.57–62); 11. *Crucem sanctam* (pp.62–66); 12. *Canite tuba in Sion* (pp.66–71; secunda pars *Rorate coeli* pp. 71–76); 13. *O beata et benedicta* (pp.77–82); 14. *Ave Trinitatis* (pp.87–92); 15. *Exi cito in plateas* (pp.92–97); 16. *Paucitas dierum* (pp.97–100; secunda pars *Manus tuae Domine* pp.101–104); 17. *Domine secundum actum* (pp.104–109); 18. *Derelinquat impius* (pp.109–114); 19. *O sacrum convivium* (pp.115–120); 20. *O admirabile commercium* (pp.120–124).

D0068 Lerner, Edward R., ed. *Study Scores of Musical Styles.* New York: McGraw-Hill, 1968. M2.L47.S9

D0069 Liliencron, Rochus Freiherr von, ed. *Chorordnung für die Sonn- und Festtage des evangelischen Kirchenjahre, entworfen und erläutert. . . .* Gütersloh, 1900. New edition, ed. Hans Joachim Moser. Kassel: Bärenreiter, 1929.

Freiherr von Liliencron was one of the outstanding scholars of his generation; among his many achievements was the editing of well over forty volumes of the *Denkmäler deutscher Tonkunst.* The *Chorordnung* contains versions of ten Palestrina works.

D0070 Lück, Stephan, ed. *Sammlung ausgezeichneter Compositionen für die Kirche.* Trier, 1859; second ed. Leipzig: P. Braun's Verlag, 1884–1885.

The first edition was published in two volumes.

Vol 1 contains *Missa Papae Marcelli.*

Vol 2 contains motets *Haec dies; Loquebantur variis linguis; O salutaris hostia; O bone Jesu; Tu es Petrus; Veni sponsa Christi; Alma redemptoris mater*; magnificat *Magnificat octavi toni.*

For the second edition, vols 1–3 were edited by Michael Hermesdorff; vol 4 was edited by Heinrich Oberhoffer. Preface by Stephan Lück dated July 1883 in French and German double-column format. In this edition, note values were halved throughout; Latin texts were underlaid; some dynamics markings and other editing added.

Vol 1 contains no.5, *Missa Aeterna Christi munera a 4* (SATB, pp.87–112).

Vol 2 contains no.5, *Missa Iste Confessor a 4* (SATB, pp.85–108); no.8, *Missa Papae Marcelli a 6* (SATTBB, pp.149–199, transposed down 1 tone).

Vol 3 contains no.3, *Dies sanctificatus a 4* (SATB, pp.9–15); no.23, *Haec dies a 6* (SSATTB, pp.82–86); no.26, *Loquebantur variis linguis a 4* (SATB, pp.95–100); no.31, *Exultate Deo a 5* (SAATB, pp.113–119): no.42, *O salutaris hostia a 4* (SATB, pp.156–158).

Vol 4 contains no.3, *O bone Jesu a 4* (SATB, pp.4–5); no.20, *Tu es Petrus a 6* (SSATTB, pp.61–67); no.29, *Veni sponsa Christi a 4* (SATB, pp.106–109); no.37, *Magnificat octavi toni a 8* (SATB SATB, two choirs arranged on one 4-stave system, pp.134–148), no.39, *Alma Redemptoris Mater a 4* (SATB, pp.155–158).

D0071 *Manoscritti musicali rari.* Rome: Studio Internationale, 1949.

Series contains no.1, Gianfranco Maselli and Virgilio Mortari, ed. *Omnis pulchritudo Domino, a 8 voci in 2 cori, da un manoscritto autografo inedito.* Rome: De Santis, 1950.

SSAT ATTB, unaccompanied. Latin text. Edition based on a manuscript in the Biblioteca del Conservatorio Santa Cecilia, Rome (*I-Bsc* Ris.B. I. I.), of which a page (cantus of chorus I) is reproduced in fascimile. Scored by Maselli; prefatory notes by Mortari.

Contains motet *Omnis pulchritudo Domine a 8.*

D0072 Marchal, André, ed. *8 [Huit] ricercari [4 vocum] dans le 8 tons.* Orgue et liturgie 3. Paris: Éditions musicales de la Schola Cantorum et de la Procure generale de musique, 1951. 24pp.

Arranged for organ. Contains prefatory notes and remarks by Marchal on registration; a preface by Joseph Samson; suggestions for execution by Joseph Bonnet.

Contains *Ricercare I del primo tono* (pp.8–9); *Ricercare II del secondo tono* (pp.10–11); *Ricercare III del tertio tono* (pp.12–13); *Ricercare IV del quarto tono* (pp.14–15); *Ricercare V del quinto tono* (pp.16–17); *Ricercare VI del sesto tono* (pp.181–19); *Ricercare VII del settimo tono* (pp.20–22); *Ricercare VIII del ottavo tono* (pp.22–24).

D0073 Margittay, Sándor, ed. *Anthologia Organi. Orgelmusik aus acht Jahrhunderten.* Mainz: B. Schott's Söhne/Budapest: Editio Musica, 1976.

Vol 3, *Die Römische Schule und ihre Nachfolger* [ED6758], contains

Ricercar del settimo tuono (pp.22–25). Preface with notes; musical edition based on Fellerer's 1933 publication of ricercari. Edited.

D0074 Merritt, Arthur Tillman. *Sixteenth-Century Polyphony. A Basis for the Study of Counterpoint.* Cambridge, MA: Harvard University Press, 1939.

A respected manual for the study of sixteenth-century style, containing numerous musical examples. Only complete works or sections (rather than phrases or cadences) are listed here. Contains *Missa Aeterna Christi munera, Kyrie* (untexted, p.103); *O bone Jesu* (motet a 4, dubious attribution, pp.105–107); *Anima mea turbata est* (motet a 4, pp.108–117); *Missa Gabriel Archangelus, Sanctus* (*Pleni sunt coeli* only, pp.157–160); *In diebus illis* (motet a 4, pp.169–183); *Dies sanctificatus* (motet a 4, pp.186–196).

D0075 Mikel, E., ed. *Lauda Sion. Sammlung von hundertfünfzig 2- 3- und 4-stimmigen Gradualien, Offertorien, Hymnen und marianischen Antiphonen für das ganze Kirchenjahr. Op.7.* Regensburg: Pustet, 1904 (Vorrede 1880).

D0076 Morris, Reginald Owen. *Contrapuntal Technique in the Sixteenth Century.* Oxford: Clarendon, 1922. 74 + 49pp. ML446. M8.

A twentieth-century counterpoint manual that rejects species counterpoint, clearly admires Palestrina, and takes numerous examples from his work. There is a large number of two- or three-measure quotations of voice leading examples, interspersed with complete or half-complete sections of several works. Editions use original note values, modern clefs. Contains no.55, part of *Missa Aeterna Christi munera* [part of *Agnus Dei*] (p.9); no.157, *Missa Petra sancta* [*Kyrie I*] (p.20); no.168, *Missa Veni sponsa Christi* [part of *Sanctus*] (p.23); no.169, *Missa De feria* [part of *Kyrie II*] (p.23); no.183, *Missa Brevis* [part of *Agnus Dei*] (p.29); no.184, *Missa Sacerdotes Domini* [*Sanctus*] (p.30); no.192, motet *Veni sponsa Christi* [complete] (pp.32–34); no.193, motet *Tu es Petrus* [to cadence on *ecclesiam meam*] (pp.35–36); no.194, motet *O bone Jesu* (p.37).

D0077 *Die Motette im Wandel des Kirchenjahres.* Heidelberg: Süddeutscher Musikverlag Willy Müller, n.d. [1960s].

A series of works designated for seasons and feasts of the liturgical year, issued separately. Latin text. Contains [M022] *Loquebantur in variis linguis* (SATB); [M040] *Salvator mundi* (SATB); [M044] *Quam pulchri sunt* (SATB); [M047] *Quae est ista* (SATB).

D0078 *Musica sacra: La settimana santa nella Cappella Sistina.* Roma: Typis Ejusdem Ephemiridis apud Typographeum R.C.A., 1870.

D0079 Ney, Joseph Napoleon [" le Prince de la Moskowa"], ed. *Recueil de musique ancienne. Recueil des morceaux de musique ancienne, éxécutés aux concerts de la Société de Musique Vocale, Religieuse et Classique, fondée à Paris en 1833 . . . sous la direction de M. Le Prince de la Moskowa. Publié par la Société.* Paris: Pacini, 1842. 11 vols.

Vol 1 contains *Missa Papae Marcelli* ["*Pape Marcel*"] (pp.1–68); *Missa*

Aeterna Christi munera (pp.69–104); sequence *Stabat mater a 8* (pp.105–130); motet *Fratres ego enim a 8* (pp.131–142); motet *Adoramus te* (pp.144–145); mass movement *Pleni sunt coeli a 3* (ATB, pp.146–147); madrigal *Alla riva del Tebro* (pp.149–152).

Vol 5 contains madrigals *Vaghi pensieri* (pp.85–91); *Là ver l'aurora* (pp.92–96).

Vol 7 contains *Tribularer si nescirem*; *Agnus Dei*; *Popule meus*; *Canite tuba*; *Vinea mea electa*; *Una hora non potuisti*; *Tantum ergo*; *Tristis est anima mea* [secunda pars *In monte Oliveti*]; *Esurientes*; *Corporis misterium*; *O bone Jesu*; *Sicut erat*; *Dei mater alma*; *Lauda anima mea*; *Hodie Christus natus est*; *Gloria Patri.*

Vol 9 contains *Missa Canonica* ["*Messe Canonique*"]; *Missa pro defunctis* ["*Messe de Requiem*"].

Vol 10 contains motets no.106, *Dies sanctificatus* (pp.1–10); no.107, *Sicut cervus* (pp.11–16); no.108, *Sicut cervus* transposed up a minor third ["*Même morceau en la bémol*"] (pp.17–22); no.109, *Laus honor virtus gloria* (pp.23–30); no.110, *Veni sponsa Christi* (pp.31–38).

D0080 Niedermeyer, Louis, ed. *La Maîtrise* [later *La Grande Maîtrise*]. Paris: Editions Publimuses, 1857–1861.

A composer who became deeply committed to religious music, Niedermeyer (1802–1861) sought to found a school which prepared church musicians through a study of chant, counterpoint, and study of the works of masters of the sixteenth through eighteenth centuries. This series was founded in 1857 with Joseph d'Ortigue as a journal of religious music with an ultimately didactic intent. Compositions by Palestrina include the following:

Year 1 (pub. 1857), no. 1. *Kyrie . . . à quatre voix* [*Missa Aeterna Christi munera*]; no. 4. *O bone Jesu. Motet à quatre voix*; no. 5. *Gloria . . . à quatre voix* [*Missa Aeterna Christi munera*]; no. 7. *Pleni sunt coeli, à trois voix* [*Missa O magnum mysterium*]; no. 8. *Dei mater alma. Motet à quatre voix* [hymn *Ave maris stella*]; no. 10. *Sicut cervus desiderat ad fontes. Motet à quatre voix*; no. 11. *Credo . . . à quatre voix* [*Missa Aeterna Christi munera*].

Year 2 (pub. 1858), no. 2. *Sanctus et Benedictus . . . a quatre voix* [*Missa Aeterna Christi munera*]; no. 3. *Agnus I . . . à quatre voix* [*Missa Aeterna Christi munera*].

Year 3 (pub. 1859), no.13. *Quae vox, à quatre voix* [hymn *Sanctorum meritis*].

D0081 Novack, Saul, ed. *Masses and Motets. Giovanni Pierluigi da Palestrina.* Based on Raffaele Casimiri's edition. New York: Dover, 1993.

Economical and attractive paperbound selection of material from the Kalmus reprint of the Casimiri edition. Contains (pp.vii–xi) "Publisher's Note" with some Gregorian incipits and "Texts and Translations" of all Latin material.

Contains *Missa Ave regina coelorum a 4* (pp.1–29); motet *Veni sponsa Christi a 4* (pp.30–32); *Missa Veni sponsa Christi a 4* (pp.33–56); motet *O magnum mysterium a 6* [seconda parte: *Quem vidistis*] (pp.57–65); *Missa O magnum mysterium a 5* (pp.66–104); motet *Ascendo ad Patrem a 5* [secunda pars *Ego rogabo Patrem*] (pp.105–113); *Missa Ascendo ad Patrem a 5* (pp.114–147); *Missa L'homme armé a 5* (pp.148–186); *Missa Papae Marcelli a 6* (pp.187–221).

D0082 Novello, Vincent, ed. *The Fitzwilliam Music, being a collection of sacred pieces, selected from manuscripts of Italian composers in the Fitzwilliam Museum, now for the first time published by permission of the University of Cambridge.* London: Pub. for the Editor, 1825. 5 vols.

Vol 1, pp.32–34 contains a "Quintetto" *Et incarnatus est*, with a reduction of the vocal parts added as organ accompaniment. It is listed as derived "from an MS Mass in A Minor by Palestrina" in the Fitzwilliam Museum, Cambridge. Preface pages iii–vii; paragraph about Palestrina on page iv.

D0083 O'Regan, Noel, ed. *Giovanni Pierluigi da Palestrina. Three Pieces for Triple Choir. Ad te levavi. Beati omnes. Salve Regina. SATB/SATB/SATB.* Edinburgh: Edinburgh Music Imprint, 1994.

Preface (pp.1–2) and editorial commentary with English translations of texts printed before each work. Noted as the first modern edition to use the recently rediscovered original choir III parts by Palestrina. Contains motets *Ad te levavi* (pp.3–10); *Beati omnes* (pp.11–19); *Salve Regina* (pp.20–28).

D0084 Palisca, Claude V., ed. *Norton Anthology of Western Music.* Third ed. New York: Norton, 1996. 2 volumes.

Vol 1, *Ancient to Baroque*, includes two movements from the *Missa Papae Marcelli* [*Credo*, pp.218–228, and *Agnus Dei I*, pp.229–231]. Reprinted from the Casimiri edition, vol 4, pp.177–187 and 194–196 respectively. Commentary on the music on pp.232–233; Latin and English texts of the *Credo* at the bottom of p.228. The first edition of this anthology (published 1980) contains the music of the *Credo* only (vol 1, pp.200–210), without printed commentary.

D0085 Pellini, Giulio, Siro Cisilino, and Charles van den Borren, eds. *Sei missae dominicales a cinque voce (1592). Celebre raccolte musicali venete del Cinquecento.* Padova: G. Zanibon, 1981. 255pp.

Note [as translated from Italian] indicates "also contains the Missa Dominicalis, unpublished, by Giov. Pierluigi da Palestrina, with whom his brother Silla and his sons Rodolfo and Angelo collaborated (from the exemplar in London, Buckingham Palace, and the manuscript in the Biblioteca Estense, Modena)."

Contains *Missa dominicalis a 5* by Palestrina; a *Missa dominicales a 5* by Palestrina in collaboration with members of his family; plus other *Missae dominicales* by Giaches de Wert, Francsco Rovigo, Giangiacomo Gastoldi, and Alesssandro Striggio.

D0086 Perinello, Carlo, ed. *Pier Luigi Sante da Palestrina. Madrigali a 4 e 5 voci, trascritti in notazione moderna con sottoposto un sunto per pianoforte.* [alternative title *Canzonette e madrigali: per canto e pianoforte*]. I Classici della musica italiana 21. Raccolta nazionale delle musiche italiane 82–84. Gen. ed. Gabriele d'Annunzio. Milano: Società anonima notari, ca. 1919. 3 vols.

Text is both printed before each work and underlaid. The piano accompaniment is equivalent to a reduction of the various vocal parts. Music is extensively edited.

Vol 82 (all selections SATB), contains *Donna, vostre mercede* (pp.3–9); *Che debbo far, che mi consigli, Amor?* (pp.10–15); *Veramente in amore* (pp.16–22); *I vaghi fiori e l'amorose fronde* (pp.23–30).

Vol 83 contains *Mori quasi il mio core* (SATB, pp.3–10); *La cruda mia nemica* (SATB, pp.11–19); *O bella Ninfa mia* (SATTB, pp.20–27).

Vol 84 contains *Placide l'acqu'e placid'era il vento* (SATTB, pp.3–11); *Soave fia il morir* (SAATB, pp.12–18).

D0087 Phillips, Peter, general ed. *Renaissance Masters. Masses.* Bury St. Edmunds: Chester Music, 1990.

General introduction by Peter Phillips; introduction by Ivan Moody; suggestions for performance by Peter Phillips.

Vol 1, ed. Ivan Moody, *Missa Dies sanctificatus: SATB.* Renaissance Masters. Motets. London: Novello Publishing, 1995.

Introductory notes by Peter Phillips (dated 1990); introduction by Ivan Moody (dated 1991); comments on individual works and suggestions for their performance by Peter Phillips (dated 1991). Includes English translations printed as text in captions; keyboard reductions for rehearsal.

Vol 2, ed. Ivan Moody, *Motets for Four Voices.* Bury St. Edmunds: Novello, 1995.

Contains motets *Ave Maria* (transposed up 1 tone, pp.8–12); *Benedicta sit sancta Trinitas* (transposed down 1 tone, pp.13–19); *In diebus illis* (transposed up minor third, pp.20–27); *Lapidabant Stephanum* (transposed down 1 tone, pp.28–33); *Loquebantur variis linguis* (transposed down 1 tone, pp.34–40); *O Rex gloriae* (transposed down 1 tone, pp.41–46); *Valde honorandus est* (transposed down 1 tone, pp.47–51).

D0088 Pirrotta, Nino, and Giuliana Gialdroni, eds. *I musici di Roma e il madrigale: Dolci affetti (1582) e Le gioie (1589).* L'Arte Armonica/Musica Palatina 1. Roma: Accademia Nazionale di Santa Cecilia/Libreria Musicale Italiana, 1993. 186pp. ISBN 88–7096–089-7.

An edition of two important madrigal collections to which the best-known composers active in Rome in the second half of the sixteenth century, including Palestrina, contributed. Contains *Dunque perfido amante* (p.2).

D0089 Powley, Harrison, ed. *Il Trionfo di Dori: The 29 Madrigals of the 1592 Collection for Mixed Voices.* Renaissance Voices series. New York: Gaudia Music and Arts, Inc., 1990.

Contains no.29, *Quando dal terzo cielo à 6* (pp.239–246). SSATTB, Italian and English translation at head of text, transposed down a fourth. With introductory notes, facsimile reproductions, and an appendix containing editorial guidelines and a list of sources.

D0090 Proske, Karl, ed. *Missa Papae Marcelli triplici concentu distincta, videlicet: I. Joannis Petri Aloisii Praenestini Missa . . . genuina sex vocum. II. Missa eadem ad quatuor voces reducta, auctore Joanne Francisco Anerio. III.*

Eademque Missa duplici choro octo vocibus concinenda, auctore Francisco Suriano . . . juxta editiones principes fidelissime in partitionem redegit . . . publicavit Carolus Proske. Mainz: B Schott's Söhne, 1850.

Includes three versions of the mass: Palestrina's original for six voices; the reworking by Giovanni Francesco Anerio for four voices; the version by Francesco Soriano for eight voices. Scored with retention of the original note values; untransposed, without tempo or dynamic markings.

D0091 Proske, Karl, ed. *Musica divina. Sive thesaurus concentuum selectissimorum omni cultui divino totius anni juxta ritum Sanctae Ecclesiae Catholicae inservientium: Ab excellentissimis superioris aevi musicis muneris harmonicis compositorum. Quos e codicibus originalibus tam editis quam ineditis accuratissime in partitionem redactos. Ad instauranam polyphoniam vere ecclesiasticam publice offert Carolus Proske. Annus 1–2.* Ratisbonae: Friderici Pustet [Regensburg: Friedrich Pustet], 1853–1876. Year 1 vol 4 and Year 2 ed. J. Schrems or Franz Xaver Haberl.

Year 1, vol 1, *Liber Missarum* (1853), contains masses *Missa Brevis* (pp.1–30); *Missa Iste Confessor* (pp.31–54); *Missa Dies sanctificatus* (pp.55–90).

Vol 2, *Liber Motettorum* (1855), contains motets *Dies sanctificatus* (pp.29–33); *Valde honorandus* (pp.59–63); *Pueri Hebraeorum* (pp.117–220); *Haec dies* (pp.134–138); *Surrexit pastor* (pp.154–158); *Loquebantur variis linguis* (pp.179–185); *Quam pulchri* (pp.271–277); *Fuit homo* (pp.313–318); *Quae est ista* (pp.346–351); *Misso Herodes* (pp.359–364); *Adoramus te* (pp.377–379); *Princeps gloriossisime Michael* (pp.382–385); *Salvator mundi* (pp.394–398); *O quantus luctus* (pp.414–418); *Congratulamini mihi a 4* (pp.423–426); *Isti sunt viri* (pp.443–447); *Veni sponsa Christi* (pp.506–510); *Exaudi Domine* (pp.519–523); *Sicut cervus* (pp.533–539; secunda pars *Sitivit anima*).

Vol 3, *Psalmodiam, Magnificat, Hymnodiam, et Antiphonas B. Mariae Virg. complectens* (1859), contains a *Magnificat octavi toni* (pp.282–289); hymns *Hostes Herodes* (pp.357–363); *Vexilla regis* (pp.363–373); *Veni Creator spiritus* (pp.378–386); motet *Alma Redemptoris mater* (pp.496–502; secunda pars *Tu quae genuisti*).

Vol 4, *Liber Vespertinus* (1863), contains *Lamentationes: In coena Domini; Parasceve; Sabbato sancto* (pp.49–104); falsobordone *Miserere* (pp.209); *Benedictus Dominus* (pp.263–268); *Improperia* (pp.295–297); litany *Litaniae BMV* (pp.362–369).

Year 2, vol 1, *Liber Missarum* (ed. J. Schrems, 1855–1857), contains masses *Missa Tu es Petrus a 6* (facs.4); *Missa Ascendo ad Patrem a 5* (facs.6); *Missa Papae Marcelli a 6* (facs.7); *Missa Aeterna Christi munera a 4* (facs.8).

Vol 2, *Liber Motettorum* (ed. J. Schrems and F. X. Haberl, 1869–1876), contains motets *Diffusa est gratia* (facs.2, pp.20–24); *Vidi turbam magnam* (facs.3, pp.60–76).

Vols 3 and 4 contain no music by Palestrina.

D0092 Proske, Karl, ed. *Selectus novus missarum praestantissimorum superioris* *aevi auctorum, juxta codices originales tum manuscriptos tum impressos editarum a Carolo Proske.* Ratisbonae [Regensburg]: Pustet, 1853–1861. 2 vols.

Vol 1 (1855–1857) contains masses *Veni sponsa Christi a 4* (pp.1–32); *Assumpta est Maria a 6* (pp.85–138).

Vol 2 (1861) contains mass *Dum complerentur a 6* (pp.401–456).

D0093 Items D0091 and D0092 reprinted as *Musica divina; Annus primus & Annus secundus. Selectus novus missarum.* Introd. Paul Henry Lang. New York: Johnson Reprint Corp., 1973. 10 vols in 8.

Reprint in one collection of the two Proske editions.

D0094 Riemann, Hugo, ed. *Musikgeschichte in Beispielen.* Leipzig: Verlag von E. A. Seeman, 1911. M2.R53.

D0095 Rimbault, Edward F., ed. *A Collection of Ancient Church Music, Printed for the Motet Society.* London: J.A. Novello, 1847. 3 vols ["Divisions"].

Each selection was printed with a keyboard accompaniment for rehearsal. The underlaid English translations are adaptations of Anglican service texts. Some music was evidently edited and adapted to fit English words smoothly. At times this apparently meant adding or removing measures or sections. The original Latin texts were not attributed in this edition, though several works are very familiar and recognizable; for example, nos.8 and 11 of volume 3 are *Sicut cervus* and *Exaltabo te*, respectively. In vol 1 ("First Division"), indications for liturgical placement/use are provided at the head of each selection.

First Division, *Anthems for Festivals.* No.4, "If thou shalt confess" [St. Andrew] (SATB, pp.14–21); no.5, "Almighty and everliving God" [St. Thomas] (SATB, pp.21–27); no.6, "O Jerusalem" [St. Stephen] (SSTB, pp.28–33); no.7, "These things have I written unto you" [St. John the Evangelist] (SSTB, pp.34–37); no.8, "These are they that follow the Lamb" [Innocents] (SATB, pp.38–40); no.9, "This shall be the Covenant" [Circumcision] (SATTB, pp.41–46); no.10, "Break forth into joy" [Epiphany]; no.28, "Behold the Lamb of God" [Easter] (SATTB, pp.160–168); no.29, "How beautiful upon the mountain" [Ascension] (SATB, pp.169–176); no.31, "Holy, holy, holy, Lord God Almighty" [Trinity] (SSATB, pp.180–188).

Second Division, *Services.* Contains *Magnificat* (SATB, pp.91–98); *Nunc dimittis* (SATB, pp.99–102).

Third Division, *Miscellaneous Anthems.* Contains no.8, "O God, thou art my God" (SATB, pp.26–29; secunda pars "My soul thirsteth for thee" pp.29–32); no.11, "I will magnify thee, O God" (SSATB, pp.39–44); no.14, "O Lord my God" (SATB, p.55); no.23, "O Lord God of our salvation" ("adapted to English words by Dr. Aldrich," SATTB, pp.93–98).

D0096 Robinson, Ray, ed. *Choral Music: A Norton Historical Anthology.* New York: Norton, 1978. M1495.C54218.

Contains selections from *Missa Papae Marcelli* (Sanctus and Benedictus) (pp.63–70) drawn from Ewerhart edition. Provides English translation of text at end.

D0097 Roche, Jerome, ed. *The Flower of the Italian Madrigal for Mixed Voices. Volume II: Monte-Willaert.* Renaissance Voices series. New York: Galaxy Music, 1988.

Assisted by Elizabeth Roche. Translations into English by Mary Ambrose.

Contains madrigals *Il tempo vola a 5* (SAATB, pp.70–76; seconda parte *Ivi vedrai la gloria* pp.76–83); *Soave fia il morir* (SAATB, pp.84–89; SAATB; transposed up minor third). Italian and English texts at head of music.

D0098 Roche, Jerome, ed. *Introduction to the Italian Madriagl for Four Voices.* Renaissance Voices series. New York: Galaxy Music, 1990.

Contains *Alla riva del Tebro* (pp.115–118). Italian and English texts (translations by Barbara Reynolds) at head of music. SATB, transposed down 1 tone. Note: "Newly revised and edited from the former *Penguin Book of Madrigals for Mixed Voices.*"

———. Rochlitz, Friedrich, ed. *Sammlung vorzüglicher Gesangstücke der anerkannt-grössten Geschichte der Tonkunst. . . .* Mainz, Paris und Antwerpen: B. Schotts Söhnen, 1835. 3 vols.

For main entry describing this early history of music in text and examples, see item E0540.

Includes the following music by Palestrina: no.A: *Adoramus te a 4* (SATB, p.1, Latin underlay only); no.B, *Gloria* (SATB SATB arranged on one 4-stave system, p. 2, Latin underlay); no.C, *Pleni sunt coeli a 3* (ATB, p.3, Latin underlay); no.D, motet *O bone Jesu a 4* (SATB, p.4, Latin underlay); no.E, *Improperia* (SATB SATB, pp.5–7, Latin underlay, some tempo markings given); no.F, madrigal *Credo gentil a 5* (SATTB, pp.8–9, Italian underlay); no.G, psalm motet *Lauda, anima mea* (SAATB, pp.10–12, Latin underlay).

D0099 Röseling, Kaspar, ed. *Musica Spiritualis. Eine Auswahl altklassischer kirchlicher a cappella Gesänge und Messen, in Verbindung mit Dr. F. Haberl, H. Hübsch, Prof. Th. B. Rehmann, Prof. Dr. Th. Schrems, Prof. H. Schroeder.* Regensburg: Franz Feuchtinger, 1950.

Series IA, *Masses*: no.2, *Missa Aeterna Christi munera* (ed. Hanns Hübsch, pub. 1952, SATTB).

Series IB, *Motets:* no.5, *Sicut cervus* [secunda pars *Sitivit anima mea*] (ed. Hanns Hübsch, pub. 1950, SATB).

D0100 Rose, Bernard, ed. *A Sixteenth-Century Anthem Book.* London: Oxford University Press, 1960.

Contains selections from *Missa Quarta* [1582] (Benedictus a 3–4, pp.23–26; Sanctus "Holy, Holy, Holy" a 4 pp.44–47). Note values halved; transposed up 1 tone.

D0101 Rutter, John, ed. *Choral Classics.* Oxford: Oxford University Press, 1999.
Contains pp.63–69, *Hodie Christus natus est* (SSAB + ATTB), based on the print in the *Motettorum liber tertius*, Venice 1575.

D0102 Saint-Réquier, Leon, ed. *Collection "Palestrina": édition populaire des oeuvres religieuses des grands maîtres de XVIme, XVIIme et XVIIIme siècles. Transcription avec clefs usuelles et indications d' interprétation. . . .* Paris: Hérelle, ca. 1913. 4 vols.
Note values halved; extensive editing.
Vol 1 contains no.1, *O bone Jesu a 4* (SATB, pp.1–2); no.8, *Salvator mundi a 4* (SATB, pp.23–28); no.9, *Missa Iste Confessor a 4* [*Kyrie, Gloria, Sanctus, Benedictus, Agnus Dei I* only] (SATB, pp.29–44); no.10, *Verbum caro a 4* (SATB, pp.45–46); no.12, *Salve Regina à 4 voix égales* (pp.49–55); no.14, *Sub tuum praesidium à 4 voix égales* (pp.58–61); no.18, *Confitemini Domino à 4 voix égales* (pp.73–75); no.20, *Lauda Sion a 4* (SATB, pp.78–81).
Vol 2 contains no.22, *Tantum ergo a 4* (SATB, pp.6–8); no.25, *Tantum ergo a 5* (SATTB, pp.15–18); no.33, *Christe lux vera a 4 voix égales* (pp.43–45).
Vol 3 contains no.46, *Missa Aeterna Christi a 4* [lacking *Credo*] (SATB, pp.5–24); no.50, motet *Jesu rex admirabilis a 3* (SAT, p.32); no.51, *O Redemptor a 4* [doubtful attribution] (SATB, p.33); no.57, *Isti sunt viri sancti a 4* (SATB, pp.47–51); no.68, *Valde honorandus est a 4* (SATB, pp.77–81).
Vol 4 is a reprint of the selections in the preceding volumes which were designated for equal voices: no.12, *Salve Regina*; no.14, *Sub tuum praesidium*; no.18, *Confitemini Domino*; no.33, *Christe lux vera.*

D0103 Schauerte, Gustav, ed. *Hymnar.* New York: Schwann, n.d.
A collection that may be derived from an earlier publication, with its respective selections also issued separately. All selections are TTBB for men's voices. Contains [1455III] *Alma redemptoris*; *Pueri Hebraeorum*; *O bone Jesu*; [1455XIII] *Nunc dimittis.*

D0104 Schering, Arnold, ed. *Geschichte der Musik in Beispielen. Dreihundertfünfzig Tonsätze aus neun Jahrhunderten*. Leipzig: Breitkopf und Härtel, 1931; repr. New York: Broude Brothers, 1951; repr. Wiesbaden: Breitkopf & Härtel, 1959. M2.S34.
Contains no.121, "Benedictus, dreistimmig, aus der Missa 'Lauda Sion' (Venedig 1582)" [*Missa Lauda Sion* (Benedictus only, 3 vv on 2 staves)] (p.120); no.122, "Aus der Hohe-Lied Motetten (Rom 1584)" [*Adjuro vos, filiae Jerusalem*, 5vv on 3 staves] (pp.121–123).

D0105 Schinelli, Achille and Giovanni Vianini, eds. *Collana di composizione polifoniche vocali sacre e profane, a due, tre, quattro e cinque voci dei secoli XV, XVI e XVII. Per gli Istituti Magistrali, scuole secondarie, Società Corali, Conservatori di Musica.* Milan: Edizioni Curci, 1958–1986. 5 vols.
Commentary in Italian, English, German. These selections were intended

to provide students with an introduction to historical styles and their performance. The music is printed *a cappella*; Schinelli's selections are extensively edited, while Vianini's suggest relatively more discreet intervention. (Vol.5 contains no music by Palestrina.)

Vol 1, *Canzone sacre, Versetti, Inni, Mottetti e brani diversi a 2, 3, 4 e 5 voci*, contains no.2a, *Pars mea a 3 voci pari* (SSAM p.23); no.2b, *Recordata a 3 voci pari* (from *Lamentations for Holy Saturday*, SSA, pp.24–25); no.3a, *Et misericordia a 3 voci pari* (from *Magnificat primi toni*, SAA, p.26); no.3b, *Deposuit potentes a 3 voci pari* (from *Magnificat octavi toni*, SAA, p.27); no.3c, *Esurientes a 3 voci pari* (from *Magnificat septimi toni*, SSA, p.28); no.4, *Jesu rex admirabilis a 3* (SABar, p.29, Latin underlaid, second verse printed below music); no.9, *O bone Jesu a 4* (SATB, p.36); no.15, *Super flumina Babylonis a 4* (SATB, pp.50–53); no.16, *Sicut cervus a 4* (SATB, pp.54–56); no.17, *Nigra sum a 5* (SATTB, pp.57–60). From a selection of *Madrigali spirituali* in the same volume, no.4, *Vergine chiara a 5* (SATTB, pp.72–78).

Vol 2, *64 Composizioni profane* (ed. Schinelli, with preface in Italian, English, and German by G. C. Paribeni; printed *a cappella*, extensively edited), contains canzonette from the *Ghirlanda* publication of 1587: no.27, *Da così dotta man à 3* (SAT, p.60, verse 1 Italian text underlaid, with texts of verses 2 and 3 at bottom of score); no.28, *Ahi, che quest'occhi miei à 3* (SAT, p.61, verse 1 Italian text underlaid, with texts of verses 2–4 at bottom of score); no.34, *Pose un gran foco nel mio petto amore à 4* (SATB, p.67, verse 1 Italian text underlaid, text of verse 2 at bottom of score); no.35, *Vedrassi prima à 4* (SATB, pp.68–69, verse 1 Italian texts underlaid, with texts of verses 2–4 at bottom of score).

Vol 3, *50 Composizioni profane (Madrigali)* (ed. Schinelli), contains no.19, *Già fu chi m'ebbe cara* (SATB, pp.54–56); no.20, *Chiare, fresche e dolci acque* (SATB, pp.57–59); no.21, *I vaghi fior e l'amorose fronde à 4* (SATB, pp.60–63); no.22, *Alla riva del Tebro à 4* (SATB, pp.64–66); no.23, *La cruda mia nemica à 4* (SATB, pp.67–69); no.31, *Vestiva i colli (in due parte) à 5* (SATTB, pp.102–110, from *Il Desiderio* [1560]); no.32, *Le selve avea d'intorno (in due parte) à 5* (SATTB, pp.111–117, from *Quarto libro delle Muse* [1574]); no.33, *Placide l'acque, e placid'era il vento à 5* (SATTB, pp.118–121, from *Mus. XIII illustri* [1576]).

Vol 4, *23 Mottetti sacri a quattro voci misti* (ed. Giovanni Vianini), contains *Ave maris stella* (SATB, pp.16–17, two voices have Latin text underlay); *Alma redemptoris mater* (SATB, pp.24–26); *Bone Pastor* [labelled "dal 'Lauda Sion' Cantico dei Cantici"] (SATB, pp.27–29); *Christus factus est* (SATB, pp.38–39); *Dies sanctificatus* ((SATB, pp.42–46); *O Domine Jesu Christe* (SATB, pp.72–73).

D0106 Schmidt-Görg, Joseph, ed. *History of the Mass.* Anthology of Music 30. General ed. Karl Gustav Fellerer. Köln: Arno Volk Verlag, 1968.

Historical introduction to the mass genre, pp.5–16; English translation by Robert Kolben.

Contains *Missa Assumpta est Maria* a 6 [*Kyrie* only] (pp.67–70). Note values halved; *Mensurstrich.*

D0107 Schöberlein, Ludwig, and Friedrich Riegel, ed. *Schatz des liturgischen Chor- und Gemeindegesangs nebst dem Altarweisen in der deutschen evangelischen Kirchen aus den Quellen vornehmlich des 16. und 17. Jahrhunderts geschöpft mit den nöthigen geschichtlichen und praktischen Erläuterungen versehen und unter der msikalischen Redaktion von Friedrich Riegel für den Gebrauch in Stadt- und Landkirchen. . . .* Göttingen: Vanderhoeck und Ruprecht, 1865–1872. 2 vols.

This formidable work is a compilation of service music for the Lutheran liturgical year, for Sunday communion services (ordinary and proper material), vespers, feast days, and special occasions. The repertory is drawn primarily from sixteenth- and seventeenth-century Lutheran composers but also contains a significant number of examples by Palestrina, Anerio, and other members of the Roman school. Three volumes were projected, but only two eventually appeared. All the material by Palestrina below contains a German text underlay, with identification of the source and Latin incipit.

Vol 1 contains no.274, "O guter Jesu, ach erbarm dich unser" [*O bone Jesu a 4*], partitura, (p.438); no.275, "O Jesu Christ, dein theures Blut" [*Ad coenam Agni providi*], partitura (pp.438–441).

Vol 2 contains no.32, "Hosanna" [not identified, SSAT] (pp.42–43); [no number] "Allgemeine Ton für die Passions-Antiphonen [after the *Improperia* for Good Friday by Palestrina, 4 voices on 2 staves] (p.397); no.260, "Gott, der Herr, der Gott Israel, sei gelobt" [for Maundy Thursday, 4 voices on 2 staves] (p.397); no.298, "O Kreuz, du einz'ger Hoffnung Zier" [*O crux spes unica*, from *Vexilla regis prodeunt*, SATB] (pp.497–498); no.309, "*Improperia*: Was hab ich dir gethan, O mein Volk? [*Popule meus*, for Good Friday, SATB on 2 staves] (pp.518–519); no.314, "Preis und Ehr, Herr Jesu" [*Adoramus te, Christe*, SATB on 2 staves] (p.527); no.323, "Wie der Hirsch schreit" [*Sicut cervus*, SATB on 2 staves] (pp.466–469); no.620, "Kyrie" [complete, not identified in source, SATB on 2 staves] (pp.928–930); no.647, "Am Ölberg in Gethsemane" [*In monte oliveti*, SATB on 2 staves] (pp.1007–1009); no.648, "Tief betrübt bis zum Tode" [*Tristis est anima mea*, SATB on 2 staves] (pp.1009–1011); no.649, "Siehe, als wir ihn sahen" [*Ecce vidimus eum*, SATB on 2 staves] (pp.1011–1014); no.650, "Einer unter euch wird heute mich verrathen" [*Unus ex discipulus*, SATB on 2 staves] (pp.1014–1015); no.651, "Alle Ältesten des Volkes haben sich versammelt" [*Seniores populi consilium*, STAB on 2 staves] (pp.1015–1016); no.652, "Alle meine Freunde haben verlassen mich" [*Omnes amici mei*, SATB on 2 staves] (pp.1017–1018); no.653, "Ausgeliefert bin ich" [*Tradiderunt me in manus impiorum*, SATB on 2 staves] (pp.1018–1020); no.654, "Ich bin ausgeschüttert wie Wasser" [*Sicut aqua effusus sum*, SATB on 2 staves] (pp.1020–1021); no.655, "Dunkel geworden sind meine Augen" [*Caligaverunt oculi mei*, SATB to SSAA, on 2 staves] (pp.1022–1023); no.656, "Finsternis ward über das Land" [*Tenebrae factae sunt*] (pp.1024–1025); no.657, "Da ward er gestraft und gemartert" [*Sicut ovis ad occisum*] (pp.1025–1027); no.658, "Auf doch, Jerusalem" [*Jerusalem surge*, SATB to SSAA] (pp.1027–1029); no.659, "Siehe, wie dahin" [*Ecce quomodo moritur*, SATB] (pp.1029–1031); no.660, "Könige stehen auf in Lande" [*Adstiterunt reges terrae*] (pp.1031–1032); no.661, "Joseph von Arimathea hat Pilatum" [*Rogavit autem Pilatum*] (pp.1032–1034).

D0108 *A Selection from the works of Palestrina, in vocal score, with an accompaniment for the organ or pianoforte.* London: Novello and Co., ca.1865.

SATB with added keyboard accompaniment: *Missa Papae Marcelli* (pp.115–140).

D0109 Soderlund, Gustave Fredric, and Samuel H. Scott, eds. *Examples of Gregorian Chant and Sacred Music of the 16th Century.* New York: Prentice-Hall, 1971.

This is a companion volume to Soderlund's *Direct Approach to Counterpoint in Sixteenth-Century Style* (New York: Appleton-Century-Crofts, 1947, with several reprintings). Uses modern clefs and original note values. Includes discussion of sources, commentary and translations of texts pp.294–303.

For examples of three-voice counterpoint: *Magnificat primi toni:* Et misericordia a 3 (pp.57–58); *Magnificat tertii toni:* Et misericordia a 3 (pp.59–60); *Magnificat quinti toni:* Et misericordia a 3 (pp.61–62); *Magnificat sexti toni:* Et misericordia a 3 (pp.63–64); *Magnificat secundi toni:* Deposuit potentes a 3 (pp.67–68); *Magnificat quarti toni:* Deposuit potentes a 3 (pp.69–70); *Magnificat octavi toni:* Deposuit potentes a 3 (pp.71–72); *Missa Iam Christus astra ascenderat,* Credo ("Crucifixus" to "non erit finis" a 3, pp.77–79); *Missa Spem in alium,* Credo ("Crucifixus" to "non erit finis" a 3, pp.80–86); *Missa Repleatur os meum laude,* Credo ("Crucifixus" to "non erit finis" a 3, pp.87–90); *Missa Inviolata,* Credo ("Crucifixus" to "ad dexteram Patris" a 3, pp.91–93); *Missa de beata Virgine,* Sanctus ("Pleni sunt coeli" a 3, pp.102–103); *Missa Ad fugam,* Sanctus ("Pleni sunt coeli" a 3, pp.104–105); *Missa Aspice Domine,* Sanctus ("Pleni sunt coeli" a 3, pp.106–108); *Missa Brevis,* Benedictus (to " . . . in nomine Domini" a 3, pp.111–113).

For examples of four-voice counterpoint: *Missa De feria,* Kyrie a 4 (complete, pp.124–128); *Missa Dies sanctificatus,* Kyrie a 4 (complete, pp.129–131); *Missa Gabriel Archangelus,* Hosanna (pp.132–133); *Missa Sine nomine,* Sanctus a 4 (pp.134–136); *Dies sanctificatus* (motet a 4, complete, pp.137–140); *Oculos in altum tollite* (hymn for the feast of the Transfiguration a 4, pp.141–145); *Magnificat quinti toni* (a 4, complete, pp.146–156); *Missa Sanctorum meritis*, Agnus Dei I and II a 4 (pp.157–161).

For examples of five- and six-voice counterpoint, and for complete works (including sections intended to complete the presentation of works already introduced): *Missa Petra sancta*, Kyrie a 5 (complete, pp.162–167); *Missa Vestiva i colli*, Kyrie a 5 (complete, pp.168–172; Gloria complete, pp.173–181); *Alleluia! Tulerunt Dominum* (motet a 5, pp.182–189); *Tu nobis dona fontem* a 3 and *Gloria Deo* (last two strophes of hymn *Ad preces nostras* for Quadragesima Sunday, pp.190–192); *Laudate Dominum* (offertory a 5, pp.193–197); *Improperium exspectavit* (offertory a 5, pp.197–202; also facsimile reproduction of original vocal parts for this work pp.211–213); *Exaltabo te* (offertory a 5, pp.202–206); *Litaniae de Beata Virgine* a 5 (pp.207–210); *Missa Ad fugam,* Kyrie a 4 (pp.214–215, together with Hosanna a 4, pp.215–216, Benedictus a 3, p.217, and Agnus Dei I a 5, pp.218–219); *Missa L'homme armé* a 5 (complete, all movements, pp.220–249); *Missa Ut re mi fa sol la a 6* (complete, all movements, pp.250–278); *Missa Repleatur os meum laude* (Kyrie, pp.279–283; Sanctus-Benedictus, pp.284–289; Agnus Dei I pp.289–291; Agnus Dei II pp.291–293).

D0110 Somma, Bonaventura, ed. *Polifonia vocale sacra e profana sec. XVI.* Roma: de Santis, c.1942–[1947]. M2.P65.

Vol 3 contains *Missa Papae Marcelli: sex vocum* (edition no. 609, SATTBB, 36 pp; cor pts 609A-B); [M2011.P157.P2+ S6].

Vol 6 (pub. ca. 1947) contains *Missa brevis quattuor vocum (1570)* (edition no. 703, SATB, 34pp; cor pts 704–705).

D0111 Stewart, Robert. *An Introduction to Sixteenth-Century Counterpoint and Palestrina's Musical Style.* New York: Ardsley House Publishers, 1994.

The author/compiler's goal was "to provide a representative cross-section of Palestrina's ecclesiastical compositions for study and analysis."

Contains Lamentation: *Feria VI in parasceve, Lectio II, Filii Sion* (p.93); *Missa Tertia Jesu nostra redemptio* [Benedictus] (p.94); *Missa Veni sponsa Christi* [Pleni sunt coeli] (p.99*); Missa Quarta L'homme armé* [Benedictus] (p.102); *Missa O Rex gloriae* [Benedictus] (p.104); *Missa Ave Maria* [Pleni sunt coeli] (p.106); *Magnificat IV toni* [Fecit potentiam] (p.109); hymn *Virgo singularis* (p.112); hymn *Lavacra puri* (p.115); *Missa Secunda* [Benedictus] (p.117); *Missa Ave Regina coelorum* [Crucifixus] (p.120); motet *Exaudi Domine* (p.124); *Magnificat V toni* [Et exsultavit] (p.129); motet *Surrexit pastor bonus* (p.132); motet *Anima mea turbata est* (p.139); *Magnificat II toni* [Sicut erat] (p.144); Hymn *Castae parentis* (p.146); offertory *Deus enim firmavit* (p.149); *Missa L'homme armé* [Kyrie excerpt] (p.155); Lamentation: *Feria VI in parasceve, Lectio III* [*Aleph, Ego vir, Aleph* (p.158); *Me minavit* (p.162); *Aleph* (p.163); *Tantum in me vertit* (p.164); *Beth* (p.165); *Vetustam fectit* (p.166); *Jerusalem* (p.167)]; *Missa Ad fugam* [Kyrie (p.170); Sanctus (p.171, *no* Pleni); *Hosanna* (p.172); Benedictus (p.174); Agnus Dei II (p.176)]; *Litaniae liber secundus: Prima pars* [condensed: *Kyrie eleison* (p.180); *Ave Maria* (p.184)].

D0112 Wennerstrom, Mary. *Anthology of Musical Structure and Style.* Englewood Cliffs, NJ: Prentice-Hall, 1983.

These examples are reprinted from the Casimiri edition.

Contains motet *Veni sponsa Christi* (pp.51–54); mass *Missa Veni sponsa Christi* [Kyrie complete (pp.54–57)].

D0113 Witt, Franz Xaver, ed. *Musica sacra.* Musikbeilage 1. Regensburg: Friedrich Pustet, 1868.

Contains arrangements of vocal music as "Praeludien für die Orgel" [preludes for the organ].

Includes *Missa Brevis* [*Kyrie II* only]; *Missa Iste Confessor* [Sanctus only].

D0114 Wolff, Hellmuth Christian, ed. *Original Vocal Improvisation from the*

16th–18th Centuries. Anthology of Music 41. Cologne: Arno Volk, 1972.

Pages 67–83 contain diminutions for *Io son ferito* and *Ave verum corpus* by Bovicelli.

The four unembellished parts have the suggested scoring for performance of viola 1, viola 2, violoncello 1, violoncello 2.

II. Individually Issued Items

A number of items listed below are associated with broader-ranging series, although issued as individual items. When possible, the publisher's reference number is supplied following the publication date, and before the number of pages.

D0115 [No editor listed] *Adoramus te.* New York: Schwann, n.d. H13. 1p. TTBB, men's voices.

D0116 [No editor listed] *Amors Pfeil.* (*Nessun visse giammai più di me lieto.*) *Das Singwerk* series. Frankfurt: C. F. Peters, ca. 1958. 11pp.

SATB, madrigal from Book I for four voices; German and Italian texts.

D0117 [No editor listed] *Come, Thou Holy Spirit, Come.* Church Music Society Reprints no.24. London: S.P.C.K., 1928; London: Oxford University Press, 1934.

Arrangement of hymn [Hab.VII.25] as anthem.

D0118 [No editor listed] *Death Is but Sleep. O Gentle Death.* New York: Carl Fischer, 1938.

SAATB *a cappella*, version of madrigal *Soave fia il morir* with English text by A. Mattulath.

D0119–D0120 [No editor listed] *Missa Aeterna Christi munera.* Amsterdam: Uitgave Annie Bank, ca. 1966. JP 6, 15pp; JP 7, 12pp.

JP 6, for TTBB, transposed down a fourth from the original. The *Credo* [JP 7] was published separately from the rest of the mass.

D0121 [No editor listed] *Missa Ascendo ad Patrem.* Church Music of the XVIth and XVIIth Centuries for unaccompanied voices no.6110. New York: J. Fischer & Bro., n.d. [early 20th century].

SATTB, extensively edited.

D0122 [No editor listed] *Missa Brevis.* Church Music of the XVIth and XVIIth Centuries for unaccompanied voices no.5040. New York: J. Fischer & Bro., n.d. [early 20th century].

SATB, extensively edited.

D0123 [No editor listed] *Missa celeberrima vulgo dicta Papae Marcelli 6 vocibus concinenda. . . . Editio nova secundum editionum Romanum anni 1567 unacum praevia vita auctoris et historia hujusce missae. . . .* Augsburg: Anton Böhm, c.1840.

D0124 [No editor listed] *Missa In festis apostolorum II quinque vocum cum populo activo*. Regensburg: Friedrich Pustet, 1961. 34pp. M2011.P25.I5.

D0125 [No editor listed] *Missa Iste confessor. SATB a cappella. Palestrina*. New York: Edward B. Marks Music Corp., 1949. 46pp.
SATB, Latin text.

D0126 [No editor listed] *Missa Papæ Marcelli, a seis voces*. Madrid, Union Musical Española, 1961. 61pp. M2011.P25.P37.
Reduction for keyboard for rehearsal. Latin text.

D0127 [No editor listed] *Missa Papae Marcelli*. [*Credo*]. Church Music of the XVIth and XVIIth Centuries for unaccompanied voices no. 6221. New York: J. Fischer & Bro., n.d. [early 20th century].
SATTBB.

D0128 [No editor listed] *Missa Regina coeli für gemischten Chor a cappella*. Graz: Styria Steirische Verlaganstalt, 1949. 28pp. M2011.P25.R4.

D0129 [No editor listed] *Motet for the Festival of Our Lord's Nativity*. Edinburgh: Paterson & Sons, 1897.

D0130 [No editor listed] *Quando dal terzo cielo*. Laaber: Laaber Verlag, n.d. AV103–03. 6pp.
SSATTB, for mixed voices. Italian text.

D0131 [No editor listed] *Sicut cervus*. Egtved: Edition Egtved, n.d. KB065.
SATB, motet *a cappella*.

D0132 [No editor listed] *Sitivit anima mea*. Egtved: Edition Egtved, n.d. KB207.
Secunda pars of *Sicut cervus*. SATB, *a cappella*.

D0133 [No editor listed] *Sicut cervus*. Williamstown, MA: Broude Brothers, n.d. MGC VII-3.
Contains also secunda pars, *Sitivit anima mea*. Latin text with English translation.

D0134 [No editor listed] *Laudate Dominum in tympanis* [a 12]. Polyphonic festival motets by XVIth century masters. New York: J. Fischer & Bro., ca. 1942.
SATB SATB SATB, with piano reduction.

D0135 Atkins, I., ed. *O bone Jesu, exaudi me. O blessed Jesus, hear Thou my prayer*. Novello's Octavo Anthems no.1141. London: Novello, 1926.
SATB SATB, Latin motet, edited with English text by I. Atkins.

D0136 Bank, J.A., ed. *Adoramus te*. Amsterdam: Annie Bank B.V., 1950. A004. 2pp.
SSAA, women's voices, or SSAT, mixed voices, ranked as of 'medium difficulty' in performance. Latin text.

———. Bank, J.A., ed. *Canticum canticorum*. Amsterdam: Annie Bank, n.d. [ca. 1950].

Each of the 29 motets of Book IV, Canticum cauticorum, was issued separately, as series H1–H29; *da cappella* with underlaid Latin text.

D0137 H1: *Osculetur me* (SATTB).
D0138 H2: *Trahe me post te* (SATTB).
D0139 H3: *Nigra sum, sed formosa* (SATTB).
D0140 H4: *Vineam meam* (SATTB).
D0141 H5: *Si ignoras te* (SATTB).
D0142 H6: *Pulchrae sunt genuae tuae* (SATTB).
D0143 H7: *Fasciculus myrrhae* (SATTB).
D0144 H8: *Ecce tu pulcher es* (SATTB).
D0145 H9: *Tota pulchra es* (SATTB).
D0146 H10: *Vulnerasti cor meum* (SATTB).
D0147 H11: *Sicut lilium inter spinas* (SATTB).
D0148 H12: *Introduxit me Rex* (SATTB).
D0149 H13: *Laeva ejus* (SATTB).
D0150 H14: *Vox dilecti mei* (SATTB).
D0151 H15: *Surge propera amica mea* (SATTB).
D0152 H16: *Surge, amica mea* (SATTB).
D0153 H17: *Dilectus meus mihi* (SATTB).
D0154 H18: *Surgam et circuibo* (SATTB).
D0155 H19: *Adjuro vos, filiae* (STTBB).
D0156 H20: *Caput ejus* (STTBB).
D0157 H21: *Dilectus meus descendit* (SATBB).
D0158 H22: *Pulchra es amica mea* (STTBB).
D0159 H23: *Quae est ista* (SATTB).
D0160 H24: *Descendi in hortum meum* (SATBB).
D0161 H25: *Quam pulchri sunt* (SSATB).
D0162 H26: *Duo ubera tua* (SATTB).
D0163 H27: *Quam pulchra es et quam decora* (SAATB).
D0164 H28: *Guttur tuum sicut* (SAATB).
D0165 H29: *Veni veni dilecte mi* (SATTB).

D0166 Bank, J.A., ed. *Confitemini Domino.* Amsterdam: Annie Bank B.V., 1950. 4pp.

SSSA, for women's voices. Latin text, from Psalm 117.

D0167 Bank, J.A., ed. *Dies sanctificatus.* Amsterdam: Annie Bank B.V., 1950. K015. 2pp.

SATB, mixed voices, Latin text.

D0168 Bank, J.A., ed. *Missa Brevis.* Amsterdam: Annie Bank B.V., 1951. JP14. 20pp.

SATB, mixed voices. Latin text.

D0169 Bank, J.A., ed. *Missa Sine nomine (Mantuana).* Amsterdam: Annie Bank, B.V., n.d. [ca.1950]. JP9. 23pp.

TTBB, men's voices. Latin text.

D0170 Bank, J.A., ed. *O admirabile commercium.* Amsterdam: Annie Bank B.V., 1950. K047. 2pp.
SATTB, mixed voices. Latin text.

D0171 Bank, J.A., ed. *Popule meus.* Amsterdam: Annie Bank B.V., n.d. [ca.1950]. GW90. 2pp.
TTBB, men's voices. Latin text.

D0172 Bank, J.A., ed. *Surrexit pastor bonus.* Amsterdam: Annie Bank B.V., n.d. P27. 2pp.
TTBB, men's voices. Latin text.

D0173 Bank, J.A., ed. *Tantum ergo.* Amsterdam: Annie Bank B.V., 1950. A015. 4pp.
TTBBB, men's voices. Latin text.

D0174 Barclay Squire, William, ed. *Stabat Mater. Motet for Double Chorus (Unaccompanied) Composed by G. Pierluigi da Palestrina.* Novello's original octave edition. London: Novello & Company, Ltd., 1898.
SATB SATB, piano accompaniment for rehearsal only, Latin text underlaid. Prefatory notes by William Barclay Squire.

D0175 Barclay Squire, William, ed. *Miserere mei Deus. Have Mercy upon Me, O God. Penitential Psalm for Two Choirs, Nine Voices. Unaccompanied.* Novello's Collection of Anthems 811. London: Novello, 1905 [Original edition ca. 1876].
Barclay Squire's adaptation using the words of the English *Book of Common Prayer.*

D0176 Barnes, R., ed. *O magnum mysterium.* London: Cathedral Music, 1978. 6pp. M2092.P25.O2.1978.
SSAATB, *a cappella.* Facsimile reproduction of transcriber's manuscript.

———. Bäuerle, Hermann, ed. *Pierluigi da Palestrina.* Leipzig: Breitkopf und Härtel, 1904. 8 vols.
These items were issued separately, in small groups and in volumes. For comprehensive listing of contents, see item D0009.

D0177 Bennett, G. J., *By the Waters of Babylon.* [*Super flumina Babylonis*]. Novello's Octavo Anthems no.1074. London: Novello, 1920.

D0178 Benson, L., ed. *I vaghi fiori. When Flow'ry Meadows. Madrigal.* Oriana series no.44. London: Novello, 1905.

D0179 Benson, L., ed. *Quando del terzo cielo. When from the Realm Supernal.* Oriana series no.42. London: Novello, 1905.
Edition of madrigal from *Il trionfo di Dori* [Venice, 1592], English translation of text by W. G. Rothery.

D0180 Benson, L., ed. *Se di pianti e di stridi. If in Lovers' Lamenting.* Oriana series no.51. London: Novello, 1905.

Edition of madrigal from *Il quatro libro delle muse* [Venice, 1574], English text by A. C. Curtis.

D0181 Bevan, Gwilym, ed. *Children of the Hebrews.* Waterloo, ON: Waterloo Music Co. Ltd., n.d.

SATB, arrangement of *Pueri Hebraeorum*, graded as "medium easy."

D0182 Boepple, Paul, ed. *Assumpta est Maria. Motet for Six Mixed Voices, or Three Women's Voices with Strings or Three Men's Voices with Strings.* Dessoff Choir Series 1. New York: Music Press, 1941. 18pp. M1495.D43. no.1.

Latin text underlay, also printed as text with English translation preceding score.

D0183 Boepple, Paul, ed. *Magnificat in the Fourth Mode. For Women's Voices a cappella SSAA. Palestrina.* Dessoff Choir Series 12. New York: Music Press, 1941. 16pp. M1495.D43. no.12.

SSAA, Latin text underlay, also printed as text with English translation preceding score.

———. Bordes, Charles, ed. *Anthologie des maîtres religieux primitifs des quinzième, seizième et dix-septième siècles.* Paris: Durand et Fils, 1893. 6 vols. Reprint New York: Da Capo, 1981.

These items were issued both in a series of six volumes, and separately, as a series entitled *Anthologie des maîtres religieux ancients pour chant et orgue, ser. 1. Répetoire des chanteurs de Saint-Gervais.* Edition populaire. Paris: Bureau d'Edition de la Schola Cantorum, ca. 1893–1912.

Each motet was published with a vocal reduction for keyboard (organ), and was extensively edited. See item D0014 for a comprehensive listing of contents.

D0184 Braune, O., ed. *Missa Assumpta est Maria in coelum für sechs Singstimmen.* Leipzig: Breitkopf und Härtel, ca.1865.

Score with piano arrangement.

D0185 de Brant, Cyr [pseudonym for Vincent Higginson], ed. *Missa Aeterna Christi munera. Giovanni Pierluigi da Palestrina.* Church Music of the XVIth and XVIIth Centuries for Unaccompanied Voices no.8127. New York: J. Fischer & Bro., 1945. 1 plate, 38pp. M2011.P25.A3.

SATB and SATB with piano reduction. Reproduced from manuscript copy.

D0186 Bridge, Sir Frank, ed. *This Is the Day. Motets by Palestrina and His School 4.* London: Bosworth and Company, 1907.

SATB arrangement of motet *Haec dies*, with texts translated from the Latin to English and adapted by the Rev. H.C. Daniell-Bainbridge. Music has English underlay only, with organ part for practice only.

D0187 Bridge, Sir Frank, ed. *With Other Tongues Spake the Apostles. Motets by Palestrina and His School* 7. London: Bosworth and Company, 1907.

SATB, arrangement of motet *Loquebantur in variis linguis*, with texts translated from the Latin to English and adapted by the Rev. H.C. Daniell-Bainbridge. Music has English underlay only, with organ part for practice only; note values halved, 3 flats in signature.

D0188 Bridge, Sir Frank, ed. *Thou Art Peter. Motets by Palestrina and His School* 8. London: Bosworth and Company, 1907.

SSATTB, arrangement of *Tu es Petrus* [prima pars only], with texts translated from the Latin to English and adapted by the Rev. H.C. Daniell-Bainbridge. Music has English underlay only; SATB, with organ part for practice only; note values halved; 2 flats in signature.

D0189 Budd, G.W., ed. *False Love, Now Shoot, and Spare Not. Madrigals for Four Voices . . . scored from the original Part Books, published by N. Yonge in 1588, by G.W. Budd.* London: Calkin & Budd, ca. 1843; reissued London: Addison, Hollier & Lucas, 1859.

Edition of the madrigal *Amor ben puoi* as it was published with an English text as no.4 in *Musica Transalpina* of 1588.

D0190 Budd, G.W., ed. *Love So Doth Fill My Heart. Madrigal for Four Voices . . . scored from the original Part Books, published by N. Yonge in 1588, by G.W. Budd.* London: Calkin & Budd, ca. 1843; reissued London: Addison, Hollier & Lucas, 1859.

Edition of the madrigal *Gioia m'abond'al cor* as it was published with an English text as no.3 in *Musica Transalpina* in 1588.

D0191 Button, H.E., ed. *Exaltabo te, Domine*. Novello's Octavo Anthems no.1135. London: Novello, 1924.

Edition based on manuscript London, British Library Add.31398.

D0192 Buxton, Ralph W., ed. *O bone Jesu.* New York: NDC Editions Inc./C.F. Peters, 1999. N10. 6pp.

SSATTB, mixed voices, ranked as of 'medium difficulty' in performance. Latin text.

D0193 Buxton, Ralph W., ed. *Peccantem me quotidie.* New York: NDC Editions Inc./C.F. Peters, 1999. N11. 7pp.

SATTB, mixed voices. Latin text.

D0194 Caillard, Marie-France, ed. *Adoramus te.* Fontenay [France]: Philippe Caillard, 1993. PC298. 2pp.

SATB, mixed voices. Latin text.

D0195 Caillard, Philippe, ed. *O Domine Jesu Christe.* Fontenay [France]: Philippe Caillard, 1994. PC0289. 2pp.

SATB, mixed voices. Latin text.

D0196 Caillard, Philippe, ed. *Pars mea/Bonus est Dominus.* Fontenay [France]: Philippe Caillard, 1995. X0069. 4pp.
SAB, mixed voices. Latin text.

D0197 Caillard, Philippe, ed. *Salve Regina.* "Répertoire de l'Ensemble Vocal Philippe Caillard." Fontenay [France]: Philippe Caillard, n.d. R42. 8pp.
SATB + SATB, mixed voices. Latin text.

D0198 Caillard, Philippe, ed. *Surge, illuminare Jerusalem.* "Répertoire de l'Ensemble Vocal Philippe Caillard." Fontenay [France]: Philippe Caillard, n.d. R41; PC0441. 8pp.
SATB + SATB, mixed voices. Latin text.

D0199 Cain, Noble, ed. *Dies sanctificatus.* New York: Boosey & Hawkes, 1948. 9pp.
SATB.

D0200 Cain, Noble, ed. *Loquebantur variis linguis.* New York: Harold Flammer, 1945. 12pp.
SATB arrangement *a cappella.*

D0201 Cain, Noble, ed. *Salvator mundi.* New York: Boosey & Hawkes, 1948. 10pp.

D0202 Cain, Noble, ed. *Surrexit pastor bonus.* New York: Boosey & Hawkes, 1955. 8pp.
SATB, *a cappella.* Latin text, with English text adapted by Noble Cain.

D0203 Cecil, Leonard, ed. *Giovanni Palestrina 1525–1594. Deh! Fuss'or qui madonna.* Cologne: Haas-Verlag, 1995. HM 294–9.
Transcription by Cecil of this madrigal for an ensemble of four brass instruments.

D0204 Clough-Leighter, H., ed. *Alla riva del Tebro. On the Banks of the Tebro.* Boston: Boston Music. 1911.
SATB, with English text by N. H. Dole.

D0205 Clough-Leighter, H., ed. *Ogni beltà, madonna. All Other Beauty, Lady.* Boston: Boston Music. 1911.
SATB, with English text by N.H. Dole.

D0206 Coates, Henry, ed. *Ah, Look upon These Eyes. Canzonet for Female Voices.* Novello's Octave Edition of Trios, etc., for Female Voices no.575. London: Novello, 1939.
Adaptation of Ahi*, che quest'occhi* for three female voices, with music and English text by Henry Coates.

D0207 Coates, Henry, ed. *Joy in My Heart Doth Dwell.* The Oriana no.109. London: Novello, 1938.

Edition of madrigal *Gioia m'abond'al cor*, with musical edition and English text by Coates.

D0208 Coates, Henry, ed. *My Heart with Grief Did Fill.* [*The Musical Times* no.1164.] London: Novello, 1940.
SATB, madrigal *Morì quasi il mio core* [Book II], with musical edition and English text by Coates.

D0209 Coates, Henry, ed. *O Radiant Glory.* Oriana series no.108. London: Novello, 1938.
SATB, madrigal *O che splendor* [Book II], with musical edition and English text by Coates.

D0210 Coates, Henry, ed. *Tell Me, What Master Hand. Canzonet for Female Voices.* Novello's Octave Edition of Trios, etc., for Female Voices no.576. London: Novello, 1939.
Adaptation of *Da così dotta man*, with musical edition and English text both by Henry Coates.

D0211 Collins, H.E., ed. *Alma redemptoris mater.* Latin Church Music of the Polyphonic Schools no.16. London: J & W Chester, 1931.
SATB, motet with Latin text underlay. English translation provided at head of music, a piano reduction for rehearsal only.

D0212 Collins, H.E., ed. *Creator alme siderum. Vesper Hymn for Advent.* London: editor, 1921.
Lithograph edition in score.

D0213 Collins, H.E., ed. *Crucem sanctam subiit. Motet for Five Voices.* London: editor, 1916.
Lithograph edition in score. Another edition of this work by Collins published in 1931 as no.22 in series Latin Church Music of the Polyphonic Schools, q.v.

D0214 Collins, H.E., ed. *Crucem sanctam subiit.* Latin Church Music of the Polyphonic Schools no.22. London: J & W Chester, 1931.
SSATB, *a cappella.* Latin text underlay. English translation provided at head of music.

D0215 Collins, H.E., ed. *De profundis a 5.* Latin Church Music of the Polyphonic Schools 36. London: J & W Chester, 1936.
SATTB, *a cappella.* Latin text underlay, with English translation provided at head of music.

D0216 Collins, H.E., ed. *Domine, quando veneris judicare terram, ubi me abscondam?* London: editor, 1918.
SATB, lithograph edition in score.

D0217 Collins, H.E., ed. *Dum complerentur dies Pentecostes. Motet for Six Voices.* London: Dinham Blyth & Co., 1916.
Lithograph edition in score. Another edition of this work by Collins published in 1934 as no.28 in series *Latin Music of the Polyphonic Schools,* q.v.

D0218 Collins, H.E., ed. *Dum complerentur a 6.* Latin Church Music of the Polyphonic Schools no.28. London: J & W Chester, 1934.
SAATTB, *a cappella.* Latin text underlay, with English translations provided at head of music.

D0219 Collins, H.E., ed. *Exaltabo te a 5.* Latin Church Music of the Polyphonic Schools 38. London: J & W Chester, 1937.
SATTB, *a cappella.* Latin text underlay, with English translations provided at head of music.

D0220 Collins, H.E., ed. *Exultate Deo. Sing with Joy and Gladness.* Ridley's New Series Classical Church Music no.3. London: A. W. Ridley, 1936.
SAATB, with English translation by W.A. Pickard-Cambridge.

D0221 Collins, H.E., ed. *The First Lamentations of the Matins of Good Friday.* London: editor, 1919.
Lithograph edition in score of *Lamentationes* [based on MS sources, later printed edition in Cas.XIII].

D0222 Collins, H.E., ed. *Peccantem me quotidie. Motet for Five Voices.* London: Dinham Blyth & Co., 1916.
SATTB, lithograph edition in score. Another edition of this work by Collins in the Ridley series.

D0223 Collins, H.E., ed. *Peccantem me quotidie. My Sins Are with Me Ev'ry Day.* Ridley's New Series Classical Church Music no.2. London: A. W. Ridley, 1936.
SATTB, with English translation by W.A. Pickard-Cambridge.

D0224 Collins, H.E., ed. *Popule meus, quid feci tibi? The Improperia for the Morning Office of Good Friday.* London: editor, 1918.
Lithograph edition in score.

D0225 Collins, H.E., ed. *Quae est ista.* Latin Church Music of the Polyphonic Schools no.23. London: J & W Chester, 1931.
SSATB, *a cappella.* Latin text underlay. English translation provided at head of music.

D0226 Collins, H.E., ed. *Quae est ista, quae progreditur.* London: Dinham Blyth & Co., 1915.
Lithograph edition in score. Another edition of this work by Collins published in 1931 as no.23 in series *Latin Church Music of the Polyphonic Schools,* q.v.

D0227 Collins, H.E., ed. *Rorate coeli desuper. Motet.* . . . London: Dinham Blyth & Co., 1915.
Lithograph edition in score. Another edition of work published in 1930.

D0228 Collins, H.E., ed. *Rorate coeli desuper.* Latin Church Music of the Polyphonic Schools 19. London: J & W Chester, 1930.
SSATB *a cappella*, motet [secunda pars of *Canite tuba*, not included here] with Latin text underlay. English translations of text provided at the head of the music.

D0229 Collins, H.E., ed. *Salve Regina.* London: editor, 1917.
SATB SATB, lithograph edition in score.

D0230 Collins, H.E., ed. *Salve Regina a 8.* Latin Church Music of the Polyphonic Schools 26. London: J & W Chester, 1933.
SATB SATB, *a cappella*, Latin text underlay.

D0231 Collins, H.E., ed. *Surge, illuminare a 8.* Latin Church Music of the Polyphonic Schools 40. London: J & W Chester, 1938.
SATB SATB, *a cappella*. Latin text underlay, with English translation at head of music.

D0232 Collins, H.E., ed. *Tu es Petrus. Motet for Six Voices.* London: editor, 1916.
Lithograph edition in score.

D0233 Collins, H.E., ed. *Tu es Petrus. Motet for Six Voices.* Polyphonic Motets no.68. London: Cary & Co., 1932.

D0234 Damrosch, Frank, ed. *Hodie Christus natus est. Now, Today, Christ the Lord Is Born.* New York: G. Schirmer, 1969. 15pp.
SATB SATB, double choir. Text with English translation by George Mead. A reworked version of an edition by Damrosch issued by Schirmer in 1899.

D0235 Damrosch, Frank, ed. *Missa brevis, for Soprano, Alto, Tenor and Bass, a capella/Giovanni Pierluigi da Palestrina.* G. Schirmer's collection of masses and vespers. New York: G. Schirmer, 1899.
SATB, piano accompaniment for rehearsal, heavily edited.

D0236 Damrosch, Frank, ed. *Pater Noster.* New York: G. Schirmer, 1903.
SSATB, motet.

D0237 Damrosch, Frank, ed. *Populе meus. For Double Chorus. Antiphonal.* New York: G. Schirmer, 1899.
SATB SATB.

D0238 Damrosch, Frank, ed. *Stabat Mater. Motet for Twelve Voice-Parts. Palestrina.* Musical Art Society of New York series 66. New York: G. Schirmer;

Boston: Boston Music Co., c. 1909.
SATB SATB SATB, piano accompaniment for rehearsal only.

D0239 Darvas, Gabor, ed. *Missa L'homme armé for Mixed Choir (S, A, TI, TII, B) a cappella.* Budapest: Editio Musica Budapest, c. 1975. Z6441. 59pp.
SATTB. In series *Missae super L'homme armé.* Preface and notes in English and Hungarian. Editorial notes, p.60.

D0240 Darvas, Gabor, ed. *Missa Lauda Sion.* Budapest: Editio Musica Budapest, n.d. [1970s]. 213192(2). 23pp.
SATB, mixed voices. Latin text.

D0241 Davison, Nigel, ed. *Assumpta est Maria. Motet for Six Voices.* London: J & W. Chester, 1971. 8881. iii + 21pp.
SSATTB with prefatory notes.

D0242 Deis, Carl, ed. *Missa Papae Marcelli for Chorus of Mixed Voices a cappella.* English adaptation by Willis Wager. New York: G. Schirmer, 1941. Ed. 1733.
SATTBB; note values halved; piano part for rehearsal; English text underlaid with Latin; heavily edited.

D0243 Deis, Carl, ed. *O bone Jesu. O Blessed Jesus. For Four-Part Chorus of Mixed Voices.* New York: G. Schirmer, 1952. 3pp.
SATB; note values halved; piano part for rehearsal. English text underlaid with Latin. Heavily edited.

D0244 Dixon, Jon, ed. *Confitebor tibi Domine.* Carshalton Beeches, Surrey: JOED Music, c. 1994. 20pp. M2092.P25M52 1994.
SATB SATB *a cappella.* Latin text, with English translation printed in captions.

D0245 Dixon, Jon, ed. *Haec dies.* Carshalton Beeches, Surrey: JOED Music, c. 1995. 6pp. M2092.P25M54 1995.
SSATTB *a cappella.* Latin text, with English translation printed in caption. Transposed into modern clefs at a pitch suitable for SATB choirs. Edited from the first edition.

D0246 Dixon, Jon, ed. *Hodie Christus natus est.* Renaissance polyphonic choral music. JOED P3. Surrey: JOED Music, 1993.
SSAB ATTB. Score based on a reworking of the Haberl edition of 1890. English preface, p.2. Note values halved; transposed down 1 tone.

D0247 Dixon, Jon, ed. *O Domine Jesu Christe.* Renaissance polyphonic choral music JOED P43. Carshalton Beaches, Surrey: JOED Music, 1994. 8pp. M2092.P25O15 1994.
SATB SATB, *a cappella*, score based on a reworking of the Haberl edition, with note values halved; transposed into modern clefs; Latin text, with English translation at head of music.

D0248 Dixon, Jon, ed. *O gloriosa Domina.* Carshalton Beeches, Surrey: JOED Music ca. 1993. 12pp. M2092.P25O16 1993.

SATB SATB SATB, *a cappella.* Latin text, with English translation printed in caption. Transposed into modern clefs at a tone down from the original pitch. Edited from the Haberl edition.

D0249 Dixon, Jon, ed. *Sicut cervus.* Carshalton Beeches, Surrey: JOED Music, 1994. 8pp. M2092.P25M57 1994.

SATB, *a cappella.* Latin text, with English translation printed in caption. Transposed into modern clefs at a pitch suitable for SATB choirs. Edited from the Venice editions of 1598 and 1604.

D0250 Dixon, Jon, ed. *Stabat Mater Dolorosa.* Carshalton Beeches, Surrey: JOED Music, 1995. 21pp. M2099.L82P3 1995

SATB SATB, *a cappella.* Latin text, with English translation printed in caption. Transposed into modern clefs at a pitch suitable for SATB choirs. Edited principally from the Haberl edition.

D0251 Dower, Catherine, ed. *Regina coeli.* New York: Broude Brothers, n.d. AB721. 11pp.

SATB, mixed voices. Latin text.

D0252 Druffel, Peter, ed. *Soave fia il morir. O Gentle Death. Madrigal for Five Voice-Parts a cappella.* New York: G. Schirmer, 1911.

SAATB, with English text version by Frank Damrosch. Probably based on Druffel's Breitkopf edition of 1887.

D0253 Dunkley, Sally, ed. *Giovanni Pierluigi da Palestrina (1525–1594). Missa Aeterna Christi Munera.* Ilkley, UK: PCA/Pro Cantione Antiqua Ltd., 1991.

SATB; note values halved; Latin text underlay only.

D0254 Dunkley, Sally, ed. *Giovanni Pierluigi da Palestrina (1525–1594). Missa Assumpta est Maria.* Ilkley, UK: PCA/Pro Cantione Antiqua Ltd., 1992.

SSATTB; note values halved; transposed down a fourth; Latin text underlay only.

D0255 Dunkley, Sally, ed. *Giovanni Pierluigi da Palestrina. Missa Brevis.* Ilkley, UK: PCA/Pro Cantione Antiqua Ltd., 1992.

SATB; note values halved; Latin text underlay only.

D0256 Ewerhart, Rudolf, ed. *Aeterna Christi Munera. Missa for Four-Part Chorus of Mixed Voices a cappella.* Wiesbaden: Breitkopf & Härtel; New York: Associated Music Publishers, 1959.

SATB; note values halved; *Mensurstrich.*

D0257 Ewerhart, Rudolf, ed. *Assumpta est Maria. Missa for Six-Part Chorus of Mixed Voices a cappella.* Wiesbaden: Breitkopf & Härtel; New York: Associated Music Publishers, 1959.

SSATTB; note values halved; transposed down major 2nd; *Mensurstrich*. Based on manuscript in the Vatican Library, Cappella Sistina MS 76.

D0258 Ewerhart, Rudolf, ed. *Assumpta est Maria. Motet for Six-Part Chorus of Mixed Voices a cappella.* Wiesbaden: Breitkopf & Härtel; New York: Associated Music Publishers, 1963.

SSATTB; note values halved; transposed down 2nd; *Mensurstrich.* Based on manuscript in the Vatican Library, Cappella Sistina MS 76.

D0259 Ewerhart, Rudolf, ed. *Ave, mundi spes, Maria. Motette für acht Stimmen.* Wiesbaden: Breitkopf & Härtel, 1993. 12pp.

SATB SATB *a cappella.*

D0260 Ewerhart, Rudolf, ed. *Confirma hoc. Motet for Six-Part Chorus of Mixed Voices a cappella.* Breitkopf & Härtel Chor-Bibliothek 3508. Wiesbaden: Breitkopf & Härtel, 1960.

SATTB; note values halved; *Mensurstrich.*

D0261 Ewerhart, Rudolf, ed. *Dies sanctificatus. Missa for Four-Part Chorus of Mixed Voices a cappella.* Wiesbaden: Breitkopf & Härtel; New York: Associated Music Publishers, 1960.

SATB; note values halved; transposed down major 2nd; *Mensurstrich.* Based on Book VI of masses [Rome, 1594].

D0262 Ewerhart, Rudolf, ed. *Dies sanctificatus. Motet for Four-Part Chorus of Mixed Voices a cappella.*

Wiesbaden: Breitkopf & Härtel; New York: Associated Music Publishers, 1961.

SATB; note values halved; transposed down major 2nd; *Mensurstrich.* Edition based on the 1590 reprint of the edition of 1563.

D0263 Ewerhart, Rudolf, ed. *Ecce ego Joannes. Missa for Six-Part Chorus of Mixed Voices a cappella.*

Wiesbaden: Breitkopf & Härtel; New York: Associated Music Publishers, 1960.

SATTBarB; note values halved; *Mensurstrich.*

D0264 Ewerhart, Rudolf, ed. *Hodie Christ natus est. Motet for Eight-Part Chorus of Mixed Voices a cappella.* Wiesbaden: Breitkopf & Härtel; New York: Associated Music Publishers, 1958.

SSAB ATTB; note values halved; transposed down down major 2nd; *Mensurstrich.* Foreword, with English translation of text. Edition based on version in Book III of motets [Rome, 1575].

D0265 Ewerhart, Rudolf, ed. *Iste Confessor. Missa for Four-Part Chorus of Mixed Voices a cappella.* Wiesbaden: Breitkopf & Härtel; New York: Associated Music Publishers, 1961.

SATB; note values halved; transposed up major 2nd; *Mensurstrich.* Based on Rome, 1590 edition.

D0266 Ewerhart, Rudolf, ed. *Lauda Sion. Missa for Four-Part Chorus of Mixed Voices a cappella.* Wiesbaden: Breitkopf & Härtel; New York: Associated Music Publishers, 1959.

SATB; note values halved (quartered in triple sections); transposed up minor 3rd; *Mensurstrich.* Based on on Venice, 1582 edition.

D0267 Ewerhart, Rudolf, ed. *Lauda Sion Salvatorem. Motet for Four-Part Chorus of Mixed Voices a cappella.* Wiesbaden: Breitkopf & Härtel; New York: Associated Music Publishers, 1961. A-539-4.

SATB; note values halved (in triple sections they are quartered); transposed up minor 3rd; *Mensurstrich.* Based on Venice, 1564 edition.

D0268 Ewerhart, Rudolf, ed. *O magnum mysterium. Motet for Six-Part Chorus of Mixed Voices a cappella.* Wiesbaden: Breitkopf & Härtel; New York: Associated Music Publishers, 1958.

SSAATB; note values halved; transposed up minor 3rd; *Mensurstrich.* Foreword, with text translation into English. Based on Rome, 1569 print.

D0269 Ewerhart, Rudolf, ed. *Pater noster. Missa for Four-Part Chorus of Mixed Voices a cappella.* Wiesbaden: Breitkopf & Härtel; New York: Associated Music Publishers, 1962.

SATB; note values halved; transposed down major 2nd; *Mensurstrich.* Based on the manuscript Biblioteca Apostolica Vaticana, Cappella Sistina 68 and Haberl's version in the comprehensive edition.

D0270 Ewerhart, Rudolf, ed. *Stabat Mater Dolorosa.* Breitkopf & Härtel Chor-Bibliothek 3146. Wiesbaden: Breitkopf & Härtel, ca.1957.

SATB SATB; note values halved; *Mensurstrich.*

D0271 Ewerhart, Rudolf, ed. *Tu es Petrus. Missa for Six-Part Chorus of Mixed Voices a cappella.* Wiesbaden: Breitkopf & Härtel; New York: Associated Music Publishers, 1959. A-535.

SSATBarB; note values halved; transposed down major 2nd. *Mensurstrich.* Based on I-Rvat Ottob. 2927/Haberl edition. This is the mass published in 1572, not the one in Book XII (1601).

D0272 Ewerhart, Rudolf, ed. *Tu es Petrus. Motet for Six-Part Chorus of Mixed Voices a cappella.* Wiesbaden: Breitkopf & Härtel; New York: Associated Music Publishers, 1959.

SSATBarB; note values halved; transposed down major 2nd; *Mensurstrich.* Edition based on the print in the second book of motets (Rome, 1572). Foreword, with English text translation.

D0273 Expert, Henry, ed. *Tantum ergo sacramentum.* "Répertoire des Maîtres Musiciens de la Renaissance Française: Collection Henry Expert." Paris: Salabert, n.d. 3pp.

SATB, mixed voices. Latin text.

D0274 Fellerer, Karl Gustav, ed. *Dies sanctificatus.* Münster: Gregorius Musikverlag, 1970. W36. 4pp.
SATB, mixed voices. Latin text.

D0275 Ferrenberg, J. G., ed. *Messe für die Verstorbenen, (Missa Requiem) nebst dem Responsorium Libera me, in der heutigen Schreibweise herausgegeben.* . . . Cologne and Bonn, 1853.
Edition of *Missa pro defunctis a 5* from the enlarged edition of *Missarum liber primus* [1591].

D0276 Fink, Hans, ed. *Missa "Qual è il più grande amor," für fünfstimmigen gemischten Chor a cappella.* Wien: Verlag Ludwig Doblinger, 1954.
SSATB, unaccompanied, transposed up a minor third. Critical report by Hans Fink. 36pp.

D0277 Fissinger, Edwin, ed. *O beata et gloriosa Trinitas.* New Berlin, WI: Jenson Publications, n.d.
Motet SSATB, a cappella.

D0278 Galloway, G., ed. *Creator Blest of Every Star.* Novello's Short Anthems no.272. London: Novello, 1936.
SATB, English paraphrase of hymn *Creator alme siderum* [Hab.XXXI.123], translation of original Latin text by H. E. Crewdson.

D0279 Galloway, G., ed. *O Blessed Jesu.* Novello's Short Anthems no.273. London: Novello, 1936.
SATB, a cappella, motet *O bone Jesu*, with English text version by Galloway.

D0280 Galloway, G. ed. *O Praise the Lord. Motet for Double Choir* [*Laudate Dominum omnes gentes*]. Novello's Octavo Anthems no.1207. London: Novello, 1936.

D0281 Goldschmidt, Otto, ed. *Missa Papae Marcelli (Six Parts).* Novello's original octavo edition. London: Novello, 1881. 52pp.
SSA(A&T)BB, introduction (pp.i–iv) by Otto Goldschmidt dated 1880.

D0282 Gray, Robert, ed. *Now Do We Behold Him* [*Ecce vidimus eum*: attributed to Palestrina; *recte* by Marc'Antonio Ingegneri]. Robert Gray Classic Choral Series. Ft. Lauderdale, FL: Tetra/Continuo Music Group, 1991. 8pp.
SATB *a cappella.* English and Latin texts; English-language arrangement by Robert Gray.

D0283 Gray, Robert, ed. *O Blessed Jesus* [*O bone Jesu*]. Robert Gray Classic Choral Series. Ft. Lauderdale, FL: Tetra/Continuo Music Group, 1991. 4pp.
SATB *a cappella.* English and Latin texts; English-language arrangement by Robert Gray.

D0284 Gregory, Eleanor C., ed. *O Holy and Glorious Trinity.* Church Music Society Reprint no.30. London: Oxford, 1955. 16pp.
SSATB, English and Latin text.

D0285 Gregory, Eleanor C., ed. *Veni Creator.* London: Oxford, 1936.
ATB, hymn based on tenth-century Latin text with English text by "Y. H."

D0286 Grote, Gottfried, ed. *Christe redemptor omnium.* Kassel: Merseburger Verlag, 1986. EM321A. 4pp.
SATB, mixed voices. Latin text with German adaptation by the editor.

D0287 Haberl, Franz Xaver, ed. *Masses, Book 6. Missa Dies sanctificatus.* Breitkopf & Härtel Partitur-Bibliothek 2786. Leipzig: Breitkopf & Härtel, 1957.
SSAAT [soloists] and SATB [chorus].

D0288 Haberl, Franz Xaver, ed. *Repertorium musicae sacrae ex auctoribus saeculi XVI. et XVII. Collectum et redactum a Franc. Xav. Haberl. Missa "O admirabile commercium" quinque vocum.* Supplement to *Kirchenmusikalisches Jahrbuch* 9 [*Cäcilienkalendar* 19] (1894): 3–44. Regensburg: Friedrich Pustet, 1896.
Edition of *Missa O admirabile commercium.* Michael Haller wrote an analysis of this mass on pages 69–76 of the same volume. Numeration separate from the volume of the journal proper, which begins again after page 44, with page 1, and was made for separate publication. This edition was evidently published in connection with the 1894 tercentenary commemorations. Original note values and cleffings observed.

D0289 Haller, Michael., ed. *Missa Brevis für Sopran, Alt, Tenor und Bass.* Regensburg: Alfred Coppenrath, 1904.
Two-staff arrangement of voices, modern clefs, extensively edited; *Benedictus* and *Agnus Dei I* are shortened.

D0290 Hanson, Howard, ed. *Missa Papae Marcelli.* New York: J. Fischer & Bro., 1937.
Vocal score arrangement of a transcription of the mass for SSATBB and orchestra.

D0291 Hasberry, Robert L., ed. *Jesu, flos matris.* Polyphonic Motets no.18. London L.J. Cary, 1960.
SATB.

D0292 Hasberry, Robert L., ed. *Pange lingua gloriosi.* Polyphonic Motets no.13. London: L. J. Cary, 1960. 3pp.
SATB, alternating verses of the plainchant hymn with Palestrina's polyphonic verses.

D0293 Hellmann, Diethard, ed. *Missa Brevis, für Chor SSATTB, zwei Trompeten*

[Cornetti], 4 Posaunen und Basso Continuo. Stuttgarter Bach-Ausgaben. Series C, Supplement, Von Johann Sebastian Bach Bearbeitete Werke. Neuhausen-Stuttgart: Hänssler Verlag, 1988 [Edition no. 35.301/01].

An edition of the *Kyrie* and *Gloria* sections of Palestrina's *Missa sine nomine a 6* (Masses, Book 5) in an arrangement made by J. S. Bach for choir, with two trumpets and four trombones colla parte and organ basso continuo, included here for its special historical interest. Prefaces in English and German; critical report; figured bass realization.

D0294 Hellmann, Diethard, ed. *Veni Creator Spiritus.* Die Motette no.96. Stuttgart: Hänssler, [1980s].

SAATB, *a cappella*; original note values, with Latin and German text underlay.

D0295 Henson, B. R., ed. *Super flumina Babylonis. Psalm 137.* Greystone Press Choral Series. Ft. Lauderdale, FL: Greystone Press, ca. 1986. 11pp.

SATB, *a cappella.*

D0296 Herrmann, William, ed. *Sanctus.* New York: G. Schirmer, 1968.

SSAA arrangement of *Sanctus* from the *Missa Aeterna Christi munera* for women's voices.

D0297 Hopkins, Bernard, ed. *Missa Papae Marcelli. Agnus Dei.* Berkeley, CA: Musica Sacra et Profana, n.d.

SATTBB, optional instrumental accompaniment, graded at medium difficulty.

D0298 Hopkins, Bernard, ed. *Missa Ut re mi. Agnus Dei.* Berkeley, CA: Musica Sacra et Profana, n.d.

Seven-part chorus, optional instrumental accompaniment, graded as easy to perform.

D0299 Hübsch, Hanns, ed. *Hodie Christus natus est.* Heidelberg: Süddeutscher Musikverlag Willy Müller, n.d. SM1961–04.

TTBB arrangement, men's voices. Latin text.

———. Hübsch, Hanns, ed. *Das Hohe Lied Salomonis.* Heidelberg: Willy Müller/Süddeutscher Musikverlag [1960s].

These items, issued separately, are all printed *a cappella*, and are graded as of medium difficulty in performance. The series is an incomplete collection of motets from *Canticum canticorum.* Latin text, some with German translations.

D0300 SM0750/01 *Osculetur me* (SATTB).
D0301 SM0750/02 *Trahe me post te* (SATTB).
D0302 SM0750/03 *Nigra sum, sed formosa* (SATTB).
D0303 SM0750/04 *Vineam meam* (SATTB).
D0304 SM0750/05 *Si ignoras te* (SATTB).

D0305 SM0750/06 *Pulchrae sunt genuae tuae* (SATTB).
D0306 SM0750/07 *Fasciculus myrrhae* (SATTB).
D0307 SM0750/08 *Ecce tu pulcher es* (SATTB).
D0308 SM0750/09 *Tota pulchra es* (SATTB).
D0309 SM0750/10 *Vulnerasti cor meum* (SATTB)
D0310 SM0750/11 *Sicut lilium* (SATTB).
D0311 SM0750/12 *Introduxit me rex* (SATTB).
D0312 SM0750/13 *Laeva ejus* (SATTB).
D0313 SM0750/14 *Vox dilecti mei* (SATTB).
D0314 SM0750/15 *Surge propera* (SATTB).
D0315 SM0750/16 *Surge, amica mea* (SATTB).
D0316 SM0750/17 *Dilectus meus mihi* (SATTB).
D0317 SM0750/18 *Surgam et circuibo* (SATTB).
D0318 SM0750/19 *Adjuro vos* (SATTB).
D0319 SM0750/20 *Caput ejus* (SATTB).
D0320 SM0750/21 *Dilectus meus descendit* (SATTB).
D0321 SM0750/22 *Pulchra es* (SATTB).
D0322 SM0750/23 *Quae est ista* (SATTB).

D0323 Jancsovics, Antal. *Canticum canticorum: 29 motetta.* Musicotheca classica 5. Budapest: Editio Musica, 1976.

This edition, which was issued as a single volume (119 pp.), was also issued as individual numbers, series 312–42000–312–42028. See itemization in item D0059.

D0324 Jarczyk, Michael. *Coenantibus illis. Motette für fünf Stimmen a cappella.* Berlin: Musikverlag Ferraresi, 1980.

Contains preface in German and English; 1 page of fascimile manuscript reproduction. SATTB (CATQB), pp.3–8, unaccompanied.

D0325 Kelley, K.G., ed. *Father Almighty, We Thy Children Pray.* Boston: Boston Music, 1935.

SATB, *a cappella*, adapted from *Credo* of the *Missa Brevis*, with English text by K.G. Kelley.

D0326 Kingsbury, John, ed. *O Have Mercy on Us (Miserere Nostri, Domine)*. Bryn Mawr: Theodore Presser Company, 1968; 1980. 312–41340.

SSATB, *a cappella*, with piano part for rehearsal only; Latin and English text both underlaid in score; note values halved.

D0327 Klein, Maynard, ed. *Alma Redemptoris Mater. Loving Mother of Our Saviour.* New York: G. Schirmer, 1974. 7pp.

SATB, *a cappella.* Latin text with English version by Maynard Klein.

D0328 Kraft, Leo, ed. *Benedictus. For Three Voices.* New York: Mercury Music, 1960. 5pp.

SSA or TTB *a cappella*, from *Missa Repleatur os meum laude* [Book III].

D0329 Kraft, Leo, ed. *Dies sanctificatus.* New York: Mercury Music, 1959. 10pp.
SATB *a cappella.*

D0340 Kraus, Egon, ed. *Alla riva del Tebro. On the bank of the Tiber.* Zürich: Pelikan, 1955. Ed 2061. 4pp.
SATB, mixed voices. Text adapted by Alicia Adler Smith.

D0341 Kreckel, Philip G., ed. *O bone Jesu.* New York: J. Fischer & Bro., 1952. 3pp.
STB arrangement.

D0342 Kruger, Katrin, and Siegfried Petrenz. *Vestivi i colli. Diminutionen uber ein Madrigal von G.P. de Palestrina für Sopranoblockflöte und Cembalo/ Francesco Rognoni.* Celle, Germany: Moeck, 1994.
An edition of Rognoni Taeggio's diminutions on the famous madrigal. Issued as score (11pp) [2547 Moeck] and one part for soprano recorder. Preface in German with English and French translations.

D0343 Lamb, Gordon H. ed. *Magnificat; in Primi Toni (XXXV) for Double Chorus of Mixed Voices, a Cappella. Giovanni Pierluigi da Palestrina.* New York: Lawson-Gould Music Publishers, 1975.
SATB SATB, with piano reduction for rehearsal. 36pp.

D0344 Laubenstein, Paul F., ed. *Tollite jugum meum. Take My Yoke.* New York: G. Schirmer, 1949. 10pp.
SATB, *a cappella.*

D0345 Lee, John, ed. *Panis angelicus.* Chicago: G.I.A. Publications, 1976. G-2003.
SATB, mixed voices, with organ accompaniment. Latin text by Thomas Aquinas, with English adaptation by the editor.

D0346 Leicht, Hans, ed. *Palestrina. Missa Iste Confessor.* Solothurn: Solothurner Musikverlag, 1946. 24pp.
SATB.

D0347 Ley, H. G., *I Beheld and Lo! A Great Multitude* [*Vidi turbam magnam*]. Novello's Octavo Anthems no. 1215. London: Novello, 1936.
SATB, arrangement of motet *Vidi turbam magnam* with English text by H.G. Ley.

D0348 Ley, H. G., ed. *Now When Was Come the Day of Pentecost.* Novello's Octavo Anthems no.1206. London: Novello, 1936.
Dum complerentur dies Pentecostes, with English text by H. G. Ley.

D0349 Ley, H. G., ed. *On This Day, the Blessed Virgin Mary.* Novello's Octavo Anthems no.1217. London: Novello, 1937.
Hodie beata virgo Maria, with English text by H. G. Ley.

D0350 Ley, H.G., ed. *The Star Which the Wise Men Had Seen.* Novello's Octavo

Anthems no.1216. London: Novello, 1937.
Stella quam viderant Magi, with English text by H. G. Ley.

D0351 Ley, H.G., ed. *Then Came Michael the Archangel.* Novello's Octavo Anthems no.1211. London: Novello, 1936.
Venit Michael Archangelus, with English text by H. G. Ley.

D0352 Ley, H.G., ed. *They Have Taken My Lord Away.* Novello's Octavo Anthems no.1222. London: Novello, 1937.
Alleluia! Tulerunt Dominum, with English text by H. G. Ley.

D0353 Liebergen, Patrick Michael, ed. *O bone Jesu.* New York: Carl Fischer, 1989. CM8299.
SATB, mixed voices. Latin text with English adaptation.

D0354 Lockwood, Lewis. *Pope Marcellus Mass: An Authoritative Score, Backgrounds and Sources, History and Analysis, Views and Comments.* Norton Critical Scores. New York: Norton, 1975.
In addition to a score of the mass (pp.39–73) derived from vol 4 of the Casimiri edition, Lockwood presents a large body of relevant documentary and critical material.

D0355 Malin, Don, ed. *City of God.* New York: Edward B. Marks Music, n.d. 00007534.
Spiritual madrigal *Città di Dio*. SSATB, *a cappella*, English and Italian texts.

D0356 Malin, Don, ed. *O Kindly Jesus.* New York: Edward B. Marks Music, n.d. 00007813.
Spiritual madrigal *O Jesu dolce.* SATTB *a cappella*, English and Italian texts.

D0357 Malin, Don, ed. *Missa Primi Toni. Benedictus.* New York: Belwin-Mills, n.d. No.2428.
SSA, *a cappella.* Latin text.

D0358 Malin, Don, ed. *Missa Primi Toni. Domine Fili Unigenite.* New York: Belwin-Mills, n.d. No.2429.
SSA, *a cappella.* Latin text.

D0359 Mandt, Heinrich, ed. *Giovanni Pierluigi da Palestrina (1524–1594). Missa Emendemus; für vierstimmigen gemischten Chor.* Düsseldorf: Schwann, 1949. 22pp.
SATB, on two staves, *a cappella.*

D0360 Mandt, Heinrich, ed. *Missa Brevis, ad quatuor voces inaequales*. Düsseldorf: Schwann, 1952. 31pp.

D0361 Marks, A.S., ed. *Missa Brevis . . . Adapted for Use in the English Church.* Modern Church Services no.192. London: Stainer & Bell, 1914.
SATB, *a cappella.* Prefatory note by A.S. Marks.

D0362 Marlhom, A., ed. *Sicut cervus. As the Hart Panteth.* New York: Harold Flammer, 1938.
SATB, *a cappella.*

D0363 Marshall, Charles, ed. *O Lord, Have Mercy.* New York: Frank Music, 1967.
SATB, *a cappella*, arrangement of the *Kyrie* from the *Missa Sine nomine* [Book VI] by Charles Marshall. English and German texts.

D0364 Marshall, Charles, ed. *This Glad Day.* New York: Frank Music, 1966. 9pp.
SSATBB, *a cappella*, version of motet *Haec dies quam fecit Dominus*, Latin text with English text adapted from psalms by Charles Marshall.

D0365 Martin, George C., ed. *Communion Service ("Assumpta est Maria"), Composed by G. Pierluigi da Palestrina.* Edited and adapted to English words by G. C. Martin. London: Novello, 1901. 65pp.
Arrangement and adaptation of the *Missa Assumpta est Maria* for the older Anglican liturgical order: *Kyrie* (pp.1–13); *Credo* (pp.14–31); *Sanctus* (pp.32–37); *Benedictus* (pp.38–43); *Agnus Dei* (pp.44–53); *Gloria* (pp.54–65). For SSAA(i.e. A or T)TB, transposed down one tone; English words only underlaid.

D0366 Martin, George C., ed. *Communion Service (Missa Papae Marcelli) Composed by G. Pierluigi da Palestrina.* English adaptation by the Rev. W. Russell. London: Novello and Company Ltd., 1898. 63pp.
Arrangement and adaptation of the *Missa Papae Marcelli* for the older Anglican liturgical order: *Kyrie* (pp.1–10); *Credo* (pp.11–29); *Sanctus* (pp.30–43); *Agnus Dei* (pp.44–50); *Gloria* (pp.51–63). Part of the *Kyrie* is adapted as the "Response to the Commandments" of the Anglican service. For SATTBB, transposed down one tone; English words only underlaid, edited.

D0367 Martin, George C., ed. *I Will Magnify Thee, O Lord.* Novello's Collection of Anthems no.886. London: Novello, 1876 [repr. 1907].
SATTB adaptation of motet *Exaltabo te, Domine.*

D0368 Martin, George C., ed. *Palestrina's Mass "Aeterna Christi munera" Adapted for Use in the English Church.* ["New Edition, with marks of expression."] London: Novello, 1917.
Arrangement and adaptation of *Missa Aeterna munera* for the older Anglican service. SATB, English words only, edited. Based on an earlier edition, one probably in conformity with the items by Martin listed above.

D0369 Mawby, Colin, ed. *Asperges me.* Westminster Series no. 6. London: L.J. Cary, 1962. 4pp.
SATB, Latin text.

D0370 Mawby, Colin, ed. *Sicut cervus.* Westminster Series no.10. London: L. J. Cary & Co, 1962. 7pp.

SATB, Latin text.

D0371 Mitterer, Ignatio, ed. *Joannes Petraloysii Praenestini. Missa celebris Papae Marcelli. Ad quattuor voces nove reducta.* Regensburg: Alfred Coppenrath/H. Pawelek, n.d. [before 1900]. 32pp.

SATB, transposed down one tone, liberally edited. The *Agnus Dei II* was newly composed out of motivic material drawn from the rest of the mass. This edition was an original reduction of Palestrina's work by the editor, not based on the early print by Anerio.

D0372 Mitterer, Ignaz, ed. *Missa Papae Marcelli. Church Music of the XVIth and XVIIth Centuries for Unaccompanied Voices* no.6904. New York: J. Fischer & Bro., n.d.

SATB, evidently a reprint or reworking of the Coppenrath 1900 edition. Extensively edited.

———. Monterosso Vacchelli, Anna Maria. *Missa L'Homme armé.* Cremona: Fondazione Claudio Monteverdi, 1979.

Modern musical edition pp.79–132. For full description of volume see item E0294.

D0373 Niven, Lewis, ed. *Quem vidistis, pastores? Shepherds, Whom Beheld Ye?* Glen Rock, NJ: J. Fischer, 1963. 15pp.

SSAT(or A)TB, Latin text, with English text derived from the Bible.

D0374 Ouvrard, Jean-Pierre, ed. *Ad te levavi.* Paris: Heugel et Cie., 1986. H33671, PJ505. 11pp.

SATB, mixed voices, ranked as of 'medium difficulty' in performance. Edition based on the Gardano edition of the second book of motets (1604).

D0375 Parkinson, John A., ed. *As the Hart Pants.* Sevenoaks, UK: Novello & Co., Ltd., 1955.

Adaptation of *Sicut cervus.* SATB, English and Latin texts.

D0376 Parratt, Walter, ed. *Super flumina Babylonis.* London, 1883; later edition London: Leonard, Gould & Bolttler, 1940. 8pp.

SATB arrangement.

D0377 Petti, Anthony G., ed. *Alma redemptoris.* London: Chester Music, 1977. J.W.C. 55096. 3pp.

SATB, mixed voices, with piano accompaniment for rehearsal. Latin text. Present edition based on print of the second book of motets for four voices (1581).

D0378 Petti, Anthony G., ed. *Canite tuba.* New York: Alexander Broude, n.d.

SSATB, *a cappella.*

D0379 Petti, Anthony G., ed. *Dum complerentur. Now When the Day.* London: J. & W. Chester, 1967. 11pp.

SAATTB, *a cappella*, motet for Pentecost, Latin text with alternative English text by Anthony Petti.

D0380 Petti, Anthony G., ed. *Dum ergo essent. When All Disciples.* London: J. & W. Chester, 1967. 8pp.

SAATTB, motet for Pentecost [secunda pars of *Dum complerentur*, but issued separately], Latin text with alternative English text by Anthony Petti.

D0381 Petti, Anthony G., ed. *O beata Trinitas.* The Italian and Spanish Schools for Five Voices. London: Chester Music, 1980. J.W.C. 55241. 7pp.

SATTB, mixed voices, with piano part for rehearsal. Latin text. Edition based on print in *Liber primus mottettorum quae partim quinis, partim senis, partim septenis vocibus concinantur* (1569).

D0382 Petti, Anthony G., ed. *Super flumina Babylonis.* The Italian School for Four Voices. London: Chester Music, 1977. J.W.C. 55096. 4pp.

SATB, mixed voices, with piano accompaniment for rehearsal. Latin text, based on Psalm 136:1. Present edition based on print of the second book of motets for four voices (1581).

D0383 Petti, Anthony G., ed. *Surge illuminare Jerusalem.* London: J. & W. Chester, 1975. 16pp.

SATB SATB, double choir, motet for Epiphany.

D0384 Pike, Lionel, ed. *Hodie Maria virgo. Magnificat Antiphon for Second Vespers of the Assumption of the Blessed Virgin Mary.* Borough Green, UK: Novello, 1976.

SSAT, *a cappella* or with organ accompaniment.

D0385 Pisano, Richard, ed. *O Domine Jesu.* Ft. Lauderdale, FL: Plymouth Music Co., ca. 1967. 4pp.

SATB, *a cappella.*

D0386 Pisano, Richard, ed. *Praise Be to Thee.* Ft. Lauderdale, FL: Plymouth Music Co., ca. 1988. 4pp.

SAB, *a cappella.*

D0387 Pizarro, David, ed. *This Is the Day.* New York: H. W. Gray, 1960. 12pp.

SSATTB, a cappella, Latin and English texts; adaptation of Latin motet *Haec dies quam fecit Dominus*, with English text adapted from Psalm 118 by Pizarro.

D0388 Procter, Michael, ed. *Missa Papae Marcelli.* Gloucester, UK: Beauchamp Press, 1994. 24pp.

SSATTB, *da cappella*. Preface in English by Michael Procter.

D0389 Reichwein, Heinz, ed. *O Domine Jesu Christe.* Möseler Verlag, 1990. 2pp.
TTBB, men's voices. Latin text.

D0390 Reynolds, G., ed. *Adoramus te Christe.* New York: J. Fischer & Bro., 1923.
Arrangement of motet for women's voices.

D0391 Richardson, [ ], ed. *Jesus Christ, Our Lord Was Crucified.* New York: Spratt Music Publishers, n.d.
SATB, adaptation of *Christus factus est.*

D0392 Richardson, [ ], ed. *Upon the Mount of Olives.* New York: Spratt Music Publishers, n.d.
SATB, adaptation of *In monte Oliveti* [work now ascribed to Ingegneri].

D0393 Roberts, J.V., ed. *Come Holy Ghost. Anthem for Unaccompanied Singing.* Novello's Collection of Anthems 829. London: Novello, 1876.
Adaptation of a *Gloria Patri* from the *Magnificat tertii toni*; edition based on a manuscript in Magdalen College Library, Oxford. This is the movement that became popular in the Anglican hymnal as the Easter melody "Victory," usually sung to words beginning "The strife is o'er, the battle done."

D0394 Rockstro, W[illiam] S[myth], ed. *Missa Assumpta est Maria (VI vocum) auctore Giovanni Pierluigi da Palestrina.* London: Novello, n.d. [ca.1882]. [also pub. New York: H. W. Gray, 1883]. 56pp. M2011.P25.A7.
SSATTB, with "reductio partiturae"; numerous suggestions for performance.

D0395 [Rockstro, William Smyth, ed.] *Missa Brevis.* London, Novello and New York: H.W. Gray, 1890. 55pp.

D0396 Rockstro, W[illiam] S[myth], ed. *Missa "O Admirabile Commercium" for Five Voices in the Mixolydian Mode (Transposed) Composed by G. Pierluigi da Palestrina.* London and New York: Novello, Ewer & Co., 1891.
Original note values; organ part for rehearsal; transposed down 1 tone; extensively edited.

D0397 Roff, J., ed. *Jesu! Rex admirabilis. Jesu! O King Most Wonderful.* New York: Edwin H. Morris, 1955.
SSA or TTB, arrangement with Latin and English texts.

D0398 Rose, Bernard, ed. *Missa Quarta.* London: Oxford, 1957.
SATB, *da cappella*. Edition of this mass (from *Missarum liber quartus*, 1582) in older Anglican liturgical format: *Kyrie, Sanctus, Benedictus, Agnus Dei, Credo, Gloria.* Partly reissued in *A Sixteenth-Century Anthem Book*, item D0100.

D0399 Rostagno, J.H., ed. *Missa Sine nomine. Super modulum Je suis desheritée. Church Music of the XVIth and XVIIth Centuries for Unaccompanied Voices* 6220. New York: J. Fischer & Bros., 1930.

D0400 Rowlands, Léo, ed. *Alma redemptoris.* Miami: McLaughlin & Reilly, 1936. 921. 4pp.
SATB, mixed voices. Latin text.

D0401 Saar, Louis Victor, ed. *O bone Jesu.* Boston: Oliver Ditson, 1928. 332–14207. 2pp.
SSA, for women's voices. Latin text with English adaptation.

D0402 Sargent, Malcolm, ed. *O admirabile commercium.* London: Oxford University Press, 1963. 7pp.
SSATB, *a cappella.*

D0403 Sargent, Malcolm, ed. *Videntes stellam.* London: Oxford, 1965. 8pp.
SSAATTBB, *a cappella.*

D0404 Schabasser, Josef, ed. *O crux ave.* Vienna: Döblinger Musikverlag, 1965. 43503/D.9139. 2pp.
SATB, for mixed voices. Latin text, hymn *Vexilla regis* (verse 6). Previously published in "Passion und Ostern," *Chorsätze alter Meister.*

D0405 Schabasser, Josef, ed. *Stabat Mater.* Vienna: Döblinger Musikverlag, 1965. 43503/D.9141. 36pp.
SATB + SATB, for mixed voices. Latin text, from sequence *Stabat Mater* by Jacopone da Todi. Previously published in "Passion und Ostern," *Chorsätze alter Meister.*

D0406 Scheel, J., ed. *Stabat Mater . . . für zwei Chöre mit gemischten Stimmen. Mit Vortragsbezeichnungen nach R. Wagner für Männerchöre.* Leipzig: Kahnt, 1887.
SATB SATB in score, bringing forward Wagner's performance suggestions from the Kahnt edition of 1878.

D0407 Schering, Arnold, ed. *Missa Papae Marcelli.* London: E. Eulenburg; New York: Eulenburg Miniature Scores, 1923. x + 52pp. E.E. 4376. Reissued in 1950s as score no. 963.
Miniature score format; preface by Arnold Schering dated 1923 in German and English; Latin text underlaid, with German translation; piano reduction also provided.

D0408 Schering, Arnold, ed. *Stabat Mater.* Edition Eulenburg 996. Leipzig: Ernst Eulenberg, 1924. Reissued London: E. Eulenburg, 1949; New York: Edition Eulenburg [1950s].
SATB SATB. Miniature score. Preface by Arnold Schering, German and English, 1924.

D0409 Scott, Cyril K., ed. *Ave Maria. For Four Female Voices.* London: Oxford, 1927.
Motet *a vocibus paribus*, with English text by B. E. Bulman.

D0410 Scott, Cyril K., ed. *Christe redemptor.* Motets of the Polyphonic School 1. London: Stainer & Bell, 1919.
Adaptation with English text by D.P. Thomas.

D0411 Shaw, Watkins, ed. *Missa Aeterna Christi munera.* Church Music Society Reprints 49. London: Oxford University Press, 1969. 16pp.
SATB, movements in older Anglican/Episcopalian liturgical sequence (*Kyrie, Sanctus, Benedictus, Agnus Dei, Gloria* [with intonation]). English translation by Henry Sandon underlaid. Piano accompaniment/reduction for practice only, some editing of parts.

D0412 Simkins, C.F., ed. *Vexilla regis prodeunt. The Royal Banners Forward Go.* London: Hinrichsen, 1968. 20pp.
SATB, hymn with Latin text (*Venantius Fortunatus*); English translation by J. M. Neale.

D0413 Smith, H.G. *et al.*, ed. *Arise, Shine, for Thy Light Is Come. Anthem for Four Voices with English Words.* York Series no.1069. York: Banks & Son, 1931.
SATB adaptation of the *Gloria* from the *Missa Ecce ego Joannes.*

D0414 Smith, H.G., ed. *As the Hart Panteth. Anthem. . . . Choir Series of Anthems* no.189. London: The Choir Office, 1924.
SATB, adaptation of motet *Sicut cervus desiderat*, with English text adapted by H.G. Smith.

D0415 Smith, H.G., ed. *Behold, and See If There Be Any Sorrow.* York Series no.922. York: Banks & Son, 1927.
Adaptation of *Kyrie* of the *Missa Ave Regina coelorum* [Book XI].

D0416 Smith, H.G., ed. *By the Waters of Babylon.* York Series no.1067. York: Banks & Son, 1930.
Adapted to English words by H.G. Smith.

D0417 Smith, H.G., ed. *Come unto Him. Introit or Short Anthem.* Dublin: H.G. Smith, 1925.
Adaptation of *Sanctus* of the *Missa De beata virgine* [Book II], English text by H.G. Smith.

D0418 Smith, H.G., ed. *God Is a Spirit. Introit or Short Anthem.* Choir Series no.245. London: J.A. Sharp, 1929.
Adaptation of *Sanctus* of the *Missa Ave Regina coelorum* [Book XI], English text by H.G. Smith.

D0419 Smith, H.G., ed. *God Shall Wipe Away All Tears. Anthem.* Dublin: H.G. Smith, 1925.
Adaptation of *Agnus Dei I* of the *Missa De beata virgine* [Book II].

D0420 Smith, H.G., ed. *God So Loved the World.* London: Cary & Co., 1933.

M2092.4.P.
SATB, with keyboard accompaniment for rehearsal only.

D0421 Smith, H.G., ed. *Hear Thou in Heaven. Introit or Short Anthem.* Dublin: H. G. Smith, 1925.
Adaptation of *Agnus Dei I* of the *Missa Ave Regina coelorum* [Book IX].

D0422 Smith, H.G., ed. *Holy, Holy. Introit or Short Anthem.* Choir Series no.242. London: J. A. Sharp, 1929.
SATB, adaptation of *Sanctus* from the *Missa Aeterna Christi munera*, with English text adapted by H.G. Smith.

D0423 Smith, H.G., ed. *I Will Arise.* Choir Series no.254. London: J. A. Sharp, 1930.
SATB adaptation of *Agnus Dei I* of the *Missa O sacrum convivium*, with music and English text adapted by H.G. Smith.

D0424 Smith, H.G., ed. *Is It Nothing to You?* Choir Series no.265. London: J. A. Sharp, 1931.
Adaptation of *Improperia. Popule meus* as anthem, with music and text adapted by H.G. Smith.

D0425 Smith, H.G., ed. *Jesu, the Very Thought of Thee.* Choir Series no.252. London: The Choir Office, 1930.
SATB adaptation of *Agnus Dei* of the *Missa Regina coeli* [Book XII]. English text adapted from an eleventh-century Latin hymn by E. Caswell.

D0426 Smith, H.G., ed. *Lamb of God. Introit or Short Anthem.* York Series no.1035. York: Banks & Son, 1920.
SATB adaptation of the *Agnus Dei* from the *Missa O admirabile commercium*, edited and with English text supplied by H.G. Smith.

D0427 Smith, H.G., ed. *Lead Thou and Guide Me. Motet.* York series no.1068. York: Banks & Son, 1931.
SATB adaptation of motet *Perfice gressus meos*, with English text version by H.G. Smith.

D0428 Smith, H.G., ed. *Let the People Praise Thee.* Choir Series no.300. London: The Choir Office, 1935.
SATB adaptation of the *Gloria* of the *Missa O admirabile commercium*, edited and with English text supplied by H. G. Smith.

D0429 Smith, H.G., ed. *Lift Up Your Heads, O Ye Gates. Anthem.* York Series no.1096. York: Banks & Co., 1932.
Adaptation of the motet *Loquebantur in variis linguis*, with adaptation of texts from Psalm 24 by H.G. Smith.

D0430 Smith, H.G., ed. *Lord, Thou Hast Been Our Dwelling Place. Anthem.* Choir Series no.209. London: J. A. Sharp, 1926.

SATB adaptation of the *Gloria* of the *Missa Brevis*, with English text adapted from Psalm 90 by H.G. Smith.

D0431 Smith, H.G., ed. *O Sacred Head Once Wounded.* Choir Series no.280. London: The Choir Office, 1933.

SATB adaptation of the *Kyrie* from the *Missa Sine nomine* [Book VI], edited and with English text by H.G. Smith.

D0432 Smith, H.G.,ed. *O Lord, Bow Down Thine Ear. Introit or Short Anthem.* York Series no.893. York: Banks & Son, 1925.

SATB adaptation of the *Kyrie* of the *Missa Aeterna Christi munera*, with English text by H.G. Smith.

D0433 Smith, H. G., ed. *O Lord God, Lamb of God. Anthem.* Choir Series no.326. London: The Choir Office, 1929.

SATB adaptation of the *Gloria* from the *Missa Papae Marcelli,* with English text by H. G. Smith.

D0434 Smith, H.G., ed. *O God, Have Mercy. Anthem.* Choir Series no.247. London: The Choir Office, 1929.

SATB adaptation of the *Kyrie* from the *Missa Papae Marcelli*, with English text derived from Psalm 51 and adapted by H.G. Smith.

D0435 Smith, H.G., ed. *O Sing Unto the Lord. Anthem.* Choir Series no.223. London: J. A. Sharp, 1927.

SATB, adapted from *Credo* of the *Missa Brevis*, with English text derived from Psalm 96 by H.G. Smith.

D0436 Smith, H.G., ed. *Praise Ye the Lord. Anthem.* Choir Series no.269. London: The Choir Office, 1931.

Motet *Ego sum panis vivus*, adapted to English text by H.G. Smith.

D0437 Smith, H.G. et al., ed. *Seek Ye the Lord. Introit or Short Anthem adapted to English Words.* York Series no.1034. York: Banks & Son, 1930.

Adaptation of *Alma redemptoris Mater.*

D0438 Smith, H.G., ed. *Thy Rebuke Hath Broken His Heart. Anthem.* York Series no.958. York: Banks & Son, 1928.

SATTB arrangement of *Improperium expectavit*, with English text adapted by H.G. Smith.

D0439 Smith, H.G., ed. *We Laud and Praise Thee. Anthem.* Choir Series no.253. London: The Choir Office, 1930.

SATN adaptation of the *Sanctus* from the *Missa Papae Marcelli*, with English text by H.G. Smith.

D0440 Smith, H.G., ed. *Why Art Thou Cast Down, O My Soul?* York Series no.1390. York: Banks & Son, 1938.

Adaptation of *Anima mea turbata est* [secunda pars of *Heu mihi*], with English text adapted by H.G. Smith.

D0441 Smith, H.G., ed. *The Wilderness Shall Be Glad.* Choir Series no.293. London: The Choir Office, 1933.

Adaptation of *Gloria* of the *Missa Regina coeli* [Book XII], with music and English text adapted by H.G. Smith.

D0442 Somma, Bonaventura, ed. *Missa Aeterna Christi munera.* Rome: de Santis, ca.1950. edition #1037/1038A-B.

SATB.

D0443 Stern, Hermann, ed. *Missa ad fugam für Chor SATB (SAATB).* Die Motette no.609. Neuhausen-Stuttgart: Hänssler-Verlag, 1983.

SATB (SAATB); original note values, with both Latin and German text underlay; plainchant intonations supplied for *Gloria* and *Credo. Mensurstrich.*

D0444 Stewart, C. Hylton, ed. *Adoramus te.* Novello's Short Anthems no.249. London: Novello, 1924.

SATB, with English text by Hylton Stewart.

D0445 Stewart, C. Hylton, ed. *We Adore Thee, Lord Jesus.* Novello's Short Anthems no.333. London: Novello, 1960. 4pp.

SATB, Latin text with English version by Hylton Stewart; transposed.

D0446 Taylor, Deems, ed. *Sub tuum* [*praesidium*]. New York: J. Fischer & Bro., 1921.

Arranged for four-part female choir.

D0447 Terry, Richard R., ed. *Bone Pastor. Very Bread, Good Shepherd, Tend Us.* Polyphonic Motets no.44. London: Cary & Co., 1931.

SATB, adaptation of motet *Lauda Sion*, with an English text by Richard Terry.

D0448 Theil, Carl, ed. *Palestrina's Missa Papae Marcelli—sechstimmig—für den praktisch-liturgischen Gebrauch.* Berlin: Sulzbach, ca.1902. [Fourth edition 1912] 27pp.

SSATTB in score. A version of part of this edition [*Kyrie, Benedictus, Agnus Dei*] is located in *Die Musik* 4 (1905), Musikbeilage, Heft 22. 8pp.

D0449 Thomas, Bernard, ed. *Divisions on Vestiva i colli: For Treble Instrument and Continuo.* Ricercari e passagi 13. London: Pro Musica Edition, ca. 1987.

Contains score and 3 parts of instrumental settings and elaborations of *Vestiva i colli* by Girolamo dalla Casa, Giovanni Bassano, Francesco Rognoni, and Bartolomeo de Selma e Salaverde.

D0450 Vervoitte, Charles Joseph, ed. *Iste confessor, messe à 4 voix avec accompag-*

nemt d'orgue ou de piano, ad libitum. Paris: Girod, ca.1865. 46pp.
SATB, with additional accompaniment for rehearsal or performance. Edited.

D0451 Wagner, Richard, ed. *Stabat Mater. Motet for Double Chorus a cappella. G. da Palestrina.* New York: G. Schirmer, ca.1900.
SATB SATB. Alternations of soli and chori marked in score, and otherwise edited. 19pp.

D0452 Wagner, Richard, ed. *Stabat mater. Motette für zwei Chöre a capella. Mit Vortrags-Bezeichnungen für Kirchen- und Conzert-Aufführungen eingerichtet von Richard Wagner.* Leipzig: Kahnt, 1878.
SATB SATB in score, edited and with suggestions for performance by Wagner.

D0453 Washington, Henry, ed. *Exultate Deo.* London: J. & W. Chester, 1958. 7pp.
SATB, motet; additional score reduction for rehearsal; note values halved.

D0454 Washington, Henry, ed. *Missa Aeterna Christi munera.* London: J. & W. Chester Ltd., 1953. 31pp.
SATB/SATTB; additional score reduction for rehearsal; note values halved. Preface by Washington with mass plainchants and commentary.

D0455 Washington, Henry, ed. and arr. *Missa Brevis for Four Voices by Palestrina.* London: J. & W. Chester, 1950. 32pp.
SATB; additional score reduction for rehearsal; note values halved. Preface by Washington.

D0456 Washington, Henry, ed. *Stabat Mater dolorosa.* London: J. & W. Chester, 1974. 36pp.
SATB SATB; additional score reduction for rehearsal; note values halved.

D0457 West, J.E., ed. *In Divers Tongues Spake the Apostles.* Novello's Collection of Anthems no.913. London: Novello, 1876.
Arrangement of motet *Loquebantur in variis linguis*, with English text paraphrased from Acts of the Apostles, ch.2, by W.G. Rothery.

D0458 Williams, W., ed. *Like as the Hart.* New York: G. Schirmer, n.d.
SATB, *a cappella*. Adaptation of *Sicut cervus*, together with its secunda pars, *Sitivit anima mea*, rendered here as *My Soul Is Athirst.*

D0459 Williamson, John Finlay, ed. *Alleluia! Tulerunt Dominum. For Five-Part Chorus of Mixed Voices a cappella.* New York: G. Schirmer, 1932.
SSATB, Latin with English text adapted by Gustave Reese.

D0460 Williamson, John Finlay, ed. *Alma redemptoris mater. Bow Down Thine Ear,*

O Lord. New York: G. Schirmer, 1933.
SATB, *a cappella.* English text adapted from Psalm 86 by Arthur Mendel.

D0461 Williamson, John Finlay, ed. *Bonum est confiteri. It Is a Good Thing to Give Thanks.* New York: G. Schirmer, 1945. 8pp.
SSATB, *a cappella.* English text adapted from Psalm 92:1 by Gustave Reese.

D0462 Williamson, John Finlay, ed. *Exultabo te. Thee Will I Extol, O My Lord.* New York: G. Schirmer, 1932.
SSATB, *a cappella.* English text adapted from Psalm 30 by Gustave Reese.

D0463 Williamson, John Finlay, ed. *Exultate Deo. Sing and Praise Jehovah.* New York: G. Schirmer, 1933.
SSATB, *a cappella.* English text version adapted from Psalm 81 of the King James version of the Bible by Arthur Mendel.

D0464 Williamson, John Finlay, ed. *Introduxit me rex. To the Cellar of Wine I Came.* New York: G. Schirmer, 1936.
SATTB, *a cappella.* English text by Arthur Mendel.

D0465 Witt, Franz Xaver. *Missa "Hodie Christus natus est" octo vocibus concinenda.* Regensburg: Pustet, 1871.

D0466 Woodworth, G. Wallace, ed. *Benedictus.* Harvard-Radcliffe Choral Music series no.9814. New York: G. Schirmer, 1949.
SSAA, *a cappella* with piano reduction for rehearsal only. Text in Latin with English translation. Adaptation of *Benedictus* from *Missa O admirabile commerium.*

D0467 Woodworth, G. Wallace, ed. *Sanctus and Osanna.* Harvard-Radcliffe Choral Music series no.9809. New York: G. Schirmer, 1949.
SSAATB, *a cappella* with piano reduction for rehearsal only. Text in Latin with English translation. Adaptation of *Sanctus* and *Osanna* from *Missa O admirabile commercium.*

D0468 Woodworth, G. Wallace, ed. *Stabat Mater.* Harvard-Radcliffe Choral Music series no.9811. New York: G. Schirmer, 1949.
SATB SATB, *a cappella* with piano reduction for rehearsal only. Text in Latin with English translation.

D0469 Woodworth, G. Wallace, ed. *Supplicationes.* Harvard-Radcliffe Choral Music series no.9798. New York: G. Schirmer, 1949.
TTBB, *a cappella* with piano reduction for rehearsal only. Arrangement of excerpts from the *Litaniae liber secundus.*

D0470 Zanon-Vené, ed. *Corporis mysterium. Sacrament of Priceless Worth.* New York: G. Ricordi, 1957. 7pp.

SATB, *a cappella*; hymn arranged as motet. Latin text from *Pange lingua*; English translation by Harold Heiberg.

D0471 Zanon-Vené, ed. *Gaude Barbara. O Sing Joyfully.* New York: G. Ricordi, 1957. 9pp.

SSAA, *a cappella*; motet, Latin text; English translation by Harold Heiberg.

D0472 Zanon-Vené, ed. *Salvete flores martyrum. Descend, Thou Heavn'ly Dove.* New York: G. Ricordi, 1957. 7pp.

SATB, *a cappella*; hymn arranged as motet. Latin text; English translation by Harold Heiberg.

D0473 Zanon-Vené, ed. *Veni sponsa Christi. The Crown Eternal.* New York: G. Ricordi, 1957.

SATB, *a cappella*; motet. Latin text. English translation by Harold Heiberg.

D0474 Zipper, Herbert, ed. *Palestrina. Missa Iste Confessor. SATB a cappella.* Arthur Jordan Conservatory of Music Choral Series 16. New York: Edward B. Marks Music Corp., 1949. 46pp.

SATB, keyboard reduction for rehearsal; Latin text. Prefatory notes on sources, particulars of edition, and editorial policy.

Chapter 6

Bibliography of Secondary Literature

I. General Background, History, and Contemporaries

E0001 Abbiati, Franco. *Storia della Musica.* 3rd ed. Milan: Garzanti, 1967. 3 vols. ML160.A224.

In vol 1 of this general history, *Dalle origini al Cinquecento*, pp.424–463 address the state of church music, the Council of Trent and the Counter-Reformation, and the music of Palestrina and his contemporaries. This section also contains a color plate with a portrait of the composer and a facsimile page from the Lateran 59 autograph. In the second edition, comparative coverage is found in vol 1, pp.491–518, with more extensive illustrations.

E0002 Abraham, Gerald, ed. *The New Oxford History of Music. Vol 4: The Age of Humanism 1540–1630.* London: Oxford, 1968. ML60.N44. vol 4.

See pp. 312–371, the chapter by Henry Coates and Gerald Abraham entitled "Latin Church Music on the Continent. 2. The Perfection of the A Cappella Style," which discusses the style of Palestrina and his contemporaries Lasso, de Monte, and others, and provides a good style overview by genre.

E0003 Agee, Richard John. "The Privilege and Venetian Music Printing in the 16th Century." Ph.D. dissertation, Princeton, 1982. 401 pp. [43/07A, p.2147 DEU82–28188].

Documents by means of an examination of archival documents the terms under which various sixteenth-century Venetian firms were licensed to print music publications. Demonstrates that licensing was an evolving process in which the nature and circumstances of a privilege changed over time.

E0004 Agee, Richard J. "The Venetian Privilege and Music-Printing in the Sixteenth Century." *Early Music History* 3 (1983): 1–42.

Distilled from the author's Ph.D. thesis; see preceding item.

E0005 Ambros, August Wilhelm. *Geschichte der Musik.* Breslau and Leipzig: Breitkopf und Härtel, 1862–1882. 5 vols. [vol 1, 1862; vol 2, 1864; vol 3, 1868; vol 4, 1878; vol 5, 1882]. ML160.A56.1887.

Volume 4 of this work, perhaps the last multivolume general history of music authored by a single person, deals with Palestrina and the Roman school. See also E0065 for Italian translation of the material on Palestrina by Giovanni Insom (ed. Lino Bianchi).

E0006 Atlas, Allan. *Renaissance Music: Music in Western Europe, 1400–1600.* The Norton Introduction to Music History series. New York: Norton, 1998. ISBN 0–393–97169-4. ML172.A84.1998.

A fine recent period history directed to serious students and early music specialists, with an unfolding of developments in style over two centuries and an interesting historiographical method. In chapter 37, "The Counter-Reformation in Italy and Spain," pp.580–605 devote particular attention to Palestrina and the genres in which he composed. An exceptional amount of judiciously chosen source documents, style examination, and reception history in the space allowed.

E0007 Bäumker, Wilhelm. "Die polyphone Musik auf dem Concile von Trient, sess. XXII." *Monatshefte für Musikgeschichte* 9 (1877): 123–125, 147–148.

Mainly provides text (in Latin, with parallel German translation) of the eighth canon debated during the twenty-second session of the Council of Trent on September 10, 1562.

E0008 Beck, Hermann. "Das Konzil von Trient und die Probleme der Kirchenmusik." *Kirchenmusikalisches Jahrbuch* 48 (1964): 108–117.

A more-than-usually careful examination of the Tridentine conciliar decretals and debate on the question of the place of music in the Roman liturgy, as well as the subsequent history of this debate in church thought and discipline, and its effects on Italian church music generally.

E0009 Bernstein, Jane. "Financial Arrangements and the Role of Printer and Composer in Sixteenth-Century Italian Music Printing." *Acta Musicologica* 63 (1991): 39–56.

Examination of the economic effects of the sixteenth-century music publishing industry on printers and composers, focused mainly on the period 1540 to 1580. Discusses issues of marketability and funding, describing how independent production, partnerships, commissions, and patronage were used in financing editions. Notes that composers clearly found advantages in publication, both in terms of financial return and in the accurate transmission of their works.

E0010 Brown, Howard Mayer, and Louise K. Stein. *Music in the Renaissance*. 2nd ed. Prentice Hall History of Music Series 2. Englewood Cliffs, NJ: Prentice-Hall, 1999. ISBN 0–134–00045–5. ML172.B86.1999.

An excellent introduction to musical style in the fifteenth and sixteenth centuries. Chapters 10 and 11 (pp. 273–329) address the Council of Trent and provide clear and elegant examinations of the styles of Palestrina, Lasso, Victoria, and Byrd. Chapters contain judicious short bibliographies.

E0011 Casimiri, Raffaele. "Annibale Zoilo (1540?–1592) e la sua famiglia. Nuovi documenti biografici." *Note d'Archivio* 17 (1940): 1–25.

Biographical material about the younger contemporary with whom Palestrina undertook the emendation of the Roman Gradual beginning in 1577. Contains appendix of Italian and Latin documents.

E0012 Casimiri, Raffaele. "I 'Diarii sistini.'" *Note d'Archivio* 1 (1924): 85–99, 149–162, 267–274; 3 (1926): 1–16, 169–192, 257–272; 4 (1927): 256–266; 9

(1932): 53–60, 150–159, 260–266; 10 (1933): 45–57, 149–164, 261–276, 326–343; 11 (1934): 76–92, 300–315; 12 (1935): 55–70, 126–141, 249–264; 13 (1936): 59–76, 147–156, 201–214; 14 (1937): 19–33, 73–88, 128–143, 298–313; 15 (1938): 281–287; 16 (1939): 74–99; 17 (1940): 65–71.

Older but still useful transcription of Sistine diary entries for the years 1535 to 1560.

E0013 Casimiri, Raffaele. " 'Disciplina musicae' e 'maestri di capella' dopo il Concilio di Trento nei maggiori istituti ecclesiastici di Roma: Seminario romano—Collegio germanico—Collegio inglese (secoli XVI–XVII)." *Note d'Archivio* 12 (1935): 1–26, 73–81; 15 (1938): 1–14, 49–64, 97–112, 145–156, 225–247; 16 (1939): 1–9; 19 (1942): 102–109, 159–168; 20 (1943): 1–17.

An early documentary study of three selected Roman seminaries in the sixteenth and seventeenth centuries. Contains details of musical organization, descriptions of duties, and numerous biographical notices of *maestri,* students, and musicians. Vols 12 and 15 in particular contain details of activities of musicians in Palestrina's orbit. Casimiri referred the reader to his 1922 documentary biography for amplification of remarks on Palestrina, the first *maestro di cappella* of the Roman Seminary (1566–1571).

E0014 Casimiri, Raffaele. "Firmin Le Bel di Noyon, maestro in Roma di Giovanni Pierluigi da Palestrina." *Note d'Archivio* 1 (1924): 64–77.

Documentary sources for Firmin, who, as *maestro di cappella* at Santa Maria Maggiore in 1540, had the juvenile Palestrina among his choristers. Includes transcription of Firmin's 6–voice motet *Puer natus est.*

E0015 Casimiri, Raffaele. " 'Il Vittoria': nuovi documenti per una biografia sincera di Tommaso Ludovico de Victoria." *Note d'Archivio* 11 (1934): 111–197.

Biographical study of Palestrina's notable contemporary, with a large quantity of documentary material, 23 items of which are reproduced. Derides in passing the description of Victoria as "the ape of Palestrina," asserting the distinctive qualities and Hispanic roots of Victoria's personal style.

E0016 *The Catholic Encyclopedia.* New York: The Encyclopedia Press, 1907–1954. 16 vols. Supplement. New York: The Gilmary Society, 1922–1951. 2 vols. BX841.C3.

Reference work addressing Catholic thought, history, liturgy, practices, and personalities for the educated layperson, with a clear post-Tridentine (and pre-Vatican II) perspective. Useful for explanations of liturgical terminology, organization, and practices relevant to Palestrina's religious music. See also item E0042.

E0017 *Ceremoniale Episcoparum Iussu Clementis VIII. Pont. Max. nouissimi reformatum. Omnibus Ecclesiis; praecipue autem Metropolitanis Cathedralibus, & Collegiatus perutile, ac necessarium.* Rome, 1600; Rome: Lepido Fatij, 1606.

Manual of liturgical ceremonial, procedure, and performance practice issued during the reign of the last pope for whom Palestrina worked.

E0018 Culley, Thomas D. *Jesuits and Music. I. A Study of the Musicians Connected with the German College in Rome during the Seventeenth Century and of Their Activities in Northern Europe.* Rome: Jesuit Historical Institute, 1970. ML 3033.8.R6C8. vol 1.

Provides valuable information on the manner in which many sixteenth- and seventeenth-century church musicians were educated in Rome, including many younger contemporaries and disciples of Palestrina. Also suggests what repertories of music were used in contemporary liturgical ceremonies and how, as well as some avenues through which the polyphonic style of the Roman school was disseminated outside Italy.

E0019 Cusick, Suzanne Gertrude. "Valerio Dorico: Music Printer in Sixteenth Century Rome." Ph.D. dissertation, University of North Carolina at Chapel Hill, 1975. [36/10A, p.6359 DDJ76–09231] Pub. as *Valerio Dorico: Music Printer in Sixteenth Century Rome*. Studies in musicology 43. Ann Arbor: UMI Research Press, 1981. ISBN 0–8357–1173–0. ML427.D7C9.

Discusses in detail the printing and editorial practices of the publisher responsible for over half the music printed in Rome ca. 1550 to 1580. Dorico published most of Palestrina's prints through 1572. In practice this *tipografo* gave composers considerable legal and editorial authority over the process of printing their own works, and music published by him has a reasonable claim to be authoritative text. Bibliographical catalog included.

E0020 Damilano, Piero. "Liturgia e musica nell' epoca palestriniana." *Atti del Convegno di Studi Palestriniani. 28 settembre-2 ottobre 1975*, ed. Francesco Luisi. Palestrina: Fondazione Giovanni Pierluigi da Palestrina, 1977. ML410.P15C77.1975. pp. 313–325.

Enumerates some of the perceived abuses present in mid-sixteenth century Roman liturgies and describes the revision of Roman service books ca. 1570 to 1615. Indicates general directives for reform and their implications for Palestrina's production, especially regarding polyphonic style, choice of text propers for setting, and his cultivation of recently approved texts, notably certain litanies.

E0021 Fellerer, Karl Gustav. "Ausdruck und Klang in der Kirchenmusik um 1600." *Kirchenmusikalisches Jahrbuch* 65 (1981): 31–44.

Discussion of the increasing verticality of harmonic conception in church music generally, which is traced through both theoretical and practical source readings that deal with the relationship of counterpoint and harmony, dating from the second half of the sixteenth century. Notes that new and expressive possibilities were also being realized ca. 1600 through chromatically colored writing, which was not inconsistent with the goals of church music provided that declamatory needs were met.

E0022 Fellerer, Karl Gustav. "Church Music and the Council of Trent." *Musical Quarterly* 39 (1953): 576–594.

Reviews writings and activities concerned with the reform of church music in the early and mid-sixteenth century. Notes that there is a recurrent emphasis on the intelligibility of text and on a spiritual attitude in the composer, rather than on specifically stylistic issues. Argues that the ideal from the church's perspective was an amalgam of the new spiritual principles with a polyphonic/harmonic compromise of texture with correct text declamation. Points out that many of the younger generation would in fact see the mandates of the council realized in monodic genres; but the demand for intelligibility also affected concertante music and even plainchant itself. The council issued little in the way of decrees, but it did mark out a path of development by offering the spiritual foundation for reform.

E0023 Fellerer, Karl Gustav, ed. *Geschichte der katholischen Kirchenmusik.* Kassel: Bärenreiter, 1972–1976. 2 vols. ISBN 3–7618–0225–0. ML3002.F43.1972.

Vol 2, *Die Kirchenmusik vom Tridentinum bis zur Vaticanum II*, pp.7–71, contains a series of seven articles by various authors constituting an overview of varieties and developments in church music in the Tridentine and immediate post-Tridentine period. Includes a discussion of Palestrina and numerous contemporaries, as well as a bibliography.

E0024 Fenlon, Iain. "Patronage, Music and Liturgy in Renaissance Mantua." In *Plainsong in the Age of Polyphony.* Cambridge: Cambridge, 1992. ISBN 0–521–40160–7. ML178.P6.1992t. pp. 209–235.

Studies the new liturgical foundation of S. Barbara in Mantua and the interests which underlay Duke Guglielmo Gongaza's creation of this musicoliturgical complex. In it the duke sought to bring together traditions of plainsong and polyphony for political and social, as well as religious, purposes. Palestrina had an important working relationship with this foundation from 1568 to 1587 through the patronage of the duke and the music he wrote for the Santa Barbara liturgy.

E0025 Fenlon, Iain, ed. *The Renaissance from the 1470s to the End of the Sixteenth Century.* Man and Music. Englewood Cliffs, NJ: Prentice-Hall, 1989. ISBN 0–13–773409-3. ML172.R6.1989t.

Presented as a series of detailed and very interesting articles designed to indicate together the contexts and sociointellectual forces that shaped the development of musical genres in this period. In addition to Fenlon's introductory essay on music and humanistic society, the book examines musical life in major Western European cultural centres. See Christopher Reynolds on Rome, item E0050.

E0026 Finscher, Ludwig, ed. *Die Musik des 15. und 16. Jahrhunderts.* Neues Handbuch der Musikwissenschaft 3. ed. Carl Dahlhaus. Laaber: Laaber, 1989–1990. 2 vols. ISBN 3–89007–043–4. ML172.M88.1989-90.

Vol 2, chapters 2–5 are style-cultural histories of the mass, motet, and liturgical *Gebrauchsmusik* in the sixteenth century, with special attention to Palestrina pp.246–252, and many mentions *passim* in the discussion of issues of style.

E0027 Gaspari, Gaetano et al. Bologna. Conservatorio di musica "G.B. Martini." Biblioteca. *Catalogo della biblioteca del Liceo musicale di Bologna.* Bologna, Libreria Romagnoli dall'Acqua, 1890–1893. Vol 4 has imprint: Bologna: Fratelli Merliani; vol 5 has imprint Bologna: Azzoguidi. ML136.B6L6.

A great store of information about early printed music and manuscript items pertaining to Palestrina (and many others), this is the catalog of the great collection located in what is now known as the Civico Museo Bibliografico Musicale, Bologna. In addition to valuable descriptions of individual items, Gaspari also frequently transcribes prefatory material which conveys much primary information on music of the sixteenth through eighteenth centuries.

E0028 Georgiades, Thrasybulos. *Musik und Sprache.* Berlin: Springer, 1954; *Music and Language: the Rise of Western Music as Exemplified in Settings of the Mass*, trans. Marie Louise Göllner. Cambridge, UK: Cambridge, 1982. 139pp. ISBN 0–521–29902–0. ML3849.G43.1982.

A study of the history of musical accentuation of text, with a section on Palestrina.

E0029 Grout, Donald Jay, and Claude V. Palisca. *A History of Western Music.* 5th edition. New York: W.W. Norton, 1996. ISBN 0–393–96904–5. ML160.G87.1996.

Chapter 8 of this well-known history, "Church Music of the Late Renaissance and Reformation" (pp.239–267), contains an introduction to the music of Palestrina (pp.250–256), including a look at the *Missa Papae Marcelli*, as well as short studies of his great contemporaries Victoria, Lasso, and Byrd.

E0030 Haberl, Ferdinand. "Jacobus de Kerle e le sue *Preces speciales* per il Concilio di Trento." *Quadrivium* 7 (1966): 31–38.

Describes the interactions of the Roman cardinals Vitelli and Borromeo with cardinal Truchsess von Waldburg, the employer of Jacobus de Kerle. Contains an analytical discussion of the music of the *Preces.*

E0031 Hayburn, Robert F. *Papal Legislation on Sacred Music 95 A.D. to 1977 A.D.* Collegeville, MN: Liturgical Press, 1979. ISBN 0–814–61012–5. ML3002.H43.

Contains English translation of texts of encyclicals and directives relating to purposes, uses, and kinds of liturgical music, as well as to the management, discipline, and privileges of church musicians and musical establishments. Arranged in chronological order by papal reign.

E0032 Hermelink, Siegfried. *Dispositiones Modorum. Die Tonarten in der Musik Palestrinas und seiner Zeitgenossen.* Münchener Veröffentlichungen zur Musikgeschichte 4. Tutzing: Schneider, 1960. ML3811.H4.

A study of the nature and use of modality in the sixteenth century, with Palestrina's music as a primary focus but encompassing that of numerous other composers. Derived from the structures of plainchant, based on examination of octave species and transpositions, twenty scales are demonstrated to be used in polyphony of the period.

E0033 Hucke, Helmut. "Die römische-katholische Kirche." In *Religiöse Authoritäten und Musik*, ed. Dorothea Baumann and Kurt von Fischer. Kassel: J. Stauda, 1984. 136pp. ISBN 3–798–2017–9. ML36.R45.1984. pp. 24–46.

Historical overview of conciliar decretals and papal documentary statements dating from ca. 600 to the Second Vatican Council regarding the nature and role of music used in the Roman Catholic liturgy.

E0034 Leichtentritt, Hugo. "The Reform of Trent and Its Effect on Music." *Musical Quarterly* 30 (1944): 319–328.

Examines some of the music specially composed in response to issues debated by the Council of Trent, notably Kerle's *Preces speciales*, as well as reviewing motets by Vincenzo Ruffo, Francesco Rosselli, and Don Fernando de las Infantas. Notes that in point of fact these composers modified their stylistic manners more significantly to meet the newly affirmed qualities for optimal church music than Palestrina did.

E0035 Lockwood, Lewis. *The Counter-Reformation and the Masses of Vincenzo Ruffo.* Studi di Musica Veneta 2. Venice: Fondazione Cini, 1970. ML 410.R898.L6.

In addition to being the principal study of Ruffo's music and activities, this is a valuable study of the environment of church music in Italy ca. 1540 to 1580 for Ruffo and his contemporaries and contains careful assessment and use of documentary sources. Indicates that provided the Tridentine mandate to respect the decorum and audibility of the liturgical text was observed, there was a greater range of and toleration for stylistic diversity and experimentation in music than had been previously realized.

E0036 Lockwood, Lewis. "Some Observations on the Commission of Cardinals and the Reform of Sacred Music." *Quadrivium* 7 (1966): 39–55.

A clearheaded reevaluation of the connection of the Commission of Cardinals with the "reform" of sacred polyphonic composition. Reviews evidence that the careful and objective Karl Weinmann did not have on this matter [*Das Konzil von Trent und die Kirchenmusik*, Leipzig 1919] that suggests there may have been some real interest on the part of some of the commission members in banning polyphony, as one had in fact briefly done so in his own diocesan cathedral in the 1530s. Also indicates some of the possible reactions by cardinals Vitelli and (in greater depth) Borromeo to the "tryouts" of "intelligible" music in 1565.

E0037 Lockwood, Lewis. "Vincenzo Ruffo and Musical Reform after the Council of Trent." *Musical Quarterly* 43 (1957): 342–371.

Insightfully examines two separate but related phases toward church music reform beginning around 1560: various opinions regarding the merits and usefulness of polyphony, and individual searches for an appropriate sacred music. Traces in particular Carlo Borromeo's association with Ruffo and others, and indicates the nature of some of their musical experiments. Notes the extraordinary flexibility in Ruffo's own stylistic stance, which, it is suggested, enabled him to embrace reform ideals (as exemplified in musical styles) to a radical degree. Concludes with an assessment of Ruffo in the context of his contemporaries, notably Palestrina.

E0038 Lightbourne, Ruth. "A Roman Procession (1583)." In *Liber Amicorum John Steele. A Musicological Tribute,* ed. Warren Drake. Festschrift series 16. Stuyvesant, NY: Pendragon, 1997. ISBN 0–945–19380–7. ML55.S82.1997. pp. 117–138.

Detailed study of a Corpus Christi procession based on a lengthy diary entry by the rector of the German College in Rome, Michele Lauretano. Addresses the scope and importance, pageantry, and musical practices of these significant devotional and social events. Includes full Italian transcription of the diary entry on which the article is based.

E0039 Ludwig, Peter. *Studien zum Motettenschaffen der Schüler Palestrinas.* Kölner Beiträge zur Musikforschung 143. Regensburg: Bosse, 1986. ISBN 3–764–9231–2. ML1403.L83.1986.

A review of repertory by younger Roman contemporaries of Palestrina, indicating some of the stylistic directions in which sacred-style composition was moving in the years between about 1580 and 1620.

E0040 Meier, Bernhard. *Die Tonarten der klassischen Vokalpolyphonie. Wesen und Bedeutung*. Utrecht: Oostheck, Scheltema and Holkema, 1974. ISBN 90–313–0009-8. ML.3811.M43; *The Modes of Classical Vocal Polyphony Described According to the Sources. With Revisions by the Author,* trans. Ellen S. Beebe. New York: Broude Brothers, 1988. ISBN 0–8450–7025–8. ML3811.M4313.1988.

Magisterial study of the behavior of modal types, melody, and cadence structures found in classical polyphony. Presents an influential method for modal analysis of Renaissance compositions, based on immersion in the writings and terminology of fifteenth- and sixteenth-century theorists and a powerful grasp of the relationships among modality, structure, and expression. To her well-informed translation of Meier's sometimes difficult prose, Beebe has added corrections and an index of musical examples.

E0041 Mercati, Angelo. "Melchiorre Major, l'autore del vibrante necrologio di Giovanni Pierluigi da Palestrina." *Note d'Archivio* 1 (1924): 57–63.

Traces Lorraine-born clerk (1539 to after 1614) associated with the confraternity of SS. Nicola e Caterina and the church of S. Luigi dei Francesi, who wrote a eulogy of Palestrina that is important evidence for his date of birth as well as a record of his death and burial.

E0042 *The New Catholic Encyclopedia.* New York: McGraw-Hill, 1967. 15 vols. Supplement 1967–1974 (vol 16). New York: McGraw-Hill, 1974. Supplement: Change in the Church (vol 17). ISBN 0–070–10235–X. BX841.N44.1967.

Younger version of *The Catholic Encyclopedia* is less close to the post-Tridentine mentality but evidently compiled with a more liberal and objective critical attitude.

E0043 O'Regan, Noel. "Processions and Their Music in Post-Tridentine Rome." *Recercar* 4 (1992): 45–80.

Examination of the role and scope of music in Rome in processions around 1575 to 1600. Holy Thursday, St. Mark's Day, the Corpus Christi, and other processions are described in detail. Archival and source evidence indicates that writing and directing music for these events were important activities of the period. The music covered a broad range of chant, alternatim settings, falsobordone, and more complex polyphony. It is often difficult to say exactly what music was used and how it was performed in a specific instance, but informed reconstructions of processional activity can be made.

E0044 O'Regan, Noel. "Music at the Roman Archiconfraternity of San Rocco in the Late Sixteenth Century." In *La musica a Roma attraverso le fonti d'archivio: atti del convegno internazionale, Roma 4–7 giugno 1992*, ed. Bianca Maria Antolini, Arnaldo Morelli, and Vera Vita Spagnuolo. Lucca: Libreria Italiana Musicale, 1994. ISBN 8–870–96050–1. ML290.8.R79M94.1994X. pp. 521–552.

An excellently documented study of the musical regulation and activities of a major Roman confraternity during the last third of the sixteenth century.

E0045 Pastor, Ludwig von. *Geschichte der Päpste seit dem Ausgang des Mittelalters. . . .* Freiburg im Breisgau, 1866–1938; *History of the Popes from the Close of the Middle Ages: Drawn from the Secret Archives of the Vatican and Other Original Sources*. London: Routledge & Kegan Paul, 1894–1961 [various publishers]. 40 vols. BX955.P35.

A central source for the history of the papacy, providing some of the essential background to Palestrina's professional and social environment.

E0046 Perkins, Leeman L. *Music in the Age of the Renaissance.* New York: Norton, 1999. 1147pp. ISBN 0–393–04608–7. ML172.P47.1999.

A history of genre and style of great breadth. The principal material on Palestrina (pp.871–897) in Chapter 25, "The Final Synthesis," is offered as illustration of "the continuities of tradition through more than a century and a half [of previous music history] and the relative coherence of the stylistic developments associated with it" [p.870]. Palestrina is understood to be at once representative of his age and exceptional for his individual creative gifts and the magnitude of his recognition by his contemporaries and posterity. Discussion of music is organized by stylistic genre.

E0047 Pirrotta, Nino, and Giuliana Gialdroni, eds. *I Musici di Roma e il Madrigale: Dolci Affetti (1582) e Le Gioie (1589).* L'arte Armonica/Musica Palatina 1. Rome: Accademia Nazionale di Santa Cecilia/Libreria Musicale Italiana, 1993. 186 pp. ISBN 88–7096–089-7.

A study and edition of two important madrigal collections to which the most famous composers active in Rome in the second half of the sixteenth century, including Palestrina, contributed. Introduction examines social background of the publications, noting that all contributors were members of the "Compagnia dei Musici di Roma," and that the patrons were noted as instrumental in the expansion of sacred music in this period.

E0048 Quadflieg, Jakob. "Über Textunterlage und Textbehandlung in kirchlichen Vokalwerke." *Kirchenmusikalisches Jahrbuch* 8 (1903): 95–138.

A detailed discussion of the problems encountered in interpreting and preparing text underlay for modern editions from pre-1600 musical sources, including ten "rules" for general procedure. Quadflieg was a major editor involved in early music publications (especially of Palestrina) issued around 1900 to 1910 by Breitkopf und Härtel, and had much opportunity to formulate his ideas. Also interesting in a slightly different context when it is remembered that questions of underlay and declamation in the "Haberl" edition were among those challenged by Casimiri.

E0049 Reese, Gustave. *Music in the Renaissance.* Rev. ed. New York: W. W. Norton, 1959. ISBN 0–393–09530–4. ML172.R42.1959.

This vast bibliographical study of music from 1400 to 1600 is still a valuable guide to scholarship before 1960. Chapter 9, "Sacred Vocal Music of the Late Renaissance" (pp.448–518), contains an overview of the Council of Trent and a survey of the music of Palestrina and a number of his important contemporaries in Rome and elsewhere. Discussion (pp.452–481) of Palestrina's background, biography, historical and stylistic position, and a general examination of his motets and masses, including numerous musical examples and work lists.

E0050 Reynolds, Christopher. "Rome: a City of Rich Contrast." In *The Renaissance from the 1470s to the End of the 16th Century*, ed. Iain Fenlon. Man and Music series. Englewood Cliffs, NJ: Prentice-Hall, 1989. ISBN 0–333–47261–6. ML172.R46.1989. pp. 63–101.

A detailed and valuable study of musical culture and institutions in Rome in this period.

E0051 Roche, Jerome. *North Italian Church Music in the Age of Monteverdi.* Oxford: Clarendon, 1984. ISBN 0–193–16118.4. ML2933.R6.1984.

Insightful study of the genres, uses, and dissemination of church music in the last years of Palestrina's life and shortly after his death. Indicates general stylistic tendencies in this period with implications for the composer's later compositions. Indicates that an ongoing major use of his smaller-scale *a cappella* music might have been for ferial observance in the larger foundations.

E0052 Rostirolla, Giancarlo. "La Cappella Giulia in San Pietro negli anni del magistero di Giovanni Pierluigi da Palestrina." In *Atti del Convegno di Studi Palestriniani. 28 settembre–2 ottobre 1975,* ed. Francesco Luisi. Palestrina: Fondazione Giovanni Pierluigi da Palestrina, 1977. ML410.P15C77.1975. pp. 99–283.

An extensive study of the organization, operations and liturgical duties, financial situation, and personnel of the Cappella Giulia for the years 1551 to 1554 and 1571 to 1594, based on archival documents. Conveys a strong sense of the chapel's working ambience during Palestrina's years there. Document transcriptions, tabulated personnel rosters, many individual biographies included.

E0053 Schaefer, Edward. "A Reexamination of Palestrina's Role in the Catholic Reformation." *Choral Journal* 35.1 (1994): 19–25.

Main interest here is in excerpts from contributors to the debate on church music reform in the years 1543 to 1563: bishop of Vienne Fridericus Blancicampianus, Emperor Ferdinand I; also specific Tridentine minutes.

E0054 Sherr, Richard. "Competence and Incompetence in the Papal Choir in the Age of Palestrina." *Early Music* 22 (1994): 607–629.

Traces fluctuating size and levels of overall vocal competence in the Sistine choir from around 1550 to 1580. Documents subversion of constitutional practices, in that certain singers were admitted without audition: some were patronage appointments of unqualified persons imposed by papal authority; some were admitted due to skill in composition although their voices were judged inadequate (including Palestrina). Other singers were older or ill, with probable effects on performance sound. Deduces that there was therefore often a substantial minority of voices unequal to producing the loud and full sonority considered ideal for a cappella singing.

E0055 Sherr, Richard. "From the Diary of a Sixteenth-Century Papal Singer." *Current Musicology* 25 (1978): 83–98.

Examines the diaries and accounts of Giovanni Antonio Merlo, a singer in the papal chapel from 1551 to 1588. A source of documentation for chapel activities, hirings, fines, and internal disputes, the diary also contains notes on works that were apparently part of the repertory of the chapel in the later 1560s.

E0056 Sherr, Richard. "A Letter from Paolo Animuccia: A Composer's Response to the Council of Trent." *Early Music* 12 (1984): 74–77.

Examines an autograph letter dated 1566 by the brother of Giovanni Animuccia. It intimates the practical way in which Paolo understood reactions in Rome to the events of the Council of Trent, and how he offered to undertake the composition of polyphony for the papal chapel in the "reformed" style. A rare item that not only documents a rather enterprising job search, but also indicates the personal sensitivity of a renaissance composer to contemporary currents in music.

E0057 Stinger, Charles. *The Renaissance in Rome.* Bloomington, IN: Indiana University Press, 1985. DG812.1.S75.1985; 2nd ed. with new preface 1998. ISBN 0–253–33491–8. 472 pp.

An outstanding study of Roman intellectual and cultural life from the reign of Eugenius IV to that of Clement VII (1443–1527).

E0058 Strunk, Oliver. "Some Motet-Types of the Sixteenth Century." In *Proceedings of the American Musicological Society*, 1939, pp.155 *et seq.*; repr. in *Essays on Music in the Western World.* New York: Norton, 1974. ISBN 0–393–02178–5. ML60.S862.E8. pp. 108–113.

An older comprehensive review of the motet genre in the sixteenth century in order to define the general character and the extent of the relationship between liturgical situation and musical style.

E0059 Ursprung, Otto. *Jacobus de Kerle. Sein Leben und Werk.* Dissertation, Munich: J. Heldwein, 1913. 115pp. ML410.K38U8.1913a.

A study of the composer of the *Preces speciales* for the Council of Trent. Notable for publishing correspondence concerning the exchanges of church polyphony between Cardinals Vitelli and Borromeo and the German court at Munich in the early 1560s.

E0060 Vita Spagnuolo, Vera. "Gli atti notarili dell'Archivio di Stato di Roma. Saggio di spoglio sistematico: l'anno 1590." In *La musica a Roma attraverso le fonti d'archivio: Atti del convegno internazionale, Roma 4–7 giugno 1992*, ed. Bianca Maria Antolini, Arnaldo Morelli and Vera Vita Spagnuolo. Lucca: Libreria Italiana Musicale, 1994. ISBN 88–709-6050–1. ML290.8.R79M94.1994X. pp. 521–552.

Emphasizes the wealth of documentary evidence to be derived from the systematic examination of notarized papers—payment statements, property payments, transfers and inventories, wedding contracts, and wills, for example—in the Archivio di Stato in Rome. As a case study, it lists abundant notices for Roman musicians, instrument makers, music printers, and publishers for one year (1590).

E0061 Weber, Edith. *Le Concile de Trente et la Musique de la Réforme et la Contre-Réforme.* Musique-Musicologie 12. Collection ed. Danièle Pistone. Paris: Champion, 1982. 301pp. ISSN 0–398–259-9. ML3003.W3.

Presents multidisciplinary documentary material on the Council of Trent and church music in an extended-outline format. Addresses the dissemination of the Protestant Reformation; the Council of Trent and its response to the Roman Church crisis (especially the 22nd and 24th sessions); the Commission of Cardinals and the reform of liturgical books, the Congregation of Rites and the actions of provincial synods. Dedicated section deals with issues of church music in this historical phrase, with its national and religious "schools," its genres and formal procedures, and the aesthetics of Tridentine music generally.

E0062 Weinmann, Karl. *Geschichte der Kirchenmusik.* Regensburg: Friedrich Pustet, 1910; *History of Church Music.* Regensburg: Friedrich Pustet, 1910 [Facs. repr. of translated edition Westport, CT: Greenwood Press, 1979. ISBN 0–8371–4363–2. ML3002.W34.1979].

Older but respected short general history of church music, informed by late Cecilian interests but also grounded in research current at the period of writing. Palestrina and the Roman school addressed on pp.108–129.

E0063 Weinmann, Karl. *Das Konzil von Trent und die Kirchenmusik.* Leipzig: Breitkopf und Härtel, 1919. [Facs. repr. Hildesheim: Georg Olms, 1980. ISBN 3–487–07006–5. ML3003.W451919a].

Probably the best work to address this issue up to its time, and still valuable. Weinmann rejected the myth of the origins of the *Missa Papae Marcelli*; although the council had condemned the admixture of secular elements with sacred music, it had not actually made a decision to ban polyphony. He also examined the activities of the persons associated with the Commission of Cardinals of 1564 to 1565, notably cardinals Vitelli and Borromeo. Notes that the interest of the cardinals was primarily in promoting an ideal of text clarity, rather than a "reform" of church music or the superimposition of any particular compositional style *per se*.

E0064 Winterfeld, Carl von. *Johannes Gabrieli und sein Zeitalter.* Berlin, 1834. 3 vols. [Facs. repr. Hildesheim: Georg Olms, 1965. ML290.2.V4.W7.1965].

Vol 1, pp.194–196 of this pioneering work on the great Venetian composer includes a comparison of Gabrieli's *cantus firmus* techniques with those of Palestrina and some of his contemporaries.

II. Biographical Literature

E0065 Ambros, August Wilhelm. "*Giovanni Pierluigi da Palestrina.* Italian trans. Giovanni Insom. ed. Lino Bianchi." *Nuova Rivista Musicale Italiana* 30 (1997): 264–322.

Italian translation of the material on Palestrina in vol 4 of Ambros's *History of Music*, originally published in 1878. P. 264 is a portrait of the composer. On p. 265 Lino Bianchi offers an introductory note on Ambros, and the translation by Insom follows.

E0066 d'Amore, Giulio, and Maria A. Morabito. "Gli esami di amissione e i concorsi per la Cappella Sistina dallo spoglio dei diari dei puntatori (1545–1607)." In *Studi in onore di Giulio Cattin*, ed. Francesco Luisi. Rome: Torre d'Orfeo, 1990. ISBN 88–851–4724–0. ML55.C288.1990. pp. 193–216.

An overview of examination and admission procedures for the Sistine Chapel, drawn from the chapel diaries dated 1545–1607.

E0067 Angoff, Charles. *Palestrina, Savior of Church Music.* New York: Ackerman, 1944. 64pp. ML410.P15.A6.

Short general biography.

E0068 Baini, Giuseppe. *Memorie storico-critiche della vita e della opera di Giovanni Pierluigi da Palestrina.* 2 vols. Rome: Società Tipografica, 1828 [Facs. repr. (lacking frontispiece portrait) Hildesheim: Georg Olms, 1966]. ML410.P15.

Although criticized for its inaccuracies of fact, its hagiographical tone, and its dearth of actual musical examples at a time when Palestrina's music in print was relatively scarce, this was nonetheless a pivotal and immensely influential biography. It was important in terms of its scope in its conscientious attempt to use the archival and manuscript material to which Baini had access, its thoughtful (though by some contested) style analysis, and its appearance during the early flourishing of the Romantic movement. Its image of the composer is also surprisingly romantic; it projects him both as spiritual visionary and solitary struggling genius.

E0069 Bandiera, Luigi, Lino Bianchi, R. Pentrella, and Giancarlo Rostirolla. *La casa di Giovanni Pierluigi da Palestrina: Cronistoria, restauro, prospettiva di utilizzazione.* Ministero per i beni culturali. Palestrina: Fondazione G. Pierluigi da Palestrina, 1986. 259pp.

Chronicles the history of the house where members of the Pierluigi family lived from the early sixteenth century until 1677, and documents its twentieth-century restoration. Includes architectural plans and many photos of the restoration process. Reports on the organization and activities of the Palestrina Foundation, which uses the house as its administrative center. Includes a general Palestrina bibliography compiled by Rostirolla.

E0070 Bandiera, Luigi. "Il Palestrina e la sua città." In *Atti del II Convegno Internazionale di Studi Palestriniani. Anno Europeo della Musica. 3–5 maggio 1986*, ed. Lino Bianchi and Giancarlo Rostirolla. Palestrina: Fondazione Giovanni Pierluigi da Palestrina/Centro di Studi Palestriniani, 1991. ML410.P15C77.1986. pp. 83–92.

Discusses the socioeconomic, professional, and ecclesiastical placement of the Pierluigi family in their native city of Palestrina for the period from 1513 to 1677.

E0071 Bandiera, Luigi. "Sulla seconda casa di Giovanni Pierluigi da Palestrina." *Studi Romani* 26 (1978): 370–374.

Identifies a house on vicolo del Duomo in Palestrina as a second house belonging to the Pierluigi family.

E0072 Bäumker, Wilhelm. "Einiges über Palestrina." *Monatshefte für Musikgeschichte* 9 (1877): 219–221.

Review of the evidence for Palestrina's date of birth, in which four points are presented in support of the author's contention [not generally accepted] that the correct date is 1514.

E0073 Bellaigue, Camille. "Giovanni Pierluigi da Palestrina." *Portraits et silhouettes des musiciens.* Paris: Delagrave, 1896.

Contains a short biographical article by a noted French late-nineteenth-century critic.

E0074 Bertini, Argia. "Palestrina e l'ambiente filippino." In *Atti del Convegno di Studi Palestriniani. 28 settembre–2 ottobre 1975*, ed. Francesco Luisi. Palestrina: Fondazione Giovanni Pierluigi da Palestrina, 1977. ML 410.P15C77.1975. pp. 367–380.

Historical overview of arguments for and against the supposition that Palestrina was acquainted with San Filippo Neri. Reviews circumstantial evidence and concludes that while their meeting does seem possible, it cannot be said conclusively that it happened.

E0075 Bertolotti, Antonio. *Musici alla corte del Gonzaga in Mantova dal secolo XV al XVIII. Notizie e documenti raccolti negli Archivi Mantovani.* Milan, 1890 [Facs. repr. Biblioteca Musica Bononiensis sec.III no.17. Bologna: Forni, 1978]. ML107.M29.B3.1969.

Pp. 47–55 print the complete correspondence of Palestrina with Guglielmo Gonzaga between 1568 and the duke's death in 1587, as well as additional diplomatic correspondence dealing with the composer. P. 48 has a facsimile signature, p. 51 an entire facsimile letter.

E0076 Bianchi, Lino. "Antoine de la Baume ultimo mecenate del Palestrina." *Nuova Rivista Musicale Italiana* 26 (1992): 85–90.

Traces the life and some of the activities of the cleric Antoine de la Baume, the warmly commended dedicatee of Palestrina's *Offertoria*, the last work published during the composer's lifetime.

E0077 Bianchi, Lino. "Due nuovi ritratti di Giovanni Pierluigi da Palestrina." *Nuova Rivista Musicale Italiana* 20 (1986): ii + 1–5.

Describes two recently located portraits of the composer, both currently in private collections. One, dated 1566 and painted on wood, is identified with the so-called Gorga–de Rensis portrait; the other is in oils on canvas and was formerly in the library of the Barberini Palace. Illustrations included.

E0078 Bianchi, Lino, and Karl Gustav Fellerer. *Giovanni Pierluigi da Palestrina.* Turin: ERI (RAI), 1971. 429pp. ML410.P15B5.

This dual volume is authored as follows. Bianchi composed "La vita" [the biography] (pp.11–255) and "I repertori liturgici e i madrigali profani e spirituali" [liturgical repertory in genres other than mass and motet, and the the secular and spiritual madrigals] (pp.371–421). Fellerer's contribution, translated into Italian here by Lorenzo Bianconi, deals with "Le messe e i motetti" (pp.263–370). Fellerer's material reappeared in German in *Palestrina-Studien*, while Bianchi's was amplified into the 1995 biography. The biographical section of the book contains 24 interesting plates of illustrations, and the book is accompanied by a recording of the *Missa Hodie Christus natus est a 8* and several motets (see Discography, item F0368).

E0079 Bianchi, Lino. *Giovanni Pierluigi da Palestrina nella vita, nelle opere, nel suo tempo.* Palestrina: Fondazione Giovanni Pierluigi da Palestrina, 1995. 945pp. ML410.P15B53.1995X [French trans. Malettra and Claudine Mela. Paris: Fayard, 1994. ISBN 2–213–59253–5. ML410.P15.B514.1994].

This second edition of Bianchi's outstanding study is a massive reworking and amplication of his portion of the 1971 dual biography with Fellerer, both in its biographical and analytical aspects. The opening section ("nella vita"), to p. 274, contains the most up-to-date and meticulous biographical documentation of the composer to date in a judicious narrative; pp.281–605 ("nelle opere") contain an examination of the sources, styles, and technical features of the masses; pp.607–788 study the motets; pp.793–907 ("nel suo tempo") examine not only the madrigals but Palestrina's general publication history in anthologies and the professional context in which he worked. Recommended.

E0080 Bianchi, Lino. *Guida alla mostra biografica Palestriniana*, ed. Lino Bianchi, design by Marta Daretti. Palestrina (Rome): Fondazione Giovanni Pierluigi da Palestrina/Centro di Studi Palestriniani, 1994. ML141.P15P34.1998.

A guide to the exhibition mounted in commemoration of the quatercentenary of the composer's death in 1994.

E0081 Bianchi, Lino, and Giancarlo Rostirolla, eds. *Iconografia Palestriniana: Giovanni Pierluigi da Palestrina, il suo tempo e la sua fortuna nelle immagini*. Arte Armonica: Serie IV, Iconografia e cataloghi 1. Lucca: Libreria Musicale Italiana, 1994. 300 p. ISBN 88–709-6100–1. ML88.P24I2.1995.

With about 300 illustrations and facsimile reproductions, together with numerous tables, the most extensive iconographic collection on Palestrina and his world to date.

E0082 Bianchi, Lino. "Il Palestrina." In *Musica e Musicisti nel Lazio*, ed. Renato Lefevre and Arnaldo Morelli. Lunario Romano 1986. XV. Rome: Palombi, 1985. ML290.2.L38M8.1985. pp. 137–143.

In the context of a simple narrative outlining Palestrina's life and work, Bianchi emphasizes the influence of the composer's education and experience, and asserts that, through all his appointments, in the wake of the Council of Trent Palestrina was called not merely to work as a *maestro di cappella*, but to express and attain the highest values of the Christian spirit.

E0083 Blume, Friedrich. "Lasso und Palestrina." *Deutsche Musikkultur* 9 (1944): 31–45.

Short consecutive biographies, continuing a tradition of contrasting the careers and reputations of the two great contemporaries.

E0084 Boetticher, Wolfgang. *Von Palestrina zu Bach. Erweiterte Neuausgabe.* Taschenbücher zur Musikwissenschaft 66, ed. Richard Schaal. Wilhelmshaven: Heinrichshofen, 1981. ISBN 3–7959-0306–8. ML194.B64.1981.

Chapter 1, pp.9–23, "Palestrina und Lasso," consists of two short consecutive biographies and some comparative assessment of the composers.

E0085 Brenet, Michel [Marie Bobillier]. *Palestrina.* Les Maîtres de la Musique. Paris: Alcan, 1906; 2nd ed. 1919. 3rd ed. 1926 [repr. Saint-Pierre-de-Salerne: G. Montfort, 1983]. ML410.P15B66.

Biography enriched by the recent publication of Cametti's researches and the author's own, some of which had appeared in the *Gazette musicale*. Sometimes spiritualized but often refreshingly clearheaded for the period. Also contains a short reception history, a review of the works and style, a catalogue of the early printed music, with references to the Haberl edition, and a bibliography.

E0086 Brumana, Biancamaria, and Galliano Ciliberti. *Orvieto: una cattedrale e la sua musica (1450–1610).* Historia Musicae Cultores Biblioteca 58. Florence: Olschki, 1990. ISBN 88–222–3776–5. ML3033.8.O9B7.1990.

Of interest in the present context because, in examining the roles of intellectuals, prelates, and patrons in the rich musical life of this cathedral, there is notice of activities of Monaldo Monaldeschi, a patron of early editions of Palestrina's music.

E0087 Cametti, Alberto. "Le case di Giovanni Pierluigi da Palestrina in Roma. La casa in Borgo San Pietro." *Rivista Musicale Italiana* 28 (1921): 419–432.

Contains facsimile of Palestrina autograph dated June 5, 1574, regarding payments and purchase of a house in Rome.

E0088 Cametti, Alberto. *Le case dei Pierluigi a Palestrina.* Rome: Tipografia Manuzio, 1925 [facs. repr. ed. L. Puliti and Giancarlo Rostirolla. I quaderni della Biblioteca Pierluigi 4. Palestrina: Fondazione Palestrina, 1996].

Documentation and discussion of the ownership histories of properties associated with the Pierluigi family.

E0089 Cametti, Alberto. *Cenni biografici di Giovanni Pierluigi da Palestrina compilati in occasione del terzo centenario della sua morte.* Milan: Ricordi, 1894. 142pp.

One of the first volumes to gather results of the new wave of archival and documentary research on the composer that was in motion by the 1880s. Contains much recently recovered material regarding the composer's biographical history and that of other members of the Pierluigi family, as well as comments on the relationships with the house of Gonzaga, the alleged connection with San Philip Neri, the composer's career aspirations, and the tercentenary commemorations. Also has a bibliography of writings about the composer dating from before 1895.

E0090 Cametti, Alberto. "Dove fa sepolto il Palestrina?" In *Annuario della Reale Accademia di Santa Cecilia* (1928/29): 351–369. Rome: Mezzetti, 1929.

Attempts to locate the site of Palestrina's grave. It is clear that he was buried in S. Peter's in what is now the Chapel of SS. Simon and Jude, which when facing the main altar is in the end of the left arm of the transept, but beyond this, the precise place is uncertain.

E0091 Cametti, Alberto. "Giovanni Pierluigi da Palestrina e le sue alleanze matrimoniali." *Rivista Musicale Italiana* 30 (1923): 489–510.

Actually a series of biographical notices about the family, drawn from census and parochial records of 1571, 1573, and 1587 to 1589. Describes the persons present in the Pierluigi household in 1571 and 1573, and documents the composer's three children, Rodolfo (his description by bishop

Odescalchi and his burial notice), Angelo (his marriage, his death, and the births and deaths of his two children), and Iginio (his marriage and the birth or baptismal records of his ten children).

E0092 Cametti, Alberto. "Un nuovo documento sulle origini di Giovanni Pierluigi da Palestrina: il Testamento di Jacobella Pierluigi (1527)." *Rivista Musicale Italiana* 10 (1903): 517–525 [repr. in *Atti del III Congresso Internazionale di scienze storiche* (Rome, 1–9 April 1903), 87–92. Rome: Reale Accademia dei Lincei, 1904, which were reprinted by Nendeln: Kraus, 1972].

Transcribes and discusses a will made by the composer's paternal grandmother, which contains the earliest known documentary evidence of Palestrina's life. He was then one or two years old.

E0093 Cametti, Alberto. *Palestrina.* Milan: Bottega di Poesia, 1925 [facs. repr. ed. Giancarlo Rostirolla. Rome: Torre d'Orfeo, 1994. xi + 394pp]. ML410.P15C24.

A full-length biography and general style appreciation representing the fruits of a number of years of documentary research. While his conception of the composer is still idealized and grounded in a certain spirituality, Cametti's many contributions did much to put the twentieth-century cultural reassessment of Palestrina on a modern basis.

E0094 Cametti, Alberto. "Palestrina pellicciaio." *Musica d'oggi* 4 (1922): 15.

Notice concerning a contract regarding Palestrina and his wife's fur business.

E0095 Cametti, Alberto. "Quale fama godesse ai suoi tempi il Palestrina." *Musica d'oggi* 10 (1928): 285–286.

Indicates that Palestrina and his music received special recognition and praise in a description written by Salvatore Torello of the procession accompanying the translation of the relics of S. Gregory Nazianzus to St. Peter's on June 10, 1580.

E0096 [Cametti, Alberto (unsigned in source)]. "La solenne inaugurazione del monumento a Giovanni Pierluigi da Palestrina." *Musica d'oggi* 3 (1921): 289.

Notice concerning the ceremonies associated with the unveiling of a monument to Palestrina in the Piazza Margherita, Rome, on October 2, 1921.

E0097 Campori, Giuseppe. *Delle relazioni di Orlando di Lasso e Gio. Pierluigi da Palestrina co'principi estensi.* Modena, 1869 [repr. *Atti e memorie delle R.R. Deputazioni di storia patria per le province Modenesi* 5 (1870): 47–54].

Noteworthy as an early source describing the working relationship of Palestrina to Cardinal Ippolito II d'Este.

E0098 Canal, Pietro. "Della Musica in Mantova. Notizie tratte principalmente dall'Archivio Gonzaga." In *Memorie del P. Istituto Veneto do Scienze, Lettere ed Arte*, 655–774. Venice 1880/1881.

Contains the earliest publication of much of the correspondence between Palestrina and Duke Guglielmo Gonzaga of Mantua. See also Bertolotti, item E0075.

E0099 Cascioli, Giuseppe. "Un ritratto del Palestrina." *Note d'Archivio* 1 (1924): 113–115.

Describes and reproduces a Palestrina portrait.

E0100 Cascioli, Giuseppe. *La vita e le opere di Giovanni Pierluigi da Palestrina principe della musica. Publicata nella ricorrenza del terzo centenario della sua morte. . . .* Rome: Tipografia Cooperativa Operaia, 1894. 124pp.

This biography provides a history of church music, describes Palestrina's family background, and offers an earnestly researched, albeit somewhat romanticized, account of the composer's life. While affected by a line of musical historiography reverting to Liberati and before, and while reminiscent of the suffering-heroic biographical stance taken by Baini, Cascioli's book also contains a significant amount of newly presented documentary material, describes the location of some important manuscript material in Roman archives, and notes the composer's ultimate connection to the Accademia Santa Cecilia. Also contains a list of quotations about Palestrina in parallel text–translation columns from a series of writers between the sixteenth and nineteenth centuries.

E0101 Casimiri, Raffaele. "La casa ospitale del Palestrina in Roma, nel 1586." *Note d'Archivio* 16 (1939): 256–257.

Transcribes a letter arranging for relatives of a papal singer to stay in Palestrina's house ("no less safe than in a monastery") in 1586.

E0102 Casimiri, Raffaele. "Un falso autografo palestriniano." *Note d'Archivio* 1 (1924): 163–175.

Further to item E0106, author reveals that, rather than having obtained evidence which established the date of Palestrina's birth, he was in fact the victim of a hoax. Reprints various newspaper items and exchanges of correspondence on this curious matter.

E0103 Casimiri, Raffaele. "Firmin le Bel e la data di sua morte." *Note d'Archivio* 3 (1926): 41–45.

While investigating the juvenile Palestrina's association with the church of Santa Maria Maggiore, Casimiri discovered that the composer's probable teacher, Firmin Le Bel, died between 27 and 30 December 1573.

E0104 Casimiri, Raffaele. *G. Pierluigi da Palestrina: nuova documenti biografici.* 2 vols. Rome: Psalterium, 1918–1922.

Extensive biographical material based on then-recent research and the author's own tireless investigation of Roman and other archives.

E0105 Casimiri, Raffaele. "Memorie musicali prenestine del sec. XVI." *Note d'Archivio* 1 (1924): 7–56.

Presents archival documents concerning activities of the organists and directors of music of the cathedral at Palestrina in the sixteenth and seventeenth centuries. Numerous biographical notices of the Pierluigi family in their home city during the same period.

E0106 Casimiri, Raffaele. "9 maggio 1525." *Note d'Archivio* 1 (1924): 1–6.

Presents a manuscript document purportedly in Palestrina's hand suggesting a precise birthdate for him of May 9, 1525. But see item E0102.

E0107 Casimiri, Raffaelo. "Il Palestrina e il Marenzio in un privilegio di stampa del 1584." *Note d'Archivio* 16 (1939): 253–255.

Contains Latin brief of Pope Gregory XIII granting a printing privilege for Palestrina motets as well as spiritual madrigals by Marenzio.

E0108 Casimiri, Raffaele. "Palestrina . . . e i più recenti dati biografici." *Note d'Archivio* 10 (1933): 70–71.

List of biographical facts and hypotheses meant to correct and annotate a history of music published in 1931.

E0109 Casimiri, Raffaele. "Palestrina e la scuola italiana del bel canto." *Note d'Archivio* 10 (1933): 69–70.

Interest here is in item derived from Casimiri's review of writings and notes by Raphael Molitor, who pointed out a report of surprisingly lukewarm remarks about Palestrina made by Giovanni Maria Nanino.

E0110 Cecconi, Luigi. *Di Pier Luigi da Palestrina; Memoria dell'avvocato L. C., dedicata all'eccellenza di d. Sigismondo de'principi Chigi.* Rome: Giunchi and Mordacchini, 1825 [*recte* 1826].

An early-nineteenth-century notice of the composer.

E0111 Coates, Henry. *Palestrina.* Master Musicians series. London: J. M. Dent and Sons Ltd., 1938 [repr. London, 1948. Italian trans. L. Panella Coggi. Milan, 1946]. ML410. P15C7. 1948.

A popular life-and-works, adulatory but also informed by then-recent research. A biography is followed by a study of style characteristics, which introduces a general survey of the music by genre. Still swayed by the myth, the author finds Palestrina's "worldly" ability to look after his professional and personal interests coupled with the "spiritual" qualities of his music to be evidence of a curiously inconsistent personality. Palestrina is a "culmination" figure in church music; it could not develop beyond him because his art was so closely aligned to plainchant in spirit and melody.

E0112 De Napoli, Giuseppe. *Deponendosi una corona alla casa di Pierluigi.* Palestrina, 1913.

E0113 De Napoli, Giuseppe. *Pierluigi da Palestrina (La vita e le opere).* Biblioteca del Popolo 35. Milan: Sonzogno, 1933.

E0114 Dixon, Graham. "Editorial." *Early Music* 22 (1994): 549.

An introduction to a special issue devoted to Palestrina, this item contains an English translation of a biographical notice about the composer in *Memorie Prenestine disposte in forma di annali* (1795) indicative of "the remarkable way in which [Palestrina's] fame was perpetuated."

E0115 Eitner, Robert. [untitled]. *Monatshefte für Musikgeschichte* 9 (1877): 221–223.

Cites contemporary documents in support of his own contention that, contrary to the image of Palestrina as impoverished throughout his life, the evidence is that (especially after the 1570s) the composer was in fact quite prosperous economically.

E0116 Felix, G[abrielle]. *Palestrina et la musique sacrée.* Société de Saint-Augustin. Bruges: Desclée, de Brouwer et Cie., 1895. 236pp. ML3003.F45.

Ostensibly a history of sacred music, this volume is written in a tone of meditative lay Catholic piety of the kind observed in the late nineteenth century, and with a sentimental enthusiasm that can easily become cloying. Text conveys ideas in the form of stories, legends, poetry, hymn texts, reworked liturgical material, and so forth, and line engravings of the kind associated with Cecilian publications, but with little in the way of chronology or historically oriented organization of material. Palestrina takes up roughly the last third of the volume, where there is some factual data derived from Baini or Fétis which then dissolves in a bath of dramatization of the Marcellus legend and of Palestrina's own artistic personality. Included here mainly as an interesting representative of one of the ways the composer's image was conceived in the later nineteenth century.

E0117 Fellerer, Karl Gustav. *Palestrina. Leben und Werk. Zweite, völlig umgearbeitete, vermehrte und verbesserte Auflage mit Kunstdruckabbildungen und zahlreichen Notenbeispielen im Text.* Düsseldorf: Schwann, 1960 [orig. pub. Regensburg, 1930]. 244pp.

An important study of the composer's life and works that systematically attempts to perceive biography in terms of the cultural currents of the period and Palestrina's own stylistic and technical development in particular. Close attention paid to his contrapuntal technique, the influence of Gregorian melody, and the interrelationships of music, language, and liturgical context, and supplies many musical examples. The aesthetic and spiritual tone, while clear, does not overtake other aspects of the text. Includes a synchronic table describing Palestrina's life and works, music history generally, cultural events and general history, and a work list.

E0118 Fétis, François-Joseph. "Palestrina." In *Biographie universelle des musiciens et bibliographie générale de la musique.* Vol 6, pp.428–436. Brussels, 1835–1844; 2nd ed. Paris: Librairie de Firmin Didot Frères, Fils et Cie., 1864. ML105.F4.

This article from the famed encyclopedia was an influential general source of information about the composer at the time in France. Provides biographical chronology, discussion of Trent and church music reform and the *Missa Papae Marcelli*, assessing the composer as "the greatest musician of his time." Mentions roles of Choron, Cherubini, and Fétis himself in reviving interest and performances of the music. Provides fairly comprehensive work list and indicates his knowledge of the Baini, Santini, Landsberg, and Proske collections.

E0119 Ferracci, Emilio. *Il Palestrina. Documenti di vita. Problemi e prospettive d'arte.* Accademia Internazionale "Giovanni Pierluigi da Palestrina." Collana di Studi Palestriniani 1. Rome: Edizioni del Centro di Studi Palestriniani, 1960. 131pp. ML410.P15F48.

Clear chronicle of Palestrina's life and activities, together with the publication and editing history of his works through 1960. Documents Pierluigi family connection with the house in Palestrina until 1677 and traces subsequent owners through the nineteenth century. Written as part of a campaign to motivate Italian government authorities to assist in restoration of the house as a center for Palestrina studies. Appends archival list of meticulous measurements and renovation cost estimates made in 1677 for the house.

E0120 Frey, Hermann Walter. "Das Diarium der Sixtinischen Sänger Kapelle in Rom für das Jahr 1594." *Analecta Musicologica* 14 [*Studien* 9] (1974): 445–505. ML5.A47.v.14.

Transcription of the Sistine diary entries made for the year 1594 by the *punctator* Ippolito Gambocci. Particularly notable here for their notices of Palestrina's death, funeral, and memorial service, they are also a valuable record of the lives of the singers, the daily services and activities of the choir, and the events associated with the appointment of new members and, in this case, a *maestro di cappella*.

E0121 Gallico, Claudio. "Guglielmo Gonzaga signore della musica." *Nuova Rivista Musicale Italiana* 11 (1977): 321–334.

A study of the compositions of Guglielmo Gonzaga, patron of Palestrina, interesting for its implications for Palestrina's critiques of the duke's work. Contains (pp.330–334) a catalog of compositions recognized as Guglielmo's, including hymns, masses, motets, and madrigals.

E0122 Gautier, Jean-François. *Palestrina, ou l'esthétique de l'âme du monde.* Arles: Actes Sud, 1994. ISBN 2742701680. ML410.P15G38.1994X.

Argues that insight into the cultural, aesthetic, and spiritual life of an epoch through various kinds of analysis enables a closer understanding of the composer, his works, and the age in which they are produced. The cultivation of counterpoint, a discipline involving both reason and the senses, is emblematic of that "musical" life and also characteristic of the musical history of the west generally. Also contains annotated discography of selected recordings of 1980s and 1990s (pp. 111–119). See Chapter 7.

E0123 Giazotto, Remo. "Giovanni Pierluigi da Palestrina, Quinzio Solini, Tarquinio Merula: cinque documenti inediti. . . . Tre documenti inediti sulla libera attività in Roma di Giovanni Pierluigi da Palestrina." *Nuova Rivista Musicale Italiana* 18 (1984): 625–630.

Cites three documents concerning Palestrina's activities in 1578. Claims that they have not been published; author is apparently unaware that they were previously transcribed by Kinsky. Notes that they were formerly part of the Heyer Collection and sold in 1927. The location of the first of the three is unspecified or unknown, but a facsimile of it is reproduced (p.629); the other two are presently in a private collection in Turin. See also item E0130.

E0124 Haberl, Franz Xaver. "Das Archiv der Gonzaga in Mantua, mit besonderer Rücksicht auf Giovanni Pierluigi da Palestrina." *Kirchenmusikalisches Jahrbuch* 1 (1886): 31–45.

Excerpts for German readers from Pietro Canal's "Della musica in Mantova" (1881) [see item E0098] for the period 1550 to 1587. Gives details about musical activities at the Mantuan court and the ducal church of Santa Barbara. Prints German translation of some of Palestrina's correspondence with Duke Guglielmo Gonzaga and reproduces numerous references to Palestrina and other composers in diplomatic exchanges and other archival sources.

E0125 Haberl, Franz Xaver. "Die Cardinalskommission von 1564 und Palestrinas Missa Papae Marcelli." *Kirchenmusikalisches Jahrbuch* 7 (1892): 82–97.

Argues from documentary evidence against positions held by Baini. Although the authorized purpose of the Commission of Cardinals of 1564 was the organizational reform of the papal bureaucracy, it did not specifically implement church music reform: the Council of Trent left this in the hands of provincial synods and diocesan bishops. Nor was Palestrina selected by this commission to compose three masses, among them the *Missa Papae Marcelli*, to exemplify correction of the misapplications of music for the mass, for the *Papae Marcelli* mass was in existence well before this time. This article was pivotal for the debunking of the Marcellus mass myth and is still valuable, especially when read in conjunction with more recent work by Jeppesen on the mass and Lockwood on the 1564 Commission.

E0126 Haberl, Franz Xaver. "Nach Palestrina wegen Palestrina." *Cäcilienkalendar* 4 (1879): 6–15.

Describes some of Haberl's explorations in Rome and in the town of Palestrina on a search for archival and biographical material, as well as some of his early work on the comprehensive edition. Contains transcriptions of [Latin] contracts: between the young musician and the cathedral of San Agapito; his and Lucrezia Gori's marriage contract; and a will detailing property division among the heirs of Francesco Gori (Lucrezia's father). Text contains four engravings.

E0127 Haberl, Franz Xaver. "Synchronistische Tabelle über den Lebensgang und die Werke von Giovanni Pierluigi da Palestrina und Orlando di Lasso." *Kirchenmusikalisches Jahrbuch* 9 (1894): 86–99.

Chronologically organized, this article gives then-known biographical information about Palestrina and Lasso in a parallel column format. Apparently meant in part to stimulate further interest in research into lesser-known areas of Palestrina's and particularly in Lasso's life; Haberl was well aware that the superb Lasso had had, up to that time, less general critical attention than Palestrina.

E0128 Heinemann, Michael. *Giovanni Pierluigi da Palestrina und seine Zeit.* Laaber: Laaber, 1994. ISBN 3–89007–292–5. ML410.P15H45.1994.

Recent German biography, strongly influenced by recent historiography on reception history. Also contains useful apparatus: a detailed chronological outline including parallel events in contemporary history, religion, and culture, a catalog of works, and an extensive bibliography.

E0129 King, Ethel M. *Palestrina, the Prince of Music.* Brooklyn, NY: Theo Gaus's Sons, 1965. ML410.P15.K5.

E0130 Kinsky, Georg. "Schriftstücke aus dem Palestrina-Kreis." In *Festschrift Peter Wagner zum 60. Geburtstag*, ed. Karl Weinmann. Leipzig: Breitkopf und Härtel, 1926. ML55.F47. pp.108–117.

Transcribes manuscript receipts purchased from Roman collector Carlo Lozzi in 1909 for the Wilhelm Heyer collection of Cologne. Includes three payment orders connected with Palestrina's professional activities in March to May 1578, one bearing an autograph statement.

E0131 Lindell, Robert. "Die Neubesetzung der Hofkapellmeisterstelle am Kaiserhof in den Jahren 1567–1568: Palestrina oder Monte?" *Studien zur Musikwissenschaft* 36 (1985): 35–52.

The story that Philippe de Monte obtained the position of *Kapellmeister* at the imperial court because Palestrina, who was previously considered for the position, had asked too high a salary, is well known. Although this is fundamentally accurate, Lindell notes that Monte and Roussel were both being considered before Palestrina entered the ranks, and that Palestrina's case moved so far along because the imperial court had had trouble communicating with Monte, who was in Naples at the time. It is also likely that Palestrina did not seriously want to relocate, whereas Monte might have found the imperial position naturally more congenial because of his Flemish ethnic and cultural background.

E0132 Lockwood, Lewis, and Jessie Ann Owens. "Palestrina, Giovanni Pierluigi da." *The New Grove Dictionary of Music and Musicians*, ed. Stanley Sadie. Vol 14, pp. 118–137. London: MacMillan, 1980.

See item E0133.

E0133 Lockwood, Lewis, and Jessie Ann Owens. "Palestrina." In *The New Grove High Renaissance Masters. Josquin, Palestrina, Lassus, Victoria, Byrd.* New York: Norton, 1984. ISBN 0–393–01689-7. ML390.H622.1984t. pp. 93–153.

A somewhat expanded and updated version of the fine article published in the *New Grove Dictionary of Music and Musicians* (see item E0132). Lockwood wrote the main text; Owens prepared the work list.

E0134 Lunelli, Renato. "Iconografia monteverdiana." *Rivista Musicale Italiana* 47 (1943): 38–45.

A portrait in the Ferdinandeum Museum, Innsbruck, once thought to be of Palestrina, is demonstrated to be Claudio Monteverdi.

E0135 Mischiati, Oscar. "Minima praenestina: un ritratto di Palestrina alla Biblioteca Casanatense." In *Atti del II Convegno Internazionale di Studi Palestriniani. Anno Europeo della Musica. 3–5 maggio 1986*, ed. Lino Bianchi and Giancarlo Rostirolla. Palestrina: Fondazione Giovanni Pierluigi da Palestrina/Centro di Studi Palestriniani, 1991. ML410.P15C77.1986. pp. 610–611.

Description of a Palestrina portrait owned by the Casanatense Library, bequeathed to it by Giuseppe Baini in 1837.

E0136 Molitor, Raphael. *Die nachtridentische Choralreform zu Rom Ein Beitrag zur Musikgeschichte des XVI. und XVII. Jahrhunderts.* Leipzig: Leuckart, 1902. 2 vols [facs. ed. Hildesheim: Georg Olms, 1977. ML3084.M72.1901A].

Vol 1, *Die Choral-Reform unter Gregor XII,* pp.216–305, deals with the period in which Palestrina and Zoilo actually worked on the reform of chant books. Vol 2, *Die Choral-Reform unter Klemens VIII und Paul V*, pp.1–57, deals with the fate of the chant books between 1585 and 1605. This includes an assessment of Palestrina's contribution to the books as of 1594, and continues with an account of the series of lawsuits brought by Iginio Pierluigi against the publisher Raimondi and members of the Camera Apostolica. The lawsuits took place in three phases between 1596 and 1602, and were decided, despite appeals, in favor of Raimondi.

E0137 Naumann, Emil. *Italienische Tondichter von Palestrina bis auf die Gegenwart. Eine Reihe von Vortragen, gehalten in 1874 u. 1875.* Berlin: R. Oppenheim, 1876. ML390.N345.

Not reviewed.

E0138 O'Regan, Noel. "Orlando di Lasso and Rome: Personal Contacts and Musical Influences." In *Orlando di Lasso Studies*, ed. Peter Bergquist. Cambridge, UK: Cambridge University Press, 1999. ISBN 0–521–59387–5. ML410.L3075. pp. 132–157.

In examining Lasso's relations with Rome, the article discusses the possibility of musical cross-fertilization between Lasso and Palestrina. This could have been effected both personally, through points of contact such as their common connections to major Roman basilicas and to the Arciconfraternita del Santissimo Crocifisso, and through the influence of compositions by Lasso on Roman style, particularly with respect to newer textural and harmonic features, especially in the areas of polychoral music and the treatment of musical imitation or parody.

E0139 O'Regan, Noel. "Palestrina, a Musician and Composer in the Market-Place." *Early Music* 22 (1994): 551–572.

Discusses changing employment conditions of church musicians in later sixteenth-century Rome. Describes Palestrina's known freelance activity, which included providing music for processions in Rome in the 1550s and for the Confraternity of SS. Trinità in 1576 and 1578.

E0140 O'Regan, Noel. "Palestrina and the Oratory of Santissima Trinità dei Pellegrini." In *Atti del II Convegno Internazionale di Studi Palestriniani. Anno*

Europeo della Musica. 3–5 maggio 1986, ed. Lino Bianchi and Giancarlo Rostirolla. Palestrina: Fondazione Giovanni Pierluigi da Palestrina/Centro di Studi Palestriniani, 1991. ML410.P15C77.1986. pp. 95–121.

English and Italian texts; Italian translation pp.109–120 by Sophie Le Castel. Documents Palestrina's responsibilities in connection with the musical life of the confraternity and oratory of SS. Trinità dei Pellegrini in the 1570s, including preparation of music for Lent, Holy Week, and for processions.

E0141 Pedrell, Felipe. "Palestrina." In *Músicos contemporáneos y de otros tempos*. Paris: Sociedade de Ediciones Literarias y Artísticas. Librería Paul Ollendorf, 1910. ML60.P373. pp. 325–330.

Item is dated 1908 in text. Refers to Brenet's new *Palestrina* (see item E0085) as putting to rest some of the legendary material about the composer by presenting documentary evidence. Reviews literature on Palestrina's date of birth, the myth of the *Missa Papae Marcelli*, the composer's alleged poverty, and other comparable material.

E0142 Pedrell, Felipe. "Palestrina y Victoria." In *Homenaje a Menendez y Pelayo en el año vigésimo de su professorado*. Madrid: Libreria General de Victoriano Suarez, 1899. PQ6004.M4. pp. 149–152.

Short comparison of styles of Palestrina and Victoria.

E0143 Pertica, Domenico. "Il Restauro della Casa del Palestrina." In *Il Palestrina. Bolletino trimestrale del Centro Internazionale di Studi Palestriniani* 3 (1963): 14–20.

Details plans for restoration of the house in Palestrina where the composer's family lived and where he is thought to have been born. Describes confirming the identity of the house, its fate over the centuries, and the planned steps to be taken during the actual renovation.

E0144 Prod'homme, Jacques-Gabriel, ed. *Écrits de musiciens (Xve-XVIIIe siècle)*. Paris: Mercure de France, 1912 [3rd ed. repr. New York: Da Capo Press, 1985]. ML90.P7.

Pp. 56–63 contain French translations of the dedications of the *First Book of Motets a 5, 6, 7* to Ippolito d'Este (1567), of the *Fourth Book of Motets* (*Canticum canticorum*) to Pope Gregory XIII (1584), and of the *Hymnus totius anni* to Pope Sixtus V (1589).

E0145 Pugliese, Annunziato. "La cappella musicale del cardinale Ippolito d'Este." In *La Cappella Musicale nell'Italia della Controriforma. Atti del Convegno (Cento 1989)*, ed. Oscar Mischiati and Paolo Russo. Quaderni della RidM 27. Florence: Olschki, 1993. ISSN 0394–4395–27. ML3033.2.C65.1989X. pp. 381–394.

Chronicles the activities and personnel of Cardinal Ippolito's chapel, for which Palestrina was *maestro* during the years 1567 to 1571.

E0146 Pyne, Zoë Kendrick. *Giovanni Pierluigi da Palestrina: His Life and Times*. London: Lane, 1922 [repr. Westport, CT: Greenwood Press, 1970]. ML410.P15.P9.

An intelligent and readable biographical narrative in English that fleshes out the then relatively recent documentary researches of Cametti, Casimiri, and numerous others working in the years from 1880 to 1920, while managing for the better part to avoid hagiographical excess. Narrative is balanced with information conveying some sense of papal, court, and cultural life in the sixteenth century.

E0147 Raugel, Félix. *Palestrina.* Les Musiciens Célèbres. Paris: Librairie Renouard/Henri Laurens, 1930. ML410.P15R38.

Biography containing an interesting blend of early twentieth-century archival research with some imaginative embroidery and "great man" historiography. Moves away from the savior myth and deals with some qualities of compositional style, but also contains imaginary conversations and other romantic vestiges.

E0148 Ramella, Carlo. "*Puer qui natus est,* mottetto a cinque voci di Guglielmo Gonzaga." *Rivista Internazionale di Musica Sacra* 15 (1994): 254–270.

Discussion and transcription of a motet preserved in the Santa Barbara *fondo* of the library of the Verdi Conservatory in Milan (numbered S.B.8), a work also printed during Duke Guglielmo's lifetime. Interesting as an examination of the musical accomplishments of Palestrina's patron, for Palestrina is known to have provided critical advice on certain of Guglielmo's compositions at the duke's particular request.

E0149 Samson, Joseph. *Palestrina ou la poésie de l'exactitude*. Geneva, 1940 [repr. Geneva: Henn, 1950. ML410.P15S15.1950].

Investigates the animating spirit of Palestrina's music, which uses church liturgy as a framework. His music's constructive elements are cantus firmus, canon, and "cyclic" themes, and its structural unity depends on a succession of related ideas brought into a just relationship with the rhythms and meanings of the text. Concludes that both spiritually and technically Palestrina was attached to the past.

E0150 Schmid, Theodor. "Principes musicae—Fürsten der Tonkunst." *Kirchenmusikalisches Jahrbuch* 20 (1895): 49–76.

Consecutive biographies and observations on Palestrina and Lasso, noted by the author as the most extensive and fitting attempt of its kind to date. In the Palestrina section is a review of his life and early reception history, and observations on the issues of Trent and church music reform, a résumé of the history of the revision and publication of the Medicean gradual, and thoughts on the composer's ability to set a text.

E0151 Schmitz, Eugen. *Palestrina.* Leipzig: Breitkopf und Härtel, 1914 [repr. 1953].

Not reviewed.

E0152 Schwartz, Rudolf. "Zur Partitur im 16. Jahrhunderts." *Archiv für Musikwissenschaft* 2 (1920): 73–78.

Noted here as it contains the transcription of Palestrina's letter of March

3, 1576, to Guglielmo Gonzaga, in which the composer mentions putting music into partitura in order to study it. The article, a study of the practice of scoring in the sixteenth century, provides context for this remark.

E0153 Sharp, Geoffrey Brinsley. *Lassus and Palestrina.* Novello Short Biographies. London: Novello, 1972. ML410 L3 S47. pp. 12–20.

Short biography, breezy in tone, intended for amateurs and audiophiles.

E0154 Simi Bonini, Eleanora. "Minima archivalia: Giovanni Pierluigi da Palestrina tra la cappella di S. Giovanni in Laterano e la cappella di S. Maria Maggiore." In *Atti del II Convegno Internazionale di Studi Palestriniani. Anno Europeo della Musica. 3–5 maggio 1986*, ed. Lino Bianchi and Giancarlo Rostirolla. Palestrina: Fondazione Giovanni Pierluigi da Palestrina/Centro di Studi Palestriniani, 1991. ML410.P15.C77.1986. pp. 65–79.

Biographical notices from archives of San John Lateran and Santa Mary Major relevant to Palestrina's adolescence and apprenticeship. Transcriptions in appendix.

E0155 Summers, William J. "*The Compagnia dei Musici di Roma* 1584–1604: a Preliminary Report." *Current Musicology* 34 (1982): 7–25.

Discusses early history of this confraternity, of which most of the preeminent Roman musicians, including Palestrina, were members. Relatively little is known about its influence on musical, academic, and court life in Italy, but its membership and activities have been somewhat clarified. Includes table of members, table of printed anthologies with music by members; discusses other published compilations where the membership of the society was strongly represented.

E0156 Super, Antoine. *Palestrina (G. Pierluigi): Étude historique et critique sur la musique religieuse. Précédée d'une lettre adressée à l'auteur par un maître en liturgie Mgr. Isard, l'éminent Éveque du diocèse de Annecy.* Paris: V. Retaux, 1892. xxiv + 82pp. ML410.P15S86.

Not reviewed.

E0157 Torrigio, Francesco Maria. *Le sacre Grotte Vaticane*. Rome: Mascardi, 1630.

Contains early information, including the note (part 2, p.166) that Palestrina was buried in St. Peter's before the altar in the chapel of SS. Simon and Jude.

E0158 Venuti, Massimo. "Inedito Palestrina nel quarto centenario della morte." *Rassegna Musicale Curci* 47.2 (1994): 10–13.

Notes that Palestrina had a much stronger and economically astute personality than is often popularly imagined. Suggests that Palestrina's artistic mandate was not so much the comprehensibility of text *per se* as the evolution of a personal *modus operandi*, where the listener would not primarily contemplate the complexities of technique and structure, but rather develop a personal rapport with text and music.

E0159 Walter, Anton. "Palestrina und Orlando. Eine kunst- und culturgeschichtliche Studie zum dritten Centenarium ihres Todesjahres." *Historisch-politische Blätter* 113 (1894): 777–804, 873–879.

A comparative study of the two composers, for the third centenary of the death of both.

E0160 Walter, Anton. "Dr. Witts Zeugnis für Palestrina und Orlando. Eine ästhetisch-liturgische Jubiläumsgabe." *Kirchenmusikalisches Jahrbuch* 9 (1894): 48–59.

A comparative study; see also item E0159.

E0161 Weidinger, Josef. "Palestrina und Lasso, zwei Classiker der Kirchenmusik." *Zeitschrift für katholische Theologie* 21 (1897): 503–511.

Another comparative study of the works and style of these two composers.

E0162 Weiss, Piero, ed. *Letters of Composers through Six Centuries*. Philadelphia: Chilton Book Company, 1967. 622pp. ML90.W44.

Pp. 16–17 contain English translations of two letters from Palestrina to Duke Guglielmo Gonzaga, dated February 2, 1568, and March 3, 1570, respectively. Comments on letters on p. 480.

E0163 Weinmann, Karl. *Palestrinas Geburtsjahr. Ein historisch-kritische Untersuchung*. Regensburg: Pustet, 1915.

A careful review of the evidence for Palestrina's date of birth—which is still not precisely known—and writings up to the publication date on the subject.

E0164 Weinmann, Karl. "Die päpstliche Kapelle unter Paul IV." *Archiv für Musikwissenschaft* 2 (1920): 54–72.

Description and history of the reform program for the Sistine Chapel under Paul IV, who is noted in this context as the pope who removed Palestrina from the roster because of his married status. Provides a list of the singers present in 1555, each of whom has a biographical chronology of activities, as well as a (Latin) transcription of the Sistine diaries from May 23, 1555, to August 18, 1559, the day Paul IV died.

III. Studies of Sources, Music, and Style

E0165 Acciai, Giovanni. "La Canzone alla Vergine del Petrarca nell' interpretazione madrigalistica di Cipriano de Rore e Giovanni Pierluigi da Palestrina." In *Atti del II Convegno Internazionale di Studi Palestriniani. Anno Europeo della Musica. 3–5 maggio 1986*, ed. Lino Bianchi and Giancarlo Rostirolla. Palestrina: Fondazione Giovanni Pierluigi da Palestrina/Centro di Studi Palestriniani, 1991. ML410.P15C77.1986. pp. 167–174.

Studies the treatment of modality, melodic design, disposition of cadences, rhetorical figures, and musical symbolism in two settings of

Petrarch's *Vergine* poetic cycle by Rore and Palestrina respectively. In both cases the verses are treated as a single great lyric scheme composed of several movements, each with its own stylistic profile. Apart from their differences in cadential treatment, Palestrina's cycle is distinguished by modal subtleties and clear perception of poetic construction, while Rore's is notable for the richness of its motivic technique, its musical-rhetorical symbolism, and stylization.

E0166 Ackermann, Peter. "Motette und Madrigal. Palestrinas Hohelied-Motetten im Spannungsfeld gegenreformatorischer Spiritualität." In *Festschrift für Winfried Kirsch zum 65. Geburtstag*, ed. Peter Ackermann, Ulrike Kienzle, and Adolf Nowak. Tutzing: Hans Schneider, 1996. pp. 49–64.

Examining the modal, sectional and the richly expressive relationships among the motets of the *Canticum canticorum* (Book IV of the motets for five voices), Ackermann perceives the use of cyclic closure in the structure of the series as a whole. He considers that all these factors emphasize the expression of a dramatic concept which causes *Canticum canticorum* to transcend the typical stylistic and structural boundaries of the motet as a genre. In the case of extraliturgical texts such as these, the rules for motets (note values, modality, text expression) can be subject to such variation, and here, in fact, Palestrina uses style elements associated with the madrigal. This bridging of genres is a response to his sense of the modified parameters the texts allow, and the works are evidence of his sensitive and dynamic conception of the relationship of genre and style.

E0167 Ackermann, Peter. "Die Werke Palestrinas im Repertoire der Cappella Sistina." In *Collectanea II. Studien zur Geschichte der päpstlichen Kapelle. Tagungsbericht Heidelberg 1989*, ed. Bernhard Janz. Capellae Apostolicae Sixtinaeque Collectanea Acta Monumenta 4. Vatican City: Biblioteca Apostolica Vaticana, 1994. ISBN 88–210–0655–7. ML3051.V3C65.1994. pp. 405–430.

Notes that 40 percent of the items listed in Llorens's Cappella Sistina catalog contain items by Palestrina. This includes nearly all the printed music published during his lifetime, as well as 101 manuscript items. Main part of the article is a study of the manuscripts and their contents, organized by date of copying or compilation. Notes that the appearance of Palestrina items falls into phases: from around 1563 to around 1616, 1616 to 1687 and the early eighteenth century, and the middle decades of the eighteenth century. Includes a list of the Palestrina motets that were assigned new texts from the 1740s to the 1760s and indicates some of their concomitant rhythmic modifications.

E0168 Ahnjeld, Paul Floyd. "The Madrigals of Horato Fáa." D.M.A. thesis, University of Illinois, Urbana-Champaign, 1988. DA 8823071.

Compares Fáa's cyclic madrigals with Palestrina's and argues that Fáa's are more like Wert's.

E0169 Allaire, Gaston Georges. "Rediscovering Modulations in the Secular and Sacred Works of Palestrina." *Recercare* 6 (1994): 5–40.

Examines the structural dimension of the hexachord system and implications for the mode system in Glarean's *Dodecachordon.* Notes the function of the Guidonian hand as a contemporary frame of reference for reading polyphonic music, and studies conventions regarding signatures and cadences in the performance practice of the music. Scores of *Vestiva i colli a 5* and *O quam suavis a 4* (printed pp.25–37) are used to discuss and illustrate the main points of discussion.

E0170 Alwes, Chester. "Palestrina's Style: the Art of Balance." *Choral Journal* 35.1 (1994): 13–17.

Discusses aspects of Palestrina's style that caused it to be considered the epitome of sixteenth-century modal counterpoint: distinctive yet carefully controlled dissonance treatment, and flexibility in use of textures and in treatment of text stresses and accents. *Missa brevis* examined as case in point.

E0171 Angelis, Lepanto de. "Musiche manoscritte inedite del sec. XVI–XVII dell'archivio del Pio Sodalizio dei Piceni in Roma." *Note d'Archivio* 16 (1939): 29–31.

Inventory of unpublished manuscripts, many anonymous, containing works by sixteenth- and seventeenth-century Roman polyphonists. Among them is a copy of Palestrina motet *Domine quando veneris a 4*.

E0172 Anglès, Higinio. "Palestrina y los 'Magnificat' de Morales." *Anuario musical* 8 (1953): 153–166.

Discusses several *Magnificat*s by Cristobal de Morales, some verses of which Palestrina elaborated with one or two *si placet* parts in a manuscript presently located in the Cappella Giulia fondo of the Vatican Library. Analyzes Palestrina's technique and compares differences in color and temperament with Morales's original.

E0173 Antonowytsch, Miroslaw. *Die Motette Benedicta es von Josquin des Prez und die Messen super Benedicta von Willaert, Palestrina, de le Hèle und de Monte*. Utrecht: J. R. van Rossum, 1951. ML3003.A58.1951.

A comparative study of how Josquin's motet *Benedicta es* was parodied in four masses by Willaert, Palestrina, de le Hèle, and de Monte. Includes analysis of the motet and its dissemination in manuscript and printed sources, and a movement-by-movement study of the relationship of the four masses to the model. Argues that in several technical aspects the influence of Josquin on Palestrina is not confined to this particular imitation mass but can be observed in other music of Palestrina's early creative period.

E0174 Apfel, Ernst. "Zur Entstehungsgeschichte des Palestrinasatzes." *Archiv für Musikwissenschaft* 14 (1957): 30–45.

Argues that the key to understanding the origin of the observant contrapuntal technique associated with Palestrina and his successors is found by examining the evolution of various kinds of two- and three-voice cadence formulas and how they served to establish the general structure of a free composition.

E0175 Auda, Antoine. "La mesure dans la messe 'L'homme armé' de Palestrina." *Acta Musicologica* 13 (1941): 39–59.

Argues vehemently against Casimiri's transcription of the problematic notation of the *L'homme armé* mass in vol 3 of the second edition of Palestrina's works.

E0176 Auda, Antoine. "La prolation dans l'édition princeps de la Messa *L'homme armé* de Palestrina et sa résolution dans l'édition de 1599." *Scriptorium* 4 (1950): 85–102.

Auda's concluding publication dealing with the contentious notation of Palestrina's *L'homme armé* mass, based on a comparison of primary source printings.

E0177 Auda, Antoine. "Le 'Tactus' dans la Messe *L'homme armé* de Palestrina." *Acta Musicologica* 14 (1942): 27–73.

Auda's response to Casimiri's *La polifonia vocale*. See also items E0195 and E0196.

E0178 Barbieri, Patrizio. "*Chiavette* and Modal Transposition in Italian Practice (c. 1500–1837)." *Recercare* 3 (1991): 5–79.

Historical survey of the use of transposition clefs, or *chiavette*, in Italy, with lucid and extensive documentation from theoretical sources. Examines their purposes and their relationship to the changing mode systems of the seventeenth century, and addresses questions of vocal tessitura and clef groupings in performance practice. Although *chiavette* largely fell out of use in the mid-seventeenth century, they were retained by academic musicians and followers of the *stile alla Palestrina* into the 1800s.

E0179 Barbieri, Patrizio. "On a Continuo Organ Part Attributed to Palestrina." *Early Music* 22 (1994): 587–606.

Documents evidence of origins of services in pontifical private apartments around 1585. Notes practice of intabulating polyphonic vocal compositions and early liturgical appearances of *basso per l'organo*, and offers hypotheses for their use; also describes the type and registration of organs used in Rome.

E0180 Barblan, Guglielmo, and Agostino Zecca Laterza. "The Tarasconi Codex in the Library of the Milan Conservatory." *Musical Quarterly* 60 (1974): 195–221.

Discussion and index of the Milan Biblioteca del Conservatorio di Musica Giuseppe Verdi MS s.s., known as the *Tarasconi* or *Clerici* codex, a mid-latter-sixteenth century MS madrigal collection of Parmesan provenance containing works by 33 composers. Provides a lengthy list of concordances and modern editions of contents. Eight madrigals (nos. 69, 71, 101–103, 116, 154, 204) are ascribed to Palestrina, the attributions of two of which (69 and 204) are noted as "G.P." and considered uncertain.

E0181 Baroffio, Giacomo Bonifacio. "Palestrina e il canto gregoriano: l'Innodia."

In *Atti del II Convegno Internazionale di Studi Palestriniani. Anno Europeo della Musica. 3–5 maggio 1986*, ed. Lino Bianchi and Giancarlo Rostirolla. Palestrina: Fondazione Giovanni Pierluigi da Palestrina/Centro di Studi Palestriniani, 1991. ML410.P15C77.1986. pp. 23–26.

Notes that Palestrina's polyphonic hymns were mostly appropriate to vespers services and were suitable for the propers of various religious orders. Suggests that Gregorian melodies, particularly hymns and sequences, were sung in a mensurally rhythmic manner, not a free oratorical one.

E0182 Belli, Antonio. "I madrigali profani del Palestrina." *Il Palestrina. Bolletino trimestrale del Centro Internazionale di Studi Palestriniani* 3 (1963): 9–13.

Traces the history of Palestrina's madrigal publications. Asks whether the works are largely neglected due to their incompatibility with Palestrina's image as a composer of sacred music, because of his own belief in their moral profanity, or due to an inability of the public to see that they are the product of a solidarity with all aspects of Christian humanist experience. Asserts that while they are not overly innovative, they exhibit refined skill, "color" and "*imitazione della natura*" in a universal sense.

E0183 Besutti, Paola. "Giovanni Pierluigi da Palestrina e la liturgia mantovana." In *Atti del II Convegno Internazionale di Studi Palestriniani. Anno Europeo della Musica. 3–5 maggio 1986*, ed. Lino Bianchi and Giancarlo Rostirolla. Palestrina: Fondazione Giovanni Pierluigi da Palestrina/Centro di Studi Palestriniani, 1991. ML410.P15C77.1986. pp. 157–164.

Discussion of music composed for the palatine basilica of S. Barbara in Mantua. "Neo-Gregorian" chant melodies expressly composed for the Mantuan liturgy demonstrate modal considerations suggesting they were conceived with possible polyphonic elaboration in mind. Palestrina's polyphonic masses for Mantua constitute a unicum within his production due to the contrapuntal treatment used, the particulars of the plainchant on which they are constructed, and their unusual alternatim manner of performance.

E0184 Bewerunge, Heinrich. "Der metrische Bau der Themen Palestrinas." *Musica Divina. Monatschrift für Kirchenmusik* 5 (1917): 72–75; 6 (1918): 133–140, 173–179, 211–221.

Not reviewed.

E0185 Bianchi, Lino, and Giancarlo Rostirolla, eds. *Atti del II Convegno Internazionale di Studi Palestriniani. [Palestrina e la sua presenza nella musica e nella cultura europeo dal suo tempo ad oggi. 3–5 maggio 1986]*. Palestrina: Fondazione Giovanni Pierluigi da Palestrina/Centro di Studi Palestriniani, 1991. ML410.P15C77.1986.

A compilation of papers presented at the conference "Palestrina and his presence in music and in European culture from his time to today," European Year of Music, May 3–5, 1986. Papers in this volume are individually indexed in the present bibliography.

E0186 Bini, Annalisa. "Catalogo della mostra bibliografica-documentaria" In *Atti* *del II Convegno Internazionale di Studi Palestriniani. [Palestrina e la sua presenza nella musica e nella cultura europeo dal suo tempo ad oggi. 3–5 maggio 1986].* Palestrina: Fondazione Giovanni Pierluigi da Palestrina/Centro di Studi Palestriniani, 1991. ML410.P15C77.1986. pp. 631–710.

Catalogue of exhibition displayed at the 1986 conference.

E0187 Blume, Jürgen. *Geschichte der mehrstimmigen Stabat-Mater-Vertonungen.* Musikwissenschaftliche Schriften 3. Munich: Emil Katzbichler, 1992. 2 vols. ISBN 3873971224. ML3090.B6.1992.

Vol 1, pp.52–66, and vol 2, pp. 29–39, contain useful studies of Palestrina's *Stabat Mater* settings as well as discussion of works that Palestrina's setting immediately influenced.

E0188 Bobbitt, Richard. "Harmonic Tendencies in the *Missa Papae Marcelli*." *Music Review* 16 (1955): 273–288.

Attempts to understand compositional processes in the *Gloria* and *Credo* of this mass in terms of an idiosyncratic theory of harmonic tonality. Appreciates some characteristic qualities of the composer's vertical structures, although analysis is historically somewhat decontextualized.

E0189 Böker-Heil, Norbert. "Der Zustand polyphoner Strukturen: ein Beispiel automatischer Stilbeschreibung." In *International Musicological Society. Report of the Eleventh Congress, Copenhagen 1972*, ed. Henrik Glahn, Søren Sørensen, and Peter Ryom. Copenhagen: Wilhelm Hansen, 1974. ISBN 87–7455–026–8. ML36.I6.1972. pp. 108–120.

Uses madrigal *Vestiva i colli* in comparison with other works to demonstrate how computer software can be used as a means of establishing style-specific formal constants in polyphonic music that are difficult to investigate and elaborate by other means.

E0190 Brenet, Michel. "L'auteur des *Répons* de Palestrina." *Gazette Musicale*, June 20 and 27, 1897.

A response to Tiersot's insistence that the set of 27 responsories in vol 32 of the "Haberl" edition, declared doubtful by Haberl, must be by Palestrina. Tiersot continued the exchange and continued to hold his view through the 1920s. See below, item E0359.

E0191 Bujic, Bojan. "Palestrina, Willaert, Arcadelt and the Art of Imitation." *Recercare* 10 (1998): 105–131.

Investigates factors which could explain some similarities between Willaert's and Palestrina's madrigal *Amor, Fortuna, e la mia mente.* A close reading of the rhetorical techniques of Petrarch's sonnet together with contemporary critical commentaries suggest that Willaert associated the sonnet conceits with musical motifs that create a system of reference throughout his composition. Palestrina's version, while sharing several musical traits and structural details with Willaert's and indicating a close reading of the text, pays less attention to refinements of rhetoric. It is impossible to ascertain that Willaert's version influenced Palestrina's directly, but similarities in the openings of both madrigals argue for their possible common knowledge of models and imitative procedures associated with this kind of setting, likely derived from Arcadelt.

E0192 Carver, Anthony F. *Cori Spezzati: The Development of Sacred Polychoral Music to the Time of Schütz.* Cambridge, UK: Cambridge University Press, 1988. 2 vols.

A study of the historical evolution of the technique of writing for separated choirs, including theoretical discussions by Vicentino and Zarlino and copious examples of its practical development. Vol 1, pp. 108–118, contains a valuable discussion of Palestrina's polychoral music in several genres; vol 2 pp. 86–92, reprints the polychoral motet *Videntes stellam Magi* from vol 33 of the Casimiri-Bianchi complete edition.

E0193 Casimiri, Raffaele. *Il "Codice 59" dell'Archivio Musicale Lateranense, autografo di Giov. Pierluigi da Palestrina.* Rome: Tipografia Poliglotta Vaticana, 1919.

A detailed inventory and study of the principal surviving Palestrina autograph: its provenance and history; observations on the composer's working process; editorial corrections of works published in the Haberl edition; editions of some previously unpublished works.

See also cross entry in Chapter 4, "Casimiri . . . Codice" for a list of the works published in the volume.

E0194 Casimiri, Raffaele. "Un dibattito musicologico a proposito della missa *L'homme armé* del Palestrina." *Note d'Archivio* 20 (1943): 18–42.

A continuing refutation of Antoine Auda's position (see item E0175) on the mensural interpretation of selected passages in the *L' homme armé* mass, in 25 points. This was the effective end of the Auda-Casimiri exchange; Casimiri died soon after completing this article, although Auda continued to publish on the subject into the 1950s.

E0195 Casimiri, Raffaele. "Il 'Kyrie' de la Messa *L'homme armè* di Giov. Pierluigi da Palestrina e una trascrizione errata." *Note d'Archivio* 10 (1933): 101–108.

Discussion of perceived errors in the Haberl transcription of this work. Also a mission statement describing the aims and purposes of Casimiri's "national edition" of Palestrina's works, which purports to modify and correct the errors of the Haberl edition in light of the rules of historical criticism and the latest discoveries of musicological research.

E0196 Casimiri, Raffaele. *La polifonia vocale del sec. XVI e la sua trascrizione musicale moderna. A proposito di un critica di Antoine Auda.* Rome: Psalterium, 1942.

A summary statement of Casimiri's views in the controversy with Auda over correct transcription of some aspects of sixteenth-century music, a debate that by this time had continued for more than ten years.

E0197 Casimiri, Raffaele. "La *Missa Cantantibus Organis Caecilia* a 12 voci di Giovanni Pierluigi da Palestrina e de'suoi scolari." *Note d'Archivio* 8 (1931): 233–244.

Discusses mass for three choirs, movements of which were composed by Palestrina (part of the *Gloria*), Annibale Stabile, Francesco Soriano, Andrea Dragoni, Ruggero Giovanelli, Prospero Santini, and Curzio Mancini, based on material from Palestrina's 5–part motet *Cantantibus organis*.

E0198 Casimiri, Raffaele. "Il sepolcro dei cantori pontifici nelle Chiesa Nuova di Roma." *Note d'Archivio* 3 (1926): 221–232.

Description, with two illustrations dated 1640 and 1792, of the monument to papal singers who were buried at Santa Maria in Vallicella (Chiesa Nuova), together with a commentary on the musical canon incised on it. Although several pre-twentieth century writers believed that the canon was composed by Palestrina, it was most likely written by Gregorio Allegri. Casimiri transcribed the resolved canon on pp.230–232.

E0199 Casimiri, Raffaele. "I 'XXVII Responsoria' di M.A. Ingegneri, attribuiti a Giov. Pierluigi da Palestrina." *Note d'Archivio* 3 (1926): 17–40, plus 4 unnumbered pages of tipped-in examples.

Examines primary sources, early prints, and internal stylistic evidence, particularly chromatic use, to argue that 27 responsories, attributed to Palestrina since about 1750, were in fact composed by Marc' Antonio Ingegneri. Another response to Tiersot's insistence that the Palestrina attribution was correct. See item E0359.

E0200 Cattin, Giulio. "Scelta di testi e 'cantus firmi' nel primo libro dei mottetti di Palestrina." In *Atti del II Convegno Internazionale di Studi Palestriniani. Anno Europeo della Musica. 3–5 maggio 1986*, ed. Lino Bianchi and Giancarlo Rostirolla. Palestrina: Fondazione Giovanni Pierluigi da Palestrina/Centro di Studi Palestriniani, 1991. ML410.P15C77.1986. pp. 141–153.

Analysis of first book of motets, with respect to liturgical placement of texts and the presence or absence of a cantus firmus in individual settings. Of 36 motets, only 7 employ a cantus firmus. Notes that use of a Gregorian cantus firmus as an element of musical structure is more frequent in Palestrina's successive motet publications.

E0201 Cavicchi, Adriano. "Appunti sulla prassi esecutiva della musica sacra nella seconda metà del XVI secolo con riferimenti alla musica del Palestrina." In *Atti del Convegno di Studi Palestriniani. 28 settembre–2 ottobre 1975*, ed. Francesco Luisi. Palestrina: Fondazione Giovanni Pierluigi da Palestrina, 1977. ML 410.P15C77.1975. pp. 295–311.

A judicious exploration, with roundtable discussion, of questions surrounding the practical performance of late sixteenth-century music, with reference to contemporary evidence: the great diversity in manner and taste from one place to another; differences in pitch levels, timbres, and phrasing and accentuation; number of players or singers per part, and solo/chorus or *concertato* alternations; improvisation of ornaments and counterpoints; accompaniment by organ and instruments; differences in approach between sacred and profane music.

E0202 Cavicchi, Adriano. "Una sconosciuta messa funebre di probabile attribuzione palestriniana." In *Atti del Convegno di Studi Palestriniani. 28 settembre–2 ottobre 1975*, ed. Francesco Luisi. Palestrina: Fondazione Giovanni Pierluigi da Palestrina, 1977. ML 410.P15C77.1975. pp. 411–414.

Notice of a funeral mass *a voci pari* (3 tenors and bass) which is ascribed to Palestrina in a manuscript located in Ferrara, Biblioteca Comunale Ariostea. States belief that attribution is correct, calls for further stylistic study, and suggests that work could have been written for the Ferrarese Accademia della Morte.

E0203 *Census-Catalogue of Manuscript Sources of Polyphonic Music, 1400–1550.* American Institute of Musicology/Neuhausen-Stuttgart, Hänssler, 1979–1988. 5 vols. ISBN 01967037. ML135.R46.1979t.

A census containing detailed descriptions and bibliography for manuscripts containing music by composers active within the dates indicated, listed by city and site of holding.

E0204 Cerone, Pedro. *El Melopeo y el Maestro. Tractado de Musica Theorica y Pratica.* Naples: J. B. Gargoni and L. Nucci, 1613 [facs. repr. Bologna: Forni, 1969]. MT6.C35.1971.

Contains (p.1013 *et seq.*) an extensive discussion of the mensuration problems presented by Palestrina's *Missa L'homme armé,* in part drawn on Zacconi's discussion.

E0205 Chambure, Alain de. *Palestrina. Catalogue des oeuvres religieuses.* Vol 1. Paris: Société Palestrina–Fondation France Télécom, 1989. 67pp.

"Provisional edition." Provides lists of the religious works by text incipit, genre, length in measures in modern transcription, scoring in parts, year of original publication, and notes on their respective locations in the Haberl, Casimiri, and Kalmus editions; a chronological list of publications 1554–1601, with the titles of the works in each; a list of feasts and occasions of the liturgical year paired with compositions by Palestrina suitable for performance on those occasions, and a list of works in manuscript presumed to be by Palestrina although unpublished. Especially useful as a reference in liturgical and concert performance preparation.

E0206 Chater, James. "Two Forgotten Madrigals by Palestrina." *Studi musicali* 11 (1982): 203–228.

Transcriptions and analysis of text and music of *Soligno e vagh'augello* (pub. 1562; the bass part here is a reconstruction) and *O pastor, dove vai così doglioso?* (pub. 1594). Chater disputes Einstein's interpretation of the latter work (see E0223), suggesting instead that *O pastor* has a metaphysical theme, and that its poetic and musical conventions reflect a meditation upon the composer's own approaching death.

E0207 Chrysander, Friedrich ["Chr."]. "Das 'Hohe Lied' von Palestrina." *Leipziger allgemeine musikalische Zeitung* 16 (1881): 99–103, 115–119, 132–134, 148–152, 166–172, 181–185, 410–411, 423–427.

Discusses vol 4 of the Haberl edition, concentrating on *Canticum canticorum* ("The Song of Songs"), although the volume contains 21 additional 5–voice motets. Examines the somewhat enigmatic text, approaches to text setting, and rationales for Palestrina's personal compositional choices. Provides critical discussion of its early publication history and analyzes the cycle's possible modal organization.

E0208 Ciliberti, Galliano. "Una nuova fonte per lo studio degli inni di Costanzo Festa e Giovanni Pierluigi da Palestrina (Cattedrale di S. Florida di Città di Castello)." *Revue Belge de Musicologie* 46 (1992): 145–62.

Discusses manuscript *Città de Castello, Cattedrale di S. Florido, Archivio Capitolare MS 2084 (olim VI C 11)*, probably redacted in late 1550s, containing 3 hymns (including the unpublished *Lauda mater ecclesia*) written by Palestrina during his tenure at St. John Lateran (1555–1560), as well as 26 hymns by Costanzo Festa. Examines its relationship to other manuscripts produced by Vatican scriptorium. Hypothesizes present location of MS due to activities of Cardinal Vitellozzo Vitelli.

E0209 Ciliberti, Galliano. "Organizzazione della Chiesa e organizzazione musicale in Umbria nel XVI secolo." In *La Cappella Musicale nell'Italia della Controriforma. Atti del Convegno (Cento 1989)*, ed. Oscar Mischiati and Paolo Russo. Quaderni della RidM 27. Florence: Olschki, 1993. pp. 337–352.

Noteworthy for indicating holdings of Palestrina material (both manuscript and printed) in the Umbrian cities of Assisi, Città del Castello, Gubbio, Orvieto, Perugia, Spello, and Spoleto.

E0210 Ciliberti, Galliano. "Jacobus Handl Gallus e la 'Scuola musicale Romana' del XVI secolo." In *Gallus Carniolus in Europska renesansa. Gallus Carniolus und die europäische Renaissance.* Internationale Tagung Ljubljana October 21–24, 1991. vol 2 ed. Dragotin Cvetko and Danila Pokorn. Ljubljana: Slovenska Akademija Znanosti in Umetnosti, 1992. ISBN 86–7131–068–X. ML410.H315G33.1991.v.2. pp. 101–131.

Notes the strong presence of Gallus in sixteenth-century Italian religious musical institutions (especially papal) and argues that his relationship to them and their stylistc influence on him are greater than has been realized. Points out strong similarities between Gallus's musical treatment of particular texts and those by Palestrina and others. Palestrina compositions particularly examined include *Tribus miraculis*, *Quem vidistis pastores*, and *Ave Maria a 4.*

E0211 Comes, Liviu. "L'importanza delle formule melodiche nello stile palestriniano," trans. Traian Sofonea and Pietro Derossi. In *Atti del Convegno di Studi Palestriniani. 28 settembre–2 ottobre 1975*, ed. Francesco Luisi. Palestrina: Fondazione Giovanni Pierluigi da Palestrina, 1977. ML410.P15C77.1975. pp. 287–294.

Contends that Palestrina's style can be comprehended in terms of its filiation to Gregorian monophony, not only in terms of mode, intervallic relationships, and rhythmic shaping, but also in the composer's tendency to express and transform formulaic melodic phrases as applied to a polyphonic context.

E0212 Comes, Liviu. *Melodica palestriniana.* Bucharest: Editions musicales de l'Union des Compositeurs, 1971. 198pp. Italian trans. by Pietro Derossi and Traiano Sofonea, *La melodia Palestriniana e il canto gregoriano*. Jucundum laudatio 1974–1975, A13. Venice: San Giorgio Maggiore, 1974–1975. 262pp.

Examines the sources and technical and structural characteristics of Gregorian melodies used by Palestrina. Notes the importance of these characteristics for understanding the underlying shaping and rhythms of the composer's melodies. Points out melodic features in his music, understood as a function of vertical musical formulas that are useful in study of style considerations.

E0213 Crawford, David. "Two Choirbooks of Renaissance Polyphony at the Monasterio de Nuestra Señora of Guadalupe." *Fontes artes musicae* 24 (1977): 145–174.

Discussion of two manuscripts of Spanish provenance, copied mainly between about 1560 and 1610, which contain several Palestrina masses. These versions contain several interesting variants from the texts which Palestrina published in Books II and III of masses; there is also a new final *Kyrie* for the *Missa sine nomine a 4* which is absent from the printed version of 1567.

E0214 Cummings, Anthony M. "Toward an Interpretation of the Sixteenth-Century Motet." *Journal of the American Musicological Society* 34 (1981): 43–59.

Examines the Sistine Chapel diaries for the years 1534–1559, 1560–1561, 1594, and 1616 for evidence to support the assumption that the liturgical uses of the motet were freer than formerly believed. Besides their performance in a variety of extraliturgical contexts, motets were clearly associated with the Offertory, Elevation, and Communion of the Mass, even though their texts might be only marginally related to the liturgical feast being sung.

E0215 Dean, Jeffrey. "The Repertory of the Cappella Giulia in the 1560s." *Journal of the American Musicological Society* 41 (1988): 465–490.

Analyzes an inventory of Cappella Giulia music books (Vatican City, Biblioteca Apostolica Vaticana, Archivio di Stato di San Pietro, Armadi XX–XXIII; fondo Cappella Giulia, Miscellanea. Busta 426, fascicolo 15, no.2) compiled between 1559 and 1566. They contain no music by Palestrina, although he was the *maestro di cappella* of the Giulia from 1551–1554. Concludes that most of Palestrina's sacred music was apparently composed after his return to the Cappella Giulia in 1571, probably in response to the Tridentine liturgical reforms of 1568 to 1570.

E0216 Dixon, Graham. "The Performance of Palestrina: Some Questions, but

Fewer Answers." *Early Music* 22 (1994): 667–675. [French version "L'interprétation des oeuvres de Palestrina. Des questions, peu des réponses." In *L'interprétation de Palestrina*. Paris: Association Palestrina, 1991. pp. 67–77.]

Deals with the conditions for performance of polyphonic music in smaller churches in sixteenth-century Rome. Addresses questions of the number of singers in a typical choir (generally one per part), the participation of organ and instruments, the use of improvised embellishment, sounding pitch, and issues of expressiveness.

E0217 Dolinar, Anton. "Die mehrstimmige Behandlung der Kirchentöne bei Palestrina." Dissertation, University of Vienna, 1927. 206pp.

Not reviewed.

E0218 Dower, Catherine Anne. "Cappella Sixtina Codices in the Catholic University of America Library." *Notes* 36 (1980): 615–623.

A history and description of four manuscript codices (MSS 201–204) presently located in the Mullen Library, Catholic University of America, originally associated with the Sistine Chapel and the Vatican Library, which were copied from 1726 to 1727. They contain numerous works by later sixteenth-century Rome-based composers, including 24 compositions by Palestrina. Three facsimiles included.

E0219 Dower, Catherine Anne. "Eighteenth-Century Sixtine Chapel Codices in the Clementine Library of the Catholic University of America." Ph.D. dissertation, Catholic University of America, 1968.

The author's doctoral dissertation, from which the material in item E0218 derives.

E0220 Dufourcet-Hakim, Marie-Bernadette. "La *Missa Veni Sponsa Christi* de Giovanni Pierluigi da Palestrina." *Ostinato rigore: Revue internationale d'études musicales* 4 (1994): 163–178.

Analyzes this parody mass, demonstrating its balance between counterpoint and homophony for the benefit of its greater intelligibility, Latin prosody, and expressive qualities. Indicative of some of the tendencies in Roman church music in the later sixteenth century.

E0221 Düwell, Klaus Ulrich. "Studien zur Kompositionstechnik der Mehrchörigkeit im 16. Jahrhundert. Dargestellt an Werken von Lasso, Palestrina, Victoria, Handl und Giovanni Gabrieli." Inaugural dissertation, Köln, 1963. ML174.D85.

A comparative study of the treatment of polychoral writing in works of the later sixteenth and early seventeenth centuries.

E0222 Einstein, Alfred. *The Italian Madrigal*, trans. Alexander H. Krappe, Roger H. Sessions, and Oliver Strunk. 3 vols. Princeton, NJ: Princeton University Press, 1949; repr. 1971. ISBN 0–691–09112–9. ML2633.E32.

Vol 1, pp.311–318, of this classic study addresses Palestrina's secular madrigals, with special attention to his first book (1555). Interprets the oeuvre as essentially moderately conservative, with its primary stylistic forebears in Festa and Arcadelt, possessing great harmonic purity and a special feeling for sonority. Somewhat limited in its appreciation of Palestrina in particular, not effectively accounting for the lasting popularity of a number of his works.

E0223 Einstein, Alfred. "Ein unbekanntes Madrigal Palestrinas." *Zeitschrift für Musikwissenschaft* 7 (1925): 530–534.

Identifies and transcribes Palestrina madrigal *O pastor, dove vai così doglioso?* in Giovanni Andrea Dragoni's fourth madrigal book (1594). Characterizes work as an occasional piece, a farewell in dialogue form with pastoral trappings. But see Chater, item E0206.

E0224 Eitner, Robert. "Palestrina als Chromatiker." *Monatsheft für Musikgeschichte* 18 (1886): 77–82.

In this older item, the author, remarking how startled he is by the opening progression of the *Stabat Mater*, notes a number of instances using similar chromatic techniques in works by Palestrina, Lassus, and Hassler.

E0225 Fellerer, Karl Gustav. "Das Credo in Palestrinas *Missa Ecce Sacerdos*. Ein kleiner Beitrag zur Stilkunde des 16. Jahrhunderts." In *Gedenkschrift für Hermann Abert von seinem Schülern*, ed. Friedrich Blume. Halle und Saale: Niemeyer, 1928. ML/55/A28B6. pp. 44–56.

See Fellerer, *Palestrina-Studien* 1982, pp. 247–257, item E0228.

E0226 Fellerer, Karl Gustav. *Die Deklamationsrhythmik in der vokalen Polyphonie des 16. Jahrhunderts*. Düsseldorf: Schwann, 1928.

See Fellerer, *Palestrina-Studien* 1982, item E0228.

E0227 Fellerer, Karl Gustav. "Zur Frage der Deklamationsrhythmik." *Zeitschrift für Musikwissenschaft* 11 (1928): 314–318.

See Fellerer, *Palestrina-Studien* 1982, item E0228.

E0228 Fellerer, Karl Gustav. *Palestrina-Studien.* Collection d'Études Musicologiques/Sammlung musikwissenschaftlicher Abhandlungen 66. Baden-Baden: Valentin Koerner, 1982. ISBN 3–87320–566–1. ML410.P15F46.

A gathering of a large number of Fellerer's earlier publications on Palestrina's music, on individual works, genres, and aspects of style; the "Palestrina style"; and the so-called *stile antico* in the eighteenth century. The chapters or selections are not literal reprints in every case; some are indeed reprints, but others represent a conflation or reworking of more than one item into a continuous text. Useful to read as a single document. Those items which have some form of reprint in the present text are individually indexed in citations documenting their original publication.

E0229 Fenlon, Iain. *Music and Patronage in Sixteenth-Century Mantua.* Cambridge, UK: Cambridge, 1980. 2 vols.

Vol 1, pp. 79–117, study the building of the basilica of S. Barbara and the development of a liturgical repertory for it, including an extended discussion of Palestrina's relationship with Duke Guglielmo Gonzaga and the music the composer produced for performance at this church.

E0230 Fischer, Klaus. "Le composizioni policorali di Palestrina," trans. Sergio Sablich. In *Atti del Convegno di Studi Palestriniani. 28 settembre–2 ottobre 1975*, ed. Francesco Luisi. Palestrina: Fondazione Giovanni Pierluigi da Palestrina, 1977. ML410.P15C77.1975. pp. 341–363.

Consideration of the composer's role in developing the polychoral idiom. Asserts that Palestrina observes universal generic requirements but in manner is closer to Romans such as Animuccia than to Lasso or the Venetians. His double-choir litanies exhibit somewhat greater contrast of material and shorter, more rapidly alternating choirs than are found in most of his other polychoral music, which typically shows longer individual choral statements, imitation in consecutive vertical blocks, and correspondence of thematic material between choirs.

E0231 Fragapane, Carlo. *Indice alfabetico per incipit verbali delle opere di Giovanni Pierluigi da Palestrina.* Florence: Author, 1981. Reprinted in *La cartellina* 8, no. 29 (1984): 80–85.

A list of works organized by text incipit.

E0232 Franke, Veronica Mary. "Palestrina's Fifteen Five-Part Imitation Masses Modelled Upon Motets: a Study of Compositional Procedures." D.Phil. thesis, Christ Church, Oxford, 1990.

Examines Palestrina's selection of models as a basis for mass composition in terms of possible motivation, how his selection compares with those of contemporaries, how choices reflect his compositional outlook. Studies Palestrina's borrowing and procedures for transformation of material. Advocates a broadened idea of *imitatio* to "elaboration upon a known polyphonic source." Endeavors to move beyond studies of line and dissonance treatment to exploration of vertical dispositions, textures, and sonority of Palestrina's masses.

E0233 Fromsen, Michele. "A Conjunction of Rhetoric and Music: Structural Modelling in the Italian Counter-Reformation Motet." *Journal of the Royal Musical Association* 117 (1992): 208–246.

In examining compositional procedures by which composers imitated formal characteristics of their models, the author studies the manner in which Palestrina's motet *Quem vidistis pastores* was used as a model for Victoria's motet on the same text.

E0234 Gallico, Claudio. "Observations on Palestrina *Vestiva i colli*." In *International Musicological Society. Report of the Eleventh Congress, Copenhagen 1972*, ed. Henrik Glahn, Søren Sørensen, and Peter Ryom. Copenhagen: Wilhelm Hansen, 1974. ISBN 87–7455–026–8. ML36.I6.1972. pp. 86–89.

Observes that in the poetic text the words, syllables, and vowels as phonemes are of great importance for the quality and color of the sound of this madrigal. Notes that the musical setting tends to cancel the peculiarly poetic dimension of the text, substituting or transposing it into a domain modified as to language and communication, and making it something unique. There may be in it a lack of invariable correpondence between the rhythmic structure and the qualitative poetic scheme, but rhythmic features may be superimposed from without from a variety of factors (generic tradition of musical formulas, for example). Notes that in this madrigal overall there is some contradiction between prosodic and architectonic structures; but the weight of values is on musical language and technique.

E0235 Godt, Irving. "A New Look at Palestrina's *Missa Papae Marcelli*." *College Music Symposium* 23.1 (1983): 22–49.

Believes assumption by some that the thematic material of *Missa Papae Marcelli* is based on *L'homme armé* tune is probably without foundation. Suggests instead that Palestrina may have followed a deliberate stylistic neutrality respecting his choice of materials. Asserts that the mass's unities derive from the functional equivalences and allusive power of cyclic and thematically transformed material. While such material can seem commonplace in itself, it is treated with great flexibility, ingenuity, and persuasive art.

E0236 Gottwald, Clytus. "Palestrina: *L'homme armé*." In *Palestrina: Zwischen Démontage und Rettung*, ed. Heinz-Klaus Metzger and Rainer Riehn. Munich: Text + Kritik, 1994. pp. 43–59.

Reviews the history of *L'homme armé* masses, the challenges to scholars and interpreters which were posed by Palestrina's two masses, and the subsequent controversies over the transcription of the composer's notation. Offers hermeneutical discussion of whether the *Missa Papae Marcelli* is based on the *L'homme armé* melody, and what messages the ambiguous similarity of themes may convey.

E0237 Haar, James. "The Early Madrigals of Lassus." *Revue Belge de Musicologie* 39–40 (1985–86): 17–32.

Argues for influence of Palestrina, among others, on Lassus's early madrigal style.

E0238 Haar, James. "*Pace non trovo:* A Study in Literary and Musical Parody." *Musica Disciplina* 20 (1966): 95–149 [Italian translation "*Pace non trovo:* una parodia letteraria e musicale." In *Il madrigale tra Cinque e Seicento*, ed. Paolo Fabbri. Bologna: Il Mulino, 1988. pp. 231–248].

An exemplary study of how a sonnet by Petrarch (which was paraphrased, parodied, centonized, and burlesqued, both as to text and text meaning) was set by a number of composers, including one Ivo (probably Ivo Barry), Ihan Gero, and indirectly by Palestrina. In one text version of uncertain authorship, one line of the Petrarch sonnet is quoted as the last line of each of fourteen verses. Palestrina set this text, creating a kind of madrigal cycle or series. In a remarkable parody, displaying a "chromatic" style not overt in his first madrigal book, Palestrina closes each stanza of his own setting of the fourteen verses with a parodied quotation of the appropriate line from the Ivo setting of the original sonnet. Each step in the evidence and argument is meticulously examined, and the article concludes with a discussion of the parody techniques used by Palestrina here.

E0239 Haar, James. "Palestrina as Historicist: the Two *L'homme armé* Masses." *Journal of the Royal Musical Association* 121 (1996): 191–205.

Argues that in his *L'homme armé* masses, Palestrina displayed a historicist sense through his choice of cantus firmus and virtuoso emulation of mensuration practices from 50 years before his time. Asserts that these gestures indicate a wish to connect himself with the professional tradition of the Cappella Sistina.

E0240 Haass, Walter. *Studien zu den "L'homme armé" Messen des 15. und 16. Jahrhunderts.* Kölner Beiträge zur Musikforschung 136, ed. Heinrich Hüschen. Regensburg: Gustav Bosse Verlag, 1984. 178 pp.

Comparative study of over two dozen masses, including both of Palestrina's, which use the famous chanson tune as a cantus firmus. Chapters deal in turn with some style characteristics and arrange material according to the approximate date of setting. Formal structure of the chanson, the structure of Mass movements relative to it and diverse methods of treating the contrapuntal material are analyzed.

E0241 Haberl, Franz Xaver. *Bibliographischer und thematischer Musik-Katalog des päpstlichen Kapellarchivs im Vatikan zu Rom.* Bausteine für Musikgeschichte. Vierteljahrsschrift für Musikwissenschaft 2. Leipzig, 1888. ML160.H98.

An early published catalog of the papal collections. See also items E0281 and E0282.

E0242 Haberl, Franz Xaver. "Die ersten drei Bände der Motetten Palestrinas." *Kirchenmusikalisches Jahrbuch* 5 (1890): 1–27.

An examination (work by work) of salient stylistic traits in Palestrina's first three books of motets (pub. 1569, 1572, 1575), with running commentary on remarks by Baini, Kandler *et al.*

E0243 Haberl, Franz Xaver [sacerdote Francesco Saverio Haberl]. *Giovanni Pierluigi da Palestrina e il Graduale Romanum Officiale dell'Editio Medicaea (1614). Contribuito alla Storia della Liturgia dopo il Concilio di Trento.* Regensburg: Friedrich Pustet, 1894. 59pp [also in German trans. as *Giovanni Pierluigi da Palestrina und das Graduale Romanum der Editio Medicaea von 1614.* Regensburg: Friedrich Pustet, 1894].

A history of the so-called Medicean edition of the Roman Gradual and efforts to revive its standard use in the 1870s. Examines some of the documents and correspondence associated with the preparation of the edition (1578–1615; a series of them printed in the appendix, pp.36 *et seq.*). Discusses Palestrina's role in the revision of the chant and offers some suggestions as to why his activity on the work was largely discontinued after about 1580 (he was sidetracked by other work; another gradual was published in

Venice; possibly inadequate methods for printing plainchant). Suggests reasons why it took this gradual so long to reach print.

E0244 Haberl, Franz Xaver. "Praefationes." In *Giovanni Pierluigi da Palestrina. Opera Omnia*. vols. 10–33. Leipzig: Breitkopf und Härtel, 1880–1907.

The series of prefaces, beginning with vol 10, found in each of the indicated volumes of the first comprehensive edition are of great value for information on and descriptions of printed and manuscript sources for Palestrina in the late nineteenth century, and for knowledge of Haberl's critical apparatus and methodology.

E0245 Haigh, Andrew C. "The Harmony of Palestrina." Dissertation, Harvard University, 1946. 324pp.

See item E0246.

E0246 Haigh, Andrew C. "Modal Harmony in the Music of Palestrina." In *Essays on Music in Honor of Archibald Thompson Davison, by His Associates*. Cambridge, MA: Harvard, 1957. ML55.D28H3. pp. 111–120.

Investigates some of the harmonic tendencies in Palestrina's music. Does statistical analysis to indicate proportionate use of various modes. Suggests that the composer tends to exhibit preferences among mode choices, and that works in the various modes show characteristic and distinctive harmonic patterns as well as patterns of modal cadences and cadence formulas. While these modal haronic patterns exist, they show certain slight unexplained irregularities that seem evidence of the pull of tonality, a feeling for which was growing in later sixteenth century music. Offers a "theory of modal harmonic gravitation" in which harmonies are attracted toward the center of the total harmonic sphere, in which modal "tonics" occupy various positions.

E0247 Hall, Alison. *Palestrina: An Index to the Casimiri, Kalmus and Haberl Editions.* MLA Index and Biography Series 22. Philadelphia: Music Library Association, 1980. xiii + 82pp. ISBN 0–914–95418–0. ML134.P26.H3

Locator for works in three editions, organized by title/incipit index and by classified (genre) index.

E0248 Haller, Michael. "Analyse der Missa: 'O admirabile commercium' von Giov. Pierluigi da Palestrina." *Kirchenmusikalisches Jahrbuch* 9 (1894): 69–76.

An analysis that partitions the motet model into its eight constituent phrase/music components and indicates how each phrase's material is distributed through the various movements of the mass. Notes as an important feature the elaboration of the adapted material through devices of imitation and inverted counterpoint, and the creation of variety and expressiveness through coloristic groupings of voices.

E0249 Haller, Michael. "Meditationen über die 'alten Schule,' nebst einer Analyse der Missa '*Iste Confessor*' von G. Pierluigi da Palestrina." *Cäcilienkalendar* 6 (1881): 36–45.

Following a discussion of "strict" and "free" contrapuntal styles, the formation of melody appropriate for strict counterpoint, note values, rhythm, and mode issues, Haller applies the discussion to an examination of the hymn *Iste confessor*, and in turn analyzes how the phrases of the hymn are used to generate melodic and imitative material for each of the movements of the polyphonic *Missa Iste confessor.*

E0250 Haller, Michael. "Motivierung des neukomponierten III. Chores in sechs 12–stimm. Compositionen Palestrina." *Kirchenmusikalisches Jahrbuch* 4 (1889): 38–44.

Discusses compositional decisions involved in the reconstruction by Haller of the missing third-choir parts of triple choir pieces published in volume 26 of the Haberl edition. Note: the original missing parts for some of these works were recently recovered and the compositions republished. See O'Regan, items E0301, E0302, and E0680.

E0251 Hamburger, Povl. *Studien zur Vokalpolyphonie*. Bd. I–II. German trans. Hans Georg Lenz. Wiesbaden, 1956. Orig. published Copenhagen: Nordisk Forlag Arnold Busck, 1956. ML446 H3.

Contains a list of Palestrina's masses (p.44).

E0252 Hanson, John R. "Enumeration of Dissonance in the Five-Voice Masses of Palestrina." *Theory and Practice* 9 (1984): 125–141.

Statistical study of the appearance and uses of various dissonances in Palestrina's five-voice masses. Hanson enumerates the numbers and distribution of these devices and combines them in a database with information acquired in his study of three- and four-voice masses and mass sections of 1983 (item E0253) in an attempt to clarify Palestrina's compositional style.

E0253 Hanson, John R. "Enumeration of Dissonance in the Masses of Palestrina." *College Music Symposium* 23.1 (1983): 50–64.

Statistical study of selected uses of dissonance, first in three-voice mass sections, then in four-voice masses, primarily for pedagogical purposes. Enumerates uses of five kinds of suspensions, accented passing tones, consonant fourth, cambiata, and 6/5 harmonic combination in order to 1) provide a list of sources with many occurrences of a particular device; 2) highlight their prototypical distribution; 3) evaluate generalizations about the style in counterpoint books; 4) provide a basis for comparison to selections in anthologies; 5) make a list of sources which illustrate rare or exceptional devices.

E0254 Hanson, John R. "Pedagogy of Sixteenth-Century Counterpoint: Selected Examples with Commentary." *Theory and Practice* 4 (1979): 5–14.

Examines dissonance treatment in works by Josquin and Palestrina found in some general anthologies, and comments on the suitability of those sources for classroom teaching.

E0255 Harran, Don. "Stories from the Hebrew Bible in Music of the Renaissance." *Musica Disciplina* 37 (1983): 235–288.

Attempts to isolate and define a repertory of Hebrew Bible (Old Testament) stories in musical settings. Among the motets selected for examination are four by Palestrina: *Aegypte noli flere a 5, Santificavit Moyses a 5, Inveni David a 5* and *Susanna ab improbis senibus a 6.* The collection is examined for the textual and musical procedures used; for their relationship to other bodies of information where parallels of Old Testament narrative exist, especially those in painting; for the relation of these biblical stories to other biblical texts (narratives, psalms, Lamentations, and the Song of Songs). Opens up consideration of these texts in terms of motives and activities of Christian Hebraicists of the Old Testament in the Renaissance.

E0256 Haydon, Glen. "The Lateran Codex 61." In *Internationale Gesellschaft für Musikwissenschaft. Bericht über den siebenten internationalen musikwissenschaftlichen Kongress Köln 1958*, ed. Gerald Abraham et al. Kassel: Bärenreiter, 1959. ML36.I6.1958. pp. 126–131.

A study of the manuscript Rome, San Giovanni in Laterano, Archivio Musicale MS61, a collection of hymns probably written around 1575, mostly by or under the direction of Annibale Stabile, and apparently copied from an earlier, lost MS. Interspersed among Festa's *Hymni per totum annum* are 27 hymns by other composers, including three by Palestrina, *Veni creator a 4*, *Pange lingua a 4*, and *Tristis erant apostoli a 4.* Compositional style of these works is analyzed in text, and a table describing the non-Festa hymns generally is provided on pp.129–131.

E0257 Hell, Helmut. "Die Vorlagen zur unechten Messe 69 in der neuen Reihe der Lasso-Gesamtausgabe." *Musik in Bayern* 20 (1980): 39–49.

Demonstrates that a mass purported to be by Lasso is actually a probable nineteenth-century conflation of material by Carl Neuner. The "mass" consists of a contrafactum of a motet by Lasso, together with a *Benedictus* by Albrechtsberger and an *Agnus Dei* by Palestrina.

E0258 Höfler, Janez. "Sui motetti a doppio coro di G.P. da Palestrina." In *L'Arte di Giovanni Pierluigi da Palestrina. Atti e Documentazione. VI Convegno Europeo sul Canto Corale. Promosso e Organizzato dalla Corale Goriziana "C.A. Seghizzi."* Gorizia: Grafica Goriziana, 1975. pp. 23–32.

Studies four motets from *Libro secondo* (1572) and seven from *Libro terzo* (1575) that are datable with relative security. Argues that the 8–part 1572 motets are based on psalmodic structures and use diverse combinations of voices without adhering to any preset bichoral scheme, while the 1575 works are more obviously antiphonal, respect verse structure, and frequently repeat text in both choirs. Following a suggestion in Cerone that Palestrina composed "in the style of Phinot," Höfler compares the 1575 pieces with double choir music in *Novus thesaurus musicum* (1568).

E0259 Hüschen, Heinrich. "Lob- und Preismotetten auf die Musik aus früheren Jahrhunderten." In *Musica Scientiae Collectanea 12. Festschrift für Karl Gustav Fellerer zum siebzigsten Geburtstag am 7. Juli 1972*, ed. Heinrich Hüschen. Köln: Volk, 1973. pp. 225–242.

Contextualizes setting of the text *Cantantibus organis Caecilia* with material about the Cecilian legend, an analysis of the text itself and its musical treatment by several Renaissance composers as well as Palestrina.

E0260 Illing, Carl-Heinz. *Zur Technik der Magnificat-Komposition des 16. Jahrhunderts.* Kieler Beiträge zur Musikwissenschaft 3. Wolfenbüttel and Berlin: Kallmeyer, 1936.

Originally a Ph.D. dissertation from the University of Kiel. About half of this book is devoted to analysis of Palestrina's magnificats.

E0261 Janz, Bernhard. "*Nativitas tua Dei genetrix virgo*. Palestrinas Motette und die gleichnamige Parodiemesse im Kodex Cappella Sistina 70." In *Aufführungs- und Bearbeitungspraxis der Werke Palestrinas vom 16. bis zum 20. Jahrhundert*, ed. Friedrich Wilhelm Riedel. Kirchenmusikalische Studien 3. Sinzig: Studio, Verlag Schewe, 1997. pp. 25–42.

Examines an anonymous mass entitled *Nativitas tua Dei genetrix* in the manuscript I-Rvat Cappella Sistina 70, which Janz recognizes as a parody mass based on a motet published by Palestrina in *Motecta festorum* (1564). Argues from a variety of inductive, circumstantial, and stylistic evidence (including the manner of disposition of the thematic material, consistent with Palestrina's methods but sometimes divergent from Pontio's theoretical instructions) that Palestrina is the author of the mass, and suggests reasons why it may have been neglected and fallen out of the Sistine repertory.

E0262 Jeppesen, Knud. "Das isometrische Moment in der Vokalpolyphonie." In *Festschrift Peter Wagner zum 60. Geburtstag*, ed. Karl Weinmann. Leipzig: Breitkopf und Härtel, 1926. repr. 1969. ML55.F47. pp. 87–99.

Contains a history of the use of note-against-note declamatory polyphony for drawing attention to particular words or phrases in vocal music from 1300 to 1600. Palestrina's uses of such text setting tend to be somewhat more inflected verbally, more natural, and more flexible than the rather mechanical and emblematic uses of such declamation in earlier Netherlandish polyphony or fourteenth-century cases such as Machaut.

E0263 Jeppesen, Knud. *Kontrapunkt. Lehrbuch der klassischen Vokalpolyphonie.* Leipzig: Breitkopf und Härtel, 1935, repr. Leipzig: VEB-Breitkopf und Härtel, 1956 [trans. *Counterpoint. The Polyphonic Vocal Style of the Sixteenth Century.* Englewood Cliffs, NJ: Prentice-Hall, 1939]. MT55.J54K.

A manual of instruction in sixteenth-century counterpoint reliant on Jeppesen's *The Style of Palestrina and the Dissonance*, E0267. See especially pp.83–97.

E0264 Jeppesen, Knud. "Marcellus-Probleme." *Acta Musicologica* 16 (1944): 11–38. ML5 A2 [trans. in *Giovanni Pierluigi da Palestrina: Pope Marcellus Mass.* Norton Critical Score. New York: Norton, 1975. M2011.P25.M38.1975].

Contains reprint of "Wann entstand die Marcellus-Messe?" [see item E0272].

E0265 Jeppesen, Knud. "Le Messe Mantovane di Giovanni Pierluigi da Palestrina." *Manifestazioni di attività culturale.* Rome: Accademia Nazionale di S. Cecilia, 1955.

See item E0266.

E0266 Jeppesen, Knud. "Pierluigi da Palestrina, Herzog Guglielmo Gonzaga und die neugefundene Mantovaner-Messe Palestrinas: ein ergänzender Bericht." *Acta Musicologica* 24 (1953): 132–179.

The expanded report on a recovery of Palestrina material of outstanding importance, namely the works the composer wrote for Duke Guglielmo Gongaza and his new liturgical foundation of Santa Barbara in Mantua. Describes the Santa Barbara collection and how it was settled in Milan; the Santa Barbara foundation itself, with its distinctive liturgy and plainchant; elaborates in depth Palestrina's working history with Duke Guglielmo, including transcriptions of much of their correspondence. Provides extensive analyses of the masses and their relationship to the unique chant they use, and discusses their alternatim manner of performance. Studied together with the extant correspondence, these works (the only ones Palestrina wrote for a liturgy other than the Roman) are of very great value for understanding the composer's working methods and aspects of style.

E0267 Jeppesen, Knud. *Palestrinastil med saerligt henblik paa dissonansbehandlingen.* Copenhagen, 1923; 2nd ed. Copenhagen: Ejnar Munksgaard, 1946 [German trans. *Die Dissonanzbehandlung in den Werken Palestrinas.* Copenhagen, 1925; German trans. *Der Palestrinastil und die Dissonanz.* Leipzig, 1925. repr. 1927, 1946. English trans. *The Style of Palestrina and the Dissonance*, 1927; 2nd. ed. intro Edward J. Dent. London: G. Cumberlege, 1946, repr. New York: Dover, 1970]. ML3003.J362.1946; ML410.P15.J5.

An exhaustive and influential study of the composer's contrapuntal technique. The approach used does not attempt to group compositions chronologically or in terms of style phases, and thus does not readily indicate how his overall style may have evolved over time, but still an impressive analysis of Palestrina's characteristic technical decisions.

E0268 Jeppesen, Knud. "Problems of the *Pope Marcellus Mass*: Some Remarks on the *Missa Papae Marcelli* by Giovanni Pierluigi da Palestrina." In *Giovanni Pierluigi da Palestrina. Pope Marcellus Mass. An Authoritative Score. Backgrounds and Sources. History and Analysis. Views and Comments*, ed. Lewis Lockwood. Norton Critical Score. New York: W.W. Norton, 1975. ISBN 0–393–02185–8; ISBN 0–393–09242–9 (pbk). M2011.P25M38.1975. pp. 99–130.

English translation of the *Acta Musicologica* article.

E0269 Jeppesen, Knud. "The Recently-Discovered Mantova Masses of Palestrina. A Provisional Communication." *Acta Musicologica* 22 (1950): 36–47.

A description of manuscript masses in the Santa Barbara *fondo* of the Conservatorio di Musica Giuseppe Verdi in Milan, which are identified with the masses known to have been composed by Palestrina and sent to Guglielmo Gonzaga of Mantua on his commission in 1578 to 1579. Also comments on Oliver Strunk's article in the 1947 *Musical Quarterly* dealing with Duke Guglielmo and a *Missa Dominicalis* ascribed to Palestrina.

E0270 Jeppesen, Knud. "Palestriniana. Ein unbekanntes Autogramm Palestrinas und einige unveröffentlichte Falsibordoni des Giovanni Pierluigi da Palestrina." In *Miscelánea en Homenaje a Monseñor Higinio Anglés* I, ed. Miguel Querol et al. Barcelona: Consejo Superior de Investigaciones Cientificas, 1958–1961. ML55.A58. pp. 417–432.

Discusses Vatican City, Biblioteca Apostolica Vaticana, MS Vat. Lat. 10776, a Palestrina autograph containing hymns and *falsibordoni*, in the context of a large amount of other affiliated manuscript and print material. Suggests some identifications for *falsibordone* material in the Guidetti 1587 publication as well.

E0271 Jeppesen, Knud. "II. Über einen Brief Palestrinas." In *Festschrift Peter Wagner zum 60. Geburtstag*, ed. Karl Weinmann, Leipzig: Breitkopf und Härtel, 1926. repr. 1969. ML55.F47. pp. 100–107.

Analyzes a letter written by Palestrina on March 3, 1570, in response to Duke Guglielmo Gonzaga's request for a critique of some of his compositions. Examines Palestrina's comments as reflecting his methods for instruction and critical assessment of music. Comments to Guglielmo indicate that Palestrina put the duke's work into score and advised the enriching of its harmonic sonorities and the polishing of its contrapuntal treatment. In the absence of any actual annotated scores, Jeppesen suggests examples from Palestrina's music as illustrations.

E0272 Jeppesen, Knud. "Wann entstand die Marcellus-Messe?" In *Studien zur Musikgeschichte: Festschrift für Guido Adler zum 75. Geburtstag*. Vienna: Universal-Edition, 1930; repr. 1971. pp. 126–136.

This article formed part of the "Marcellus-Probleme" article by Jeppesen that appeared in *Acta Musicologica* in 1944–1945. The *Acta* version, translated into English by Lewis Lockwood, appears in the Norton Critical Score edition of the *Missa Papae Marcelli*, item E0268.

E0273 Killing, Joseph. *Kirchenmusikalische Schätze der Bibliothek des Abbate Fortunato Santini. Ein Beitrag zur Geschichte der katholischen Kirchenmusik in Italien.* Düsseldorf: Schwann, 1910.

A history and description of the great collection of Fortunato Santini (1778–1861). He spent more than half a century collecting and scoring music from before 1800, much of which was from then-inaccessible libraries and archives. A number of his original sources have since disappeared. The collection of nearly six thousand items—manuscripts, prints, and scorings of parts—eventually came to reside at the Episcopal Seminary in Münster. An important location for early prints of Palestrina's music and for investigating manuscript traditions, otherwise untraceable works, and *opera dubia*.

E0274 Klassen, Johannes. "Zur Modellbehandlung in Palestrinas Parodiemessen." *Kirchenmusikalisches Jahrbuch* 39 (1955): 41–55.

Examines how thematic material from polyphonic models is integrated into Palestrina's mass movements. Discusses the sectionalization of models and argues for the composer's careful attention to adapting word-rhythm relationships, metrical phrase treatments, and text assonance and alliteration in the models to particular mass passages. Finds evidence of symbolic allusions between portions of model text and passages in masses suggested through melodic shaping and affective parallels.

E0275 Klassen, Johannes. "Die Parodiemesse bei Palestrina." Dissertation, Bonn, 1950. 123pp. (typescript).

See items E0274, E0276, E0277.

E0276 Klassen, Johannes. "Das Parodieverfahren in der Messe Palestrinas." *Kirchenmusikalisches Jahrbuch* 38 (1954): 24–54.

A more detailed statistical study of the distribution and modification of the material of a polyphonic model within the various movements of Palestrina's parody masses. Examines direct and symbolic text-music relationships, as well as thematic and rhythmic modifications of preexistent material when adapted from one context to another.

E0277 Klassen, Johannes. "Untersuchungen zur Parodiemesse Palestrinas." *Kirchenmusikalisches Jahrbuch* 37 (1953): 53–63.

Investigation of 41 parody masses by Palestrina, of which 23 use models derived from his own work, while 18 are based on models by others. The non-Palestrina sources tend to be representative of the post-Josquin, Italianized Netherlandish style.

E0278 Kuhn, Max. *Die Verzierungs-Kunst in der Gesangs-Musik des 16.–17. Jahrhunderts (1535–1650).* Beihefte der Internationalen Musikgesellschaft 7. Leipzig: Breitkopf und Härtel. 1902. ML1403.K96.

An early and influential study of printed sources on diminution and ornamentation technique and their practical application to music of the late Renaissance and early Baroque. Reviews the relevant texts, examines their suggestions, and reproduces a large number of examples from various books. See entry in Chapter 5, "Modern Editions" for a description of the Palestrina examples transcribed in this text, under section I, cross-listing "Kuhn."

E0279 Kurtzman, Jeffrey G. "Tones, Modes, Clefs and Pitch in Roman Cyclic Magnificats of the 16th Century." *Early Music* 22 (1994): 641–664.

Derived from a study of relationships between *Magnificats* of Palestrina and those of sixteenth-century predecessors in the Sistine chapel. Hypothesizes that the practical origin and purposes of so-called *chiavette* and other related clef combinations derived from a wish to create a notational correspondence (whatever the sounding pitch may have been) between the reciting tones of antiphons and their psalms or canticles.

E0280 Leichtentritt, Hugo. *Geschichte der Motette.* Leipzig: Breitkopf & Härtel, 1908 [facs. repr. Hildesheim: G. Olms, 1967]. ML3090.L52.

Chapter 6, pp.142–207, deals with "Palestrina and the Roman School." Influenced by the newly completed Haberl edition, this is a survey of salient features of many of Palestrina's better-known motets, emphasizing both their technique and the interdependence of their rhetorical and affective qualities.

E0281 Llorens, Josephus M. *Capellae Sixtinae Codices musicis notis instructi sive manu scripti sive praelo excussi.* Studi e testi 202. Vatican City: Biblioteca Apostolica Vaticana, 1960 [repr.1972].

Highly detailed catalog (in Latin) of the Biblioteca Apostolica Vaticana's Sistine *fondo*, one of the most important sources for Palestrina works in early manuscript copies and the central custodian of the earlier performance tradition.

E0282 Llorens, José M. [Josephus]. *Le opere musicali della Cappella Giulia I: manoscritti e edizioni fino al '700.* Studi e testi 265. Vatican City: Biblioteca Apostolica Vaticana, 1971.

Catalog of the Cappella Giulia musical *fondo*, another of the most important sources for primary Palestrina material.

E0283 Llorens, José M. "Tres ignoradas antífonas de Giovanni Pierluigi da Palestrina, identificadas en el fondo musical de la Cappella Giulia." *Anuario musical* 22 (1967): 1–19.

Discusses three unattributed antiphon motets, *Sancta Dei genetrix a 4*, *Petrus apostolus a 4,* and *Da pacem Domine a 4,* in Rome, Biblioteca Apostolica Vaticana, Cappella Giulia VIII.39, ff.190v–193, together with documentary evidence pinpointing Palestrina's authorship. (This is the same MS containing Morales *Magnificats* with *si placet* parts by Palestrina.) Contains transcriptions of these three works (pp.13–17), plus four pages of plates with facsimiles of the three works and the receipt from Archivio Capitolare di San Pietro, vol 150, f.23, that proves that Palestrina was their composer.

E0284 Lockwood, Lewis, ed. *Giovanni Pierluigi da Palestrina. Pope Marcellus Mass. An Authoritative Score. Backgrounds and Sources. History and Analysis. Views and Comments,* ed. Lewis Lockwood. Norton Critical Score. New York: W.W. Norton, 1975. ISBN 0–393–02185–8; ISBN 0–393–09242–9 (pbk). M2011.P25M38.1975. pp. 99–130.

In addition to a score of the mass (pp.39–73) derived from vol 4 of the Casimiri edition, Lockwood presents English translations of a large body of relevant contemporary documents and critical reception material. Also included is Lockwood's article "Notes on the Text and Structure of the *Pope Marcellus Mass"* (pp.77–98) and his English translation of Knud Jeppesen's "Problems of the *Pope Marcellus Mass*: Some Remarks on the *Missa Papae Marcelli* by Giovanni Pierluigi da Palestrina" (pp.99–130) [see item E0268].

E0285 Luisi, Francesco. "Le alterazioni nella musica di Palestrina." In *Atti del Convegno di Studi Palestriniani 28 settembre–2 ottobre 1975*, ed. Francesco Luisi. Palestrina: Fondazione Giovanni Pierluigi da Palestrina, 1977. ML 410.P15C77.1975. pp. 51–98.

Relying on sixteenth-century theoretical sources dicussing *musica ficta*, it is argued that alteration of pitches at cadences to "modernize" the language beyond what is found in contemporaneous sources of Palestrina's sacred vocal music is appropriate more often than is assumed.

E0286 Marshall, Robert L. "The Paraphrase Technique of Palestrina in his Masses Based on Hymns." *Journal of the American Musicological Society* 16 (1963): 347–372.

Study of nine masses using techniques of polyphonic construction derived from preexistent material belonging to a specific monophonic genre. Palestrina first derives a subject suitable for imitation by imposing a rhythmically distinct and concise form upon the model, then distributes it according to the sequence of phrases found in the original hymn. In polyphonic elaboration he achieves variety through a constantly changing order of voice entries in the presentation of the borrowed material, but the disposition of the hymn phrases over the course of a movement depends on the design both of the hymn and the particular mass section. Each mass represents individual solutions to these problems.

E0287 McCray, James E. "A Survey of Published *Magnificats* for Treble Voices." *Choral Journal* 28 (1988): 5–11.

Surveys and describes a selection of *Magnificats* for the period from 1450 to 1980. Palestrina's are among the earliest represented.

E0288 Meier, Bernhard. "Modale Korrektur und Wortausdeutung im Choral der Editio Medicaea." *Kirchenmusikalisches Jahrbuch* 53 (1969): 101–132.

After reviewing the foundations of the reform, this study examines how the "reformed" chant of the Medicean edition was reshaped modally and had its "superfluities" and "barbarisms" removed for the sake of enhancing both musical and textual clarity. Concludes that the edition is actually better than its reputation, and that the editing work was relatively rationally based, not so very far off the mark, and certainly not done in blind ignorance or silly pedantry. Article does not directly mention Palestrina for obvious reasons, but presumably at some level his handiwork is present among the examples studied here.

E0289 Meier, Bernhard. "Zu den 'in mi' fundierten Werken aus Palestrinas Offertoriums-Motettenzyklus." *Die Musikforschung* 37 (1984): 215–220.

In examining Palestrina's offertory cycle (pub. 1593), Meier argues against Harold Powers's interpretation of the first 32 motets of the collection as being organized in series according to the eight traditional church modes. Argues that in considering the "in mi" group (nos. 9–16, founded on modes III and IV), Palestrina actually seems to have transposed the order of the mode presentation (i.e. III follows IV). Suggests that this is because the affective character of the texts and their liturgical placement were better served through the choices of mode that were actually made here, even if there was a seeming inconsistency in the pattern of the cycle as a result.

E0290 Mies, Paul. "Stabat mater dolorosa. Probleme und Grundlagen für eine Untersuchung über das Verhältnis von textlicher und musikalischer Struktur." *Kirchenmusikalisches Jahrbuch* 27 (1932): 146–153.

Comparisons of structure and declamation in Palestrina's musical treatment of the *Stabat mater* text with those found in settings by Josquin, Anerio, and Pergolesi.

E0291 Mischiati, Oscar. "Il manoscritto corsiniano dei 'Ricercari' di Giovanni Pierluigi da Palestrina." In *Atti del II Convegno Internazionale di Studi Palestriniani. Anno Europeo della Musica. 3–5 maggio 1986*, ed. Lino Bianchi and Giancarlo Rostirolla. Palestrina: Fondazione Giovanni Pierluigi da Palestrina/Centro di Studi Palestriniani, 1991. ML410.P15C77.1986. pp. 177–201.

A study, inventory of and concordance list for Rome, Biblioteca Corsiniana Ms. M 14 (olim 2490), the source for the *Ricercari* attributed to Palestrina. Mainly a large collection of vocal music in partitura, the MS was probably written out around 1600 for compositional study and for the practice of basso continuo/basso seguente accompaniment by an organist.

E0292 Mischiati, Oscar. "'Ut verba intelligentur': circostanze e connesioni a proposito della *Missa Papae Marcelli*." In *Atti del Convegno di Studi Palestriniani (28 settembre–2 ottobre 1975)*, ed. Francesco Luisi. Palestrina: Fondazione G.P. da Palestrina, 1977. ML 410.P15C77.1975. pp. 415–426.

Notes that the demand for intelligibility of the text in polyphony was the function of a broader humanistic and Renaissance aesthetic. Its direct implications for the Tridentine deliberations are evident in correspondence which preceded and was contemporary with the council, and the practical results of such attitudes are clearly observed in the stylistic formulation of the *Missa Papae Marcelli*.

E0293 Monterosso, Raffaello. "La prassi esecutiva palestriniana nella prospettiva del pensiero teorico rinascimento." In *L'arte di Giovanni Pierluigi da Palestrina. Atti e documentazione. VI Convegno europeo sul canto corale. Promosso e organizzato dalla Corale Goriziana "C.A. Seghizzi."* Gorizia: Grafica Goriziana, 1975. pp. 41–54.

Addresses problems in reading sixteenth-century notation, questions of rhythmic organization, and aspects of interpretive expression. Discusses notational problems of the *L'homme armé* mass and cites numerous sixteenth- and seventeenth-century theorists on the changing nature, speed, and treatment of the tactus. Traces Haberl/Casimiri/Auda controversies over *L'homme armé* notation. Reviews theorists' remarks on differences between manners of singing church and chamber polyphony with respect to physical deportment, number and fullness of voices, and application of ornaments to music.

E0294 Monterosso Vacchelli, Anna Maria. *La Messa 'L'homme armé' di Palestrina: Studio paleografico ed edizione critica.* Istituta e Monumenta, Serie II, Instituta 7. Cremona: Fondazione Claudio Monteverdi, 1979. M2011.P25.H6.1979.

Introduction, pp.13–41, reviews the long and controversial history dealing with the interpretation of the notation in this work; pp.42–47 present a critical apparatus; pp.51, 52–61, and 62–75 reproduce in facsimile the editions of 1570 and 1599 respectively, and pp.79–132 present Monterosso Vacchelli's transcription of the mass.

E0295 Morelli, Arnaldo. "Intorno a un codicetto polifonico del primo Seicento (I-Rsc, G.389)." *Recercare* 1 (1989): 97–109.

Discussion of provenance and function of this MS, drawn up in 1617 by organist Alessandro Nison. Besides containing four other Palestrina motets, it is the only known source for his 6-part motet *Congratulamini.*

E0296 Moser, Hans Joachim. "Vestiva i colli." *Archiv für Musikforschung* 4 (1939): 129–156. Reprinted in Hans Joachim Moser. *Musik in Zeit und Raum. Ausgewählte Abhandlungen*. Berlin: Merseburger, 1960. pp. 34–58.

Discusses adaptation of the material of Palestrina's popular secular work in a series of imitation masses by the composer himself and by several of his contemporaries, namely Nanino, Giovanelli, Belli, Biondi da Cesena, Nucius, and Lasso. Also examines arrangements, diminutions, reworkings, and even burlesques of the original madrigal.

E0297 Novack, Saul. "Tonality and the Style of Palestrina." In *Music and Civilization: Essays in Honor of Paul Henry Lang*, ed. Edmond Strainchamps, Maria Rika Maniates, and Christopher Hatch. New York: Norton, 1984. ISBN 0–393–01677–3. ML55.L213.1984. pp. 428–443.

Describes how problematic it has been to speak of the operations of modality in sixteenth-century polyphony music, and that identification of specific modes in terms of the church modes or Glarean's extension of them has been inadequate. Notes that studies of Palestrina's style have not reflected his considerations of tonality as a unifying force. Points out that the composer uses various kinds of harmonic function, both internally and at final cadences, and in the large-scale projection of various chords, especially IV and V. Such chords not only function as structural harmonic chords but are also themselves prolonged harmonically. Functioning chords combine with the directions of voices and repetitions of design to create inner form and a strong sense of tonal direction.

E0298 Ollikkala, Debra Margaret. "G.P. da Palestrina: A Study of His Paraphrase Masses Based on Antiphons." D.M.A. thesis, University of Illinois at Urbana-Champaign, 1993. DA932912.

Studies the structural and stylistic features of nine mass settings based on antiphons. Explores paraphrase procedures, namely the transformation of the antiphon into material suitable for polyphony and the use of that material throughout the mass.

E0299 Ollikkala, Debra Cairns. "The Use of Cadences to Define Structure in Selected Masses of Palestrina." *Choral Journal* 35.1 (1994): 27–32.

Discusses cadential hierarchies serving to articulate segments of musical structure as an aspect of Palestrina's compositional procedure. Four categories of cadence types are described according to their general contrapuntal features and their relative strength. Analysis of *Credo* from *Missa Regina coeli a 5* illustrates how cadences define syntactical units together with various levels of musical structure. Notes on communicating these qualities in performance are offered.

E0300 O'Regan, Noel. "The Early Polychoral Music of Orlando di Lasso—New Light from Roman Sources." *Acta Musicologica* 56 (1984): 234–251.

Contains information on a number of 8-voice motets by Palestrina in sources of Roman origin, particularly MS partbooks with a provenance of Santa Maria in Vallicella (Chiesa Nuova) and Cappella Giulia. Evidence indicates that some of these motets were reworked by Palestrina or others in order to be sung by spatially separated choirs.

E0301 O'Regan, Noel. "The Introduction of Polychoral Music into the Papal Chapel in the Late Sixteenth and Early Seventeenth Centuries." In *Collectanea II. Studien zur Geschichte der päpstlichen Kapelle. Tagungsbericht Heidelberg 1989*, ed. Bernhard Janz. Capellae Apostolicae Sixtinaeque Collectanea Acta Monumenta 4. Vatican City: Biblioteca Apostolica Vaticana, 1994. ISBN 88–210–0655–7. ML3051.V3C65.1994. pp. 431–450.

Polychoral music does not seem to have been adopted in Rome before the 1570s, but Palestrina was the first Roman composer to publish such music in 1575. This study examines eleven Cappella Sistina manuscripts which contain such music (a significant amount of which is by Palestrina) to understand the extent of the repertory, the composers associated with it, its stylistic evolution, and its important uses. Notes that it was relatively slow to be introduced into the chapel, not becoming fully established until the 1590s, and it remained in regular use but was being composed in an idiom already retrospective by the 1620s. It was used especially for Vespers and for motets during mass on feast days.

E0302 O'Regan, Noel. "The Performance of Palestrina: Some Further Observations." *Early Music* 24 (1996): 145–154.

Responds to articles by Dixon (item E0216) and Sherr (item E0054) in 1994 *Early Music*. Suggests that performance practice changed between the late fifteenth and late sixteenth centuries with respect to the number of vocalists per part in polyphonic music, and that singing by single and multiple singers on each part coexisted throughout the period, although there was an increase in one-per-part singing as the sixteenth century progressed.

E0303 Ouvrard, Jean-Pierre. "Le tempo chez Palestrina." In *L'interprétation de Palestrina. Journées d'étude.* Royaumont: Société Palestrina, 1990. pp. 45–65.

Questions the presence both of *tempus imperfectum integrum* in *Vestiva i colli* and the *tempus imperfectum diminutum* in the mass on that madrigal, which would make possible an execution in equalized values. This is consistent with Casimiri's position in the debate with Antoine Auda on this subject.

E0304 Owens, Jessie Ann. "Palestrina as Reader: Motets from the Song of Songs." In *Hearing the Motet. Essays on the Motet of the Middle Ages and Renaissance*, ed. Dolores Pesce. New York: Oxford, 1997. ISBN 0–195–09709-2. ML3275.H4.1997. pp. 307–328.

Notes the unusual qualities of Palestrina's fourth motet book for five voices (*Canticum canticorum,* or the "Song of Songs"): a single source, the Bible, provided all its texts, which the composer himself probably selected and arranged; the motets themselves made a unified whole, individually similar in length and structure and probably composed within a short period of time. Musically and conceptually the texts are divided into four large sections, each with a particular tonality or tonal type. The composer created a large-scale motet cycle by interrelating these sections through a variety of thematic and refrainlike techniques. He musically reinforced his "reading" of the texts by accentuating particular aspects of their meaning and structure, and by treating them in a somewhat "livelier" manner than was typical for motets.

E0305 Paccagnella, Ermenegildo. *Palestrina, il linguaggio melodico e armonico.* Biblioteca Historiae Musicae Cultores 7. Florence: Olschki, 1957. 126 pp. ISBN 3–87397–122–4. ML3090.B6.1992.

E0306 Phillips, Peter. "Reconsidering Palestrina." *Early Music* 22 (1994): 574–585.

A consideration of Palestrina's *cori spezzati* writing as found in motet publications of 1572 and 1575. Argues that Palestrina refined his use of the idiom from one involving imitative writing, diverse textures, and somewhat limited choral separation to one demonstrating a more sharply focused separation of two answering choirs, together with scoring which is more clearly homophonic than polyphonic.

E0307 Pike, Lionel. "New Palestrina Sources." *Musical Times* 117 (1976): 685–688.

Discusses arrangement by Peter Phillips of two works by Palestrina: the 5-voice *Quanti mercenarii* (itself a contrafactum of *Io son ferito*) for cantus, bassus, and bassus generalis in *Paradisus sacris* of 1628, and the 4-voice motet *Hodie Maria virgo* found in a publication dated 1616 (ascribed to Palestrina but not in the collected editions). Argues that study of these works, especially *Hodie Maria virgo*, gives valuable insights into matters of style; discusses performance issues at length.

E0308 Pike, Lionel. "The Opening of Palestrina's *Stabat Mater*." *Consort* 42 (1986): 29–34. ML5 C65 MUSI.

Examines opening progression as vehicle for close interpretation of the text and as harnessing of techniques of "new music" to increase directness of musical approach. Notes that the composer chose solmization syllables similar to sound of text, as well as *molle* hexachords to convey ideas of suffering and sweetness. Suggests methods employed here are similar to those used in madrigal *La ver l'aurora*.

E0309 Poos, Heinrich. "Saggio sul vero metodo di analisi della musica palestriniana [Versuch über die wahre Art, Palestrina zu analysieren]." In *L'arte di Giovanni Pierluigi da Palestrina. Atti e Documentazione. VI Convegno Europeo sul Canto Corale. Promosso e Organizzato dalla Corale Goriziana "C.A. Seghizzi."* Gorizia: Grafica Goriziana, 1975. pp. 65–77.

Admonishes the deficient aesthetic perception of Palestrina as stylistically undifferentiated, which Poos ascribes to the nineteenth-century emphasis on instrumental music. Claims that writings which seriously analyze Palestrina are statistical in method and without context. Using the *Kyrie I* of the *Missa Quem dicunt homines* as an example, he proposes an analytical procedure which addresses the subtle and intricate affinities of parts, as well as the overall contrapuntal conception, asserting that this will improve insight into individual style formation in sixteenth-century music generally.

E0310 Possiedi, Paolo. "Intavolature di musiche vocali. Note per l'esecutore." *Il Fronimo* 7.4 (1980): 5–14.

Uses contemporary intabulations of Palestrina's popular madrigal *Vestiva i colli* by Terzi and Galilei to illustrate various principles and techniques for the intabulation of sixteenth-century vocal music for the lute.

E0311 Powers, Harold S. "The Modality of *Vestiva i colli*." In *Studies in Renaissance and Baroque Music in Honor of Arthur Mendel*, ed. Robert L. Marshall. Kassel: Bärenreiter, and Hackensack, NJ: Joseph Boonin, 1974. ISBN 0–193–57426–0. ML55.M415.S7. pp. 31–46. [also published in International Musicological Society, *Report of the Eleventh Congress—Copenhagen 1972*. Copenhagen, 1974. pp. 89–103. Italian trans as "La modalità di *Vestiva i colli*." In *Il madrigale tra Cinque e Seicento,* ed. Paulo Fabbri. Bologna: Il Mulino, 1988. pp. 189–206].

Insightful and influential article offering modal and structural analysis of Palestrina's famous madrigal, based on a study of sixteenth- and early-seventeenth-century theoretical writings and a review of some twentieth-century authorities on Renaissance mode theory. Additionally examines cleffing and mode structure in Palestrina's *Vergine* madrigal cycle (1581) and the *Offertoria* (1593).

E0312 Powers, Harold S. "Modal Representation in Polyphonic Offertories." *Early Music History* 2 (1982): 43–86 [Cambridge: Cambridge University Press, 1982].

Examination of modal practices in Palestrina's offertories supports the contention that the offertory cycle was intended to bring the tradition of singing freestyle motets (without plainchant referents) meant to accompany the action around the Offertory more in line with the official language of the divine service. This was done by providing free motets with texts not merely appropriate to the day but proper to the liturgy. Notes also that collection shows the innovation of arranging the first 32 items in order of the eight church modes.

E0313 Powers, Harold S. "Tonal Types and Modal Categories in Renaissance Polyphony." *Journal of the American Musicological Society* 34 (1981): 428–470 [repr. in *Garland Library of the History of Western Music. Renaissance Music*, Part 2, ed. Ellen Rosand. New York: Garland Publishing, Inc., 1985. pp. 98–140].

Study of correlation of tonal types in Renaissance polyphonic compositions with modal categories according to traditional schemes. Notes contrasting patterns in systems, cleffing, and final sonorities as objective criteria minimally marking off certain tonal types from one another. But while they may represent a concept of church modes, they are not church modes *per se*; church modes are culture-contextual "emic" musical concepts, while tonal types are objectively marked "etic" musical entities.

E0314 Quereau, Quentin W. "Aspects of Palestrina's Parody Procedure." *Journal of Musicology* 1 (1982): 198–216.

Discusses normative parody procedures in masses based on motets published by Moderne in the 1530s and '40s. Considers the factors which play a part in the selection and distribution of model material through the sections of a particular mass. Examines Palestrina's transformational procedures, pointing out both similarities and differences between the model and the composer's reworking.

E0315 Quereau, Quentin W. "Palestrina and the Motetti del Fiore of Jacques Moderne: a Study of Borrowing Procedure in Fourteen Parody Masses." Ph.D. dissertation, Yale University, 1974. DDJ75–01392.

Examines five aspects of models drawn from Moderne's 1532 anthology on which Palestrina based masses, namely melody, harmonic vocabulary, rhythmic procedure, stability of motivic content, and dissonance treatment. Finds strong stylistic resemblances between Palestrina's models and his compositional techniques in the masses based on those models. Concludes that there is a good possibility the composer knew the Moderne publication.

E0316 Quereau, Quentin W. "Sixteenth-Century Parody: An Approach to Analysis." *Journal of the American Musicological Society* 31 (1978): 401–441.

Analyzes contrapuntal relationships between overlapping motivic entries in passages working with borrowed motifs.

E0317 Radole, Giuseppe. "Tematica gregoriana in Palestrina." In *L'arte di Giovanni Pierluigi da Palestrina. Atti e Documentazione. VI Convegno Europeo sul Canto Corale. Promosso e Organizzato dalla Corale Goriziana "C.A. Seghizzi."* Gorizia: Grafica Goriziana, 1975. pp. 79–88.

Discusses the rhythmic and structural modifications Palestrina made to cantus firmus melodies so as to endow them with free declamatory qualities and to render them suitable for imitative requirements and useful generally as the basis for a contrapuntal structure. Discussion is grouped according to the strict or free use of the chant and by compositional genre.

E0318 Rahe, Heinrich. "*Die Motette Palestrinas*." Dissertation, Münster, 1943 (typescript).

Not reviewed, but clearly the basis for items E0319, E0320.

E0319 Rahe, Heinrich. "Der Aufbau der Motetten Palestrinas." *Kirchenmusikalisches Jahrbuch* 35 (1951): 54–83.

Examines the construction of Palestrina's motets. Finds that local contrasts in melodic and textural treatment are organized in terms of polar symmetries, and that such organization extends to large-scale sections of the motet text. Observes that a sense of symmetry underlying a principle of contrast is consistent with the larger aesthetic sensibility of the sixteenth century.

E0320 Rahe, Heinrich. "Thema und Melodiebildung der Motetten Palestrinas." *Kirchenmusikalisches Jahrbuch* 34 (1950): 62–81.

Analysis of the intervallic makeup, linear shaping, and imitative qualities, together with their interrelationships, in the melodies and countermelodies in Palestrina's motets. Observes that not only does Palestrinian melody fulfill the Renaissance search for symmetry and balance of tensions and contrasts, but that through its qualities is projected a sense of the language being set.

E0321 Reardon, Colleen. "Two Parody *Magnificats* on Palestrina's *Vestiva i colli*." *Studi musicali* 15 (1986): 67–99.

Points out that virtually every genre of sixteenth-century music was affected by the parody process. Discusses two *Magnificats* parodies of Palestrina's madrigal by Joseph Ascanio (fl. 1581–1589) and Carlo Berti (ca.1561–1602), comparing transformative and compositional decisions made by two different composers who adopted the same model. Parody/imitation process *per se* comes under review, and it becomes evident that parody technique as applied to the *Magnificat* is distinctly different from that for polyphonic masses.

E0322 Rees, Owen. "Roman Polyphony at Tarazona." *Early Music* 23 (1995): 410–419.

Discussion of Tarazona, Archivo Capitular, MS16, an isolated manuscript cantus partbook (the first of a set for a group of 8-part works) containing late-sixteenth-century Roman polychoral repertory. Two works are attributed to Palestrina. One, a *Magnificat sexti toni*, is unlikely to be his, but stylistic examination of the other work, a *unica* motet *Petre amas me*, supports an attribution to Palestrina. This manuscript suggests there is scope for further investigation of the influence of large-scale Roman polyphony on sacred music in Spanish institutions, whether through Neapolitan connections or through the existence in Rome of an Aragonese confraternity. *Petre amas me* is transcribed (p.413), as well as examples of other work.

E0323 Rees, Owen. "Triple-Choir Works by Palestrina and Victoria." *Early Music* 26 (1996): 170–172.

A review of Noel O'Regan's 1994 edition of three triple-choir works (item D0083), but with interesting additional material. Comments on the origin of the music, with the suggestion that these works may have been written for the confraternity of Trinità dei Pellegrini in 1576 and 1578, when Palestrina is known to have been connected with the institution.

E0324 Reese, Gustave. "The Opening Chant for a Palestrina Magnificat." In *A Musical Offering. Essays in Honor of Martin Bernstein*, ed. Edward Clinkscale, and Claire Brook. New York: Pendragon Press, 1977. ML55.B384.1977. pp. 239–241.

Brief note supporting a correction made by Paul Boepple in 1941 to the plainchant verses sung alternatim with a Palestrina *Magnificat* on the fourth tone. Boepple's edition differed from those of Haberl and Casimiri.

E0325 Reese, Gustave. "The Polyphonic Magnificat of the Renaissance as a Design in Tonal Centers." *Journal of the American Musicological Society* 13 (1960): 68–78.

Outlines some characteristic procedures for this genre: liturgical practices and psalm tone formulae, use of psalm tone as a melodic element, investigation of tonal schemes, orchestration of polyphony. Observations are claimed to be compatible with over 200 settings by composers of various nationalities, including 35 *Magnificats* by Palestrina.

E0326 Respighi, Carlo [monsignor]. *Giovanni Pierluigi da Palestrina e l'emendazione del Graduale Romano.* Società di San Giovanni Evangelista. Rome: Desclée, 1899.

A study of the so-called Medicean edition of the Roman Gradual, in which it is concluded that Palestrina cannot be regarded as an important editor of Gregorian chant, much less of the edition that was published some twenty years after his death.

E0327 Respighi, Carlo [monsignor]. *Nuovo Studio su Giovanni Pierluigi da Palestrina e l'emendazione del Graduale Romano con Appendice di Documenti.* Società di San Giovanni Battista. Rome: Desclée, 1900.

Another treatment of the origins and history of the Medicean edition, published not long after the preceding item. Disputes Haberl's assumptions and suggestions about why the work was not completed during the reign of Gregory XIII or during Palestrina's lifetime.

E0328 Riedel, Friedrich Wilhelm, ed. *Aufführungs- und Bearbeitungspraxis der Werke Palestrinas vom 16. bis zum 20. Jahrhundert.* Kirchenmusikalische Studien 3. Sinzig: Studio, Verlag Schewe, 1997. ISBN 3–89564–037–9. ML410.P15A84.1997.

Papers fron the international symposium held July 1–2, 1994, at the Musikwissenschaftliches Institut, Johannes—Gutenberg–Universität, Mainz. A collcction of nine essays dealing with issues of performance and with editorial and transcription practice in Palestrina's music ranging chronologically from his lifetime to the present. Individually indexed.

E0329 RISM. *Répertoire Internationale des Sources Musicales. Recueils Imprimés, XVI–XVII Siècles. 1. Liste Chronologique*, ed. François Lesure. Munich: G. Henle, 1960.

Chronological list of published collections of music by more than one composer ranging from 1501 to 1700. Citations include composers represented but do not list works by title.

E0330 RISM. *Répertoire Internationale des Sources Musicales. Series A/I. Einzeldrucke vor 1800.* Kassel: Bärenreiter, 1975.

Volume 6 pp. 396–404 list publications dedicated entirely to works by Palestrina but do not list the individual works within each by title.

E0331 Ritter, Gottfried August von. "Die *Ricercari sopra li toni* von G.P. Palestrina (?)" *Monatshrifte für Musikgeschichte* 6 (1874): 134–138.

An early description of each of the eight presumably instrumental ricercari attributed to Palestrina, presumably unknown to or overlooked by Baini. Palestrina's authorship is not confirmed here, but it is concluded that the pieces are in fact of excellent workmanship and can readily be related to the style of writing for the genre as it existed in the late sixteenth century.

E0332 Robertson, Alec. "A Practical Edition of Palestrina." *The Chesterian* 25, no.163 (1950): 106–108.

Nominally a review of an edition of the *Missa Brevis*, this item also contains a few interesting comments on sixteenth-century scoring practices in manuscript and early printed music, including some notes on the Lateran 59 Palestrina autograph.

E0333 Roche, Jerome. *Palestrina.* Oxford Studies of Composers 7. London: Oxford University Press, 1971. ISBN 0193141175. ML410 P15R6.

A study that conceives Palestrina's oeuvre in terms of an actual development over the course of a creative career. Works are examined both by genre and through their division into three style periods, encompassing successive phases that indicate connections with a late Netherlandish style, with a particular concern for textual clarity, and one when more "progressive" tendencies—interest in large-scale writing, sonorous colors, and more vertical sonorities—became increasingly evident.

E0334 Roche, Jerome. "Prefigurazioni del barocco nelle ultime opere del Palestrina [Prefigurings of the Baroque in the Late Works of Palestrina]." In *L'arte di Giovanni Pierluigi da Palestrina. Atti e documentazione. VI Convegno europeo sul canto corale. Promosso e organizzato dalla Corale Goriziana "C.A. Seghizzi."* Gorizia: Grafica Goriziana, 1975. In English, with outline of contents in Italian. pp. 89–95.

Asserts that Palestrina's later works differ significantly from his earlier ones and have forward-looking characteristics associated with the Baroque: respect for the text, remarkable attention to vertical sonority, harmonic color, groupings, and textural contrasts. Notes that the late *Missa Assumpta est Maria* features these qualities. Suggests such works may be judiciously embellished by the singers and accompanied by the organ.

E0335 Rogers, Rachel Ratliff. "Palestrina's Use of Triple Meter in Four-Voice Counterpoint." Ph.D. dissertation, Louisiana State University and Agricultural and Mechanical College, 1979. DDJ79–27544.

Computer-assisted analysis of all four-voice passages in triple meter. Compiles typical "rules" or procedures for such passages, apparently as a guide for student replication of the style, dealing with imitation, intervallic and part movement, treatment of passing tones, and suspensions. Of limited usefulness: the statistics have neither a historical nor a chronological style context, there is no citation of other contemporary composers or theorists, and the bibliography is anemic.

E0336 Rostirolla, Giancarlo. "Les éditions de Palestrina du XVI siècle à nos jours." In *L'interprétation de Palestrina. Journées d' étude*. Royaumont: Société Palestrina, 1990. pp. 1–11.

Palestrina prints (excluding modern editions and those authored by the composer himself) are found in sources of various types, such as anthologies and instrumental reductions, to which are added the examples printed in counterpoint treatises and theoretical works of the eighteenth century. For an optimal modern edition, the editor should collate sources close to the author with those not reviewed by the author, as well as later prints, in order to assess variants and corrections.

E0337 Roth, Joachim. "Zum Litaneischaffen G.P. Palestrinas und O. di Lassos." *Kirchenmusikalisches Jahrbuch* 44 (1960): 44–49.

A comparative study of Palestrina's and Lasso's litanies. Examines the peculiarities of litany texts and the compositional methods to which they lend themselves. While Lasso's litanies are mostly *falsobordoni*, liturgical *Gebrauchsmusik* that play a small role in his overall output, Palestrina's are much more carefully through-composed, with modeling and shaping of sections leading to an integrated and somewhat differentiated work. The Lauretan litanies of both composers for eight-voice double choir are compared. Lasso uses two sonically dissimilar choirs, texturally and metrically consistent, in which the forces of both unite only near the conclusion; Palestrina uses two similar high-voiced choirs organized by a ritornello-type structure, often changing textures and combinations of voices. Suggests on the one hand that for Lasso these are minor compositions which, however, do not harm his reputation; for Palestrina they may reflect a greater interest and even confidence in handling a particular kind of liturgical text.

E0338 Roth, Joachim. *Die mehrstimmigen lateinischen Litaneikompositionen des 16. Jahrhunderts*. Kölner Beiträge zur Musikwissenschaft 14. Regensburg: Bosse, 1959. ML3093.R68.

A study of the litany as a genre in the sixteenth century, with an examination of the text and its potential for musical setting and a survey of the extant repertory and its composers, Palestrina among them.

E0339 Samson, Joseph. "Le symbolisme dans les messes palestriniennes." *Revue Musicale* 20 (1939): 18–28.

Extract from author's book (see item E0149). Argues that Palestrina attempts to establish a kind of ideal relationship between particular mass material and the model (including its text gestures) on which it is based. When musical materials are removed from their earlier context and enter the mass, themes *per se* acquire a larger, more totally musical significance and give each work its unique character. Music is no longer merely text ornament but has a being of its own which participates in the liturgical celebration.

E0340 Schering, Arnold. "Takt und Sinngliederung in der Musik des 16. Jahrhunderts." *Archiv für Musikwissenschaft* 2 (1920): 465–498.

Study of the interpretation of the tactus in sixteenth-century music, with extensive references to Palestrina's compositions.

E0341 Schmidt-Görg, Joseph. "Vier Messen aud dem XVI. Jahrhundert über die Motette *Panis quem ego dabo* des Lupus Hellinck." *Kirchenmusikalisches Jahrbuch* 25 (1930): 77–93.

After an introductory analysis of Hellinck's motet *Panis quem ego dabo* (pub. 1532 by Moderne), the author discusses imitation masses by Lupus, Bartholomeo le Roy, Clemens non Papa, and Palestrina modeled on the motet. From analysis of cadence structures and uses of melodic and imitative material, it is concluded that Lupus and Palestrina imitate the model fairly closely (though not necessarily literally, and in Palestrina's case with a distinctive tonal color and freer counterpoint), while le Roy's and Clemens's masses are more freely composed and imitate the model only selectively. Each mass has its own personal style manner.

E0342 Schnürl, Karl. "Die Variationstechnik in den Choral-Cantus-Firmus-Werken Palestrinas." Dissertation, University of Vienna, 1949. 187pp.

E0343 Schnürl, Karl. "Die Variationstechnik in den Choral-Cantus-Firmus-Werken Palestrinas." *Studien zur Musikwissenschaft* 23 (1956): 11–66.

E0344 Schubert, Peter N. "The Fourteen-Mode System of Iluminato Aiguino." *Journal of Music Theory* 35 (1991): 175–210.

Exposition of Aiguino's system which, unlike Glarean's 12–mode ordering, was designed to explain all modal phenomena in terms of the eight church modes. Includes discussion of mode in Palestrina's offertories of 1593, especially *Jubilate Deo.*

E0345 Schubert, Peter N. "Mode and Counterpoint." In *Music Theory and the Exporation of the Past*, ed. Christopher Hatch, and David W. Bernstein. Chicago and London: University of Chicago Press, 1993. ISBN 0226319016. MT6.M96205.1993. pp. 103–136.

Palestrina's 4–voice motet *Dies sanctificatus* is used to illustrate a method of analysis which relates contrapuntal technique to mode, cadence structure, and text phrases, based on the principles offered in two treatises by Illuminato Aiguino: *La illuminata di tutti i tuoni di canto fermo* (Venice 1562) and *Il tesoro illuminato di tutti i tuoni di canto figurato (*Venice 1581).

E0346 Schuler, Manfred. "Werke Palestrinas in Orgeltabulaturen des 16. Jahrhunderts." In *Aufführungs- und Bearbeitungspraxis der Werke Palestrinas vom 16. bis zum 20. Jahrhundert*, ed. Friedrich Wilhelm Riedel. Kirchenmusikalische Studien 3. Sinzig: Studio, Verlag Schewe, 1997, pp. 13–23.

Discussion of particulars of transposition, voice leading, and ornamentation used in intabulations of Palestrina motets as found in a number of later sixteenth-century sources, notably publications issued by Jacob Paix in 1583 and 1589, as well as in a number of manuscript sources from Breslau and elsewhere. Notes that intabulations of Palestrina's music were already disappearing in favor of those of younger composers by the end of the sixteenth century.

E0347 Schwartz, Rudolf. "Zu den Texten der weltlichen Madrigale Palestrinas." *Jahrbuch der Musikbibliothek Peters* 13 (1906): 95–97.

Early, preliminary attempt to identify some of the authors of the texts of Palestrina's secular madrigals. Discusses poets associated with items in vol 28 of the Haberl edition: Nicolo Amanio, Pietro Bembo, Giacopo Sannazaro, Francesco Coppetta, Giovambattista Strozzi, and Ippolito Capilupi.

E0348 Sibley, David J. "The Sixteenth-Century Parody Mass." Ph.D. dissertation, University of Nottingham, 1990.

Comparative analysis of 33 masses, compiled by common titles into eight groups. Analysis performed 1) of different composers using the same model, and 2) by comparing one group with another. Each of the eight groups contains a mass by Palestrina. Argues that the characters of the parody masses selected for discussion are in large part determined by the purely musical content of their models. Palestrina masses studied include *O rex gloriae; Virtute magna; Panis quem ego dabo; Quem dicunt homines; Benedicta es; Io son ferito; Quando lieta sperai; Je suis desheritée.*

E0349 Sivec, Joseph. "Lamentatiònes Ieremiae prophetae Jakoba Gallusa." In *Gallus Carniolus in Europska renesansa. Gallus Carniolus und die europäische Renaissance.* Internationale Tagung Ljubljana, October 21–24, 1991. Vol 2, ed. Dragotin Cvetko and Danila Pokorn. Ljubljana: Slovenska Akademija Znanosti in Umetnosti, 1992. ISBN 86–7131–068–X. ML410.H315G33.1991.v.2. pp. 80–99.

An examination of the similarities and differences between the *Lamentations* of Gallus and those of Palestrina and others of the Roman school. Gallus not only chose a different breviary text for his *Lamentations* (from the 1517 Prague Breviary), he set the text for two four-voiced choirs, a texture very seldom used in his work. The polyphony of the letter-intonations ("Aleph," etc.) is less intense, shorter, and simpler thematically than Palestrina's. But like Palestrina's, Gallus's setting is close to homophonic in texture. [Based on summary in following German article.]

E0350 Snow, Robert J. "An Unknown *Missa pro defunctis* by Palestrina." In *De musica hispana et aliis: Miscelánea en honor al Prof. Dr. José López-Calo, S.J., en su 65 cumpleaños*, vol 1. Santiago da Compostela: Universidad de

Santiago da Compostela, 1990. 2 vols. pp. 387–430.

Examines a *Requiem a 4* preserved in two Spanish sources: Barcelona, Biblioteca Orfeó Catalá, MS10 (dated late-seventeenth to early-eighteenth century, in which the work is ascribed to Palestrina) and Alquézar, Colegiáta (Huesca) MS1 (where it is anonymous). Internal style analysis suggests that the material—introit, *Kyrie*, offertory, and communion in the case of the Barcelona MS, the *Sanctus* and *Agnus Dei* in the Alquézar source—may derive from Palestrina. Further stylistic comparison with the *Requiem* in the *Missarum liber primus* (2nd edition) reveals strong similarities and supports the attribution of the previously unknown work to the Roman master.

E0351 Stefani, Gino. "Gli Offertori di Palestrina. Aspetti musicali e liturgici." *Musica Sacra* 90 (1966): 82–89 [German version "Die Offertorien Palestrinas. Musikalische und liturgische Aspekte." *Musik und Altar* 1 (1967): 7–23].

A study of the offertories with respect to their liturgical context, melodic treatment, and modal arrangement. Note that the compositions are arranged according to classical mode series rather than according to their position in the church year.

E0352 Stevenson, Robert. "Sixteenth and Seventeenth Century Resources in Mexico." *Fontes artis musicae* 1 (1954): 69–77; 2 (1955): 10–14.

Includes discussion of the "Valdés Codex," bearing watermarks datable to Spain from 1561 to 1571, which contains five masses attributed to Palestrina. In addition to the masses *Aeterna Christi munera, Ave regina coelorum, Quem dicunt homines,* and *Già fu chi m' ebbe cara*, one, *Missa Christus resurgens* (modeled on a Richafort motet), has not been found in any European manuscript. Stevenson lists arguments for its authenticity.

E0353 Straus, Joseph. "The Motivic Structure of Palestrina's Music." *In Theory Only* 7.4 (Nov.1983): 3–23.

Argues that Schenkerian perceptions can be applied to pretonal music. Describes four possible sources of motivic and thematic unity in a composition: repetition, thematic varying, thematic transformation, and hidden repetition; argues that the last two are common in Palestrina's music and have an important influence on middleground and cadential structures. Analyzes motet *Sicut cervus, Kyrie* from the *Missa Papae Marcelli, Pleni* from *Missa Gabriel archangelus*, and the motets *Dies sanctificatus* and *Veni sponsa Christi.* Notes that for the composer, plainchant and melody provided motivic germs, which might not only be transformed in subtle ways but suggest middleground and background shapes as well.

E0354 Strunk, Oliver. "Guglielmo Gonzaga and Palestrina's *Missa Dominicalis*." *Musical Quarterly* 33 (1947): 228–239.

Examines Palestrina's working relationship with Duke Guglielmo through their correspondence, a large part of which is translated into English here. Strunk argues that a disputed *Missa Dominicalis* was in fact written by Palestrina for Mantua probably in 1578 to 1579, citing particularly the peculiar version of the plainchant on which it is based.

E0355 Strunk, Oliver. "Guglielmo Gonzaga and Palestrina's *Missa Dominicalis.*" In Strunk's *Essays on Music in the Western World.* New York: Norton, 1974. ISBN 0–393–02178–5. ML60.S862.E8. pp. 94–107.

Reprint of item E0354, above, but see also pages xvii–xx in the *Preface*, which contain a follow-up with historical notes about Duke Guglielmo and describing Knud Jeppensen's discovery of Palestrina's Mantuan masses in Milan. Notes that the *Missa Dominicalis* was not among them, but Strunk continued to claim its authenticity, which is now in fact generally presumed.

E0356 Tacaille, Alice. "L'emprunt au *corpus* grégorien dans les motets de Palestrina. Une approche quantitative." *Ostinato Rigore: Revue Internationale d'Études Musicales* 4 (1994): 185–191.

Examination of 251 liturgical motets and 66 of the 79 hymns of Palestrina, concluding that these works have a continuity with the Gregorian tradition.

E0357 Tiersot, Julien. "Un oeuvre contestée de Palestrina." *Le Ménéstrel* 63 (1896): 113–123.

See below, item E0359.

E0358 Tiersot, Julien. "Les 27 Répons de Palestrina." *Le Ménéstrel* 64 (1897).

Another part of the Tiersot-Brenet exchange; see item E0359.

E0359 Tiersot, Julien. "Pour le Centenaire de Palestrina. Les Répons de la Semaine-Sainte." *Rivista Musicale Italiana* 32 (1925): 381–411.

Elaborately argued, stubborn, but rationally shaky (and at times unconsciously funny) attack on the declaration that the 27 responsories printed in Haberl's collected edition as an *opus dubium* were not by Palestrina, but rather by Marc' Antonio Ingegneri. Tiersot was shocked and appalled at this conclusion, and not only decried Haberl's judgment of the sources (or lack of them for Palestrina's authorship), but, confronted with the recovered Ingegneri print of 1588 containing these works, assumed that they could only have been the result of something like plagiarism on Ingegneri's part. Tiersot had been arguing his position for years in the face of much evidence: he had had a series of exchanges with Michel Brenet in French reviews in 1896–1897 on this issue and remained unconvinced; Casimiri would publish an article in *Note d'Archivio* in 1926 in response to the present item; see E0199.

E0360 Tovey, Donald Francis. *Essays in Musical Analysis. Volume 5: Vocal Music.* London: Oxford University Press, 1937. MT90.T7.6.

Pp. 12–19 contain examinations of the motets *Paucitas dierum meorum, Exaltabo te,* and *Dum complerentur dies pentecostes.* Sensitive general analyses intended for intelligent amateurs and concert audiences not necessarily familiar with the style.

E0361 Ultan, Lloyd. *Music Theory: Problems and Practices in the Middle Ages and Renaissance.* Minneapolis: University of Minnesota Press, 1977. 267pp.

ISBN 0–8166–0802–4. ML174.U47.

A textbook designed to assist students in developing analytical and compositional techniques by studying works in historical sequence. Palestrina's style is treated in two chapters, pp. 208–227. Chapter 16 ("Palestrina: Part One") deals with general aesthetic considerations, linear contour, intervallic use, rhythmic characteristics, text treatment, and other observations on the materials of the composer's style. Chapter 17 ("Palestrina: Part Two") addresses the practices of counterpoint and dissonance treatment in two, three, or more voices.

E0362 Vale, Giacomo. "La Cappella musicale del Duomo di Udine dal sec. XIII al XIX." *Note d'Archivio* 7 (1930): 87–175.

Registers receipts and purchases of sixteenth- and seventeenth-century prints of Palestrina's music in the cathedral at Udine.

E0363 Virgili, Lavinio. "La Cappella musicale della Chiesa metropolitana di Fermo dalle origini al 1670." *Note d'Archivio* 7 (1930): 1–86.

Registers sixteenth-century prints of Palestrina's music mentioned in lists of library holdings in Fermo.

E0364 Vriees, Adriaan Bruce de. "Cadential Procedures in the Four-Part Masses of Palestrina." Ph.D. dissertation, McGill University, Montréal, 1976.

Offers a detailed method of analysis for cadence structures in late Renaissance music generally and in Palestrina in particular, based on the analytical method and terminology of Bernhard Meier. Analyses 509 cadences from all of Palestrina's four-part masses, finding in the late publications a tendency toward the sound of the full chord even at the expense of a *clausula vera*. Considers this evidence for a growing tendency toward vertical thinking in the composer's later music, a finding which may contribute to the attempt to date the posthumous works by stylistic means.

E0365 Wagner, Peter. *Geschichte der Messe. I. Teil: Bis 1600.* Leipzig: Breitkopf und Härtel, 1913. Only 1 vol published [facs. repr. Hildesheim: Georg Olms, 1972. ISBN 3–487–04249-5. ML3088.W2.1972].

This volume concludes with a general style survey of Palestrina and his contemporaries.

E0366 Wagner, Peter. "Palestrina als weltlicher Komponist." Dissertation, Strassburg, 1890. 63pp.

In this, perhaps the earliest modern study dedicated to Palestrina's secular madrigals, the great historian of Gregorian chant conveyed a high regard for these works. He described them as demonstrating a fine balance between organic compositional technique and form and an immersion in the expressive particulars of the text. See also item E0367.

E0367 Wagner, Peter. "Das Madrigal und Palestrina." *Vierteljahrsschrift für Musikwissenschaft* 8 (1892): 423–498.

To some extent a reworking of his doctoral dissertation. Presents a rough chronology of the madrigals based on their methods of composition. While admiring their technique and craft, he also concludes that Palestrina was not an innovator in the development of the madrigal, and that in terms of everything that is stylistically characteristic of the genre, other composers achieved more. Prints a series of madrigals by older contemporaries of, and influences upon, Palestrina, including works by Willaert, Verdelot, Barré, Gero, Festa, and Rore.

E0368 Weinmann, Karl. "Zur Geschichte von Palestrinas Missa Papae Marcelli." *Jahrbuch der Musikbibliothek Peters* 23 (1916): 23–42.

Notes that Baini perpetuated erroneous ideas about the origin of the mass. Weinmann suggests that the "new art" described by Palestrina in the preface to the *Missarum liber secundus* may have been mentioned not so much because of a radically new style, but to distance himself from his earlier "worldly" madrigal publication where he names himself as a papal singer. Notes that there is no evidence of what works of "intelligible music" were tried out for the Commission of Cardinals of 1564 and 1565, and that they were interested more in text clarity than in a particular musical style. There is also manuscript evidence that the mass existed before 1563. Although it is clear that Pope Marcellus II was generally reform-minded, and that he did admonish the papal singers to observe decorum in the performance of liturgical music, it is most improbable that he ever heard this mass during his brief pontificate.

E0369 Weinmann, Karl. "Palestrinas *Missa Papae Marcelli* und ihre Ausgaben." *Musica Sacra* 44 (1911): 227–231.

Describes the various editions and arrangements of the mass from the sixteenth and seventeenth centuries.

E0370 Weinmann, Karl. "Eine zwölfstimmige *Missa Papae Marcelli* von Stefano Nasimbeni." *Kirchenmusikalisches Jahrbuch* 21 (1908): 159–160.

Gives a history of early printed arrangements of this mass. Examines a 12–part arrangement in a manuscript located at Santa Maria in Vallicella, and notes its close resemblance to a printed mass dated 1610 published under the name of Stefano Nascimbeni [spelled here Nasimbeni].

E0371 Westergaard, Peter. "Linear Operations Necessary to Generate a Palestrina Foreground." In *International Musicological Society. Report of the Eleventh Congress, Copenhagen 1972*, ed. Henrik Glahn, Søren Sørensen and Peter Ryom. Copenhagen: Wilhelm Hansen, 1974. ISBN 87–7455–026–8. ML36.I6.1972. pp. 103–107.

Westergaard states (p.104): "For any Palestrina piece there is a middleground structure consisting of lines in breves or semibreves from which these operations [i.e. segmentation, rearticulation, embellishment by neighbors, borrowing, step motion, delay, and anticipation] will generate the actual foreground. However, there is no deeper structure from which these rules will generate that middleground structure. On the contrary, we would need an essentially different set of rules to generate such a middleground structure. Such a set of rules would, I believe, closely resemble the set of rules we would need to generate most pre-polyphonic Western music."

E0372 Widmann, Wilhelm. "Motette und Messe *Dies sanctificatus* von Palestrina." *Kirchenmusikalisches Jahrbuch* 21 (1908): 72–90.

Phrase-by-phrase study of thematic and imitative elaboration in the motet *Dies sanctificatus*, with a shorter section on the adaptation of this material in the mass of the same name.

E0373 Widmann, Wilhelm. "Die sechstimmige Messen Palestrinas. Ein Beitrag zur Stilkritik." *Kirchenmusikalisches Jahrbuch* 25 (1930): 94–106; 26 (1931): 59–72; 27 (1932): 110–119; 28 (1933): 10–34.

An older but meticulous analysis of melodic and textural treatment in a number of six-part masses (in greatest detail with reference to their *Kyrie* sections, although most other sections are examined as well), with comparison with their motet models when applicable. Masses examined include *Missa Papae Marcelli; Missa Ecce ego Joannes; Missa Alma Redemptor; Missa Assumpta est Maria; Missa Illumina oculos meos.*

E0374 Wolff, Hellmuth Christian. "Die Variationstechnik in den frühen Messen Palestrinas." *Acta Musicologica* 27 (1955): 59–70.

Asserts that Palestrina shows a close affinity with the Netherlanders in the techniques used in his early masses. Two masses from his first book (pub. 1554), *Ecce sacerdos magnus* and *O regem coeli*, are studied. *Ecce sacerdos magnus* uses a cyclic-variation technique, in which collected thematic material based on the *cantus firmus* is presented in the *Kyrie*, and successive movements then take this *Kyrie* material and provide a working-out of one or more of its voices. *O regem coeli* demonstrates a "free motivic variation" technique, where motivic material is drawn from the cantus firmus and associated with imitation in all the voices.

———. Zacconi, Lodovico. See item E0459; see also Haar, item E0420.

E0375 Ziino, Agostino. "Testi laudistici musicati da Palestrina" In *Atti del Convegno di Studi Palestriniani. 28 settembre–2 ottobre 1975*, ed. Francesco Luisi. Palestrina: Fondazione Giovanni Pierluigi da Palestrina, 1977. ML 410.P15C77.1975. pp. 383–408.

Examines two cycles of spiritual madrigals based on laude, *Spirito santo amor* and *O Jesu dolce*, from the *Primo libro de madrigali a cinque voci* (1581). Although primarily madrigalistic in treatment, they exhibit structural and tonal characteristics suggesting the influence of the lauda tradition: harmonic and contrapuntal simplification, homorhythmic writing, limited word or phrase reiteration, and repriselike cadence repetition.

E0376 Ziino, Agostino. "La tradizione musicale dello *Stabat Mater* fino a Palestrina." In *Atti del II Convegno internzationale di Studi Palestriniani. Anno Europeo della Musica. 3–5 maggio 1986*, ed. Lino Bianchi and Giancarlo Rostirolla. Palestrina: Fondazione Giovanni Pierluigi da Palestrina/Centro di

Studi Palestriniani, 1991. ML410.P15C77.1986. pp. 29–61.

Argues that historically the place of the *Stabat Mater* in the liturgy was ambiguous. (Palestrina's own setting was apparently used as an offertory substitute.) Although usually described as a sequence, the *Stabat Mater* in fact had a largely autonomous development heavily influenced by the lauda tradition, hymnody, and Flemish motet polyphony. Palestrina's compositional approach to it was different from that observable in his settings of other older medieval sequences. He used a double choir to differentiate single verses and to heighten poetic sense, rhythmic symmetries, and inherent drama.

IV. Reception History

1. From the Sixteenth Century to 1750

E0377 Ackermann, Peter. "Zur Frühgeschichte der Palestrinarezeption: die zwölfstimmige *Missa Cantantibus organis* und die Compagnia dei Musici di Roma." *Kirchenmusikalisches Jahrbuch* 78 (1994): 7–25.

Based on the Palestrina motet *Cantantibus organis* (pub. 1575), this mass was a collaboration by seven musicians: Annibale Stabile, Giovanni Andrea Dragoni, Francesco Soriano, Ruggero Giovanelli, Curzio Mancini, Prospero Santini, and Palestrina himself. Article explores the different ways each composer adapted material from the motet, uniting Palestrina's practices with individual compositional solutions to create a progressive compendium of possibilities. Also contains detailed information about the Palestrina manuscript tradition within the Sistine Chapel before around 1600.

E0378 Ackermann, Peter. "Palestrina-Bearbeitungen der Cappella Sistina im 18. Jahrhundert." In *Aufführungs- und Bearbeitungspraxis der Werke Palestrinas vom 16. bis zum 20. Jahrhundert*, ed. Friedrich Wilhelm Riedel. Kirchenmusikalische Studien 3. Sinzig: Studio, Verlag Schewe, 1997. pp. 43–53.

A particular group of Palestrina works was established repertory of the Sistine by the mid-seventeenth century. Copies of these works continued to be renewed for the next century even though new items were not added. In the mid-eighteenth century, more than a dozen of the "standard" motets were assigned contrafacta, which gave them new applications in the liturgical repertory. Also beginning in the mid-seventeenth century, adaptation of some of Palestrina's music was practiced, which was apparently meant to give the material a wider performing base: motets were adapted as mass movements, the polyphonic scoring of some motets was rearranged to create double-choir effects, and rhythmic rewriting which suggested accelerated tempi was done.

E0379 Ackermann, Peter. "Palestrina und die Idee der absoluten Musik." In *Palestrina: Zwischen Démontage und Rettung*, ed. Heinz-Klaus Metzger and Rainer Riehn. Munich: Text + Kritik, 1994. pp. 28–42.

Argues that Palestrina reception history up to the early nineteenth century flowed in two streams—the model of contrapuntal perfection, and the "legend." They united in the writings of E. T. A. Hoffmann, who found in Palestrina's vocal art the same transcendent romantic spirit as was manifested in absolute symphonic music. Ackermann analyzes in detail the formal processes used in the offertory motet *Illumina oculos meos* to suggest some rationale for the aesthetic appeal of the Palestrina style to the Romantics.

E0380 Ackermann, Peter. "Tradition und Fortschritt. Zur römischen Wirkungsgeschichte Palestrinas im 16. und 17. Jahrhundert." In *Musica Divina. Ausstellung zum 400. Todesjahr von Giovanni Pierluigi da Palestrina und Orlando di Lasso und zum 200. Geburtsjahr von Carl Proske*. Bischöfliches Zentralarchiv und Bischöfliche Zentralbibliothek Regensburg Kataloge und Schriften 11. ed. Paul Mai. Regensburg: Schnell & Steiner, 1995. pp. 109–116.

Notes that Palestrina reception in the seventeenth century was two-branched: on the one hand was a tradition of counterpoint and theory manifested in a particular style practice; on the other was a transfigured image of the liturgical composer and "the legend." Argues that Agazzari saw Palestrina as the initiator of a renewal in church practice rather than as an *antico*. Notes that certain of Palestrina's pupils and disciples, in compiling the *Missa Cantantibus organis* and other works, were indicating some of the modern directions in which composition in Palestrina's manner could go. Also argues that in the seventeenth century there developed an almost canonical repertory of Palestrina's works as performed in the Sistine, as evidenced in dated manuscript evidence, the late parodies of his music found in such items as dal Pane's masses of 1687, and Adami da Bolsena's *Osservazioni* (item E0381).

E0381 Adami da Bolsena, Andrea. *Osservazioni per ben regolare il coro dei cantori della Cappella Pontificia.* Rome: Antonio De' Rossi, 1711 [facs. rep. ed. Giancarlo Rostirolla. Musurgia I. Lucca: Libreria Musicale Italiana, 1988. ISBN 8870960005. ML290.8.V28A43.1711a].

A manual for liturgical ceremonial in the Sistine Chapel in the early eighteenth century. Testifies to frequency and occasions for established performance of numerous Palestrina works. Includes iconography and biography of Palestrina (pp.169–174) as well as other musicians of the Roman school, much material of which is derived from Liberati.

E0382 Agazzari, Agostino. *Del sonare sopra 'l basso con tutti li stromenti e dell'uso loro nel conserto. . . .* Siena: Domenico Falcini, 1607 [repr. Milano: Bolletino bibiografico musicale, 1933].

Included here as probably the earliest published source (p.11) for the legend that Palestrina "rescued" polyphony from being banned in the church by producing the *Missa Papae Marcelli*.

E0383 Amann, Julius. *Allegris* Miserere *und die Aufführungspraxis der Capella Sixtina nach Reiseberichten und Musikhandschriften.* Freiburger Studien zur Musikwissenschaft, Reihe 2, Heft 4. Regensburg: Pustet, 1935.

Principally a history of performance and ornamental practices associated with the Allegri work dating from the 1640s through the early nineteenth century, this book deals by extension with a cluster of other compositions by Palestrina also traditionally performed in the chapel during Holy Week, including the *Improperia*, the *Stabat Mater*, and the motet *Fratres ego enim accepi.*

E0384 Asola, Giovanni Matteo, ed. *Sacra omnium solemnitatum Psalmodia vespertina cum Cantico B. Virginis a diversis in arte musica praestantissimis viris notulis musicis exornata.* Venice: Ricciardo Amadino, 1592.

Thirteeen colleagues and students of the sexagenerian Palestrina compiled this work, introduced with an adulatory Latin dedication indicating the high esteem in which he was held. In response, Palestrina would publish the motet *Vos amici mei estis* in the Conforti psalm collection of 1592.

E0385 Banchieri, Adriano. *Conclusioni nel suono dell'organo novellamente tradotte et dilucidate in scrittori et organisti cellebri.* Bologna: heirs of Gio. Rossi, 1609 [facs. ed. in Monuments of music and music literature in facsimile. Second series, 101 New York: Broude Bros., 1975. ISBN 0845023012. MT180.B3.1975].

Another important early source for the Marcellus mass story (p.19), closely related to Agazzari's comments on the subject.

E0386 Banchieri, Adriano. *Lettere armoniche. . . .* Bologna: Girolamo Mascheroni, 1628 [facs. repr. Bologna: Forni, 1968].

In a letter to Giovanni Maria Artusi written around 1600, Banchieri exempted "modern imitators of the good Roman school" from being "destroyers of the good rules," and he cites Palestrina as a preeminent practitioner of church music (p.94), enumerating salient features of his style manner.

E0387 Basso, Alberto. "Bach e Palestrina." In *Atti del II Convegno Internazionale di Studi Palestriniani. Anno Europeo della Musica. 3–5 maggio 1986*, ed. Lino Bianchi and Giancarlo Rostirolla. Palestrina: Fondazione Giovanni Pierluigi da Palestrina/Centro Studi Palestriniani, 1991. ML410.P15C77.1986. pp. 407–419.

Describes the general interest of eighteenth-century German composers in the older style, the uses it had in seventeenth- and eighteenth-century (Protestant) countries, and the *antico* repertories available to J. S. Bach and his predecessors through anthologies and *florilegia*. Discusses Bach's virtually emblematic use of the older style (with *colla parte* instrumental accompaniments) in a number of his works, as well as his adaptation of certain older works, including Palestrina's *Missa Sine nomine a 6*. Suggests this was not simply as a matter of using old music in a new context, but done in terms of his own rethinking and exploration of the style.

E0388 Berardi, Angelo. *Ragionamenti musicali*. Bologna: Giacomo Monti, 1681.

Palestrina and Palestrina style pp.77–78 *et passim*. Berardi, a pupil of Marco Scacchi and the best-known posthumous representative of Scacchi's ideas, was perhaps the most distinguished of the later seventeenth-century Italian theorists of the techniques of the Roman school, admiring it while not giving it an exclusive ideological commitment of the Liberati-Pitoni type.

E0389 Bianconi, Lorenzo. *Il Seicento.* Turin: Edizioni di Torino, 1982. *Music in the Seventeenth Century*, trans. David Bryant. Cambridge, UK: Cambridge University Press, 1987. ISBN 0–521–26290–9. ML290.2.B513.

Excellent style history with narrative approach based on an interplay of sociocultural and stylistic insights, leaning to a somewhat diluted Marxist viewpoint. In the Bryant translation, Section III, "Sacred Vocal Music," pp.105–109, especially discuss the place of Palestrina's music and image on the seventeenth-century scene. Notes that the composer is venerated more by the theorists as the ultimate musicoliturgical ideal than as the author of a rigid stylistic code, and that the *stile alla Palestrina* by no means accounts for the totality of Italian sacred music or solves all its various post-Tridentine problems and conflicts, even from the perspective of the period itself. Good source for review of general tendencies in church music in the seventeenth century.

E0390 Bonini, Severo. *Discorsi e regole sopra la musica*, ed. Leila Galleni Luisi. Instituta et monumenta: Serie 2, Instituta 5. Cremona: Fondazione Claudio Monteverdi, 1975. ML194.B64.

An Italian edition of a seventeenth-century treatise containing interesting observations on the relationship of compositional styles. See item E0391 for further information.

E0391 Bonini, Severo. *Discorsi e regole*, trans. Mary Ann Bonino. Provo, UT: Brigham Young University Press, 1979.

Treatise (Firenze, Biblioteca Riccardiana 2218, dated ca.1650) which advocates a special place for the Palestrina style while seeking to reconcile it with the conflicting claims of monody. Attempts to integrate both into a typology for modern composition of the period. Palestrina is cited as being one of those who removed error from composition and restored the honor it once possessed, a "sublime genius" and a high authority for *da cappella* composition. Mary Ann Bonino's edition is bilingual, with Italian and English parallel texts and an extensive introduction about Bonini and his manuscript.

E0392 Celani, Enrico. "I cantori della Cappella Pontifician nei secoli XVI–XVII." *Rivista Musicale Italiana* 14 (1907): 83–104, 752–790; 16 (1909): 55–112.

A narrative history of the Sistine Chapel ranging from the reigns of Leo X to Benedict XIV, drawn from the manuscript compiled by Matteo Fornari in 1749 (Biblioteca Corsiniana, MS F.6).

———. Cerone, Pedro. *El Melopeo y el Maestro. Tractado de Musica Theorica y Pratica.* Naples: J. B. Gargoni and L. Nucci, 1613 [facs. repr. Bologna: Forni, 1969]. MT6.C35.1971.

See item E0204.

E0393 Ciliberti, Galliano. "Organizzazione musicale e orientamenti stilistici nello Stato Pontificio post-Tridentino." *Rivista Internazionale di Musica Sacra* 11.4 (1990): 343–355.

Describes the changing professional role of the Roman *maestro di cappella* in the first half of the seventeenth century. The mythologizing of Palestrina which grew during that period served in part to orient musical style and practice toward papal Rome as a Catholic cultural epicenter.

E0394 Ciliberti, Galliano, and F. Rambotti. "La produzione musicale e gli scritti teorici di Antimo Liberati, cantore della cappella pontificia (Foligno 1617–Roma 1692)." In *Annali della Facoltà di Lettere e Filosofia. Università degli Studi di Perugia.* 2 Studi storico-antropologici 25, new ser. 9 (1987–1988): 85–131.

An overview of the work of Liberati, best known as the historian and theorist who championed the style of Palestrina and the Roman school as the epitome of true church music in his critical writings. Includes a catalog of compositions (with known but lost items), the texts of his 16 extant cantatas, as well as transcriptions of the *Ragguaglio dello stato del coro de'cantori nella Cappella Sistina* (ca. 1662–1663) and the correspondence dealing with the "Corelli fifths" controversy (1685).

E0395 Cresolles, Louis de [Ludovicus Cresolles Armorici]. *Mystagogus de sacrorum hominum disciplina.* Paris: Cramoisy, 1629.

Book III, section 4, page 627, is an important early retelling of the Marcellus mass story. Cresolles adds that Palestrina himself related the tale to a member of the Jesuit order, from whom the author heard it.

E0396 Day, Thomas Charles. "Echoes of Palestrina's *Missa ad fugam* in the 18th century." *Journal of the American Musicological Society* 24 (1971): 462–469.

Notes some canonic masses by Fux and Scarlatti influenced by Palestrina's *Missa ad fugam.*

E0397 Day, Thomas. "Palestrina in History: a Preliminary Study of Palestrina's Reputation and Influence Since His Death." Ph.D. dissertation, Columbia University, 1970. 201pp.

Traces commentary on Palestrina from the sixteenth through nineteenth centuries.

E0398 Day, Thomas. "A Renaissance Revival in the Eighteenth Century." *Musical Quarterly* 57 (1971): 575–592.

Describes the continued cultivation of sixteenth-century polyphony in England from 1650 to 1780, both that of native masters and that of certain Italians such as Palestrina. Discusses Henry Aldrich's copying and emendation of Palestrina compositions in the later seventeenth century; the work of various historians; activities of the Academy of Ancient Music and the Madrigal Society.

E0399 Dixon, Graham. "The Origins of the Roman 'Colossal Baroque.'" *Proceed-*

ings of the Royal Musical Association 106 (1979–1980): 115–128.

An examination of large-scale vocal music in Rome from 1600 to 1650, which is situated in part as an extension of stylistic tendencies already present in the later music of Palestrina.

E0400 Dixon, Graham. "Progressive Tendencies in the Roman Motet in the Early Seventeenth Century." *Acta Musicologica* 53 (1981): 105–119.

Examines how some of the more progressive tendencies in Palestrina's music—notably treatment of textures and use of polychoral technique—developed in the works of his successors, notably Agazzari, Nanino, Anerio, and Cifra. Small-scale sacred works by these composers are also discussed.

E0401 Della Valle, Pietro. *Della musica dell'età nostra, che non è punto inferiore, anzi è migliore di quella dell'età passata. Al Sig. Lelio Guidiccioni. Discorso di Pietro della Valle* [1640]. Essay printed in vol 2, pp.249–264, of Giovanni Battista Doni, *Lyra Barberina Amphichordos. . . .* ed. Antonio Francesco Gori. Florence: Imperial Printer, 1763 [facs. repr. of *Lyra Barberina*, Bologna: Forni, 1974]; Della Valle essay ed. in Angelo Solerti, *Le origini del melodramma* (Turin: Fratelli Bocca, 1903, pp.148–179); partial English translation by Margaret Murata in *Source Readings in Music History, Volume 4: The Baroque Era*, ed. Oliver Strunk; rev. ed. Leo Treitler (New York: Norton, 1998, pp. 36–43).

A multifaceted traveler, linguist, and aristocratic connoisseur, della Valle's comments on the contemporary musical scene in Rome betray a modernist aesthetic sensibility and a keen awareness of style issues. He admired Palestrina's craft and taste, but he also decried contrapuntal artifice as "inexpressive" and could not justify admiration of older music for oldness's sake. He praised *Vestiva i colli* but thought the *Missa Papae Marcelli* should be relegated to a museum along with other "beautiful curiosities."

E0402 Dixon, Graham. "Tradition and Progress in Roman Mass Settings after Palestrina." In *Atti del II Convegno internzationale di Studi Palestriniani. Anno Europeo della Musica. 3–5 maggio 1986*, ed. Lino Bianchi and Giancarlo Rostirolla. Palestrina: Fondazione Giovanni Pierluigi da Palestrina/Centro di Studi Palestriniani, 1991. In English, with Italian translation. ML410.P15C77.1986. pp. 311–324.

Explores *prima prattica* mass composition during the period 1608 to 1635. As a musical genre the mass was ceasing to occupy the primary composition in Roman compositional production, as it was being overtaken by vesper settings and small-scale motets. However, this generation acknowlegded Palestrina's preeminence, and his true followers continued to explore the polychoral writing, increasing textural verticalization, and more "tonal" approach of Palestrina's late work.

E0403 Deniseau, Gérard. "Palestrina, Vignole et le Concile de Trente." *Ostinato Rigore: Revue Internationale d'Études Musicales* 4 (1994): 193–197.

Studies the effects of the mandates of the Council of Trent upon creative artists through parallel study of two exactly contemporaneous works (1567 and 1568): the *Missa Papae Marcelli* of Palestrina, and the Chiesa di SS. Nome di Gesù ("Il Gesù") in Rome, built by the architect Giacomo da Vignola (Giacomo Barozzi).

E0404 Feil, Arnold. "Zum Gradus ad Parnassum von J. J. Fux." *Archiv für Musikwissenschaft* 14 (1957): 184–192.

Scrutinizes this famous manual of counterpoint long looked upon as a homage to the Palestrina style. Notes that it is neither a generalbass treatise (as would be typical of its time), nor really a manual for vocal polyphony or the church style, and that it is fundamentally different from the manuals of Berardi or others descended from the sixteenth-century type. It isolates aspects of technique in exercises and does not teach the making of a composition in any style, and to say that *Gradus* teaches the Palestrina style almost demeans the style. What is new about the text is that it is a kind of technical finishing school for those who have already learned composition, whether through generalbass or polyphonic writing.

E0405 Fellerer, Karl Gustav. "Allgemeine geistliche Grundlagen des Palestrinastil." *Monatshrifte für katholische Kirchenmusik* 10 (1928): 1–7.

See *Palestrina-Studien,* 1982, item E0228.

E0406 Fellerer, Karl Gustav. "Instrumentale Begleitung der Werke Palestrinas im 18. Jahrhundert." *Musica Sacra* 55 (1925).

See item E0228, Fellerer, *Palestrina-Studien*, pp.355 *et seq*. Describes *bassus ad organum, basso continuo*, and *colla parte* practices in the seventeenth and eighteenth centuries, used both for the instrumental accompaniment of contemporaneous compositions in the older style and for the performance of the music of Palestrina himself. Notes that in the nineteenth century, under the romantic *a cappella* ideal, the practice of accompanying and embellishing such music was greatly reduced.

E0407 Fellerer, Karl Gustav. "J. S. Bachs Bearbeitung der Missa *Sine nomine* von Palestrina." *Bach-Jahrbuch* 24 (1927): 123–132.

See item E0228, Fellerer, *Palestrina-Studien*, p. 361 *et seq*. Describes Bach's adaptation of the Palestrina *Missa sine nomine a 6* for Lutheran performance: he excerpted the Lutheran *Missa* [*Kyrie* and *Gloria* only] and added *colla parte* and *basso continuo* instruments to the vocal parts [two cornetti, four trombones, violone, cembalo, and organ]. Bach's transcription indicates the difference in understanding of his own time in matters of the beat and measure, text declamation, and tonal harmony.

E0408 Fellerer, Karl Gustav. "Zur Kirchenmusik Roms in 17. Jahrhundert." In *Logos Musicae. Festschrift für Albert Palm*, ed. Rüdiger Görner. Wiesbaden: Franz Steiner, 1982. pp. 71–82.

Discussion of papal mandates for church music and the activity of church musicians, particularly Palestrina's successors and those working in the Roman *alla Palestrina* style. The writings of Liberati are used as an important source.

E0409 Fellerer, Karl Gustav. "Palestrina in 17. und 18. Jahrhundert." *Musica Sacra* 55 (1925).

See item E0228, Fellerer, *Palestrina-Studien*, p. 315 *et seq*. Describes the increasingly strict conceptual division of church music styles from theatrical and chamber music that occurred during the seventeenth century, and the manner in which the strict or observant church manner underwent subtle changes in harmonic and metrical technique. Examines the work of a number of practitioners. Indicates ways in which the imitators of the Palestrina style, though emphasizing that theirs was an unbroken tradition, nonetheless tended to depart from the literal features of Palestrina's manner in their own actual work.

E0410 Fellerer, Karl Gustav. *Der Palestrinastil und seine Bedeutung in der vokalen Kirchenmusik des achtzehnten Jahrhunderts. Ein Beitrag zur Geschichte der Kirchenmusik in Italien und Deutschland.* Augsburg: Dr. Benno Filser, 1929 [repr. Walluf bei Wiesbaden: Sändig, 1972]. 365pp.

See also item E0228, Fellerer, *Palestrina-Studien*. Study of material features of the Palestrinian style and the transformations which came over the late sixteenth-century manner in the course of the seventeenth and especially eighteenth centuries. Systematically surveys both theoretical and didactic writings and the strict-style music of a large number of Neapolitan, Roman, Bolognese, German, and Austrian composers. Concludes with a summary of the shifts in rhythmic, harmonic and melodic treatment, declamatory manner, and use of instrumental accompaniment which had taken place in *stile antico* emulations of late Renaissance style.

E0411 Fellerer, Karl Gustav. "Zur Palestrina-Nachahmung im 18. Jahrhundert." *Gregoriusblatt* 52 (1982): 8–13, 17–21.

See *Palestrina-Studien*, item E0228.

E0412 Fellerer, Karl Gustav. "Der stile antico in der katholischen Kirchenmusik des 18. Jahrhundert." *Musica Divina: Monatschrift für Kirchenmusik* 15 (1927), repr. Kongressbericht Wien. *Beethoven-Zentenarfeier Wien. Internationaler Musikhistorischer Kongress (Wien, 28. bis 31. März 1927).* Vienna: Universal 1927, pp. 244–246.

See *Palestrina-Studien*, item E0228.

E0413 Fellerer, Karl Gustav. "Zur Übertragung und Aufführung von Werken altklassischer Polyphonie." *Gregoriusblatt* 53 (1929).

See *Palestrina-Studien*, item E0228.

E0414 Fellerer, Karl Gustav. "Die vokalen Kirchenmusik des 17./18. Jahrhunderts und der altklassischen Polyphonie." *Zeitschrift für Musikwissenschaft* 11 (1929): 354–364.

See *Palestrina-Studien*, item E0228.

E0415 Fischer, Klaus. "Zur Palestrinarezeption in der italienischen Musiktheorie des 16. und 17. Jahrhunderts." *Kirchenmusikalisches Jahrbuch* 78 (1994): 27–39.

Valuable examination of Palestrina's reputation as found in printed theoretical sources dating from about 1570 to 1685. Provides perspective on the shifting coloration of his image—from authoritative master of his craft and excellent source for instruction to "prince of music."

E0416 Fux, Johann Joseph. *Gradus ad Parnassum sive manuductio ad compositionem musicae regularem. . . .* Vienna: Johann Peter van Ghelen, 1725; 2nd ed, 1742. [Partial Eng. trans. by Alfred Mann, *Steps to Parnassus: the Study of Counterpoint* (New York: Norton, 1943; 2nd rev. ed. 1965 as *The Study of Counterpoint*), MT55.F9. Facsimile of 1725 edition in *Sämtliche Werke, Serie VII: Theoretische und pädagogische Werke,* ed. Johann-Joseph-Fux-Gesellschaft, Graz. Kassel: Bärenreiter, 1959. M3.F97].

The famous manual of instruction in species counterpoint in which Fux pays homage to the Palestrina style, as the early eighteenth century understood it, on several levels. Constructed in a traditional dialogue format, the treatise personifies Palestrina as the master Aloysius, who instructs the student Josephus, that is, Fux.

E0417 Gaillard, Pierre. "Histoire de la légende palestrinienne." *Revue de Musicologie* 57 (1971): 11–22.

Traces the historiography of the Palestrina "legend" from the seventeenth through the nineteenth centuries. Suggests that it evolved in shifting phases (in turn ecclesiastical, nationalistic, poetic, and artistic) which were colored by the various interests and biases of generations of writers. The legend gained impetus from Agazzari and Banchieri; Baini made Palestrina a virtual national hero; the Romantics used him to evoke the past; oratorios and operas had him as a principal character.

E0418 Giustiniani, Vincenzo. *Discourse on Modern Music* [*Discorso sopra la musica de'suoi tempi. 1628*], trans. and ed. Carol McClintock. Musicological Studies and Documents 9. American Institute of Musicology, 1962. pp. 65–80.

Writing around 1628, Giustiniani comments on why the music of Palestrina continued to appeal to his contemporaries, and on the aesthetic and style techniques on which such music was based: namely, the union of a beautiful, uncomplicated flow of ideas with sound compositional principles (see especially pp.68–72 of McClintock's translation).

E0419 Gmeinwieser, Siegfried. "Girolamo Chiti (1679–1759) maestro di cappella in S. Giovanni in Laterano." *Nuova Rivista Musicale Italiana* 4 (1974): 665–677.

Assessment of the life and activities of Chiti. Musician and composer, he was also a theorist of the Roman church music style and a significant eighteenth-century collector of Palestrina's music, on which subject he also carried on an extensive correspondence with Padre Martini. Reviews Chiti's assessment of Palestrina's style and historical importance, and the influences on his thinking and its development.

E0420 Haar, James. "A Sixteenth-Century Attempt at Music Criticism." *Journal of the American Musicological Society* 36 (1983): 191–209.

Discussion of terminology in a passage from Lodovico Zacconi's *Prattica di musica* reporting remarks of Zarlino's which describe criteria by which the quality of a composition can be assessed, and noting the particulars of style in which certain composers excelled. Haar discusses what Zarlino and Zacconi meant when they indicated that Palestrina was esteemed for "arte, contrapunto, ottima dispositione," and a flowing "modulatione."

E0421 Haberl, Franz Xaver. "Das traditionelle Musikprogramm der Sixtinischen Kapelle nach den Aufzeichnungen von Adami Adami da Bolsena." *Kirchenmusikalisches Jahrbuch* 21 (1897): 36–58.

Relates travel reports on appearance and performance practice in the Sistine Chapel during Holy Week by several eighteenth- and nineteeth-century German visitors, particularly Goethe, Christoph Kayser, and Ludwig Spohr. Then reverts for the main part of the article to earlier descriptions of the chapel and its liturgical ceremonial for the church year cycle as performed around 1700, based on Adami's then generally unavailable *Osservazioni per ben regolare il coro dei cantori della Cappella Pontificia.*

E0422 Heinemann, Michael. " ' . . . alla Palestrina.' Zur Etablierung eines satztechnischen Ideals im 17. Jahrhundert." In *Palestrina: Zwischen Démontage und Rettung*, ed. Heinz-Klaus Metzger and Rainer Riehn. Munich: Text + Kritik, 1994. pp. 9–27.

Establishes that Palestrina managed his personal and professional lives astutely, and holds that his fame related in part to a new independence of Roman musical institutions after their long domination by Netherlanders. Traces the crisis in counterpoint around 1600 and how some of the subsequent controversies over contrapuntal and generic theory were argued from the point of view of an "authoritative" Roman school. Repeats seventeenth-century rules for composing church music in the strict Roman manner as developed in the writings of Marco Scacchi and Angelo Berardi.

E0423 Horn, Wolfgang. "Der 'antique Kirchen-Stylus' und die Musik Palestrinas. Bemerkungen zur Palestrina-Pflege und zur Komposition im 'gebundenen Allabreve-Stil' am Dresdner Hof zur Zeit Heinichens und Zelenkas." In *Aufführungs- und Bearbeitungspraxis der Werke Palestrinas vom 16. bis zum 20. Jahrhundert*, ed. Friedrich Wilhelm Riedel. Kirchenmusikalische Studien 3. Sinzig: Studio, Verlag Schewe, 1997. pp. 55–79.

Discusses the relevance of Palestrina's music, as well as the "stile antico" or the "alla-breve" style, to two of the best-known composers associated with the eighteenth-century Dresden court chapel. Jan Dismas Zelenka, more conservative, studied and apparently admired Palestrina's music, and he may have reworked some of it for performance, adding *basso continuo* and *colla parte* instrumental accompaniment. Johann David Heinichen, however, seemed less inclined to give the Palestrina style a dominant aesthetic role, and his own treatment of "alla breve" music suggests at least partial accommodation to late baroque style, including issues of tempi and metric accentuation. Zelenka and Heinichen had different relationships to the older tradition; neither, however, really attempted a practical close imitation of Palestrina's style.

E0424 Hucke, Helmut. "Palestrina als Authorität und Vorbild im 17. Jahrhundert." In *Congresso Internazionale sul temo Claudio Monteverdi e il suo tempo. Relazioni e communicazioni*, ed. Raffaele Monterosso. Verona: Stamperia Valdonega, 1969. pp. 253–261.

Notes that by the mid-seventeenth century two divergent views of Palestrina as master composer had already developed. One, which Hucke associates particularly with Italy, held that Palestrina's music embodied an ideal of audible expression of the text; the other, especially prevalent in Germany but also found in Italy, posits the composer as a model of technical perfection in the practice of advanced counterpoint.

E0425 João IV [John IV, king of Portugal]. *Defensa de la musica moderna contra la errada opinion del Obispo Cyrillo Franco. Al señor Juan Loreço Rabelo, Portugues de nacion, Fidalgo de la Casa del Serenissimo Rey. D. Juan el Quarto de Portugal. . . .* Lisbon, 1649.

See item E0426.

E0426 João IV [John IV, king of Portugal]. *Difesa della musica moderna contro la falsa opinion del vescovo Cirillo Franco, tradotta di spagnuolo in italiano.* Venice: A. Laurenzi, 1666.

Contemporary Italian translation of item E0425.

King John refutes the position of Bishop Franco, who in 1549 attacked what he considered to be the unintelligibility, abuses, and indecorum of contemporary church music, invoking humanistic principles and the music of the ancients. John responded that music can either express the mood of a text or expound words with musical coloration, and that music's effectiveness in part depends on addressing the changing situations of humans over time. He noted that Palestrina in particular with his polyphony demonstrated that contrapuntal means could meet the need for an intelligible text, and that judicious modern composers like him had produced effects on their listeners as great as the ancient Greeks did on theirs.

E0427 João IV [John IV, king of Portugal]. *Respuestas a las dudas que se puzieron á la Missa "Panis quem ego dabo" del Palestrina, impressa en el Libro Quinto de sus missas.* Lisbon, 1654.

Reproduced in fascimile; see item E0429.

E0428 João IV [John IV, king of Portugal]. *Risposte alli dubii proposti sopra la Messa "Panis quem ego dabo" del Palestrina, stampata nel Quinto Libro delle sue Messe. Tradotte di spagnuolo in italiano.* Rome: Mauritio Balmonti, 1655.

Contemporary Italian translation of E0427. Reproduced in facsimile; see item E0429.

E0429 João IV [John IV, king of Portugal]. *Respuestas a las dudas que se puzieron á la Missa "Panis quem ego dabo" del Palestrina, impressa en el Libro Quinto de sus missas*, ed. Mario de Sampayo Ribeiro. Rei Musicae Portugaliae Monumenta 1. Lisbon: Ramos, Afonso & Moita, 1957. ML410.P15J6 [in Portuguese and Italian].

In a dialogue format, King John raises questions regarding the mode and structure of the Palestrina *Missa Panis quem ego dabo* (from Book V of 1590) and how well it corresponds to the Lupus motet on which it is based. He reasons that the mass belongs to a mixed Mode II, as the finals are dissonant with the beginnings and antecedent cadences. But while in the king's view the movements may not articulate the mode optimally, he considers that they behave in conformity with the structure of the model, and Palestrina's fault was not one of skill but in choice of the model. Even if the finals are not concordant with the openings, at least the mode is stated at the beginning. He says it is not his intention to condemn Palestrina, however, and that the composer is in fact very learned. A revealing document with respect to the changing and more rigid qualifications for establishing mode evolving by the mid-seventeenth century.

This book has some handsome presswork but its pagination can be confusing. It runs thus: a plate with an engraving of John IV; preface (pp.vii–viii); introduction (pp.xi–xxvii), including 4 unnumbered tipped-in plates; a facsimile reproduction of *Repuestas a las dudas* of 1654 (pp.ii + 19); a facsimile reproduction of the Italian translation, *Dubii quali furono proposti . . .* of 1655 (pp.1–32); "preliminary notes" (pp.3–11); notes to the Portuguese edition (pp.13–32, in Portuguese); indices (pp.33–43). The two fascimile editions use their own respective internal pagination.

E0430 Kircher, Athanasius. *Musurgia universalis sive ars magna consoni et dissoni in X libros digesta. . . .* vol 1 Rome: Heirs of Francsco Corbelleti, 1650; vol 2 Rome: Ludovico Grignani, 1650. [repr. Hildesheim: Georg Olms, 1970].

Refers several times in vol 1 to Palestrina as marvelously accomplished both in harmony and in affective representation of words. Quoted examples include the *Crucifixus* from the *Missa Papae Marcelli* and the motet *Introduxit me rex*. See print anthology for location of printed examples.

E0431 Kolaczkowski, Jerzy. "Il culto di Palestrina in Polonia." In *L'arte di Giovanni Pierluigi da Palestrina. Atti e Documentazione. VI Convegno Europeo sul Canto Corale. Promosso e Organizzato dalla Corale Goriziana "C.A. Seghizzi."* Gorizia: Grafica Goriziana, 1975. pp. 33–40.

Traces Palestrina's music and influence in Poland from his death to the present day. An unusually large number of pre-1600 prints in archives indicate early seventeenth-century diffusion of Palestrina's music, which was also aided by the presence of a number of his immediate disciplines among the Italian musicians living in Warsaw and Krakow. His style and authority also affected indigenous composers of the period. The nineteenth-century Palestrina renaissance flourished in Poland, and its effects persisted well into the twentieth century.

E0432 Liberati, Antimo. *Lettera scritta in risposta ad una del Sig. Ovidio Persapegi, che gli fa istanza di voler vedere, ed'esaminare i componimenti di musica fatti dalli cinque concorrenti nel concorso per il posto di maestro di cappella della Metropolitana di Milano, fatto sotto il dì 18. agosto 1684 . . . e voler dare il suo parere, quale de'cinque concorrenti sia il migliore.* Rome: Mascardi, 1685. 63 pp.

After describing the evolution of church music to his own day and providing a carefully detailed list of the criteria which are to be observed for composing in the Roman style, which was "founded on Palestrina," Liberati critiques a group of compositions written for a competition held in 1684 for the post of *maestro di cappella* at the Milan cathedral. This text has been best known for its biographical sketch of Palestrina, who was pivotal to Liberati's musical historiography, as well as those of numerous other sixteenth- and seventeenth-century Roman musicians.

E0433 Lionnet, Jean. "Palestrina e la cappella pontificia." In *Atti del II Convegno Internazionale di Studi Palestriniani. Anno Europeo della Musica. 3–5 maggio 1986*, ed. Lino Bianchi and Giancarlo Rostirolla. Palestrina: Fondazione Giovanni Pierluigi da Palestrina/Centro di Studi Palestriniani, 1991. ML410.P15.C77.1986. pp. 125–137.

Documents use of Palestrina's music in Cappella Sistina liturgies for the period from 1590 to 1665. How often it was used depended in part on the personal wishes and tastes of the reigning pope and how seriously the Tridentine mandates were being implemented. While his music was respected throughout this period, evidence of its being cited as an ideal model for emulation is not readily available from Sistine sources until the 1660s.

E0434 Lionnet, Jean. "Performance Practice in the Papal Chapel During the Seventeenth Century." *Early Music* 15 (1987): 4–15.

Lucid account of the nature and purposes of Sistine chapel diaries, from which is derived an account of the duties of the *maestro*, the internal chapel administration, and the singers. Notes that the major restriction upon singers was that they performed without instruments; reviews evidence indicating that they frequently sang with one person per part, and that use of *ripieno* singers emerges only near the end of the seventeenth century. Evidence also indicates that Palestrina's work was important for mass music. An appendix of music for papal ceremonies in the year 1616 is provided, which indicates that Palestrina's music had an important place in the repertory (pp.13–15).

E0435 López-Calo, José. "Palestrina e la Controrifroma musicale in Spagna." In *Atti del II Convegno Internazionale di Studi Palestriniani. Anno Europeo della Musica. 3–5 maggio 1986*, ed. Lino Bianchi and Giancarlo Rostirolla. Palestrina: Fondazione Giovanni Pierluigi da Palestrina/Centro di Studi Palestriniani, 1991. ML410.P15C77.1986. pp. 241–250.

Describes the powerful and distinctive national tradition of Spanish religious music in the sixteenth century, one with a pronounced mystical strain heightened but not fundamentally altered by the mandates of Trent. Palestrina was virtually the only Italian composer whose music was continuously found in important Spanish churches; it was used from the late sixteenth century well into the eighteenth. The publisher Casiano López Navarro printed several volumes of Palestrina's music as late as 1728 to 1730.

E0436 Marvin, Clara. "Two Practices, Three Styles: The Evolution of Typologies of Compositional Genre in Sixteenth- and Seventeenth-Century Italian Writings on Music." Ph.D. dissertation, University of Toronto, 1998.

Chapter 4 deals with Palestrina's reputation during his lifetime and in the century after his death, as well as the evolution of the compositional style associated with his name. A feature of the discussion is the pairing of Antimo Liberati's 1685 treatise on the Palestrina style with the group of compositions the treatise was designed to critique, together with analysis of Liberati's critical method.

E0437 Montanos, Francisco de. *Arte de musica theorica y pratica. . . .* Valladolid: Fernandez de Cordova y Obiedo, 1592.

Probably the first Spanish writer on music to indicate a deep appreciation of Palestrina's music. His work was another major source for Cerone, who seems to have not only followed his text but borrowed a number of his musical examples.

E0438 Morelli, Arnaldo. "Antimo Liberati, Matteo Simonelli e la tradizione palestriniana a Roma nella seconda metà del Seicento." In *Atti del II Convegno Internazionale di Studi Palestriniani. Anno Europeo della Musica. 3–5 maggio 1986*, ed. Lino Bianchi and Giancarlo Rostirolla. Palestrina: Fondazione Giovanni Pierluigi da Palestrina/Centro di Studi Palestriniani, 1991. ML410.P15C77.1986. pp. 297–307.

Argues that it was primarily in the second half of the seventeenth century that the myth of Palestrina and an authoritative Roman school founded in his idiom gained strength. Liberati and Simonelli, working in the wake of a series of papal decretals, were perfect models of reversion to the "buoni maestri antichi." Liberati represented the ideological theorizing of a Roman school; Simonelli was the practical composer who had observant-style compositions inserted into the pontifical ceremonials of the time.

E0439 Natale, Pompeo. *Libro secondo de'solfeggiamenti a due, a tre voci, per cantare, suonare con diversi stromenti. . . . Nel fine si è posto il modo per intendere il tempo della Messa de l'homme armé del Palestrina. Il Rincontro delle Chiavi. La valuta delle Legature per intendere li libri antichi sì del Palestina* [sic], *come d'altri. . . .* Rome: Mascardi, 1681.

A volume of didactic exercises meant to instruct in the elements of practical music, but also to instruct the student in how to deal with notational and proportional issues in older printed music. Uses Palestrina's *L'homme armé* mass (already famous in the literature for its challenges in this area) as a case study.

E0440 Palisca, Claude V. "Marco Scacchi's Defense of Modern Music (1649)." In *Words and Music: The Scholar's View. Festschrift A. Tillman Merritt*, ed.

Laurence Berman. Cambridge, MA: Harvard, 1972. pp. 88–145 [repr. in Claude V. Palisca, *Studies in the History of Italian Music and Music Theory.* Oxford: Clarendon, 1994. ISBN 0–198–16167–0. ML290.1.P35.1994].

Contains a bilingual text (Italian and English) of Scacchi's short treatise, in which he was primarily concerned with defending modern music against those who considered it devoid of sound principles. His comments testify to the increasing separation of strict and free composition, and they also respond to the increasing attitude held by some that the style represented by Palestrina and his music was the only true church music style.

E0441 Pisa, Agostino. *Breve dichiaratione della battuta musicale. . . .* Rome: Bartolomeo Zanetti, 1611.

Contains (pp.86, 124 in particular) early praise of Palestrina as "most wise, most famous, and never sufficiently to be praised." He was the "prince of musicians" because due to him, the church did not abandon [polyphonic] music owing to abuses in the practice of other composers.

E0442 Pitoni, Giuseppe Ottavio. *Notitia de'contrappuntisti e de'compositori di musica*, ed. Cesarino Ruini. Studi e testi per la storia della Musica 6. Florence: Olschki, 1988. L + 389pp. ISBN 88–222–3557–6. ML105.P586.1988.

This edition of the biographical notes made by the staggeringly industrious Pitoni, *maestro* of the Cappella Giulia, is based on his two-volume manuscript of around 1725 (Biblioteca Apostolica Vaticana, Cappella Giulia, MS I/1,2). His material on Palestrina derives to some extent from Liberati but also from other Vatican sources, and was cited in its turn by Baini and others. He considered the works of Palestrina and Benevoli to be "perfect" examples of the true Roman style, and virtually everything else to be imperfect, merely tolerable, or out-and-out "corrupt" (confused or mixed stylistically).

E0443 Riedel, Friedrich Wilhelm. "Johann Joseph Fux und die römische Palestrina-Tradition." *Die Musikforschung* 14 (1961): 14–22.

In examining the formation of Fux's ideas on the strict style, studies evidence from various manuscript traditions. They indicate that there were significant associations between mid- and late-seventeenth-century Italian advocates of the *stile alla Palestrina*, notably Bernardo Pasquini (1637–1710), who was for a time connected with the Viennese imperial court, and Johann Joseph Fux and members of his school.

E0444 Roche, Jerome. " 'The Praise of It Endureth For Ever': the Posthumous Publication of Palestrina's Music." *Early Music* 22 (1994): 631–639.

Examines publication of Palestrina's music from 1594 to 1644 in all genres, including madrigal contrafacta and works in anthologies. Treats firms in Rome (Alessandro Gardano), Venice (Amadino, Angelo Gardano, Vincenti), Milan (Coppini), and various locations outside Italy, including Antwerp (Phalèse) and several German centers.

E0445 Rostirolla, Giancarlo. "*Giovanni Pierluigi da Palestrina, compositore della*

Cappella Pontificia e principe della musica: la sua produzione basilicale e palatina per un calendario/repertorio per celebrativo del quarto centenario." *Recercare* 5 (1993): 33–85.

Focuses on the distinctive organizational and musical features of the Sistine Chapel, aiming to define the role of singer-composers at that institution. These are examined in relation to Palestrina's duties in the Cappella Giulia as well as the more private papal activities involving music. On pp.56–84, Rostirolla provides a detailed calendar/repertory of Palestrina's music performed on liturgical occasions throughout the year during the composer's lifetime and in the years shortly after his death (through 1616 or 1617). Included in the calendar is the feast day/occasion, the item of repertory and its liturgical function, whether this information was established from the diary of tenor Carlo Vanni, where the referenced work is found in early published or manuscript sources, as well as its location in the modern comprehensive editions ("Haberl," "Casimiri") and in Alain Chambure's 1989 catalog.

E0446 Rostirolla, Giancarlo. "Palestrina 'ridotto' per quartetto d' archi. Una inedita testimonianza musicale per la storia della ricezione palestriniana nel Settecento." In *Atti del II Convegno Internazionale di Studi Palestriniani. Anno Europeo della Musica. 3–5 maggio 1986*, ed. Lino Bianchi and Giancarlo Rostirolla. Palestrina: Fondazione Giovanni Pierluigi da Palestrina/Centro di Studi Palestriniani, 1991. ML410.P15C77.1986. pp. 361–405.

For much of the eighteenth century, manuscript copies of music in the older style, including arrangements and transcriptions, were circulating in Rome and Bologna, suggesting serious interest in such music. This article studies an MS transcription containing 45 Palestrina hymns plus movements and sections from several masses, arranged for string quartet. The transcription is generally faithful to sources but also brings music somewhat more into line with eighteenth-century string literature styles and aesthetic sensibilities. Contains inventory of MS, transcription of examples, and MS facsimile reproductions (pp.381–405).

E0447 Rubio, Samuel. "Palestrina e la Spagna." In *L'arte di Giovanni Pierluigi da Palestrina. Atti e Documentazione. VI Convegno Europeo sul Canto Corale. Promosso e Organizzato dalla Corale Goriziana "C.A. Seghizzi."* Gorizia: Grafica Goriziana, 1975. pp. 97–106.

Describes Palestrina's interaction with music of Morales, Gabriel Galvez, and Victoria. Discusses Palestrina's representation in the writings of Spanish theorists from 1592 to 1800 and in prints and manuscripts of his music located in Spanish libraries, religious houses, and archives.

E0448 Rubsamen, Walter. "The International 'Catholic' Repertoire of a Lutheran Church in Nürnberg, 1574–1597." *Annales musicologiques* 5 (1957): 229–327.

Discusses collection of 17 codices assembled by Friedrich Lindner, cantor of St. Aegidien, Nuremberg, from 1574 to 1597, who copied chiefly from printed polyphonic sets of contemporary late Netherlandish and Italian provenance. Through examining liturgical, sociocultural, and musical factors, this item indicates how such ostensibly "Catholic" music (Palestrina's among it) was disseminated in Lutheran Germany in this period despite the tense religious climate.

E0449 Ruhnke, Martin. "Francesco Gasparinis Kanonmesse und der Palestrinastil." In *Musicae Scientiae Collectanea: Festschrift Karl Gustav Fellerer zum 70. Geburtstag am 7. Juli 1972*, ed. Heinrich Hüschen. Cologne: Arno Volk, 1973. ML55.F35M8.1972. pp. 494–516.

A detailed statistical analysis of dissonance treatment in the *a cappella Missa canonica* (1705) of Gasparini and the *Missa ad fugam* (1718) of Fux, the *Missa ad fugam* and the *Missa Virtute magna* of Palestrina, and the *Missa Virtute magna* of Clemens non Papa, to examine how the *stile alla Palestrina* was used by two baroque composers as compared with the stylistic manner of the later sixteenth century.

E0450 Schnoebelen, Anne. "The Growth of Padre Martini's Library as Revealed in His Correspondence." *Music and Letters* 57 (1976): 379–397.

Notes that Martini's gradual acquisition of a rich collection of Palestrina primary materials was a frequent topic of his correspondence with Girolamo Chiti and others. Palestrina references are discussed in some detail. Martini's painstakingly gathered library of manuscripts, prints, and theoretical treatises is now the nucleus of the Civico Museo Bibliografico Musicale, Bologna, one of the world's outstanding musical collections.

E0451 Schnoebelen, Anne. *Padre Martini's Collection of Letters in the Civico Museo Bibliografico Musicale in Bologna. An Annotated Index.* Annotated reference tools in music 2. New York: Pendragon, 1979. ISBN 0–918728–11–8. ML134.M438S3.

Presents individual summaries of letters in Martini's vast correspondence, several hundred of which refer to his search for Palestrina materials and make comments on the composer and his work. See item E0450, Schnoebelen's observations on this material.

E0452 Shay, Robert. "'Naturalizing' Palestrina and Carissimi in Late Seventeenth-Century Oxford: Henry Aldrich and His Recompositions." *Music and Letters* 77 (1996): 368–400.

Discusses the manuscript and print collections associated with Henry Aldrich (d.1710), composer as well as canon and dean of Christ Church, Oxford, and probably the primary transmitter of Palestrina's music and reputation in England before Charles Burney. Contains a highly interesting study of Aldrich's "translating" or "naturalizing" Italian music, that is, not only assigning English text to such works but recomposing their music to create a more updated and "English" idiom. Among works studied are the Palestrina-Aldrich motets "We Have Heard with Our Ears"/*Doctor bonus* and "Hold Not Thy Tongue"/*Nativitas tua.*

E0453 Stefani, Gino. "Miti barocchi: Palestrina *princeps musicae*." *Nuova Rivista*

Musicale Italiana 8 (1974): 347–355.

Examines the growth of the Palestrina mythology in the seventeenth century. The story of the composer as the rescuer of church music acquired an added layer of meaning with Rome's assertion of itself in this period as *caput orbis* in all things and Palestrina as the pivotal composer of the Roman school.

E0454 Stefani, Gino. *Musica e religione nell' Italia barocca*, ed. Antonino Buttitta. Uomo e cultura—Testi 14. Palermo: S.F. Flaccovio, 1975. 261 pp. ML3033.S73.

Insightful and richly documented examination of the cultural position of the Roman church, church-secular relations, the ecclesiastical style and the place of music *per se* in post-Tridentine church reform, the sociological position of the composer, the place of instruments, and extraliturgical devotional genres. Highly recommended for the study of Palestrina reception in seventeenth-century Italy.

E0455 Steinschulte, Gabriel M. "Palestrina und Deutschland." In *Atti del II Convegno Internazionale di Studi Palestriniani. Anno Europeo della Musica. 3–5 maggio 1986*, ed. Lino Bianchi and Giancarlo Rostirolla. Palestrina: Fondazione Giovanni Pierluigi da Palestrina/Centro di Studi Palestriniani, 1991. ML410.P15C77.1986. pp. 613–630.

An overview of historical and social factors which favored reception of Palestrina's music in Germany (both Catholic and Protestant areas) in the seventeenth through twentieth centuries. Discusses the dissemination of his style as a basis for theoretical and practical musical education, especially through Fux and a series of connections among other eighteenth-century theorists and composers. Reviews the important role of Germans in the collection, editing, and publication of Palestrina's music, especially in the nineteenth century.

E0456 Ursprung, Otto. "Palestrina und Palestrina-Renaissance." *Zeitschrift für Musikwissenschaft* 7 (1925): 513–529.

Reviews Palestrina's accomplishments in the context of the Council of Trent, the liturgical reforms taking place in the 1560s, and the interest in textual clarity evinced by members of the Commission of Cardinals. Continues as a short history of Palestrina reception, touching on new tendencies in church music in the early seventeenth century and the consequent narrowing of style focus within the so-called Palestrina style; seventeenth- and eighteenth-century strict-style cultivation that looked to Palestrina as an authority; and tendencies in the nineteenth-century revival (early Romantics, Baini, and Cecilians), with some final comments on research in his own time.

E0457 Wolff, Christoph. "Bach and the Tradition of the Palestrina Style." In *Bach: Essays on His Life and Music*. Cambridge, MA: Harvard University Press, 1991. ISBN 0–674–05925–5. ML410..B1.W79.1991. pp. 84–104.

Argues that movements from Bach's *B-minor mass*, *Clavier-Übung III*, and *Well-Tempered Clavier* exhibit his strongest connections to the Palestrina style. Finds considerable evidence for Bach's awareness of the style by way of his access to treatises and music dating from the sixteenth through eighteenth centuries. Some of Palestrina's work exists in Bach's autograph. Describes qualities of this stylistic texture and traces it in Bach's own music, concluding that its presence was an expression of genre consciousness. Bach's generic references served goals of didacticism, architectonic design, and the expression of *majestas* and *gravitas* in liturgical contexts.

E0458 Wolff, Christoph Johannes. *Der stile antico in der Musik J.S. Bachs. Studien zu Bachs Spätwerk.* Beihefte zum Archiv für Musikwissenschaft 6. Wiesbaden: Franz Steiner, 1968.

An insightful examination of *stile antico*, the strict observant style as it was cultivated in early-eighteenth-century Germany, and its significance and practice in the late music of Johann Sebastian Bach. Bach owned a copy of Palestrina's *Missa Sine nomine a 6 (Nasce la gioia mia)* which he transcribed, adding *colla parte* instruments and *basso continuo*. Text contains comments and a style analysis (p.20, table after p.160, pp.166–172), as well as a printed example, from the *Kyrie I* of the mass.

E0459 Zacconi, Lodovico. *Prattica di mvsica vtile et necessaria si al compositore per comporre i canti suoi regolatamente, si anco al cantore per assicurarsi in tutte le cose cantabili. Divisa in qvattro libri. Ne i qvali si tratta delle cantilene ordinarie, de tempi de prolationi, de proportioni, de tuoni, et della conuenienza de tutti gli istrumenti musicali. S'insegna a cantar tvtte le composizioni antiche, si dichiara tutta la Messa del Palestina titolo Lomè Armè, con altre cose d'importanza & diletteuole. . . .* Venice: G. Polo, 1592; Venice: B. Carampello, 1596. *Prattica di musica seconda parte. . . .* Venice, 1622. MT40.A2.Z34.

Vol 1, Book II, ch.xxxviii, ff.115–122, and *passim* contains an extensive and historically important discussion of questions of mensuration as presented by the notation of Palestrina's *Missa L'homme armé*. As he featured a discussion of the mass in the title of his book, Zacconi clearly considered it a significant matter.

E0460 Zanolini, Bruno. "Il 'cantus firmus' nell' opera di Palestrina, Buxtehude e Froberger." In *Atti del II Convegno Internazionale di Studi Palestriniani. Anno Europeo della Musica. 3–5 maggio 1986*, ed. Lino Bianchi and Giancarlo Rostirolla. Palestrina: Fondazione Giovanni Pierluigi da Palestrina/Centro di Studi Palestriniani, 1991. ML410.P15C77.1986. pp. 421–437.

Comparison of the techniques with which two Gregorian hymns, *A solis ortus cardine* and *Creator alme siderum*, were polyphonically elaborated by Palestrina, Froberger, and J. S. Bach respectively. (Notwithstanding the title, Buxtehude's music is not discussed; the article is labeled more accurately in the book's index.) While Palestrina's settings were vocal and characterized by subtle manipulations of particular modal features, Froberger created an instrumental capriccio in four sections based on a single varied subject and full of instrumental figurations, while Bach created a chorale prelude characterized by a continuum of melodic and rhythmic figures, linear dissonance, and transposition of the modality of the original tune.

2. From 1750 to 1914

E0461 Ackermann, Peter. "Ästhetische und kompositionstechnische Aspekte der Palestrina-Rezeption bei Franz Liszt." In *Palestrina und die Idee der klassischen Vokalpolyphonie im 19. Jahrhundert. Zur Geschichte eines kirchenmusikalischen Stilideals*, vol 1. ed. Winfried Kirsch. Regensburg: Gustav Bosse, 1989. pp. 243–256.

Argues that while Liszt admired the accomplishments of the Cecilians, he did not think they would be able to evolve a truly progressive church style. In his own sacred music, notably the oratorio *Christus* but in much else as well, Liszt inserted reworked quotations of structural material originally by Palestrina, combining gestures of the older style with a modern expressive idiom in synthesis. He seems to have sought a subjectively expressive church style dependent on connecting a heterogenous variety of influences and techniques, ultimately deriving from his Franciscan-influenced aesthetic of letting things speak for themselves.

E0462 Ackermann, Peter. "Klassische Vokalpolyphonie im Werke Michael Hallers." In *Palestrina und die Klassische Vokalpolyphonie als Vorbild kirchenmusikalischer Kompositionen im 19. Jahrhundert*, ed. Winfried Kirsch. Palestrina und die Kirchenmusik im 19. Jahrhundert 3. Kassel: Gustav Bosse Verlag, 1995. pp. 143–157.

Examines how Palestrina's style and certain compositions influenced the compositions of this Cecilian. Includes a number of comparative examples by both composers.

E0463 Arcais, F. d'. "Le onoranze a Palestrina." *Nuova antologia di scienze, lettere ed arti* 51, nr.3 [series II, vol 21], 15 giugno 1880, 762–769.

Reflections prompted by a Palestrina celebration held by the Società Musicale Romana. Calls for a new biography of the composer and pleads for the opening of papal and basilica archives to facilitate research. Says that his own age witnesses a church music situation similar to that out of which Palestrina refounded sacred music—"a bad imitation of theatrical music"—and advocates a restoration to music of that quality of religious purity associated with the composer. Views Palestrina as the first to make counterpoint serve the expression of sentiments and affections and, in this sense, as the founder of all modern music which has this goal.

E0464 Baecker, Carlernst. "Zum Palestrina-Bild in den deutschsprächigen Musikgeschichten um 1800." In *Palestrina und die Idee der klassischen Vokalpolyphonie im 19. Jahrhundert. Zur Geschichte eines kirchenmusikalischen Stilideals*, ed. Winfried Kirsch. Palestrina und die Kirchenmusik im 19. Jahrhundert 1. Regensburg: Gustav Bosse, 1989. pp. 55–63.

Notes that by around 1800 Palestrina's reception history in German-speaking countries was already divided into two streams. One, represented by writers such as Busby (in translation), Reicha, Rochlitz, and others, was historically and style-critically oriented, and was appreciative but slightly distant. The other stream, including writers such as Reichardt, Orloff, Lewald, and Krause, was oriented in a more aesthetic, philosophical, or literary direction. They hailed the composer as a central figure and "rescuer" of music and tended to a more specifically aesthetic feeling for the past.

E0465 Baini, Giuseppe. "Analysis 14. Giuseppe Baini (1775–1844): *Memorie storio-critiche della vita e delle opere di Giovanni Pierluigi da Palestrina (1828)*" ["The Ten Styles of Palestrina"]. In *Music Analysis in the Nineteenth Century. Volume I: Fugue, Form and Style*, ed. Ian Bent. Cambridge, UK: Cambridge, 1994. ISBN 052125969X . MT90.M88.1994 v.1. pp. 263–280.

Bent offers an insightful and carefully contextualized introduction (pp.263–268) to Baini's biography, using a critical approach attempting to set the composer into the context of music history. Suggests that Baini's division of Palestrina's creative practices into ten "styles" has a similarity to methodology of Vasari's *Lives*. Pp.269–280 are a translation by Jonathan Shiff of vol II, pp.420–434, of Baini's book, which deals with the "ten styles" of Palestrina.

E0466 Bauer, Hans-Joachim. "Franz Liszts Reformen zur Kirchenmusik." *Kirchenmusikalisches Jahrbuch* 73 (1990): 63–70.

Describes Liszt's wish to "rescue" church music of his own time. He envisioned a blending of the Palestrina style with contemporaneous means of expression.

E0467 Bäumker, Wilhelm. *Palestrina. Ein Beitrag zur Geschichte der kirchenmusikalischen Reform des 16. Jahrhunderts.* Sammlung historischer Bildnisse. Vierte Serie, I. Freiburg im Breisgau: Herder' sche Verlagshandlung, 1877. 76 pp.

An interesting little book with biographical information derived largely from Baini, Kandler, and Winterfeld. Most interesting for insights it offers the reader into the mind-set and forces then shaping the Cecilian movement. Traces the history of church music up to and through Tridentine events and Palestrina's place in them. Notes with disapproval the subsequent use of instruments, theatricality, and subjectivity of eighteenth- and early nineteenth-century church repertory. Implicit in the text is the suggestion that the best generally known Palestrina repertory was the *Missa Papae Marcelli* and what was heard during Holy Week at the Sistine Chapel. Describes the Palestrina revival in German singing societies, court, and churches, and cites the work of Proske and his successors to revive the *da cappella* ideal and to inspire others to create music in the "spirit" of the composer.

E0468 Bäuerle, Hermann. *Palestrina muss populärer werden. Einladung an strebsame Dirigenten und eifrige Anhänger einer heiliger Musik.* Regensburg: Pustet, 1903.

A Cecilian-influenced advocacy of the Palestrina style in a current liturgical context.

E0469 Beer, Axel. "Der Stellenwert der Kirchenmusik in ausgewählten theologischen Periodika." In *Palestrina und die Idee der klassischen Vokalpolyphonie im 19. Jahrhundert. Zur Geschichte eines kirchenmusikalischen Stilideals*, vol 1. ed. Winfried Kirsch. Regensburg: Gustav Bosse, 1989. pp. 171–179.

Evaluation of the place of church music as found in selected Catholic theological periodicals of the earlier nineteenth century. Containing a strong component of polemic and advocacy, the writings commonly stress that church music (polyphony, chant, and religious song, as simplified and improved and even with "folkish" qualities) needed to revert to its original mandate as one of the greatest liturgical ancillaries of the Roman rite.

E0470 Bellermann, Heinrich. *Der Kontrapunkt, oder Anleitung zur Stimmführung in der musikalischen Composition.* Berlin: J. Springer, 1862. MT55.B44.

Probably the standard textbook on classical polyphony *alla Palestrina* between its publication date and the appearance of Jeppesen's counterpoint book in 1927. Went through two more editions before Bellermann's death in 1903.

E0471 Bellermann, Heinrich. "Die Schlüssel im ersten Buch der vierstimmigen Motetten von Palestrina." *Leipziger Allgemeine Musikalische Zeitung* 5 (1870): 388–390, 395–397.

A discussion of clefs used in sixteenth-century music, their function, advantages, and how to read them, without much overt reference to material within the motet book referenced in the title. (This seems to refer not to vol 5 in the "Haberl" edition edited by Espagne, but to Bellermann's edition of 1869–1870 in the apparently abandoned *Denkmäler* series.) Although somewhat peripheral here, it is interesting to note that when this volume of Palestrina's music was printed with the original clefs, there was apparently such a general sense of discomfort on the part of prospective users that a primer was considered necessary.

E0472 Biba, Otto. "Der Cäcilianismus." *Bruckner-Symposium.* Linz: Anton Bruckner Institut, 1988. pp. 123–128.

Assesses the influence of the Cecilian movement on the sacred music of Anton Bruckner. Argues that the movement was not strong in Austria, and that although there is some evidence of an influence from the Palestrinian style in his work, Bruckner was basically opposed to Cecilianism.

E0473 Bonghi, Ruggero. *Pochi parole di esordio al Concerto del 2 febbraio 1895 in onore di Giovanni Pierluigi da Palestrina.* Rome: Tipografia della Pace di F. Cuggiani, 1895 [repr. in *Annuario della R. Accademia di S. Cecilia 1895/96*. Rome: Tipografia della Pace di F. Cuggiani, 1897, pp. 31–34].

E0474 Boursy, Richard. "The Mystique of the Sistine Chapel Choir in the Romantic Era." *Journal of Musicology* 11 (1993): 277–329.

Features excerpts from travelers' diaries and memoirs from around 1800 to 1850 which contain reflections on contemporaneous performance practice, religious and aesthetic image, and sociological phenomena of the Sistine Chapel. Focuses on reports about Holy Week liturgies and repertory, especially Palestrina's *Improperia* and Allegri's *Miserere.*

E0475 Burney, Charles. *A General History of Music from the Earliest Ages to the Present Period, to Which Is Prefixed a Dissertation on the Music of the Ancients.* 4 vols. London: Printed for the Author, 1776–1789 [Repr. ed. Frank Mercer. New York: Dover, 1935. repr. 1957]. ML159.B9.

Based on 1935 reprint of Burney's 1789 text. Palestrina's contribution is discussed in vol 2, chapter 2, "Of the State of Music in Italy during the Sixteenth Century . . ." (pp.128–200). Burney also demonstrates some reliance on Liberati and Adami da Bolsena, and discusses in particular the question of Palestrina's teachers and antecedents. [Reprinted musical examples cited in chapter 2, part IV, *Prints in Books* under citation in "Burney."]

E0476 Carli Ballola, Giovanni. "Il mito di Palestrina nell' Ottocento." *Chigiana: Rassegna annuale di studi musicologici* 29/30, n.s. 9/10 (1975): 115–119. ML38.S4C4.

Even while many of the leading composers of the mid-to-later nineteenth century continued to write in a grand modern idiom, the Palestrinian style was held in increasingly special regard. Causes for this include the early-nineteenth-century aesthetic and antiquarian orientation of Romanticism, a growing sense of musical history, and the retrospective and nostalgic attitude of musicians within the Catholic Church orbit. With the issue of *Moto proprio*, a new interest in church music in a modest conservative idiom increased.

E0477 Celler, Ludovic ["L. Leclercq"], ed. *La Semaine sainte au Vatican: étude musicale et pittoresque: texte et musique.* Paris: Hachette et Cie., 1867. xii + 120pp.

This text is divided into two parts. The verbal part describes events during Holy Week, including notes on performance practice of the Palestrina *Lamentations* and the history of the Sistine Chapel. The musical section contains works by Palestrina, Victoria, Allegri, and others. For a full listing of musical contents, see Chapter 5, "Modern Editions," under "Celler."

E0478 Choron, Alexandre. *Principes de Composition des Ecoles d'Italie. Adoptés par le Gouvernement Français pour servir à l'instruction des Élèves des Maîtrises de Cathedrales.* 3 vols. Paris: Le Duc, 1808.

A massive treatise on composition by the person who perhaps contributed most to the revival of practical knowledge of Palestrina's music in France in the early nineteenth century, and who was responsible for adding study of the style and performance of early music to the curriculum of the Paris conservatory. Book 6 represents a compendium of examples in church, chamber, and theatrical styles, in which both church and chamber music are represented by works by Palestrina. For a full listing of contents, see Chapter 5, "Modern Editions," under "Choron."

E0479 Coltellacci, Francesco. *Album ricordo del monumenti prenestini pubblicato in occasione del terzo Centenario del Principe della Musica Giovanni Pierluigi da Palestrina per Francesco Coltellacci, segretario del commune di Palestrina (Roma).* Rome: Stabilimento Tipografico Italiano, 1895.

E0480 Darbellay, Étienne. "L'*Esemplare* du Padre Martini: Une exégese musicologique moderne du *stile osservato*?" In *Padre Martini: Musica e cultura nel Settecento europeo. Atti del Convegno di Studi (Bologna, 15–18 settembre 1985).* Florence: Olschki, 1987. pp. 137–171.

Examines Padre Martini's remarkable *Esemplare o sia saggio fondamentale pratico di contrappunto sopra il canto fermo* (1774), a treatise on composition in which he sought to adapt principles of sixteenth-century counterpoint and the actual creation of compositions to the musical language of his own time. Martini presented heavily annotated examples from Palestrina, Morales, and a number of other composers of that period, meant to serve as teaching models from which students could learn the art of composition themselves. (The larger volume from which this article comes is also recommended as a source for studying Martini's multifarious activities related to earlier music.)

E0481 Dehn, Siegfried. *Lehre von Contrapunkt, dem Canon und der Fugue. Nebst Analysen von Duetten, Terzetten, Fugen, etc. von Orlando di Lasso, Marcello, Palestrina u.a. Neu bearbeitet von Bernhard Scholz.* Berlin: W. Weber, 1882. 192pp. MT55.D31.1882 [original edition 1859].

Manual of species counterpoint, double counterpoint, and canon, including a review of theorists of counterpoint from Zarlino to Kirnberger and Marpurg (pp.70–74) on aspects of double counterpoint. Contains a series of examples meant to be studied in conjunction with the text; for an enumeration, see Chapter 5, "Modern Editions," series section, under "Dehn."

E0482 Eximeno y Pujader, Antonio. *Delle origini e della regole della musica. . . .* Rome: Michel'Angelo Barbiellini, 1774 [facs. ed. Hildesheim: Georg Olms, 1983. ISBN 3–487–07137–1. ML159.E9.1983].

Discusses Palestrina and the *stile alla Palestrina* in Book 3, Chapter 8, "Verificazione della teorica" (pp.253–257) *et passim.* Cites Palestrina's music as an authority verifying his own statements on dissonance treatment, melodic shaping, and so forth, but this text is also of interest because of the way in which Eximeno's judgment of the style is suffused with eighteenth-century aesthetic language: Palestrina is "most worthy to study and imitate to acquire the simplicity, naturalness and elegance of the stile a cappella," and so forth.

Plate 9, intended to be studied with this section of the text, contains the *Missa Papae Marcelli* (*Kyrie* and beginning of the *Gloria*, both with added *basso continuo*).

E0483 Féderoff, Yvette and Wallon, Simone. "Choron et ses Essais de Réforme Musicale a l'Église de la Sorbonne. Un point d'histoire de la musique religieuse en France sous la Restauration." In *Logos musicae. Festschrift für*

Albert Palm, ed. Rüdiger Görner. Wiesbaden: Franz Steiner, 1982. pp. 63–70.

Description of Alexandre-Étienne Choron's revisions in the curriculum of musical education at his "Royal Institute of Religious Music." Among these were early nineteenth-century performance revivals of music by Palestrina, as well as by composers who worked in the *stile alla Palestrina*, and of sacred music of seventeenth- and eighteenth-century Italy and Germany.

E0484 Fellerer, Karl Gustav. "Zum Bild der altklassischen Polyphonie im XVIII. Jahrhundert." In *Festschrift für E. H. Meyer zum sechzigsten Geburtstag*, ed. G. Knepler. Leipzig: Deutsche Verlag für Musik, 1973. pp. 243–252. [repr. in *Palestrina Studien*, pp.341 *et seq.*].

Discusses the attitudes of some eighteenth-century writers on music toward older polyphony. Useful in particular for its listing of the compositions which would have been available in publications in that period, not only for Palestrina but also for a significant number of other fifteenth- and sixteenth-century composers.

———. Fétis, François-Joseph. "Palestrina." In *Biographie universelle des musiciens et bibliographie générale de la musique.* Brussels, 1835–1844.

See item E0118.

E0485 Gerber, Ernst Ludwig. "Palestrina." In *Historisch-Biographisches Lexicon der Tonkünstler.* Leipzig: J. G. J. Breitkopf, 1790–1792. 2 vols. Second edition as *Neues historisch-biographisches Lexicon.* Lepizig: A. Kühnel, 1812–1814. 4 vols [facs. repr. of both editions together in one 4-volume set, Graz: Akademische Druck, 1966–1969]. ML105.G475.1966.

In the first edition (1790–1792), part 3, cols. 644–646, Palestrina is assigned a sketchy biographical entry of about a quarter of a column; most of the entry gives a list of works, derived mainly from Burney, and a list of critical writings (theoretical or historical texts) where examples of Palestrina's music can be found.

In the second edition (1812–1814), part 3, cols. 65–69, the biographical entry has greatly expanded to three full columns, and adds a short list of works, followed by a list of seven works currently for sale by Breitkopf under Palestrina's name. The masses seem mostly to be arranged as Lutheran *missae* (i.e. *Kyrie* and *Gloria* only).

E0486 Gerbert, Martin. *De cantu et musica sacra a prima ecclesiae aetate usque ad praesens tempus.* 2 vols. St. Blasien: Typis San-Blasianus, 1774. 2 vols [facs. repr. ed. Othmar Wessely. Graz: Akademische Druck, 1968. ML3002A2 G3].

This great eighteenth-century research scholar had little conceptual use for *any* polyphony in church music, but suggested that insofar as such music was tolerated in fact, the polyphonic manner of Palestrina, with its careful atttention to language, was probably the most suitable.

E0487 Gerhards, Albert. "Der liturgische Hintergrund der Palestrina-Renaissance im 19. Jahrhunderts." In *Palestrina und die Idee der klassischen Vokalpolyphonie im 19. Jahrhundert. Zur Geschichte eines kirchenmusikalischen Stilideals*. vol 1. ed. Winfried Kirsch. Regensburg: Gustav Bosse, 1989. pp.181–194.

Discussion of questions of church music as an ornamental servant of liturgy; the impulses behind the nineteenth-century Palestrina renaissance and the Cecilian movement; how the concept of a "Palestrina style" was understood in a liturgical context; and conclusions on the relationship between church music and liturgical elements—how music functions both as ancillary and to engage the emotion of the liturgical participant.

E0488 Gmeinwieser, Siegfried. "Die *Missa L'homme armé* als Beispiel einer Palestrina-Bearbeitung aus dem 19. Jahrhundert." In *Palestrina und die Idee der klassischen Vokalpolyphonie im 19. Jahrhundert. Zur Geschichte eines kirchenmusikalischen Stilideals*, vol 1, ed. Winfried Kirsch. Regensburg: Gustav Bosse, 1989. pp. 223–225.

A study of how a Palestrina mass was edited in the 1830s: it was noticeably shortened, its longer melismas were removed, and textures were altered to clarify vertical sonorities.

E0489 Gmeinwieser, Siegfried. "Zum Palestrina-Stil in München." In *Palestrina und die Idee der klassischen Vokalpolyphonie im 19. Jahrhundert. Zur Geschichte eines kirchenmusikalischen Stilideals*, vol 1, ed. Winfried Kirsch. Regensburg: Gustav Bosse, 1989. pp. 215–222.

Munich had a virtually unbroken tradition of cultivating sixteenth-century polyphony from the days of Lasso to the nineteenth-century church music restoration. The article chronicles the activities of a series of nineteenth-century musicians who advocated or implemented either a modified symphonic church style or a form of the "Palestrina style" in various Munich churches, notably Caspar Ett, Johann Kaspar Aiblinger, and Joseph Rheinberger.

E0490 Haar, James. "Music of the Renaissance as Viewed by the Romantics." In *Music and Context: Essays for John M. Ward*, ed. Anne Dhu Shapiro and Phyllis Benjamin. Cambridge, MA: Harvard University Press, 1985. ISBN 0–674–58888–6. ML3735.M77.1985. pp. 126–144.

Intriguing study of the relationship of the misapprehensions of Romantic historiography to the perception of significant Renaissance musical figures and their music, as well as the effect of such images on nineteenth-century musical and literary creations. Consideration of Palestrina among others. Argues that it is due in part to highly subjective early-nineteenth-century conceptions of the composer as symbol of a lost golden age of pure and simple religious sensibility that a truly balanced picture of Palestrina's undoubtedly great but hardly unique stature has taken so long to emerge.

E0491 Haberl, Franz Xaver. "Zum 50. Todesjahre von Joseph Baini. Eine biographische Skizze." *Kirchenmusikalisches Jahrbuch* 9 (1894): 77–85.

Notes the great stimulus Baini provided to Palestrina research and the many sources reliant upon his work. Even while Haberl points out the serious problems and lacunae which fifty subsequent years have exposed in Baini's work, he nonetheless credits him with great accomplishments given the circumstances in which he worked. Continues with anecdotes and renewed appreciation of Baini's life and activities.

E0492 Haberl, Franz Xaver. "Die Gesammtausgabe der Werke Palestrinas." *Cäcilienkalendar* 5 (1880): 66–74.

Presents a report on the plan for the comprehensive Palestrina edition: includes the publisher's prospectus and lists of subscribers, as well as a letter from Pope Leo XIII on the "instauration of ecclesiastical music" and Haberl's own statement of the belief that this edition would contribute to the restoration of church music.

E0493 Hancock, Virginia. "Brahms's Performances of Early Choral Music." *Nineteenth-Century Music* 8 (1984): 125–141.

Examines performance materials in the library of the *Gesellschaft der Musikfreunde*, many of which have personal annotations and performance articulations in Brahms's hand. These materials, including works by Palestrina as well as numerous other composers of the period from 1550 to 1750, document his activities as a director of Renaissance and Baroque choral music, and directly or indirectly indicate his views on its nature and manner of performance.

E0494 Hawkins, Sir John. *A General History of the Science and Practice of Music*, 5 vols. London, 1776 [repr. as *A General History of the Science and Practice of Music, by Sir John Hawkins. A New Edition, with the Author's Posthumous Notes.* London: J. Alfred Novello, 1853]. ML159.H3.

Annotation based on 1853 reprint. Palestrina is discussed in vol 1, pp. 420–429; Hawkins's primary sources were Antimo Liberati and Andrea Adami da Bolsena, whose comments are analyzed and several of whose mistakes are corrected.

E0495 Hoffmann, Ernst Theodor Amadeus. "Alte und neue Kirchenmusik." *Allgemeine musikalische Zeitung* 16 (1814), cols. 577–584, 593–603, 611–619. repr. in *Schriften zur Musik. Aufsätze und Rezensionen.* Munich: Winkler, 1977, 2nd edition, ed. Friedrich Schnapp, 1980. ISBN 3–538–05277–8. ML60.H728.S3.1977t. pp. 209–235.

The notable essay in which Hoffmann argued for a restoration of church music predicated on the purity and genius of the transcendant Palestrina style.

E0496 Hoffmann, Wolfgang. "Zur Aufführungs- und Bearbeitungspraxis der Werke Palestrinas in Trier im 19. Jahrhundert." In *Aufführungs- und Bearbeitungspraxis der Werke Palestrinas vom 16. bis zum 20. Jahrhundert*, ed. Friedrich Wilhelm Riedel. Kirchenmusikalische Studien 3. Sinzig: Studio, Verlag Schewe, 1997. pp. 129–142.

Focuses on the *Sammlung ausgezeichneter Compositionen für die Kirche* edited by Stephan Lück (pub. 1859 in two volumes), of which a much-expanded revised edition appeared in 1884–1885 (four volumes). Discusses the important differences between the two editions and how they reflect changed perceptions of the Palestrina style and how it was to be performed.

E0497 Hohlfeld, Christoph. *Schule musikalischen Denkens: der Cantus-firmus-Satz bei Palestrina.* Wilhelmshaven: F. Noetzel, "Heinrichshofen Bucher," 1994. Text 406pp; supplement, 94pp. ISBN 3–7959-0649-0 [for solutions to examples, ISBN 3–7959-0650–4]. ML410.P15H64.1994X.

Text by Christoph Hohlfeld; section of musical examples by Reinhard Bahr. A modern examination of methods for teaching counterpoint in the sixteenth-century and "Palestrina" style, with particular reference to eighteenth- and nineteenth-century sources.

E0498 Hohn, Wilhelm. *Der Kontrapunkt Palestrinas und seiner Zeitgenossen. Eine Kontrapunktlehre mit praktischen Aufgaben.* Sammlung "Kirchenmusik" 17, ed. Karl Weinmann. Regensburg: Friedrich Pustet, 1918. 24pp. MT55.H74.

A chapbook-type manual of counterpoint, with a separate notebook of musical examples, which in some ways resembles a catechism. Part I contains instruction in the elements of species counterpoint; Part II deals with imitative counterpoint. Noted here also for the Cecilian tone and for the prefatory admonition to heed Pius X's *Moto proprio* in attitude and approach to church music composition.

E0499 Hucke, Helmut. "Palestrina als Klassiker." In *Gattungen der Musik und ihre Klassiker*, ed. Hermann Danuser. Publikationen der Hochschule für Musik und Theater Hannover 1. Laaber: Laaber, 1988. ML55.G215.1988, pp. 19–34.

Describes how a specific style for church music developed during the sixteenth century. Discusses the Council of Trent and notes that Palestrina's music was accepted as suitable for use by the papal choir. Notes also some of the recurrent eras of Palestrina's popularity in the eighteenth and nineteenth centuries.

E0500 Janitzek, Martina, and Winfried Kirsch, eds. *Palestrina und die klassische Vokalpolyphonie als Vorbild kirchenmusikalischer Komposition im 19. Jahrhundert.* Palestrina und die Kirchenmusik im 19. Jahrhundert 3. Kassel: Gustav Bosse, 1995. 196ff. ISBN 3–7649-2377–6. ML2906.P34.1995.

Collection of papers from a symposium held from May 30 to June 6, 1991, in Frankfurt am Main. Papers by Janz, Konrad, Lüttig, and Krombach are individually indexed, as they contain direct comparisons of style, describe quotations of Palestrina's music, or deal with actual traditions of Palestrina performance. Some of the unindexed but interesting papers in this collection belong more specifically to scholarship on the Cecilian movement and on compositions based on emulation or reworkings of classical polyphony than to Palestrina studies *per se*, but are worth examination.

E0501 Janitzek, Martina. "Palestrina-Editionen im 19. Jahrhundert—dargestellt an ausgewählten Beispielen." In *Aufführungs- und Bearbeitungspraxis der Werke Palestrinas vom 16. bis zum 20. Jahrhundert*, ed. Friedrich Wilhelm Riedel. Kirchenmusikalische Studien 3. Sinzig: Studio, Verlag Schewe, 1997. pp. 115–128.

Studies some transcriptions and reworkings of Palestrina works in the nineteenth century together with contemporary notices of how these editions were received. Contains printed musical examples from arrangements of the *Stabat Mater*; organ arrangements of movements from *Missa Brevis* and *Missa Iste Confessor*; Michael Haller's edition of the *Missa Brevis*; and Ignaz Mitterer's version of the *Missa Papae Marcelli*.

E0502 Janz, Bernhard. "Das editorische Werk Carl Proskes und die Anfänge der kirchenmusikalischen Reformbewegung." In *Palestrina und die Idee der klassischen Vokalpolyphonie im 19. Jahrhundert. Zur Geschichte eines kirchenmusikalischen Stilideals*, vol 1, ed. Winfried Kirsch. Regensburg: Gustav Bosse, 1989. pp. 149–169.

Discussion of activities of canon Dr. Carl Proske (1794–1861), compiler and editor of the influential *Musica divina* and *Selectus novus missarum*. Proske's ultimate goals involved liturgical revival, restoration of older polyphony, and the formation of quality church musicians. Yet he also availed himself of contemporary research and editorial techniques, so his publications function as scientifically produced editions with unaltered, precise, and authentic musical texts. Inventory of Palestrina's music in *Musica divina* and *Selectus novus missarum* included.

E0503 Janz, Bernhard. "Legende und Wirklichkeit—Die Kompositionen Giuseppe Bainis und die Tradition des Palestrina-Stils in der Päpstliche Kapelle." In *Palestrina und die Klassische Vokalpolyphonie als Vorbild kirchenmusikalischer Kompositionen im 19. Jahrhundert*, ed. Winfried Kirsch. Palestrina und die Kirchenmusik im 19. Jahrhundert 3. Kassel: Gustav Bosse Verlag, 1995. pp. 13–32.

Examines Baini's perception of the style as revealed in his own compositions for the papal choir. Includes four musical examples from Baini's compositions.

E0504 Kandler, Franz Sales. *Über das Leben und die Werke des G. Pierluigi da Palestrina genannt der Fürst der Musik, Sängers, dann Tonsetzers der päpstlichen Kapelle auch Kapellmeisters an den drei Hauptkirchen Roms. Nach dem Memorie storico-critiche des Abbate Giuseppe Baini, Sängers und Direktors der päpstlichen Kapelle, verfasst und mit historisch-Kritischen Zusätzen begleitet von Franz Sales Kandler, Mitgleid mehrerer gelehrten Gesellschaften und Kunstakademien Deutschlands und Italiens. Nachgelassenes Werk, herausgegeben mit einem Vorworte und mit gelegentlichen Anmerkungen von R.G. Kiesewetter.* Leipzig: Breitkopf und Härtel, 1834.

Abbreviated and annotated translation of Baini's recently published biography, highly influential in German-speaking countries.

E0505 Kirsch, Winfried. "Aspekte der Palestrina-Rezeption." In *Palestrina und die Idee der klassischen Vokalpolyphonie im 19. Jahrhundert. Zur Geschichte eines kirchenmusikalischen Stilideals*, vol 1, ed. Winfried Kirsch. Palestrina und die Kirchenmusik im 19. Jahrhundert. Regensburg: Gustav Bosse, 1989. pp. 17–34.

The church music restoration movement was closely related to the renewal of Roman Catholicism and the collective historical situation of early-nineteenth-century Germany. Emphasizes continuity of ideas of Cecilians with artistic, aesthetic, literary, and philosophical ideas of early Romantics. Palestrina reception was part of a renaissance of older music (and one component of a complex of church reform tendencies) where the renewal of church music was to be done by examining the spirit of old music rather than church institutions *per se*.

E0506 Kirsch, Winfried. " 'Non clamor, sed amor clangit in aure Dei'—Palestrina—Lasso—Proske in Geschichte und Gegenwart." In *Musica Divina. Ausstellung zum 400. Todesjahr von Giovanni Pierluigi da Palestrina und Orlando di Lasso und zum 200. Geburtsjahr von Carl Proske*. Bischöfliches Zentralarchiv und Bischöfliche Zentralbibliothek Regensburg Kataloge und Schriften 11. ed. Paul Mai. Regensburg: Schnell & Steiner, 1995. ISBN 3–7954–1067–3. ML141.R43P34.1994. pp. 53–63.

Examination of the comparative reception histories of the church music of Palestrina and Lasso. Describes the differing ideological attitudes and levels of intensity with which they were regarded, and notes that Proske's approach was typical: he held that Palestrina's role as church musician was the "ideal," whereas Lasso was a "great composer" and "genius." In 1894, these attitudes were still held, but by 1994 there had been a change in perspective, and the "ecclesiastical" aspect of the music of the two composers was no longer as important to an assessment of their contribution.

E0507 Kirsch, Winfried, ed. *Palestrina und die Idee der klassischen Vokalpolyphonie im 19. Jahrhundert. Zur Geschichte eines kirchenmusikalischen Stilideals.* Palestrina und die Kirchenmusik im 19. Jahrhundert 1. Regensburg: Gustav Bosse, 1989. ISBN 3–7649-2375–X. ML2906.P34.1989.

Compilation prepared in conjunction with an interdisciplinary symposium "Church Music" of the Gesellschaft für Musikforschung, held at the Johann-Wolfgang-Goethe University in Frankfurt am Main on January 16 and 17, 1987. Focus is the aesthetic, musicological, and technical/compositional aspects of Palestrina reception from 1750 to 1900 and their implications for the literature, art, and philosophy of that period; the theological and church-historical assumptions of Palestrina reception; and repertory documentation of the compositional reflections of Palestrina's style during this time. Articles individually indexed.

The preface announced a series of three titles. Vol 3, a collection of articles examining the Palestrina style as a model for nineteenth-century church composition, was published in 1995. Vol 2, projected as a bibliography of primary literature from the nineteenth century with commentary on writings from 1750 to 1900, has not appeared as of date of writing.

E0508 [Kirsch, Winfried, ed]. "Schlussdiskussion. Zur Palestrina-Rezeption in Frankreich. Zur Aufführungspraxis alter Musik im 19. Jahrhundert. Zum Bekanntheitsgrad Palestrinas in 19. Jahrhundert." In *Palestrina und die Idee der klassischen Vokalpolyphonie im 19. Jahrhundert. Zur Geschichte eines kirchenmusikalischen Stilideals*. Palestrina und die Kirchenmusik im 19. Jahrhundert 1. Regensburg: Gustav Bosse, 1989. pp. 257–260.

A series of concluding roundtable discussions on Palestrina reception in the nineteenth century by participants in the symposium held in Frankfurt in 1987.

E0509 Kirsch, Winfried. "Zur Vortragsweise der Werke Palestrinas im 19. Jahrhunderts." In *Aufführungs- und Bearbeitungspraxis der Werke Palestrinas vom 16. Bis zum 20. Jahrhundert*, ed. Friedrich Wilhelm Riedel. Kirchenmusikalische Studien 3. Sinzig: Studio, Verlag Schewe, 1997, pp. 89–114.

Examines a wide selection of excerpts from nineteenth-century writings which discuss various aspects of the performance of Palestrina's music: fundamental approaches, parameters such as dynamics, phrasing and text declamation, tempo, and rhythm.

E0510 Konrad, Ulrich. "Klassische Vokalpolyphonie in den Oratorien Carl Loewes." In *Palestrina und die klassische Vokalpolyphonie als Vorbild kirchenmusikalischer Komposition im 19. Jahrhundert*. Palestrina und die Kirchenmusik im 19. Jahrhundert 3. Kassel: Gustav Bosse, 1995. pp. 81–99.

Examines the use of the *stile da cappella, stile alla Palestrina,* and strict canonical types in the historically oriented oratorios of Carl Loewe (1796–1869). Contains comments on his oratorio *Palestrina* (ca. 1841), noting that it dramatizes the legend of Palestrina's rescue of polyphonic church music and that it quotes a number of passages from the *Missa Papae Marcelli* and an *Ave Maria.* Article concludes with several musical examples of Loewe's writing in the "older" style.

E0511 Konrad, Ulrich. "Otto Nicolai und die Palestrina-Renaissance." In *Palestrina und die Idee der klassischen Vokalpolyphonie im 19. Jahrhundert. Zur Geschichte eines kirchenmusikalischen Stilideals*, vol 1, ed. Winfried Kirsch. Regensburg: Gustav Bosse, 1989. pp. 117–142.

Discusses Nicolai's involvement with older polyphony: his activities in Rome, where he was captivated aesthetically by the Sistine choir repertory even while critiquing its musicianship; his theoretical reading and studies in the older style with Baini; an analysis of Nicolai's antiphon *Assumpta est Maria*; his collection of older music. Appendix contains selective inventory of Nicolai's collection.

E0512 Krombach, Gabriela. "Aufführungen von Werken Palestrina am Wiener Hof in der zweiten Hälfte des 19. Jahrhunderts." In *Palestrina und die Idee der klassischen Vokalpolyphonie im 19. Jahrhundert. Zur Geschichte eines kirchenmusikalischen Stilideals*, vol 1, ed. Winfried Kirsch. Regensburg: Gustav Bosse, 1989. pp. 199–213.

Notes some revival of classical vocal polyphony took place at the Viennese imperial chapel after the mid-nineteenth century. Its main impulse seems to have been less due to the Palestrina renaissance *per se* than to an element of nostalgia toward an older liturgical tradition when musical instruments were disallowed in seasons of fasting and penitence. A table of performances of works by Palestrina and his school in the court liturgies between 1858 and 1900 is appended.

E0513 Krombach, Gabriela. "Die Kirchenmusikwerke von Peter Piel und der Palestrina-Stil." In *Palestrina und die klassische Vokalpolyphonie als Vorbild kirchenmusikalischer Komposition im 19. Jahrhundert*. Palestrina und die Kirchenmusik im 19. Jahrhundert 3. Kassel: Gustav Bosse, 1995. pp. 113–125.

Chiefly an analytical comparison of the *Missa in honorem B.M.V. consolatrix afflictorum* by Peter Piel (1835–1904), a composer who had close relationships with Cecilians and their activities. Its style features relate to Palestrina's *Missa Brevis* and (to a lesser extent) *Missa Lauda Sion* and other works. Rhythmic and melodic treatment, tonality/modality, harmony, dissonance treatment and textures are compared. Concludes that while Piel's compositional style was very competent, it had little in common with Palestrina; Piel's style more closely resembles a blend of *a cappella* mass techniques of the late-eighteenth and early-nineteenth centuries.

E0514 Kromolicki, Joseph. "Palestrina und Bach in der evangelischen und katholischen Kirchenmusik." In *Festschrift Peter Wagner zum 60. Geburtstag*, ed. Karl Weinmann. Leipzig: Breitkopf und Härtel, 1926. ML55.F47. pp. 124–127.

Argues that the music of Palestrina, the greatest Roman Catholic composer, adapts well to the Lutheran liturgy with a German translation of the text, but that the music of Bach, the greatest Lutheran composer, may have only limited application to the Roman liturgy. Bach's Latin compositions (*Missae*, *Magnificat*) might adapt well, but the cantatas less so, because of their texts and the preeminence of the Lutheran chorale in them. There is also reduced room in the Roman liturgy for the kind of organ music produced by Bach, which can also be of considerable technical difficulty; but chorale preludes with melodies common to both confessions might be used in liturgical contexts.

E0515 LaFage, Adrien de [Juste-Adrien-Lenoir de]. "Avertissement." In *Vingt motets tirées du répetoire de la chapelle sixtine à Rome composés par Jean Pierluigi de Palestrina. Edition revue et corrigée avec le plus grand soin.* Paris: Mme. Ve. Launer, n.d. [1842], 2 unnumbered pages [repr. as "Avis sur l'exécution de la musique palestrinienne" in *Miscellanées musicales*. Paris: Compoir des Imprimateurs Unis, 1844. pp. 499–504.

Discussion of tempi, *musica ficta*, and particulars of notation and durations, and provides nine general admonitions to assist in the correct and stylish performance of this repertory.

E0516 La Fage, Adrien de [Juste-Adrien-Lenoir de]. *Essais de diphthérographie* *musicale, ou notices, descriptions, analyses, extraits et reproductions de manuscrits relatifs à la pratique, à la théorie, et à l'histoire de la musique*. Paris, 1864 [facs. repr. Amsterdam: Frits A.M. Knuf, 1964]. ML55.L2.1864a.

In addition to the long biographical notice about Baini (see item E0520), La Fage cites Baini in numerous other places in this work. Item 100 (pp.499–535) is a long catalog and résumé of Baini's surviving correspondence, which had been bequeathed to a friend.

This book also prints a series of musical examples in a separately numbered appendix at the back of the book. Included are no.5, *Rex virtutum a 3* (p.15); no.6, *Jesu rex admirabilis a 3* (pp.15–16); and no.7, *Giesu sommo conforto a 3* [labeled "Lauda"] (p.16).

E0517 La Fage, Adrien de [Juste-Adrien-Lenoir de]. *Miscellanées musicales*. Paris: Comptoir des Imprimateurs Unis, 1844.

Contains three items relevant to Palestrina, individually indexed.

E0518 La Fage, Adrien de [Juste-Adrien-Lenoir de]. "Précis sur la vie et les ouvrages de G. Pierluigi da Palestrina." In *Cinq messes tirées du répetoire de la chapelle sixtine à Rome*. Paris: Mme. Ve. Launer, n.d. [1842]. pp. 3–8. [repr. in La Fage, *Miscellanées musicales,* item E0517. pp. 479–498.

Clearly written biographical outline of the composer's life, following Baini in presentation of documented material, and also possessing a certain high romantic sentiment.

E0519 La Fage, Adrien de [Juste-Adrien-Lenoir de]. "III. Notice sur Joseph Baini." In *Miscellanées musicales*. Paris: Comptoir des Imprimateurs Unis, 1844, pp. 505–523.

A commemoration of Joseph Baini (1775–1844), who had died shortly before this publication was issued. Describes his early gifts as a singer; his initial acquaintance with Palestrina's music around 1804; the unsuccessful attempts by Emperor Napoleon to employ Baini in Paris in 1810; his work on the Palestrina biography; his own compositions for the pontifical chapel and his teaching; his personality and his abstemious lifestyle, and his final illness.

E0520 La Fage, Adrien de [Juste-Adrien-Lenoir de]. "Notice sur la vie et les ouvrages de Joseph Baini." In *Essais de diphthérographie musicale, ou notices, descriptions, analyses, extraits et reproductions de manuscrits relatifs à la pratique, à la théorie, et à l'histoire de la musique*. Paris, 1864 [facs. repr. Amsterdam: Frits A.M. Knuf, 1964]. ML55.L2.1864a. pp. 17–66.

This is an amplified version of the biographical article in *Miscellanées musicales*, both as to content and its appendices, which include a transcription of Baini's lengthy will, a list of his writings and musical compositions, and a listing of notices, obituaries, and eulogies about him.

E0521 Lang, Paul Henry. "Palestrina across the Centuries." In *Festschrift Karl Gustav Fellerer zum sechzigsten Geburtstag*, ed. Heinrich Hüschen. Regensburg: Bosse, 1962 [repr. in *Musicology and Performance. Paul Henry Lang*, ed. Alfred Mann and George J. Buelow. New Haven: Yale, 1997. pp. 57–65. ISBN 0–300–06805. ML60.L2362.1997.

Begins and ends with appreciation of Fellerer's *Palestrina*, noting Fellerer's work as a refreshingly objective and informative study of Palestrina's style. Compares this approach (directly and indirectly) with the idealized and noncritical veneration afforded him by a number of nineteenth-century composers and scholars, for several of which Lang offers details.

E0522 Lüttig, Peter. "Das Palestrina-Bild bei Hawkins und Burney." In *Palestrina und die Idee der klassischen Vokalpolyphonie im 19. Jahrhundert. Zur Geschichte eines kirchenmusikalischen Stilideals*, vol 1, ed. Winfried Kirsch. Palestrina und die Kirchenmusik im 19. Jahrhundert. Regensburg: Gustav Bosse, 1989. pp. 65–76.

Examines the different ways in which Burney and Hawkins evaluated Palestrina in terms of late-eighteenth-century counterpoint and composition. For the present-oriented Burney, Palestrina evolved a personal compositional speech and was a genius of progressiveness in music-text relation issues. For the antiquarian and rationalist Hawkins, Palestrina was the epitome and father figure of a specific church style.

E0523 Lüttig, Peter. *Der Palestrina-Stil als Satzideal in der Musiktheorie zwischen 1750 und 1900.* Frankfurter Beiträge zur Musikwissenschaft 23. Tützing: Hans Schneider, 1994. ISBN 3–7952–0804–1. ML446.L88.1994.

Examination of how the Palestrina style as a pedagogical ideal became identified with species counterpoint, as found in treatises of the eighteenth and nineteenth centuries, especially in the works of Fux, Heinrich Bellermann, Michael Haller, and others. Study of the influence of Palestrina's authority on Cecilianism and Cecilians. Contains lengthy analyses by Lüttig of Palestrina's *Lamentationes Feria V, in coena Domini*, and Michael Haller's nineteenth-century analyses of the Palestrina masses *O admirabile commercium* and *Iste confessor*.

E0524 Lüttig, Peter. "Wesen und Bedeutung der Kirchenmusik in Sulzers *Allgemeine Theorie der Schönen Künste.*" In *Palestrina und die Idee der klassischen Vokalpolyphonie im 19. Jahrhundert. Zur Geschichte eines kirchenmusikalischen Stilideals*, ed. Winfried Kirsch. Palestrina und die Kirchenmusik im 19. Jahrhundert 1. Regensburg: Gustav Bosse, 1989. pp. 87–103.

Investigates Sulzer's writings on "church music" (1774) for their antecedents and parallels to the vocabulary of the nascent Palestrina renaissance of the early nineteenth century. Sulzer anticipated later attitudes in his views of the necessary aesthetic qualities of church music and its specific social functions. He also paralleled later writers in his critical attitude toward the church music of his own time, which he considered too mixed stylistically, too theatrical, and lacking in appropriate emotional qualities. He longed for a past ideal and wished to retrieve older music.

E0525 Lüttig, Peter. "Zwischen Theorie und Praxis: Die Motette *Wie der Hirsch schreiet* von Heinrich Bellermann." In *Palestrina und die klassische Vokalpolyphonie als Vorbild kirchenmusikalischer Komposition im 19. Jahrhundert*. Palestrina und die Kirchenmusik im 19. Jahrhundert 3. Kassel: Gustav Bosse, 1995. pp. 101–112.

In the first edition of his landmark 1862 text on classical polyphony, Bellermann included several works by Palestrina, as well as a motet of his own composition, *Wie der Hirsch schreiet* ("As the Hart Pants"), in emulation of the style. This article compares salient features of the Palestrina compositions with those in *Wie der Hirsch schreiet*, concluding that Bellermann sought not so much a philologically exact replication of Palestrina's style and technique as its "spirit." Reprints Bellermann's motet (pp.109–112).

E0526 Mai, Paul, ed. *Musica Divina. Ausstellung zum 400. Todesjahr von Giovanni Pierluigi da Palestrina und Orlando di Lasso und zum 200. Geburtsjahr von Carl Proske.* Bischöfliches Zentralarchiv und Bischöfliche Zentralbibliothek Regensburg Kataloge und Schriften 11. ed. Paul Mai. Regensburg: Schnell & Steiner, 1995.

A collection of articles dealing with the understanding of the Palestrina image and also with Carl Proske's work as a Palestrina editor. Individually indexed.

———. Martini, Giovanni Battista. *Esemplare o sia saggio fondamentale pratico di contrappunto sopra il canto fermo. . . . Parte prima.* Bologna: Lelio della Volpe Impressore dell'Instituto delle Scienze, 1774.

———. Martini, Giovanni Battista. *Esemplare o sia saggio fondamentale pratico di contrappunto fugato. . . . Parte seconda.* Bologna: Lelio della Volpe Impressore dell'Instituto delle Scienze, 1774.

See items A0244 and A0245 for main entries.

E0527 Mayr, Johann Simon. "Osservazioni di un vecchio suonatore di viola intorno ad un articolo del signor De Sevelignes, e sulla vita ed opere di Pier Luigi da Palestrina," *Gazzetta di Milano* 1835; reprinted in the *Gazzetta di Milano* I (1842), no. 42, pp. 182–184; nos. 43–44, pp. 186–188; no. 45, pp. 193–194.

Observations on Palestrina and current state of music for the church in early nineteenth-century Italy. Mayr (1763–1845), an Italianized German, is best known to posterity for his operas, but he was also *maestro di cappella* at Santa Maria Maggiore in Bergamo from 1803 to his death and produced more than 600 sacred compositions. This text was republished in Bergamo in 1853 in conjunction with the inauguration of a monument to Mayr's memory.

E0528 Meloncelli, Raoul. "Palestrina e Mendelssohn." In *Atti del II Convegno Internazionale di Studi Palestriniani. Anno Europeo della Musica. 3–5 maggio 1986*, ed. Lino Bianchi and Giancarlo Rostirolla. Palestrina: Fondazione Giovanni Pierluigi da Palestrina/Centro di Studi Palestriniani, 1991. ML410.P15C77.1986. pp. 439–460.

Examines the influence of the Palestrinian style on Mendelssohn's early development and in a number of unpublished youthful compositions. Discusses his early studies in polyphonic technique in the strict style with Zelter; his early travels to Rome and church music compositional activity there; and his fusion of the Italian manner of the late sixteenth century into his overall manner and into an idealized version of the style adaptable for Protestant musical contexts.

E0529 Müller-Blattau, Joseph. "Palestrina—ein Meister der abendländischen Musik." *Universitas: Zeitschrift für Wissenschaft und Kultur* 16 (1961): 989–996.

Short general biography and reception history which treats in particular German music historians and writers of the eighteenth and nineteenth centuries. Concludes with some notes on image of the creative artist in Pfitzner's *Palestrina.*

E0530 Nicolai, Otto. "Über die sixtinische Kapelle." *Neue Zeitschrift für Musik* 6 (1837): no.11, pp.43–45; no.12, pp.47–48; no.13, pp.51–53; no.14, pp.55–56. Excerpts reprinted in *Palestrina: Zwischen Démontage und Rettung*, ed. Heinz-Klaus Metzger and Rainer Riehn. München: Edition Text + Kritik, 1994, pp. 6–8.

Description of the Sistine Chapel as it existed in the early nineteenth century: number and physical disposition of the singers, as well as features of performance practice such as improvisation to a cantus firmus, falsobordone, discant, and special ornamentation.

E0531 Paolucci, Giuseppe. *Arte prattica di Contrappunto dimostrata con esempi di varj autori e con osservazioni di F. Giuseppe Paolucci minor Conventuale.* Venice: Antonio de Castro, 1765–1772. 3 vols. xv + 269pp., 315pp., vii + 247pp.

For list of musical examples, see chapter 2, "Prints in Books, Theoretical Treatises," "Paolucci."

E0532 Petrini, Pierantonio. *Memorie prenestine disposte in forma di annali. . . .* Rome: Pagliarini, 1795 [facs. repr. ed. Paolo Fancelli. Palestrina: ITL, 1990].

Contains biographical passage of interest for Palestrina's reception history in the later nineteenth century. English translation in Dixon, "Editorial," item E0114.

E0533 Pfitzner, Hans. "Palestrina." In *Hans Pfitzner. Reden, Schriften, Briefe, Unveröffentliches und bisher Verstreutes*, ed. Walter Abendroth. Berlin-Fröhnau: Luchterhand, 1955.

Pfitzner discusses his interest in and use of archaizing elements in his music and the use of motivic material from Palestrina's masses, especially the *Missa Papae Marcelli*, in his own "musical legend," the opera *Palestrina.*

E0534 Pozzi, Raffaele. "L'immagine ottocentesca del Palestrina nel rapporto tra Franz Liszt e il movimento ceciliano." In *Atti del II Convegno Inter-*

nazionale di Studi Palestriniani. Anno Europeo della Musica. 3–5 maggio 1986, ed. Lino Bianchi and Giancarlo Rostirolla. Palestrina: Fondazione Giovanni Pierluigi da Palestrina/Centro di Studi Palestriniani, 1991. ML410.P15C77.1986. pp. 461–478.

Examination of Liszt's later sacred compositions in light of his relations with the Cecilian movement and certain of its members. Argues that the Liszt-Cecilian relationship was essentially one of misunderstanding. While Liszt lent his support to the Cecilians, Witt and Haberl were closer in style to the actual compositional goals of Cecilian reform than he was; Liszt sought a closer rapport between music "inside the temple" and "outside" it in his own harmonic language and style

E0535 Rectanus, Hans. "'Ich kenne dich, Josquin, du Herrlicher. . . .' Bemerkungen zu thematischen Verwandtschaften zwischen Josquin, Palestrina und Pfitzner." In *Renaissance-Studien. Helmuth Osthoff zum 80. Geburtstag*, ed. Ludwig Finscher. Tutzing: Hans Schneider, 1979. ISBN 3–7952–0256–6. ML55.O8R4. pp. 211–222.

Studies some relationships, particular aural similarities, and similar thematic contours among the Josquin motet *Benedicta es*, Palestrina's mass on that motet, and other musical materials associated with Josquin, Palestrina, and Pfitzner. Ultimately makes a case for some resonance and resemblance among aspects of the creative process between Palestrina and Pfitzner.

E0536 Regia Accademia di S. Cecilia. *Festa musicale in commemorazione del fondatore G. Pierluigi da Palestrina, organizzata dalla Regia Accademia di S. Cecilia il 2 febbraio 1895, direttore m^{o} cav. Raffaele Terziani, coadiuvato da m^{o} cav. Remigio Renzi.* Rome: Tipografia della Pace di F. Cuggiani, 1895.

E0537 Riedel, Friedrich Wilhelm. "Hat Palestrina in der kirchenmusikalischen Praxis des 19. Jahrhunderts eine Rolle gespielt?" In *Palestrina und die Idee der klassischen Vokalpolyphonie im 19. Jahrhundert. Zur Geschichte eines kirchenmusikalischen Stilideals*, vol 1, ed. Winfried Kirsch. Regensburg: Gustav Bosse, 1989. pp. 195–198.

Focusing on Austrian institutions, suggests that practical performances of Palestrina's works before the mid-nineteenth century were largely confined to elite circles and special historical concerts. In the course of the century, church music establishments were also more likely to perform arrangements of seventeenth- and eighteenth-century works, while Palestrina's music played a very minor role.

E0538 Riedel, Friedrich W. "Maximilian Stadlers Bearbeitung der Hohelied-Motetten von Palestrina." In *Aufführungs- und Bearbeitungspraxis der Werke Palestrinas vom 16. bis zum 20. Jahrhundert*, ed. Friedrich Wilhelm Riedel. Kirchenmusikalische Studien 3. Sinzig: Studio, Verlag Schewe, 1997. ISBN 3–89564–037–9. ML410.P15A84.1997. pp. 81–87.

Located at Göttweig is a manuscript reworking by Maximilian Stadler of the motets from Palestrina's *Canticum canticorum*, in an arrangement consisting of a figured bass part and an upper vocal part virtually identical to the top voice in early prints of the motets. The result is somewhat reminiscent of

Viadana's ecclesiastical concerti or of sixteenth-century intabulation practice. The existence of this version (dated around 1815 to 1833), perhaps meant to serve as devotional house music, has interesting implications for nineteenth-century Palestrina reception that diverge from Romantic *a cappella* ideology.

E0539 Riethmüller, Albrecht. "Zu den Bemühungen im 19. Jahrhundert um Palestrinas Platz in der Geschichte." In *Palestrina und die Idee der klassischen Vokalpolyphonie im 19. Jahrhundert. Zur Geschichte eines kirchenmusikalischen Stilideals*, ed. Winfried Kirsch. Palestrina und die Kirchenmusik im 19. Jahrhundert 1. Regensburg: Gustav Bosse, 1989. pp. 43–54.

In the early nineteenth century, certain German Protestant writers on music initially expressed an unenthusiastic view of Palestrina, perhaps colored by national and religious biases brought to the debate on the question: Who is the greater composer of religious music—Palestrina or Bach? Remarks in the writings of Moritz Hauptmann, Franz Bendel, and Georg Gervinus are traced. The initial somewhat negative attitude to Palestrina softened as early as the 1830s and by late in the century became notable praise. But the "Bach or Palestrina" debate raises historiographical questions: where the "beginning" of music history is placed, what facts are deemed important, and how value judgments are made. Notes that it is important to differentiate and question both critiques and apologias, whether comment is from literature, from editorial work, or from composers, and whether the writer has immediate knowledge of Palestrina's music or of the "spirit" of Palestrina.

E0540 Rochlitz, Friedrich, ed. *Sammlung vorzüglicher Gesangstücke der anerkannt-grössten Geschichte der Tonkunst. . . .* Mainz: B. Schotts Söhnen, 1835. 3 vols.

This is an early and thoughtful history of music by a distinguished music critic and journalist, presented through representative examples. Title pages and preface in German and French on opposing pages (3ff.); introduction in German and French on opposing pages (4ff). This is followed by an "Ideen zu einer Geschichte der Kirchen- und höhern Kammer-Musik in Deutschland und Italien," tracing music history through a series of great personages. The three volumes are organized chronologically overall, and each has an extensive preface dealing with its respective material. Palestrina is treated in the "Zweite Periode" at the beginning of the second part of the first volume (pp.4/5–6/7 out of pp.2–24). Short annotations regarding liturgical use are often given as footnotes. In this edition, original rhythmic values are respected, and the music is presented *a cappella* (that is, without an arranged accompaniment). For full enumeration of examples, see chapter 5, "Modern Editions," entry under "Rochlitz."

E0541 Rohan-Csermak, Henri de. "La canonisation de Palestrina et la mutation de la musique sacrée en France au XIX siècle." *Ostinato Rigore: Revue Internationale d'Études Musicales* 4 (1994): 198–214.

Argues that in France Palestrina was "rediscovered" during the 1830s and made a symbol of the return to an aesthetic ideal of musical purity. Later he became the center of debate on the nature and mission of church music, which was as much about the people carrying on the debate and the times in which they lived as about church music as such.

E0542 Rostirolla, Giancarlo. "Busti ottocenteschi di Giovanni Pierluigi da Palestrina nel "templi" Romani dell'arte e della musica." In *Musica senza aggetivi. Studi per Fedele d'Amico*, ed. Agostino Ziino. Quaderni della Rivista Italiana di Musicologia 25. Florence: Olschki, 1991. 2 vols. ML55.D22. pp. 423–461.

Documentation of some of the efforts of early-nineteenth-century enthusiasts and musical organizations to honor Palestrina, centered around the creation and display of two busts of the composer. Contains interesting insights into the personalities and the interrelationships of musical organizations in Rome and elsewhere at that time.

E0543 Schlecht, Raymund. *Geschichte der Kirchenmusik. Zugleich Grundlage zur vorurtheilslosen Beantwortung der Frage: Was ist echte Kirchenmusik*? Regensburg: Coppenrath, 1871. ML3000.S38.

A history of music extending from the period of the early Christians to around 1600, with some attention to instrumental and vocal forms from 1600 to 1800, and then refocusing on the early Cecilians and the church music "restoration" of the nineteenth century. Historiography obviously contains a strong Cecilian influence. Palestrina discussed pp.98–101. Also contains a series of musical examples: no.52, *Jesu rex admirabilis a 3* (p.351); no.53, an intabulation for "das Cimbal" of the preceding item; no.54, *Adjuro vos, filiae Hierusalem a 5* (p.353–360); no.63, *O beata et benedicta a 5* in Jacob Paix's intabulation, in score with a keyboard part and lines of the motet (pp.396–403).

E0544 Schöberlein, Ludwig, and Friedrich Riegel, ed. *Schatz des liturgischen Chor- und Gemeindegesangs nebst dem Altarweisen in der deutschen evangelischen Kirchen aus den Quellen vornehmlich des 16. und 17. Jahrhunderts geschöpft mit den nöthigen geschichtlichen und praktischen Erläuterungen versehen und unter der musikalischen Redaktion on Friedrich Riegel für den Gebrauch in Stadt- und Landkirchen.* . . . Göttingen, 1865–1872. 3 vols.

This formidable work is a compilation of service music for the Lutheran liturgical year, for Sunday communion services (ordinary and proper material), vespers, feast days, and special occasions, drawn primarily from sixteenth- and seventeenth-century Lutheran composers but also containing a significant number of examples by Palestrina, Anerio, and other members of the Roman school. Testifies to the interest in Palestrina and his colleagues in nineteenth-century Lutheran circles. For a full list of contents, see item D0107.

E0545 Schuhmacher, Gerhard. "Zur Rezeption altklassischer Vokalpolyphonie in der evangelischen Kirchenmusik des 19. Jahrhunderts." In *Palestrina und die Idee der klassischen Vokalpolyphonie im 19. Jahrhundert. Zur*

Geschichte eines kirchenmusikalischen Stilideals, vol 1, ed. Winfried Kirsch. Regensburg: Gustav Bosse, 1989. pp. 143–148.

Describes the movement by a few historically and aesthetically oriented Lutherans to introduce some Renaissance vocal polyphony, particularly Palestrina's, into choral collections intended for the use and improvement of Lutheran liturgical choirs.

E0546 Schuler, Manfred. "Zur Palestrina-Pflege im Kloster Einsiedeln." In *Palestrina und die Idee der klassischen Vokalpolyphonie im 19. Jahrhundert. Zur Geschichte eines kirchenmusikalischen Stilideals*, vol 1, ed. Winfried Kirsch. Regensburg: Gustav Bosse, 1989. pp. 227–230.

Notes that the performance of Palestrina's music becomes evident at this cloister in the 1850s. Its two apparent stimuli were the efforts of Cecilians, and the inheritance of a number of musical transcriptions made by Robert Pearsall (1791–1856), an Englishman resident in eastern Switzerland who intensely studied and wrote at length on aspects of the Palestrina style.

E0547 Seidel, Elmar. "Zur Kontrapunktlehre von Heinrich Bellermann." In *Palestrina und die Idee der klassischen Vokalpolyphonie im 19. Jahrhundert. Zur Geschichte eines kirchenmusikalischen Stilideals*, vol 1, ed. Winfried Kirsch. Regensburg: Gustav Bosse, 1989. pp. 231–241.

Examination of history, influences on, and layout of Bellermann's text on strict counterpoint in the Palestrinian style, the most influential one between Fux's *Gradus ad Parnassum* of 1725 (on which it is modeled in some important ways) and Jeppesen's text, which appeared in German translation in 1935. Notes how the conception of counterpoint and polyphony betrays a sense of tension between voice-leading and harmonic considerations.

E0548 Stenzl, Jürg. "Palestrina als Komponist in der deutschen Musikgeschichte des 19. Jahrhunderts." In *Palestrina und die Idee der klassischen Vokalpolyphonie im 19. Jahrhundert. Zur Geschichte eines kirchenmusikalischen Stilideals,* vol 1, ed. Winfried Kirsch. Palestrina und die Kirchenmusik im 19. Jahrhundert. Regensburg: Gustav Bosse, 1989, pp. 35–42.

Examines various aspects of Palestrina's image as a contrapuntist in the nineteenth century: as the composer who opened up a new era of higher art; as one who created contained, serious music; and as one who created liturgically functional music, considered at a time when such music was not central to contemporary composition; and looks at the need for Palestrina myths or mythologies.

E0549 Tafelmayer, Wolfgang. "Das Palestrina-Bild im ausgewählten Musiklexika des 18. und 19. Jahrhunderts." In *Palestrina und die Idee der klassischen Vokalpolyphonie im 19. Jahrhundert. Zur Geschichte eines kirchenmusikalischen Stilideals*, vol 1, ed. Winfried Kirsch. Palestrina und die Kirchenmusik im 19. Jahrhundert. Regensburg: Gustav Bosse, 1989. pp. 77–86.

Systematic overview of Palestrina reception as represented by 28 selected musical lexicons of the eighteenth and nineteenth centuries. Evaluations of the composer and use of his name as a metaphor for excellence in church music. Entries studied include "a cappella," "alla Palestrina," "Palestrina style."

E0550 Tebaldini, Giovanni. "Memorie: Giovanni Pierluigi da Palestrina." *Rivista Musicale Italiana* 1 (1894): 213–239.

A general style appreciation published for the third centenary of the composer's death, interesting principally for its tone and perspective. Author views Palestrina as a last great representative of the Christian art of the Middle Ages, before music was overwhelmed by paganistic melodrama. Uses language (both original and paraphrased from others) suggesting the aesthetic of sublimity found in writings from earlier in the century, both with regard to fragments of the composer's biography and to aspects of his melodic technique. In defending the merits of the *da cappella* style, the text also implicitly criticizes both the hegemony of (Italian) opera and that of (German) music generally.

E0551 Unverricht, Hubert. "Ablehnende Bewertung der orchesterbegleiteten Kirchenmusik der Klassik. Voraussetzungen und Parallelitäten der Palestrina Renaissance um 1800?" In *Palestrina und die Idee der klassischen Vokalpolyphonie im 19. Jahrhundert. Zur Geschichte eines kirchenmusikalischen Stilideals*, vol 1, ed. Winfried Kirsch. Palestrina und die Kirchenmusik im 19. Jahrhundert. Regensburg: Gustav Bosse, 1989. pp. 105–115.

Traces German-language writings from 1750 to 1820, suggesting a moralistic and aesthetic reaction against features of certain mass settings—instrumental accompaniments, concertizing performances, inappropriate sentiments. These writings sought improvement in church music, not a propagation of the older style *per se*. But the aesthetic shift they represent prepared the ground for early Romantics, who envisioned *a cappella* polyphony as a "true" and "ennobled" church style, ideal for promoting liturgical devotion.

E0552 Unverricht, Hubert, ed. *Der Cäcilianismus: Anfänge—Grundlagen—Wirkungen. Internationales Symposium zur Kirchenmusik des 19. Jahrhunderts.* Eichstätter Abhandlungen zur Musikwissenschaft 5. Tutzing: Schneider, 1988.

A collection of essays which assess the principles, activities, chief personalities, dissemination and impact of Cecilianism, the nineteenth-century Roman Catholic reform music (chiefly associated with Germany) that advocated church music reform based on renewal of Gregorian chant and a polyphonic vocal style based on Palestrina.

E0553 Unverricht, Hubert. "Carl von Winterfelds Einschätzung des Palestrina-Stils." In *Festschrift für Winfried Kirsch zum 65. Geburtstag*, ed. Peter Ackermann, Ulrike Kienzle, and Adolf Nowak. Tutzing: Hans Schneider, 1996. pp. 228–237.

Evaluation of Winterfeld's remarkable studies of Palestrina and his commentary on the then-recent publication of Baini's biography. Having himself visited Italy, observed the music at St. Peter's in Rome, scored a number of then-unavailable Palestrina works, and held conversations with Baini personally in the 1810s, Winterfeld would decry the fact that Baini did not supply musical examples in his book, and criticized Baini's division of Palestrina's works into ten style phases. Winterfeld, though in fact better-acquainted with Palestrina's music than most of his German contemporaries and an admirer of his style, did not take an overwhelmingly adulatory tone on the composer and was not closely involved with the church music reform movement in Germany advocating Palestrina's music as a model.

E0554 Unverricht, Hubert. "Die Choralreformbemühungen unter den Cäcilienern." In *Die Cäcilianismus: Anfänge—Grundlagen—Wirkungen*. Tutzing: Schneider, 1968, pp. 109–123.

Study of efforts to revive Gregorian chant, inside and outside of Cecilianism. Useful as background when considering the sudden group of publications from 1895 to 1900 dealing with Palestrina's association with the *Editio Medicaea.*

E0555 Ursprung, Otto. "Palestrina und Deutschland. Beilage: Zwei Briefe zur Vorgeschichte der Gesamtausgabe der Werke Palestrinas." In *Festschrift Peter Wagner zum 60. Geburtstag*, ed. Karl Weinmann. Leipzig: Breitkopf und Härtel, 1926. ML55.F47. pp. 190–221.

Considering its length and format, a thorough history of Palestrina's reception in German-speaking countries. Contains manuscript and print survey of pre-1620 sources in numerous cities and libraries; traces dissemination of some print material through examination of book catalogs and school manuals of the sixteenth and seventeenth centuries; outlines the extent of knowledge and cultivation of *stile alla Palestrina* through the eighteenth century; provides overview of the nineteenth-century Cecilian movement; discusses early-nineteenth-century performances of Palestrina's music. Also describes efforts to publish a collected edition of the composer's works taking place before the commencement of the "Haberl" edition, together with an appendix of correspondence relevant to this last matter.

E0556 Ursprung, Otto. *Restauration und Palestrina-Renaissance in der katholischen Kirchenmusik der letzten zwei Jahrhunderte. Vergangenheitsfragen und Gegenwartsaufgaben.* Augsburg: Dr. Benno Filser, 1924. 80pp. ML3029.U7.1924a.

Offers a detailed, perceptive outline of activity associated with Palestrinian reception history from 1780 to 1914. Describes rethinking of church music style in the late classical period and among early Romantics (Catholic and Protestant); surveys conception and practice of *stile alla Palestrina* in that period; describes in its scholarly and practical aspects the Cecilian movement for church music "restoration." Notes both Cecilians who perceived the Palestrina style as the single correct lineage for new polyphonic composition, and modernist late Romantics who strove to reconcile the

Palestrinian aesthetic with a contemporary musical idiom. Argues that the complex crosscurrents and tendencies associated with the Palestrina restoration offer a future for church music in author's own time. (This text was written after World War I and the subsidence of the Cecilian movement, in part to reenergize German Roman Catholic lay interest in church polyphony.) A remarkable work in which the roots of much late twentieth-century scholarship on nineteenth-century Palestrina reception are visible.

E0557 Waldersee, Paul Graf von. "Giovanni Pierluigi da Palestrina und die Gesammtausgabe seiner Werke." In vol 5, no.52 of *Sammlung musikalischer Vorträge.* Leipzig: Breitkopf und Härtel, 1883–1899. 5 vols [repr. Nendeln: Kraus, 1976]. ML55.W16.1976t.no.49–63.

A narrative history, with the biographical information still heavily reliant on Baini, integrated with the publication history of Palestrina's masses and motets as they had appeared in the "Haberl" edition up to that time. Interesting as a period effort, with much quotation from the prefatory materials and some attempts to deal with style. Comments on Baini's division of Palestrina's music into ten style manners, and notes (without further citation) Moritz Hauptmann's countersuggestion of three styles, namely, a manner showing Netherlandish influence; one where both melody and harmony are subordinate to text declamation; and one where the elements of the second manner are united and in balance.

E0558 Weinmann, Karl. "Die proskesche Musikbibliothek in Regensburg." *Kirchenmusikalisches Jahrbuch* 24 (1911): 107–131.

A narrative of the life and activities of the highly gifted Proske and an appreciation of his outstanding library, a rich source of Palestrina-related materials, now housed in the Episcopal Central Library, Regensburg. Proske assembled his collection of about 20,000 volumes, including both theoretical and practical music and much other material, partly through acquisition and partly by scoring much otherwise inaccessible or distantly housed music. Describes the posthumous organization, cataloguing, care, and settlement of the collection, and includes (pp.120–131) a listing of names of the composers represented in it.

E0559 Widmann, Wilhelm. "Die Gesamtausgabe der Werke Palestrinas." *Kirchenmusikalisches Jahrbuch* 21 (1908): 149–155.

A history of the then-just-completed first comprehensive edition of Palestrina's music, describing its assembly and subscriber support, as well as noting some of the major editorial questions that confronted Franz Xaver Haberl and others in its compilation.

E0560 Winterfeld, Carl von. *Johannes Pierluigi von Palestrina, seine Werke und deren Bedeutung für die Geschichte der Tonkunst, mit Bezug auf Bainis Forschungen.* Breslau: Georg Philipp Aderholz, 1832. ML410.P15W4.1832.

Winterfeld encountered Baini's biography on Palestrina while researching his own great work on Giovanni Gabrieli. He responded by publishing a work which was partly an abbreviated translation, partly a critique, in which he took Baini to task for not supplying musical examples and for aspects of Baini's grasp of Palestrina's style development. A powerful stimulus to serious interest in Palestrina in nineteenth century Germany, an important source for later German-speaking authors, and more objective regarding Palestrina's significance than some contemporary literary authors.

E0561 Witzenmann, Wolfgang. "Echi palestriniani nei mottetti di Anton Bruckner." In *Atti del II Convegno Internazionale di Studi Palestriniani. Anno Europeo della Musica. 3–5 maggio 1986*, ed. Lino Bianchi and Giancarlo Rostirolla. Palestrina: Fondazione Giovanni Pierluigi da Palestrina/Centro di Studi Palestriniani, 1991. ML410.P15C77.1986. pp. 513–525.

Notes that while Bruckner apparently had little use for Cecilians, he nonetheless esteemed Palestrina's music itself; studies the influence of Palestrina works on certain of Bruckner's smaller-scale church music. Examines in particular Bruckner's *Ave Maria*, which in the 1880s was critically evaluated in comparison with Palestrina's music; it was then noted that Bruckner responded to the influence of Palestrina in an original way and was not another empty epigone.

E0562 Zanetti, Emilia. "Victor Hugo palestriniano 'en grandeur.'" In *Atti del II Convegno Internazionale di Studi Palestriniani. Anno Europeo della Musica. 3–5 maggio 1986*, ed. Lino Bianchi and Giancarlo Rostirolla. Palestrina: Fondazione Giovanni Pierluigi da Palestrina/Centro di Studi Palestriniani, 1991. ML410.P15C77.1986. pp. 479–512.

Study of Hugo's attitudes toward older music and the formative influences from which they sprang. Reprints his poem "*Que la musique date du seizième siècle*" (pp.488–494), which hails Palestrina as the "father of harmony." Extensive appendix (pp.495–512) with reports of Choron's concerts of early music in the 1820s and 1830s, lists of their repertory, and comments on Palestrina by Fétis and others.

3. From 1914 to the Present

E0563 Albrecht, Hans. "Ein kritischer Neudruck von Haberls Palestrina-Ausgabe?" *Zeitschrift für Musikgeschichte* 16 (1934): 41–42.

Responds to Casimiri's 1933 *Note d'Archivio* article and the problematic issues posed by the Haberl collected edition, especially text underlay and the manner in which uncovered errata should be presented. An interesting example of critical bias informed by the nationalist perspective of 1930s Germany and, indirectly, Italy as well.

E0564 Anonymous. "Informazioni: Il Centro Internazionale di Studi Palestriniani." *Il Palestrina* 1 (1961): 12–16.

Contains the statutes of the *Accademia Internazionale "G.P. da Palestrina"* which constitute it as a center for Palestrina studies based in Rome and Palestrina.

E0565 *L'arte di Giovanni Pierluigi da Palestrina. Atti e documentazione. VI Con-*

vegno europeo sul canto corale. Promosso e organizzato dalla Corale Goriziana "C.A. Seghizzi." Gorizia: Grafica Goriziana, 1975.

Proceedings of a conference, dealing chiefly with issues of performance practice and reception in the music of Palestrina. Individually indexed.

E0566 Aristirov, Cristo. "Alcuni aspetti dell'opera di Palestrina." In *L'arte di Giovanni Pierluigi da Palestrina. Atti e documentazione. VI Convegno europeo sul canto corale. Promosso e organizzato dalla Corale Goriziana "C.A. Seghizzi."* Gorizia: Grafica Goriziana, 1975. pp. 119–120.

General remarks to the effect that, notwithstanding its religious and mystical vein, Palestrina's music is penetrated by a profoundly humane vitality.

E0567 Bartolucci, Domenico. "La pratica esecutiva palestriniana nella Cappella Sistina. (schema della relazione)." In *L'arte di Giovanni Pierluigi da Palestrina. Atti e documentazione. VI Convegno europeo sul canto corale. Promosso e organizzato dalla Corale Goriziana "C.A. Seghizzi."* Gorizia: Grafica Goriziana, 1975. pp. 121–122.

Outline of a talk given by the longtime director of the Sistine Chapel. Describes differences between Renaissance polyphony and present-day choirs with respect to types, qualities, and ranges of voices. Advises against excessive warmth, coolness, or contrasts of tempo in performance.

E0568 Bianchi, Lino, and Giancarlo Rostirolla, eds. *Atti del II Convegno Internazionale di Studi Palestriniani. Anno Europeo della Musica. 3–5 maggio 1986.* Palestrina: Fondazione Giovanni Pierluigi da Palestrina/Centro di Studi Palestriniani, 1991. ML410.P15C77.1986.

Proceedings of a conference on the composer held in 1986. Papers are individually indexed.

E0569 Bianchi, Lino. "Relazioni introduttiva." In *Atti del Convegno di Studi Palestriniani. 28 settembre–2 ottobre 1975*, ed. Francesco Luisi. Palestrina: Fondazione Giovanni Pierluigi da Palestrina, 1977. ML410.P15C77.1975. pp. 23–32.

Description of the mission and planned projects of the Palestrina Foundation, with an overview of the state of research in Palestrina studies as of 1975. Indicates directions for further needed research and examines recent attitudes toward the composer.

E0570 Birtner, Herbert. "Renaissance und Klassik in der Musik." In *Theodor Kroyer—Festschrift zum 60. Geburtstag.* Regensburg: Bosse, 1933. ML55.K76Z4. pp. 40–53.

Discusses the historiography and distinguishing characteristics of "Renaissance" and the identification of "classically" Renaissance composers. Names Josquin as a culminating figure in Renaissance music, while in Palestrina Birtner detects a quality akin to a "mannerist" spirituality. Palestrina is understood to be not a culmination, but an initiator of a certain fundamental distancing from the world-centered Renaissance ideology, a composer in the service of a new "churchliness."

E0571 Blumenstihl, Paolo. "Parole pronunciate dal vice presidente . . . per lo scoprimento della lapide a Giovanni Pierluigi da Palestrina, il 3 gennaio 1926." *Annuario della R. Accademia di S. Cecilia 1925/1926*. Rome: Manuzio, n.d., pp. 129–130.

E0572 Boyd, Malcolm. *Palestrina's Style. A Practical Introduction*. London: Oxford, 1973. ISBN 0–19-315224–X. ML410 P15 B685 [Italian trans. *Lo stile di Palestrina: Introduzione pratica*, trans. A.M. Morazzoni. Milan: Ricordi, 1981].

Rejects species method and uses Palestrina's sacred music as foundation for progressive discussion by topic of technical features of sixteenth-century style and musical culture. Presents teaching exercises of increasing complexity which approximate sixteenth-century methods: students are instructed to add new music to melodic lines and to parts extracted from sixteenth-century masterworks.

E0573 Cametti, Alberto. "Bibliografia palestriniana." *Bolletino Bibliografico Musicale* 1 (1926): 3–14.

Expansion of the bibliography in the 1925 *Palestrina*, item E0093.

E0574 Cametti, Alberto. "Parole . . . pronunciate quale introduzione al concerto da lui diretto nella Sala Accademica il 20 febbraio 1925, in commemorazione del quarto centenario di Giovanni Pierluigi da Palestrina." *Annuario della R. Accademia di S. Cecilia 1924/1925*. Rome: Manuzio, n.d., pp. 122–128.

E0575 Cavallini, Ivano. "Non solum princeps sed principis memoria. Vent' anni di studi su Giovanni Pierluigi da Palestrina." *Acta Musicologica* 67 (1995): 1–19.

A judicious overview of research on Palestrina between about 1975 and 1995, with discussion of a number of publications.

E0576 Cobasnian, Boris. "Alcuni problemi d' interpretazione dell' opera palestriniana." In *L'arte di Giovanni Pierluigi da Palestrina. Atti e documentazione. VI Convegno europeo sul canto corale. Promosso e organizzato dalla Corale Goriziana "C.A. Seghizzi."* Gorizia: Grafica Goriziana, 1975. pp. 115–118.

Holds that there can be significant diversity in the interpretation of Palestrina's music. Stylistic observations suggest the interpreter needs not to aim at originality for its own sake, but to make evident the profundity of the internal creative process in the compositions to be performed.

E0577 Cohen, Dalia. "Birdcalls and the Rules of Palestrina Counterpoint: Towards the Discovery of Universal Qualities in Vocal Expression." *Israel Studies in Musicology* 3 (1983): 96–123.

Claims that there are basic and universal features of vocal expression common to speech and music, and finds a resemblance between some fundamental rules controling states of tension and relaxation in the theory of "Palestrina counterpoint" and those governing certain aspects of the vocalization of birdcalls.

E0578 Cohen, Dalia. "Palestrina Counterpoint: a Musical Expression of Unexcited Speech." *Journal of Music Theory* 15 (1971): 84–111.

Examines relationship between the Palestrinian contrapuntal style and the musical aspects of speech. Describes five speech qualities which produce "tension" (including various acoustical properties as well as a sense of uncertainty or a departure from expectations) and concludes that virtually all of these are lacking in Palestrinian counterpoint, as they would introduce too great an excitement into the music. Principles of such counterpoint are like "unexcited" speech; thus some of its rules are based on factors other than musical convention or academic organization.

E0579 Comes, Liviu. "L'attualità dello studio palestriniano per i musicisti contemporanei," trans. Traian Sofonea and Pietro Derossi. In *Atti del Convegno di Studi Palestriniani. 28 settembre–2 ottobre 1975*, ed. Francesco Luisi. Palestrina: Fondazione Giovanni Pierluigi da Palestrina, 1977. In Italian, translated from Roumanian. ML 410.P15C77.1975. pp. 427–431.

Argues that while the Palestrina style unites to the highest degree the stylistic attributes of its own epoch, its polyphonic linearity (not based on functional tonality), rhythmic flexibility, and local structural asymmetries offer contemporary composers options for the reinvigoration of more recent musical language. Asserts compatibility of the idiom and its pedagogy with serialism and linear polyphonic conceptions.

E0580 Comes, Liviu. *Palestrina et son héritage après 400 ans.* Bucharest: Uniunea Compozitorilor si Muzicologilor, 1994. 87pp. [Italian translation "Palestrina e la sua eredità dopo 400 anni. I," trans. Marco Boschini. *La cartolina: Musica corali e didattica* 19, no.99 (1995): 36–45; 20, no.101 (1996): 35–44].

A commemorative review published in conjunction with the four hundredth anniversary of Palestrina's death.

E0581 Costa, Othmar. "Palestrina und seine Zeit." *Singende Kirche* 41.4 (1994): 162–168.

Discusses contemporary realization in performance of the Palestrina style, noting that since the composer's melodic style is derived from Gregorian chant, each part in the texture plays an essential role and has its own profile and personality.

E0582 Day, Thomas. "Palestrina Redivivus." *American Choral Review* 14.3 (1972): 23–29.

Practical admonitions useful for revitalizing the performance of Palestrina's works, cast in a humorous dialogue format.

E0583 De Rensis [Raffaelo]. "L'edizione italiana delle *Opere Complete* di Palestrina." *Rivista Musicale Italiana* 42 (1938): 600–604.

Relates events leading to the publication of the "Casimiri" edition.

E0584 Donato, Giuseppe. "Palestrina negli scritti di Alberto Favara." In *Atti del II*

Convegno Internazionale di Studi Palestriniani. Anno Europeo della Musica. 3–5 maggio 1986, ed. Lino Bianchi and Giancarlo Rostirolla. Palestrina: Fondazione Giovanni Pierluigi da Palestrina/Centro di Studi Palestriniani, 1991. ML410.P15C77.1986. pp. 569–585.

Favara published a series of articles and other items between 1901 and 1912 on Renaissance music and on Palestrina in particular. Favara's interest in a "return to the old" was associated with a burgeoning movement amongst the Italian intelligentsia for a rediscovery of an Italian national identity. He believed that the music of Palestrina embodied the "distinctive qualities of the race," and the study of his works would help to enable the "redemption" of Italian music. This stance was in part a nationalist counterpose against the perceived hegemony of German music, especially instrumental music, in this period.

E0585 Donella, Valentino. "Palestrina e la musica al Concilio di Trento (con un insegnamento per l'oggi)." *Rivista Internazionale di musica sacra* 15.3–4 (1994): 254–270.

Assesses the contributions made by Palestrina through the *Missa Papae Marcelli* to an understanding of reformed liturgical style in the wake of the Council of Trent. Traces the myth in some of the historical literature, and suggests the relevance of the Tridentine mandate for creation of liturgical music in a late-twentieth-century context: keep a spirit of equilibrium, and keep it functional.

E0586 Dupont, Jacques. "Notes musicologiques. En marge d'une édition complète, critique des oeuvres de Palestrina." *Revue musicale* 20 (1939): 224–228.

Asked to comment generally upon Palestrina's style by Casimiri in anticipation of the forthcoming new comprehensive edition, the author finds a sensitivity to the nuances of text setting in Palestrina similar to that of a composer like Claude Debussy. Notes however that Palestrina's compositions are characterized by an aesthetic objectivity driven by liturgical requirements and by an essentially architectural concept which circumscribes their liberty of text interpretation. This is true whether the compositions are of a lyrical and relatively formally free type on the one hand, or based on techniques such as *cantus firmus* and canon on the other.

E0587 Fano, Fabio. "Intorno al Palestrina." *Musica d'oggi* (n.s.) 1 (1958): 300–301.

Voices concern over a perceived contemporary tendency to objectify and even devalue Palestrina's music because it is not considered "progressive" or "revolutionary." Calls for reversion to the high regard in which the composer was held historically.

E0588 Fano, Fabio. "Problemi e orientamenti di critica Palestriniana." *Nuova Rivista Musicale Italiana* 29 (1995): 92–133.

Republication of an article which originally appeared in *Vichiana* in 1968 (pp.251–296). The first part profiles some of the reception history and critical approaches to Palestrina, as well as how his works inspired both subsequent composers and literary personalities. The second part is a far-ranging and perceptive style appreciation, relating Palestrina's personal manner and choices to requirements of the genres and forms in which they were used. Numerous works are examined, and penetrating comparative comment on works by Victoria, Gabrieli, Monteverdi, and others are made.

E0589 Fano, Fabio. "Richezze spirituale e stilistica dell'arte palestriniana." In *L'arte di Giovanni Pierluigi da Palestrina. Atti e documentazione. VI Convegno europeo sul canto corale. Promosso e organizzato dalla Corale Goriziana "C.A. Seghizzi."* Gorizia: Grafica Goriziana, 1975. pp. 7–15.

Notes how in recent years writers have somewhat demythologized Palestrina, virtually suggesting that the image was tiresome and monotonous in its very perfection. Argues instead that even while Palestrina maintained a superior stylistic coherence, he was richer and more intense in his dramatic sense and affective use of dissonance than is generally acknowledged, particularly in his madrigals but also in much of his church music as well.

E0590 Federhofer, Hellmut. "Ist Palestrina ein Manierist?" In *Convivium Musicorum. Festschrift Wolfgang Boetticher zum sechzigsten Geburtstag am 19 August 1974*, ed. Heinrich Hüschen and Dieter-Rüdiger Moser. Berlin: Merseburger, 1974. pp. 44–51.

Evaluates some definitions of "mannerism" in sixteenth-century music in the secondary German literature from 1930 to 1970 in light of the question whether Palestrina might be considered a mannerist because of his particular association with a Counter-Reformation sensibility. Mannnerism is associated here with traits such as the free handling of expressive dissonance or harmonic change, diminution practices, chromaticism, or radical textural change. Notes that while in certain works Palestrina does seem to strive for a kind of intensified expression through the use of dissonance and sudden harmonic shifts, these traits are characteristic generic and conventional language for certain types of works, and they are much less characteristic of Palestrina generally than of a composer like Lasso.

E0591 Ferracci, Emilio. "Il Palestrina—Il Concilio Ecumenico Vaticano II e il Concilio di Trento." *Il Palestrina. Bolletino trimestrale del Centro Internazionale di Studi Palestriniani* 3 (1963): 1–8.

Tandem narratives relating the activities, concerns, and deliberations on music in the liturgy at the Second Vatican Council in 1962 and the Council of Trent respectively. Includes a reprinted item from *L'Osservatore Romano* describing performances of Palestrina's music for various celebrations during the first session of Vatican II.

E0592 Fischer, Klaus. "Historische Bedeutung und kritische Würdigung der Gesamtausgaben im Hinblick auf Palestrinas erstes Messenbuch und andere moderne Transkriptionen seiner Werke." In *Aufführungs- und Bearbeitungspraxis der Werke Palestrinas vom 16. bis zum 20. Jahrhundert*, ed. Friedrich Wilhelm Riedel. Kirchenmusikalische Studien 3. Sinzig: Studio, Verlag Schewe, 1997. pp. 143–166.

A critical comparison of the Haberl and Casimiri editions of Palestrina's collected works, focusing on their respective editions of the First Book of Masses. Contrasts Haberl's and Casimiri's working and scholarly methods and evaluates both the virtues and problems in each edition.

E0593 Franklin, Peter. "*Palestrina* and the Dangerous Futurists." *Musical Quarterly* 70 (1984): 499–514.

A study of how the image of the composer in Pfitzner's opera is used as a vehicle on which to project early-twentieth-century debates on futurism versus conservatism, on political progressiveness versus reactionarism, and on the nature of the creative artist. Notes that while the opera is ostensibly built around the myth of the Marcellus mass, its actual drama revolves around the aging artist, who seems to have lost his creative power and sense of belonging to the world. Against the odds and through reawakened veneration for the ancient masters of the musical tradition, Palestrina here becomes a vessel of divine inspiration. While the *Marcellus* mass "saves" the tradition, he himself greets his personal twilight with a "mystical acceptance" as he keeps a necessary distance from the world. Item included here as indicating the logical extension of the image of Palestrina as solitary spiritual genius reverting back to Baini and beyond.

E0594 von Gersdorff, Dagmar. "Der Komponist Palestrina im Bewusstsein E. T. A. Hoffmanns, Thomas Manns und Pfitzners." *Mitteilungen der Hans Pfitzner-Gesellschaft* n.f. 42 (1981): 50–63.

Examines ideas about Palestrina embedded in writings by Hoffmann, Mann, and Pfitzner. For Hoffmann, Palestrina took symbolic form as the musician of spiritual simplicity and power, the renewer of church music and its rescuer from the decline into which it had fallen. For Mann's characters, Palestrina could be perceived both as the model of "polyphonic objectivity" and as a participant in its incipient decadence, effeminacy, and disintegration, which could serve to deliver humanity into Satan's hands. For Pfitzner, Palestrina was the symbol who wrestled with the existential issues facing humanity: mortality versus immortality, good versus evil, humanity's purpose, inspiration, creativity.

E0595 Ghiglione, Natale. [Editorial]. "Giovanni Pierluigi da Palestrina (1525–1594)." *Rivista Internazionale di musica sacra* 15.3–4 (1994): 3–12.

Describes how the pronouncements of the Roman church on music in liturgy have always emphasized the primacy of text, and how Palestrina, the prolific musician's musician and great exemplar of this teaching, has maintained a historical centrality and continuously influenced the greatest Western composers from his own time right through the twentieth century. Followed (pp. 9–12) by publication of a letter of benediction from Pope John Paul II to Domenico Bartolucci, life director of the Sistine Chapel, on the fourth centenary of Palestrina's death.

E0596 Ghislanzoni, Alberto. "Considerazioni e nuovi principi valutativi dell'arte palestriniana." In *L'arte di Giovanni Pierluigi da Palestrina. Atti e documentazione. VI Convegno europeo sul canto corale. Promosso e organizzato* *dalla Corale Goriziana "C.A. Seghizzi."* Gorizia: Grafica Goriziana, 1975. pp. 17–22.

Describes a view of Palestrina which likens him to other creative personalities in the Western tradition whose work appears dominated by a sense of its "perfect equilibrium of values."

E0597 Kapp, Reinhard. "Von der Sprache der Seele." *Österreichisches Musikzeitschrift* 42 (1987): 292–300.

Traces what is discerned as an emotive expressive component in the musical evolution of the West, arguing that the "language of the soul" emerged with Palestrina and had its full flowering in the period from Haydn to Webern.

E0598 Krenek, Ernst. "Giovanni Pierluigi da Palestrina." *Enciclopedia della Musica*, ed. Claudio Sartori. Milano: Ricordi, 1964. vol 3. ML100 E45. pp. 362–363.

The distinguished composer characterizes Palestrina's style as one of perfect equilibrium, based on rigorous control and maintained through delicate and invariable alternation of forces, and manifested in a complex intermingling of disciplined movement. Alludes to changing perception of Palestrina's style in the mid-twentieth century and offers a view of his place among the major composers of his time. Final reflections deal with Palestrina's usefulness for the study of counterpoint.

E0599 Luisi, Francesco, ed. *Atti del Convegno di Studi Palestriniani. 28 settembre–2 ottobre 1975*. Palestrina: Fondazione Giovanni Pierluigi da Palestrina, 1977.

Proceedings of a conference marking the 450th anniversary of Palestrina's birth. Papers are individually indexed.

E0600 Morris, Reginald Owen. *Contrapuntal Technique in the Sixteenth Century.* Oxford: Clarendon, 1922. 74 + 49pp. ML446.M8.

A manual of counterpoint that rejects the species method and seeks to teach the subject as it was done in the sixteenth century, namely through examination of the modal system, rhythm, melody, harmonic structures, canon and fugue, design, and the imitation of good models. Palestrina is still regarded as an outstanding model, and the text is suffused with examples from his works. Text includes analyses of motets *Veni sponsa Christi a 4* (pp.53–57) and *O bone Jesu a 4* (p.52). See D0076 for enumeration of examples.

E0601 Osthoff, Wolfgang. "Palestrina e la leggenda musicale di Pfitzner." In *Atti del II Convegno Internazionale di Studi Palestriniani. Anno Europeo della Musica. 3–5 maggio 1986*, ed. Lino Bianchi and Giancarlo Rostirolla. Palestrina: Fondazione Giovanni Pierluigi da Palestrina/Centro di Studi Palestriniani, 1991. ML410.P15C77.1986. pp. 527–568.

Investigation of why Pfitzner chose Palestrina as a vehicle for his own meditations on the nature of artistic genius; how Pfitzner responded to the music and figure of the earlier composer; and the types of nineteenth-century philosphical and aesthetic coloration with which Palestrina was associated in this case. Article includes reprint of pp. 228–253 of the Schott edition of Pfitzner's score.

E0602 Paccagnella, Ermengildo. "La problematica degli Studi Palestriniani e il programma del Centro." *Il Palestrina: Bolletino trimestrale del Centro Internazionale di Studi Palestriniani* 1 (1961): 2–6.

Proclaims the need for a new initiative in Palestrina studies, and that the composer and his works deserve a major reevaluation. Declares that the corpus needs a new technical analysis and historical contextualization; that its relative conservative and progressive aspects need reassessment; that the musical language needs new aesthetic appreciation; and that the problems of authentic performance of the works should be addressed. (This call has been heeded, considering the major rethinking and expansion of studies in Palestrina and Palestrina reception in the last third of the twentieth century.)

E0603 Paccagnella, Ermengildo. "Ritrovare il vero Palestrina." *Il Palestrina: Bolletino trimestrale del Centro Internazionale di Studi Palestriniani* 2 (1962): 9–15.

Elaboration of ideas regarding potential areas for renewal in Palestrina studies [see item E0602]. Asserts that understanding of the original style of the composer, not his modernizing successors and editors, has to be regained. Although only one autograph is extant, it is possible to rely on early editions as well as modern text-critical and analytical methods to establish authentic and historically accurate stylistic insights.

E0604 Pass, Walter. "Su un' estetica della sonorità vocale nelle composizioni di G. P. da Palestrina." In *L'arte di Giovanni Pierluigi da Palestrina. Atti e documentazione. VI Convegno europeo sul canto corale. Promosso e organizzato dalla Corale Goriziana "C.A. Seghizzi."* Gorizia: Grafica Goriziana, 1975. In German, with outline of contents in Italian. pp. 55–64.

Proclaims need for new systematic research into Palestrina's style. Offers overview of the composer's reception history, emphasizing misunderstandings and misuses of the style in the nineteenth century. Indicates that within certain parameters Palestrina's music demonstrates much foreground asymmetry and inconsistency. Asserts that it is the relation between style and sonority, more than that of melody, harmony, or rhythm, which needs fresh scrutiny, the result of which will improve insight into the evolution in Western music toward the major-minor tonal system.

E0605 Phillips, Peter. " 'Fürst der Musik aller Zeiten'. (On the 400th Anniversary of Palestrina's Death, Peter Phillips Goes in Search of the Real Composer Behind the Myth.)" *Musical Times* 150 (1994): 74–79.

Review and reappraisal of the Palestrina image, reaffirming that his music possesses great variety of mood, compositional method, and scoring.

E0606 Poos, Heinrich. "Saggio sul vero metodo di analisi della musica palestriniana [Versuch über die wahre Art, Palestrina zu analysieren]." In *L'arte di Giovanni Pierluigi da Palestrina. Atti e documentazione. VI Convegno europeo sul canto corale. Promosso e organizzato dalla Corale Goriziana "C.A. Seghizzi."* Gorizia: Grafica Goriziana, 1975. In German. pp. 65–77.

Admonishes the deficient aesthetic perception of Palestrina as stylistically undifferentiated, which Poos ascribes to the nineteenth-century emphasis on instrumental music. Acknowledges that those works which seriously analyze Palestrina are statistical in method and without context. Using the *Kyrie I* of the *Missa Quem dicunt homines* as an example, he proposes an analytical procedure which addresses the subtle and intricate affinities of parts as well as the overall contrapuntal conception. He asserts this will improve insight into individual style formation in sixteenth-century music generally.

E0607 Ricci, Corrado. "Il Palestrina." *Musica d'oggi* 7 (1925): 281–284, 313–316.

Text of an address delivered to the Accademia di S. Cecilia; reprinted as item E0608, below.

E0608 Ricci, Corrado. *Il Palestrina: discorso tenuto da Corrado Ricci alla R. Accademia di S. Cecilia, il 6 febbraio 1925.* Rome: G. Glingler, 1925. 26 pp. ML410 P15R53.

An address by the noted historian and sometime Italian director-general of fine arts, nationalist-flavored, arguing that, like Raphael's Santa Cecilia, Palestrina disdained instruments and used voices alone for they had a greater and purer expressive power. He freed vocal music from the cold intricacies of the Netherlanders and, with an intense religious sense, shaped and tailored it to ornamenting the liturgy.

E0609 Ronga, Luigi. "Nota sulla vocalità Palestriniana." In *Atti del congresso internazionale di musica sacra organizato dal Pontificio Istituto di musica sacra e dalla Commissione di Musica Sacra per l'Anno Santo* (Roma, 25–30 maggio 1950), ed. Higini Anglès. Tournai: Desclée, 1952. ML35.R7P5. pp. 327–329.

After describing the music of Palestrina as a rare balance of religious intensity and superbly normative technique, the author suggests that its expressive power in performance is not only a matter of variety in timbre and register but also of variety in the most subtle and intimate articulations of the voices, without any straining or striving for special effect.

E0610 Rostirolla, Giancarlo. *Bibliografia degli scritti su Giovanni Pierluigi da Palestrina (1568–1996).* Assisted by Luciano Luciani and Elena Zomparelli. I Quaderni della Biblioteca Pierluigi 3. Palestrina: Fondazione Giovanni Pierluigi da Palestrina, 1997.

A listing of nearly 1,400 items (not annotated) arranged chronologically by year of publication since 1568, including book, pamphlet, and journal items, works in course of publication, and sound recording liner notes, plus extensive indexes. Introduction, pp.5–8. Particularly useful to the specialized researcher as it includes publications in certain dailies and other difficult-to-locate items of interest (such as Italian commemorative programs) that for various reasons are outside the parameters of the present work and not included here. Item E0069 contains an early version of this bibliography.

E0611 Schlötterer, Reinhold. "Lehrmethoden des Palestrinas-Kontrapunkts." In *Gesellschaft für Musikforschung. Bericht über den internationalen musikwissenschaftlichen Kongress Basel 1962*, ed. Georg Reichert and Martin Just. Kassel: Bärenreiter, 1963. ML36.I64.1962. pp. 361–362.

Argues that at least three methods of teaching counterpoint in the style of Palestrina in use in the mid-twentieth century were unsatisfactory in terms of giving practitioners a true feeling for musical structure in the style.

E0612 *Nel VII [settimo] cinquantenario della morte do Giovanni Pierluigi da Palestrina 1594–1944.* Turin: A & C, 1944.

Not reviewed, but listed in Rostirolla's bibliography as a collection of essays on sacred music with an appendix of compositions by Palestrina and others. Title indicates it is a commemorative volume. Authors of essays represented include "P. G. B." [D.G.B.?], Pompeo Borghezio, D. G. Boyer, Arnaldo Furlotti, and M. Carignano. [G. Rostirolla].

E0613 Sherman, Bernard D. *Inside Early Music: Conversations with Performers.* New York: Oxford, 1997. ISBN 0–19-509708–4. ML457.S52.

Chapter 6, "Other Kinds of Beauty: Peter Phillips on the Tallis Scholars and Palestrina" (pp.117–132) is a conversation between Sherman and Phillips on considerations of performing Renaissance liturgical music and Palestrina in particular, featuring questions of tempo and choral sound quality. Notes the forward-looking tendencies in Palestrina's style and suggests that two or three style phases are audible over the range of his work. Includes a discussion of some recordings dating from the early 1990s.

E0614 Szabò, Tibor. "L'influenza dell' arte palestriniana sulle opere corali ungheresi nel secolo XX." In *L'arte di Giovanni Pierluigi da Palestrina. Atti e documentazione. VI Convegno europeo sul canto corale. Promosso e organizzato dalla Corale Goriziana "C.A. Seghizzi."* Gorizia: Grafica Goriziana, 1975. pp. 107–113.

Suggests the Palestrinian idiom affected Franz Liszt's later religious style with respect to the use of vertical sonorities and progressions affected by modal structures. Liszt's choices became part of the heritage of twentieth-century Hungarian sacred music and are evident in the choral works of such composers as Zoltán Kodály and Ferenc Farkas, some of which are examined here.

E0615 Venuti, Massimo. "Inedito Palestrina nel quarto centenario della morte." *Rassegna Musicale Curci* 47.2 (1994): 10–13.

Notes that Palestrina had a much stronger and economically astute personality than is often popularly imagined. Suggests that Palestrina's artistic mandate was not so much the comprehensibility of text *per se* as the evolution of a personal *modus operandi*, where the listener would not primarily contemplate the complexities of technique and structure, but rather develop a personal rapport with text and music.

E0616 Wolff, Hellmuth Christian. "Palestrina und Schönberg—zwei Extreme der europäischen Musik." In *Bericht über den internationalen musikwissenschaftlichen Kongress Wien, Mozartjahr 1956 (Wien, 3–9 juni 1956)*, ed. Erich Schenk. Graz/Cologne: Böhlau, 1958. pp. 749–753.

In an approach informed by nineteenth- and early twentieth-century philosophical attitudes, Wolff considers Palestrina and Schönberg as types supporting the historiographical thesis that, if European music history is perceived as a great unity, then one can find the overall consistency in the series of polar opposites in style and approach which have characterized it. The contrast, for instance, of "formal beauty" and expressive restraint (Palestrina) with extreme expression and affective "truth" (Schönberg) has been a long-range historical constant. Oppositions such as form/expression, static/dynamic, introverted/extroverted have been features of the tradition since Palestrina's time.

Addendum: Forthcoming Publications

The present author is indebted to Giancarlo Rostirolla's *Bibliografia degli scritti su Giovanni Pierlugi da Palestrina (1568–1996)* (Palestrina, 1997) for much of the following list (particularly for ascertaining the items in *Atti del III more Convegno*). The enumeration is supplemented by additional items and cross-reference information.

[E0617] *Atti del III Convegno di Studi Palestriniani. Palestrina e l' Europa in occasione del Quarto Centenario della morte di Palestrina. Palestrina, 6–9 ottobre 1994*, ed. Giancarlo Rostirolla and Stefania Soldati.

A major item, not yet issued. A complete list of the papers announced for this publication, slightly different from the original series of presentations made at the 1994 conference, is given below as items E0618–E0673. It will be noted that some of these items (presumably the same or similar, with matching authors and titles) have already been published in other media, some in languages other than Italian, in which case a cross-reference is provided. The internal organization of the forthcoming book is not known to the present author.

[E0618] Acciai, Giovanni. "Aderenza all'elemento prosodico e retorico nelle opere mottetistiche del Palestrina."

[E0619] Ackermann, Peter. " 'Genere' e 'stile'. Alcuni note sulle Lamentazioni del Palestrina."

[E0620] Annibaldi, Claudio. "Girolamo Frescobaldi e il Palestrina: un autografo misconosciuto, un filo riannodato."

———. Barbieri, Patrizio. "Su di basso continuo attribuito al Palestrina (ca.1580–1590)." Apparently an Italian version of E0179.

[E0621] Bernstein, Jane A. "The Publishing of Palestrina's Music in Sixteenth-Century Rome and Venice."

[E0622] Besutti, Paola. "Giovanni Pierluigi da Palestrina e la liturgia mantovana (II)." See E0183, of which the present item is apparently a second part.

[E0623] Bianchi, Lino. "Perduti il Palestrina di Johann Melchoir Ernst Sachs (1843–1927) e di Johann Gottfried Loewe?"

[E0624] Bianchi, Lino. "Raffaello de Rensis e l'Edizione Nazionale delle opere di G. Pierluigi da Palestrina."

[E0625] Bongiovanni, Carmela. "La polifonia sacra e profana intavolata: due tradizioni a confronto."

[E0626] Boschini, Marco. "La 'terza riempita' in Palestrina e Lasso. Alcuni aspetti di statica e dinamica contrappuntistica."

[E0627] Bressan, Gino. "A proposito di alcune esecuzioni integrali del 'Cantico dei Cantici.'"

[E0628] Bryant, David and Michele Pozzobon. "Alcuni contrafacta di Mottetti del Palestrina nel' archivo del Duomo di Treviso."

[E0629] Chambure, Alain de. "Problemi di prassi esecutiva palestriniana."

[E0630] Ciliberti, Galliano. "Il Palestrina e il mondo musicale controriformistaico nello Stato pontificio."

[E0631] Cornaz, Marie. "La redécouverte de Palestrina en Belgique à partir de 1830."

[E0632] Cumino, Renata. "Il trattamento del cantus firmus negli Inni del Palestrina."

[E0633] D'Ambrosio, Wilma. "Le Messe di Domenico Dal Pane su Mottetti del Palestrina (1687); un capitolo emblematico della ricezione palestriniana nel tardo Seicento."

[E0634] De Salvo, Salvatore. "Il repertorio palestriniano eseguito nella Cappella Papale nel secolo XX."

[E0635] Dubrawskaja, Tat'jiana. "Melody: the Mirror of the Palestrina's Style [*sic*]."

[E0636] Franke, Veronica Mary. "Borrowing and Transformation Techniques in Palestrina's Parody Masses."

[E0637] Freis, Wolfgang. "Palestrina's 'Harmonic Institutions.'"

[E0638] Fromsen, Michèle. "Palestrina and the Musical Canon: His Influence on Motet Composition in Northern Italy during the Post-Tridentine Era."

[E0639] Gargiulo, Piero. "Palestrina e Monte nelle antologie madrigalistiche: il caso di 'Perch'al viso d' amor portava insegna.'"

[E0640] Giuliani, Roberto. "La recezione del Palestrina nel Novecento: edizioni e fonti sonore."

[E0641] Guletsky, Irina. "The Types of Composition Proportions in Palestrina's Masses."

[E0642] Iesuè, Alberto. "Progretto per una discografia palestriniana."

———. Janitzek, Martina. "La recezione del Palestrina nell'editoria musicale dell' Ottocento." Apparently an Italian version of E0501.

[E0643] Janz, Bernhard. "Reflessioni sull'attribuzione della Messa 'Nativitas tua Dei genetrix' nel Cod.70 del fondo Cappella Sistina." See item E0261, of which this item is either a version or a supplement.

[E0644] Keil, Klaus. "RISM Handschriftendokumentation: ein klein Beitrag zu einem Werkverzeichnis."

[E0645] Krause, Ralph. "La recezione dell stile 'alla Palestrina' nella scuola napoletana del Settecento."

[E0646] Kurtzman, Jeffrey. "Palestrina's Magnificats."

[E0647] Lamla, Michael. "Osservazioni sulle Messe canoniche di J. Desprez, del Palestrina e del Francesco Suriano."

[E0648] Lindell, Robert. "The Search for the Imperial Chapelmaster (1567–1568). Why Palestrina Was Not the First Choice."

[E0649] Luciani, Luciano. "Palestrina nella biblioteca e nelle miscellanee di G. B. Martini."

[E0650] Meloncelli, Raoul. "La tradizione palestriniana nella scula polifonica romana dell'ultimo Ottocento."

[E0651] Miller, Stephen. "Palestrina and the Seventeenth-Century Mass at Rome: Re-Use, Reference and Synthesis."

[E0652] Mischiati, Oscar. "Testimonianze palestriniane nel 'Mystagogus' del Cresollio."

[E0653] Monson, Craig. "Another Look at Musical Reform at the Council of Trent."

[E0654] Nugent, George. “Jaquet, Palestrina and Strategies of Patronage: Some Reflections.”

[E0655] O’Regan, Noel. “Palestrina’s Polychoral Works: A Forgotten Repertory.”

———. Owens, Jessie Ann. “Palestrina as Reader: Motets from the Song of Songs.” See item E0304.

[E0656] Pachowsky, Angela. “La prassi esecutiva dei mottetti del Palestrina nel periodo ottocentesco della Cappella Pontificia: testimonianze dai Diari sistini.”

[E0657] Pozzi, Egidio. “Il problema della grande forma nelle Messe-parodia del Palestrina (primi due libri).”

[E0658] Pugliese, Annunziato. “Dizionario dei musicisti attivi nella corte di Ippolito II d’ Este.”

[E0659] Rice, John A. “Palestrina’s St. Cecilia Motets and the Missa ‘Cantantibus Organis.’”

[E0660] Rosato, Paolo. “Un contribuito semiotico allo studio delle relazioni tra testo e musica in Palestrina. Analisi del Mottetto ‘Beatus Laurentius’ (1563) e del Madrigale ‘La cruda mia nemica’ (1586).”

[E0661] Rostirolla, Giancarlo. “Note in margine al Codice 59 autografo del Palestrina.”

[E0662] Sawkins, Lionel. “Some Eighteenth-Century Perspectives of Palestrina.”

[E0663] Schloetterer, Reinhold. “Contemporaneità: il Palestrina e O. di Lasso.”

———. Sherr, Richard. “Competence and Incompetence in the Papal Chapel in the Age of Palestrina.” See item E0054.

[E0664] Simi Bonini, Eleonora. “Il Mottetto ‘Dum complerentur’ studiato da Girolamo Chiti.”

[E0665] Skulj, Edo. “Presenza di Palestrina in Slovenia all’ inizio del Seicento.”

[E0666] Soldati, Stefania. “ ‘Nessun vissi giammai’: Palestrina, Lasso. Marenzio.”

[E0667] Summers, William John. “Music Confraternal Life in Rome, 1584–1680: Some Observations on the Careers of Palestrina and the Roman School as Members of the Compagnia dei Musici di Roma.”

[E0668] Talamo Emilia, Anna. “Le immagini nei codici della Cappella Sistina contenenti musiche del Palestrina.”

[E0669] Toffetti, Marina. “Alcune considerazioni sulla ricezione palestriniana a Milano fra ‘500 e ‘600.”

[E0670] Uvietta, Marco. " 'Das Hohelied Salomonis' di L. Lechner e il 'Cantico dei Cantici' del Palestrina: un confronto sul pianto della retorica musicale."

[E0671] Vanhulst, Henri. "La diffusion de la musique de Palestrina dans les anciens Pays-Bas au XVIIe siècle."

[E0672] Wyn Jones, David. "The 'a cappella' Masses of the Viennese Classic School: Palestrina Honoured and Transformed."

[E0673] Zakrzewska-Nikiporczyk, Barbara. "Performances and Editions of Palestrina's Music in Poznan and Great Duchy of Poznan in the Years 1870–1918."

[E0674] *La fortuna di Palestrina in Europa fino al XIX secolo. Società Italiana di Musicologia*, ed. Rodobaldo Tibaldi. A collection of eleven papers, listed as items E0675–E0683 and cross-listed materials.

[E0675] Fabris, Dinko. "Il primo trascrittore di Palestrina in Francia nell' Ottocento: André Eler (1764–ca.1821)."

[E0676] Ferrandis, Antonio Andrés. "Presencia y pervivencia de la obra de Palestrina en una iglesia de cultos reformados: La Capilla del real Colegio-Seminario de Corpus Christi de Valencia (España)."

[E0677] Gargiulo, Piero. "Da Banchieri a Berardi: la ricezione di Palestrina nei trattati di scuola bolognese (1609–1693)."

[E0678] Giacomelli, Gabriele. "Palestrina nel repertorio musicale della cattedrale di Firenze (1638–1677)."

[E0679] Gmeinwieser, Siegfried. "Palestrina und Palestrinastil in Bayern."

———. Haar, James. "Palestrina 'historicus': le due messe '*L'homme armé*.'" Apparently an Italian version of E0239.

———. Miller, Stephen R. "Palestrina and the Seventeenth-Century Mass at Rome: Re-Use, Reference and Synthesis." See item E0651.

[E0680] O'Regan, Noel. "The Transmission of Palestrina's Triple-Choir Music: Michael Haller's Nineteenth-Century Reconstruction in the Light of Some Recently Re-Discovered Originals."

[E0681] Tibaldi, Rodobaldo. "'Alla Palestrina': una Messa di Giacomo Gozzini autografa di Giovanni Simone Mayr."

[E0682] Vacchelli Monterosso, Anna Maria. "Palestrina nei trattori teorici del primo Seicento."

[E0683] Zórawska-Witkowska, Alina. "Il Palestrina e la Polonia."

Rostirolla has also announced an eight-volume project to be entitled *Storia della Cappella Musicale Pontificia*, to be produced by the Fondazione Giovanni Pierluigi da Palestrina with the support of the Banca di Credito Cooperativo di Palestrina. Volumes of note are to include the following.

[E0684] Sherr, Richard. *Il Cinquecento: da Giulio II a Sisto V.*

[E0685] Lionnet, Jean. *Il Seicento.*

[E0686] Luisi, Francesco with Maria Adelaide Morabito Iannucci, Federico Pirani, and Giancarlo Rostirolla. *Il Settecento.*

[E0687] Kantner, Leopold M. and Angela Pachovsky. *L'Ottocento.*

[E0688] De Salvo, Salvatore. *Il Novecento.*

[E0689] Nielsen, Kirin. "The Spiritual Madrigals of Giovanni Pierluigi da Palestrina." Ph.D. dissertation, University of Illinois, Champaign-Urbana, 1998.

[E0688] Owens, Jessie Ann. "Palestrina at Work." In *Papal Music and Musicians in Late Medieval and Renaissance Rome*. ed. Richard Sherr. Oxford: Clarendon, 1998. 339pp. ISBN 0-19-816417-3. ML3033.8.R763.P2. pp. 270–300.

Chapter 7

Discography

Literature and Sources Consulted

Clough, Francis F., and G.J. Cuming, eds. *The World's Encyclopedia of Recorded Music.* London: Sidgwick & Jackson Ltd, 1952.
First Supplement April 1950–May-June 1951. London: Sidgwick & Jackson Ltd, 1952.
Second Supplement 1951–1952. London: Sidgwick & Jackson Ltd, 1953.
Third Supplement 1953–1955. London: Sidgwick & Jackson Ltd, 1957.
A major guide to recordings through 1955.

Coover, James. *Medieval and Renaissance Music on Long-Playing Records.* Detroit: Information Service, 1964. 122pp. ML156.2.C67.
A guide to recordings from the early LP era.

Croucher, Trevor. *Early Music Discography. From Plainsong to the Sons of Bach. Vol.1: Record Index. Vol. 2: Composer, Plainsong, Anonymous Work and Performer Index.* London: Library Associated Publishing, 1981. ML156.2.C76.

Darrell, R. D., with Lawrence Gilman. *The Gramophone Shop Encyclopedia of Recorded Music.* New York: The Gramophone Shop, Inc., 1936. Revisions: 2nd ed., New York: Simon and Schuster, 1942; 3rd ed. revised and enlarged, New York: Crown Publishers, 1948.
Major source for identification of 78 rpm LPs.

Gautier, Jean-François. *Palestrina, ou l'esthétique de l'âme du monde.* Actes Sud, 1994.
Discography. pp. 111–119. Recent short discography which annotates most of the items listed and offers a few review-style comments on various recordings.

Modugno, Maurizio. "Discografia di Giovanni Pierluigi da Palestrina." *Atti del II convegno internazionale di studi palestriniani*, ed. Lino Bianchi and Giancarlo Rostirolla. Palestrina: Fondazione Giovanni Pierluigi da Palestrina/Centro di Studi Palestriniani, 1991. pp. 589–607.
Offers useful overview of the history of recording Palestrina's music in this century. Notes the difficulty in dating many of these recordings, the more regrettable given the peculiar performance practice history of Palestrina's oeuvre. Does not indicate original recording technology (acoustic, electrical) or recorded medium.

Roche, Elizabeth. "Early Music on Records in the Last Twenty-Five Years." *Musical Times* 120 (1979): 34–36, 215–217.
Discusses improved presence of music before 1800 on recordings.

Numerous monthly or annual issues of the *Schwann*, *Gramophone*, and *Bielefelder* recording catalogs were also consulted, as well as various library catalogs. Discs were personally examined whenever possible.

Citation Format Used in this Discography

Recording company and number. Medium. Title of recording where indicated ["//" if title is equivalent to the name of the recorded work(s) or is otherwise not evident or ascertained]. Performer(s). Director or conductor. Date of recording [place]. Note regarding program notes, translations of texts, special information or comments. [Reissue or alternative issue information when available.]

Works by Palestrina on recording [timings when available].

Tracing the history of a recording through reissues over time, through subsidiaries, in various countries is a very difficult and time-consuming task. The citation in bold refers to the issue that has been verified, to which the author had access, or which would be the most immediately accessible to a user of this discography. Alternative citations for a performance (which can be reissues of a recording at a different time, in different countries, through different companies, or in different formats) are indicated when they can be established. These have been transcribed as they occur on the recording or in catalogs, without attempting to organize them chronologically or otherwise regularize them.

In the case of anthologies, only selections by Palestrina are listed. A rationale for the few exceptions to this procedure will be evident. Usually it is because the recording contains a model for an imitation mass if the composer of the model was other than Palestrina, or uses relevant plainchant material. To assist teachers and students of style, I have noted such items.

Works that were unavailable to me for examination and that have only limited references in catalogs and other sources, are listed in an appendix, beginning page 435. It is understood that such citations are incomplete and contain unverified and possibly inaccurate information, or are recordings which are indicated as containing Palestrina's music but the titles of the works included are not known.

F0001 Abbey APR 306. LP. *The Choirs of Bradford Cathedral.* Choirs of Bradford Cathedral. Early 1970s.

Contains motet *Haec dies quam fecit Dominus a 6.*

F0002 Abbey CACA542. Cassette. *Music for Worship. A Year at Southwark Cathedral.* Southwark Cathedral Choir. John Scott, H. Bramma. ca. 1985.

Contains motet *Dum complerentur a 6.*

F0003 Abbey LPB 663. LP. *Liverpool Cathedral Choir.* Liverpool Cathedral Choir. 1970.

Contains offertory motet *Recordare mei a 5.*

F0004 Abbey LPB 686. LP. *In Quires and Places, 2.* Leeds Parish Choir. Donald Hunt. 1970. Notes by Donald Hunt; Latin texts with English translations.

Contains motet *Tu es Petrus a 6.*

F0005 Abbey LPB 750. LP. *In Quires and Places, 15.* Choir of the Priory Church of St. Bartholomew the Great, Smithfield, London. Andrew Morris. 1975. Notes by Andrew Morris and N. E. Wallbank.
Contains motet *O beata et gloriosa Trinitas a 5.*

F0006 Abbey LPB 772. LP. *Three Cathedral Choirs.* Cathedral Choirs of Gloucester, Hereford and Worcester. Roy Massey. 1978.
Contains motet *Exultate Deo a 5.*

F0007 Abbey LPB 783. LP. *Gloucester Cathedral Choir.* Gloucester Cathedral Choir. 1977.
Contains motet *Dum complerentur dies Pentecostes a 6.*

F0008 Abbey LPB 789. LP. *Paisley Abbey Choir.* Paisley Abbey Choir. George McPhee. 1978.
Contains motet *Dum complerentur dies Pentecostes a 6.*

F0009 Abbey LPB 804. LP. *Music for Holy Week and Easter.* Choir of the London Oratory. John Hoban. 1979. Program notes by Patrick Russell.
Contains motets *Sicut cervus a 4*; *Haec dies quam fecit Dominus a 6.*

F0010 Acanta DC 21303. LP. *Gallus. Mass and Motets of the Masters.* Vienna Boy's Choir, Chorus Viennensis. Hans Gillesberger. ca. 1971. Program notes by Gerhard Schuhmacher in German and English [reissued as Acanta DC 41303 on CD in 1988; also listed as RCA RL 30379, on LP in 1979, and BASF BB 21302/3 on LP ca. 1972].
Contains motet *Hodie Christus natus est a 8.*

F0011 Acanta DC 21 841. LP. *Coro della Cappella Sistina/The Choir of the Sistine Chapel.* Sistine Chapel Choir. Domenico Bartolucci. 1979 [also listed as RCA 40 21 841 AW, and on cassette DF 31 841].
Contains motets *Cantabo Domino a 6*; *Vox dilecti mei a 5*; *Improperium exspectavit a 5*; *Paucitas dierum a 5*; *Vulnerasti cor meum a 5.*

F0012 Accent ACC 8861. CD. *Music of the Italian Pifari. North Italian Music for Cornetts and Trombones.* Concerto Palatino. 1989 (rec. April 1989, Beginjnhofkerk, Sing-Truiden, Belgium). Program notes in English, French, German.
Contains motets *Tota pulchra es amica mea* [arr. Bassano]; *Benedicta sit* [arr. Bassano].

F0013 Accent ACC 9173. CD. *"Qual lascivissimo cornetto. . ."/Virtuoso solo music for cornetto.* Bruce Dickey [cornett], Tragicomedia. 1991 (rec. Jan and Apr 1991). Case contains booklet (20pp) with notes by Bruce Dickey in English, French, German; also list of primary sources for works performed.
Contains motet *Pulchra es amica mea* [diminutions by Francesco Rognoni Taeggio] [4:27]; madrigal *Io son ferito* [diminutions by Giovanni Bovicelli] [6:13].

F0014 Accent ACC 96115D. CD. *Works for Organ. Giovanni de Macque. Giovanni*

Pierluigi da Palestrina. Liuwe Tamminga [organ]. 1996 (rec. San Petronio, Bologna, May 1996).
Contains *Ricercari primi toni–ottavi toni* (nos.1 through 8, complete).

F0015 Ace of Diamonds ADD 196 [SDD 196]. LP. *Choral Tapestry, volume 2.* Ambrosian Singers. John E. McCarthy. ca. 1968–1969 [also listed as Avant Garde AVS 129].
Contains motet *Verbum caro.*

F0016 Accord ACC 140031. LP. *Canticum canticorum. Motets à Cinque Voix.* Società Cameristica di Lugano. Edwin Loehrer. 1980.
Contains motets from *Canticum canticorum* (selections); *Adoramus te Christe a 4*; hymn *Vexilla regis.* Additional music [by Marc'Antonio Ingegneri, formerly ascribed to Palestrina]: *Quinque salutationes in Passione Domini.*

F0017 Accord ACD 201562. CD. *Thirteenth and Sixteenth Century Music.* Lugano Chamber Society Instrumental Ensemble, Lugano Chamber Society Choir (soloists L. Ticinelli-Fattori [sop], M. Minetto [mezzo], L. Malaguti [bar], J. Loomis [bass]). Edwin Lohrer. 1980.
Contains motets *Adoramus te a 4*; *Stabat Mater a 8*; hymns *Vexilla regis prodeunt a 4*; *Vexilla regis a 5*; *Vexilla regis (paschali).*

F0018 Accord 202162. CD. *Musiques pour Saint Michel.* Ensemble Sagittarius, Ensemble La Fenice. Michel Laplénie. 1992. Program notes (5pp) by Alain de Chambure.
Contains mass *Missa secunda* (1582); motet *Venit Michael archangelus a 5*; *Venite exultemus a 5*; hymn *Tibi Christe splendor Patris*; magnificat *Magnificat primi toni.*

F0019 Accord 202462. CD. *Musiques pour Saint Laurent.* Ensemble Sagittarius. Michel Laplénie. 1993 (rec. June and Sept. 1992, Abbaye de Saint-Michel in Thiérache). Program notes (6pp) by Alain de Chambure, ca. 1993.
Contains mass *Missa Beatus Laurentius a 5*; motets *Beatus Laurentius a 5*; *Confessio et pulchritudo a 5*; hymn *Deus tuorum militum*; magnificats *Magnificat octavi toni a 4; Magnificat a 4.*

F0020 Accord 203572. CD. *Palestrina. Musique pour la Vierge Marie. Music for the Virgin Mary.* Ensemble Sagittarius, Ensemble La Fenice. Michel Laplénie. 1995 (rec. June and Sept. 1992, Abbaye de Saint Michel in Thiérache).
Contains mass *Missa Salve Regina a 5*; motets *Assumpta est Maria a 6*; *Salve Regina a 5*; litany *Litaniae de BVM a 4*; hymn *Ave maris stella a 4*; magnificat *Magnificat primi toni a 4.*

F0021 Accord 203662. CD. *Musiques pour Saint Jean.* Ensemble Sagittarius, Maîtrise de Paris. Michel Laplénie. 1994 (rec. June and Sept. 1992, Abbaye de Saint Michel in Thiérache).
Contains mass *Missa Ecce ego Johannes a 5*; motets *Hic est discipulus ille a 5*; *Valde honorandus est a 5*; *Justus ut palma a 5*; *Haec dies a 6*; hymn *Exsultet coelum laudibus*; magnificat *Magnificat* [unspec]; ricercar *Ricercare sexti toni* [organ].

F0022 Alba NCD 8. CD. *Mary in the Land of Snow and Light.* Lumen Valo. Titta Lampela. 1996.
Contains motet *Stabat Mater a 8.*

F0023 Allegro AL 70. 10-inch LP (2). *Missa Ascendo ad Patrem. Missa Brevis.* Welch Chorale. James B. Welch. ca. 1950–1951. Program notes on sleeve [reissued on 12-inch LP as Allegro Elite 3097].
Contains masses *Missa Ascendo ad patrem a 5;Missa Brevis a 4.*

F0024 Allegro ALG 3016. LP. *Masses "Iste Confessor" and "Sine Nomine."* Welch Chorale. James B. Welch. 1952 [also issued as Allegro ALX 3016].
Contains masses *Missa Iste confessor a 4***;** *Missa Sine nomine* ["*Je suis désheritée*"].

F0025 Allegro ALG 3029. LP. *Italian Madrigal—Ars Nova and XVIth Century.* Vassar Madrigal Singers. Geer. ca. 1951–1952.
Contains madrigals *Da così dotta man a 3*; *Ahi che quest'occhi miei a 3.*

F0026 Allegro ALG PCD 863. CD *Missa Papae Marcelli. Stabat Mater.* Pro Cantione Antiqua. Mark Brown. 1987 (rec. January 31 to February 1, 1987, St. Alban's Church, Brooke Street, London). Program notes in English in container [also listed as PCD 863 IMP/Allegro, PK 515 IMP/Allegro].
Contains mass *Missa Papae Marcelli a 6*; motet *Stabat mater a 8.*

F0027 Allegro ALG PCD 952. CD. Masses "L'Homme Armé" and "Assumpta est Maria." Pro Cantione Antiqua of London. Mark Brown. 1990.
Contains masses *Missa Assumpta est Maria a 6*; *Missa L'homme armé a 5*; motets for Epiphany and the Assumption.

F0028 Allegro ALG PCD 973. CD. *Lamentations of Jeremiah the Prophet*. Pro Cantione Antiqua of London. Bruno Turner. ca. 1992.
Contains Lamentations *Feria V in coena Domini*; *Feria VI in Parasceve*; *Sabbato Sancto.*

F0029 Allegro ALG PCD 1076. CD. *Missa Brevis. Missa "Lauda Sion." Motets.* Pro Cantione Antiqua. Mark Brown. 1994.
Contains masses *Missa Brevis a 4* [27:00]; *Missa Lauda Sion a 4* [28:00]; motets *Super flumina Babylonis a 4* [3:52]; *Sicut cervus a 4* [secunda pars *Sitivit anima mea*] [5:52].

F0030 Allegro IMP PCD 1111. CD. *Missa Aeterna Christi munera. Missa L'homme armé.* Pro Cantione Antiqua. Mark Brown. 1992 (November 1–3), St. Jude's Church, Hampstead Garden Suburb.
Contains masses *Missa Aeterna Christi munera a 4*; *Missa L'homme armé.* Additional music, plainchant hymn *Aeterna Christi munera.*

F0031 Alpha APS 347. LP. *Music from Gibraltar.* Choir of the Cathedral of St. Mary the Crowned. Michael Davis, Steven Landrell. n.d.
Contains motet *O bone Jesu a 4.*

F0032 Alpha APS 349. LP. *The Choir of the Metropolitan Cathedral of St. David, Cardiff.* Metropolitan Cathedral Choir, Cardiff. David Neville. 1983.
Contains mass *Missa Aeterna Christi munera a 4* [*Kyrie* and *Agnus Dei* only].

F0033 Alpha DB 252. LP. *Motetti.* Collegium Vocale, Ghent. Phillippe Herreweghe. 1979. Program notes by Jerome Lejeune.
Contains motet *Sicut cervus a 4.*

F0034 Alpha DB 254. LP. *Luxembourg Madrigal Choir.* Luxembourg Madrigal Choir (Ton Koopman [organ]). Daniel Schertzer. Before 1981.
Contains madrigal *Ogni beltà, madonna a 4.*

F0035 Alpha LPA 0028. LP. *New College Choir.* New College Choir. 1963 [also issued as Alpha avme 008, 7-inch LP, withdrawn before 1965].
Contains motet *Confitemini Domino a 4.*

F0036 American Recording Artists ARA 2001. 12-inch 78 rpm. *Vatican Choir.* Sistine Chapel Choir. Lorenzo Perosi. Date not listed [also issued in ARA set AA 1].
Motet: *Confitebor tibi Domine a 8* [II, 1572]; *Super flumina Babylonis a 4* [V, 1581]

F0037 Analekta FL 23013. CD. *Italian Instrumental Music from the Renaissance.* De Serres [dulm], Michaud [rec], Soly [org], Trudel [sackb]. 1990s.
Contains madrigal *Vestiva i colli a 5* [with diminutions by Bartolomeo da Selma].

F0038 Analekta FL 23120. CD. *Palestrina: Missa Ut re mi fa sol la and other sacred works.* Le Choeur de Studio de Musique Ancienne de Montréal. Christopher Jackson. 1997 (rec. June 1997, Chappelle du Grand Séminaire, Montréal). Booklet (14pp) contains program notes by Marcel de Hêtre and François Filiatrault and Latin texts with English and French translations.
Contains mass *Missa Ut re me fa sol la* (*Kyrie* [4:17]; *Gloria* [3:49]; *Credo* [6:46]; *Sanctus* [5:01]; *Benedictus* [3:31]; *Agnus Dei I* [3:27]; *Agnus Dei II* [3:06]); motets *Omnes pulchritudo a 8* (attributed to Victoria on this recording) [5:25]; *Ecce, nunc benedicite Dominum a 12* [2:40].

F0039 Angel 36013. LP. *Echoes from a Sixteenth-Century Cathedral.* Roger Wagner Chorale. Roger Wagner. 1967 [orig. issue ca. 1960] [also issued as Capitol SP8460].
Contains mass *Missa Brevis a 4* [*Agnus Dei*]; motet *Alma redemptoris Mater a 8.*

F0040 Angel S-36022. LP. *Palestrina: Pope Marcellus Mass. Victoria: Three Motets.* Roger Wagner Chorale. Roger Wagner. 1969. [Reissued on CD as *Pope Marcellus Mass with Fauré Requiem.*] Anonymous program notes included.
Contains mass *Missa Papae Marcelli a 6.*

F0041 Angel S-37512. LP. *Palestrina. Missa Hodie Christus natus est & six motets.* Choir of King's College, Cambridge. Philip Ledger. 1978. Sleeve notes by Iain Fenlon; English translations of texts in liner [also listed as EMI ASD 3559; EMI 2C 069-03272; EMI 1C 065–03272].

Contains mass *Missa Hodie Christus natus est a 8* [27:11]; motets *Hodie Christus natus est* [2:42]; *Canite tuba* [6:10]; *Ave Maria* [4:16]; *Tui sunt caeli* [2:37]; *Jubilate Deo* [3:35]; *O magnum mysterium* [6:25].

F0042 L'Anthologie Sonore AS 47. 12-inch 78 rpm. *L'Anthologie Sonore.* "Motet and Madrigal" Group. Heinrich Opienski. ca. 1937 [this disc is vol. 5 in series issue, dated ca.1935; reissued on LP as Haydn Society AS 9 (vol. 2, set AS-B), ca. 1953–1955].

Contains motet *Vulnerasti cor meum a 5*; hymn *Vexilla regis . . . o crux ave*; madrigals *Alla riva del Tebro a 4*;*La cruda mia nemica a 4.*

F0043 Archiv ARC 3074. LP. *IV. Research Period: The High Renaissance (16th Century). Series F: Palestrina and His School. Giovanni Pierluigi da Palestrina: Missa Papae Marcelli. Stabat Mater. Improperia.* Aachener Domsingknaben, Aachener Domchor. Theodor B. Rehmann. 1955–1956. Contains two leaflets with historical notes, notes on sleeve by Karl Gustav Fellerer, recording information, and Latin texts with English translations [also issued as Archiv AP 13032; APM 14526].

Contains mass *Missa Papae Marcelli a 6* [27:23]; motet *Stabat Mater a 8* [7:30]; Improperia *Ecce lignum crucis* [2:45]; *Popule meus* [2:45]; *Quid ultra debui* [2:56]; *Ego te exaltavi* [1:06]; *Crucem tuam* [2:00]; *O crux ave* [1:10] [12:42 total].

F0044 Archiv ARC 3182. LP. *IV. Research Period: The High Renaissance (16th Century). Series F: Palestrina and His School. Giovanni Pierluigi da Palestrina: Missa Papae Marcelli. Eight Motets.* Regensburger Domspatzenchor. Theobald Schrems. 1961. Contains liner notes by Karl Gustav Fellerer, as well as Latin texts with English translations [also issued as ARC 73182; ARC 198 182, DG 410 596–1].

Contains mass *Missa Papae Marcelli a 6* [3:24; 4:38; 7:33; 3:19; 2:53; 4:48] [26:35 total]; motets *Laudate Dominum a 5* [2:42]; *Terra tremuit a 5* [2:13]; *Ascendit Deus a 5* [2:03]; *Illumina oculos meos a 5* [2:57]; *Ego sum panis vivus a 5* [3:02]; *Pueri Hebraeorum a 4* [1:44]; *Jubilate Deo a 5* [3:54]; lamentation *Incipit oratorio Jeremiae* [7:45].

F0045 Archiv ARC 3241. LP. *IV. Research Period: The High Renaissance (16th Century). Series F: Palestrina and His School. Giovanni Pierluigi da Palestrina: Missa Tu es Petrus. Missa Assumpta est Maria.* Regensburger Domchor. Hans Schrems. 1965 (rec. July 3–8, 1965, St. Emmeran's, Regensburg. Contains program notes by Karl Gustav Fellerer; Latin texts with English translations inserted into sleeve [also issued as ARC 73241; ARC 198 341].

Contains masses *Missa Tu es Petrus a 6* [25:00]; *Missa Assumpta est Maria a 6* [24:20].

F0046 Archiv ARC 3243. LP. *IV. Research Period: The High Renaissance (16th Century). Series F: Palestrina and His School. Giovanni Pierluigi da Palestrina. Missa Hodie Christus natus est. Improperia.* Regensburger Domchor. Hans Schrems. 1964. Liner notes provide texts with English translation, recording information. Notes indicate that primary sources for the *Improperia* were the MSS I-Rvat CS 205 and 206, probably composed ca. 1555 to 1560 [reissued as Archiv 198 343].

Contains mass *Missa Hodie Christus natus est a 8* [3:21; 4:57; 7:29; 4:10 (*Sanctus*); 2:20 (*Benedictus*); 5:12]; improperia *Ecce lignum crucis etc. a 8* [23:45, Hab.xxxi.175–80].

F0047 Archiv 3283. LP. *IV. Research Period: The High Renaissance (16the Century). Series F: Palestrina and His School. Giovanni Pierluigi da Palestrina. Missa Dum Complerentur. Motets*. Regensburger Domspatzenchor. Hans Schrems. 1966 (rec. July 2–7, 1966, St. Emmeran's, Regensburg) [also issued as ARC 73283; ARC 198 383].

Contains mass *Missa Dum complerentur a 6*; motets *Tu es Petrus a 6*; *Assumpta est Maria a 6*; *Ave Regina coelorum a 8*; *Hodie Christus natus est a 8*; *Dum complerentur a 6*.

F0048 Archiv 198 434. LP. *IV. Research Period: The High Renaissance (16th Century). Series F: Palestrina and His School. Madrigali e ricercari.* Regensburger Domspatzenchor. Hans Schrems; Musica Antiqua. Rene Clemencic. 1967. Based on Haberl edition, vol. 28.

Contains madrigals [in vocal versions] *Il tempo vola a 5; Se fra quest'erb'e fiore; Ahi che quest'occhi miei a 3; Vestiva i colli a 5*; *Il dolce sonno a 5; Da così dotta man sei a 3; Io son ferito a 5*; also madrigals [in instrumental arrangements] *Da così dotta man*; *Vestiva i colli*; *Ahi che quest'occhi miei*; *Io son ferito*; *Il dolce sonno*; *Se fra quest'erb'e fiore*; ricercari *Ricercare quarti toni*; *Ricercare sexti toni*; *Ricercare octavi toni.*

F0049 Archiv 2533 322. LP. *Missa Aeterna Christi munera.* Pro Cantione Antiqua London. Bruno Turner. 1976 (rec. July 8–9, 1974, All Saints, Petersham). Program notes in German, English, French, Italian by M. H. Schmid [also issued as cassette 3310 322. Motets and Lamentation material reissued as Archiv 2723 070; also on ARC 437072–2 on LP and in Collectio Argentea on CD; also on CD as ARC 445 667–2, *Geistliche Musik der Renaissance*].

Contains mass *Missa Aeterna Christi munera a 4*; motets *O bone Jesu a 4*; *Sicut cervus a 4*; *Super flumina Babylonis a 4*; lamentation *Incipit oratio Jeremiae.*

F0050 Archiv 415 517-1. LP. *Missa Papae Marcelli. Tu es Petrus.* Choir of Westminster Abbey. Simon Preston. 1985 (rec. Feb 1985, All Saint's Church, Tooting, London). Program notes by Jean-Pierre Ouvrard in French, English, German, and Italian; Latin texts with translations in English, French, German [reissued on CD as ARC 415 517–2].

Contains mass *Missa Papae Marcelli a 6* [32:00]; motet *Tu es Petrus a 6* [6:34].

F0051 Archiv 437 833-2 AH. CD. *Missa Hodie Christus natus est*. Gabrieli Consort and Players. Paul McCreesh. 1993 (rec. Santa Maria Maggiore, Rome, Dec. 1992, and All Saints' Church, Tooting, London, Feb. 1993). Notes indicate that this recording is a liturgical re-creation of the third mass for Christmas Day as it might have been celebrated at Santa Maria Maggiore around 1620, including appropriate

Roman plainchant to link the polyphonic items. Program notes by Graham Dixon and Paul McCreesh. Contains list of sources and texs with English translations.

Contains mass *Missa Hodie Christus natus est a 8* (*Kyrie* [2:41]; *Gloria* [3:57]; *Credo* [6:05]; *Sanctus* [5:22]; *Agnus Dei* [3:02]); motet *Hodie Christus natus est a 8* [1:47].

F0052 Archiv 439 961-2. LP (2). *Palestrina. Masses and Motets.* Regensburger Domchor, Hans Schrems; Theobald Schrems; Pro Cantione Antiqua, Bruno Turner; Westminster Abbey Choir, Simon Preston. Notes by Jessie Ann Owens [reissued on 2 CDs in 1994 as Archiv 439962–2, 439963–2].

Contains masses *Missa Dum complerentur a 6*; *Missa Tu es Petrus a 6*; *Missa Papae Marcelli a 6*; motets *Dum complerentur a 6*; *Tu es Petrus a 6*; *Illumina oculos meos a 5*; *Jubilate Deo a 5*; *Laudate Dominum omnes gentes a 8; Pueri Hebraeorum a 4*; lamentations *Incipit oratio Jeremiae prophetiae.*

F0053 Archiv 445 667-2 (445 668-2-445 674-2). CD (7). *Geistliche Musik der Renaissance/The Flowering of Renaissance Choral Music.* Pro Cantione Antiqua of London, Hamburger Bläserkreis für alte Musik, London Cornett and Sackbut Ensemble, Early Music Consort of London. Bruno Turner. 1995. Program notes by Ludwig Finscher in German, English, and French [reissue of recordings on various Archiv discs 1973 to 1978. Palestrina selections on CD 6 (ARC 445 673 2)].

Contains motets *Sicut cervus a 4; Super flumina Babylonis a 4; O bone Jesu a 6*; lamentation *Incipit oratio Jeremiae [a 4–8].*

F0054 Argo CD 410 005-2ZH. CD. *Allegri: Miserere. Victoria, Palestrina, Monteverdi.* Choir of Westminster Cathedral. Stephen Cleobury. 1983. Notes by John Whenham; contains Latin texts with English translations [also issued on LP as Decca 410 005–2 ZK; as Argo XRDL 1013; also on cassette KZDC 1013 or ZRDL 1013 AZ].

Contains motets *Exsultate Deo a 5*; *Peccantem me quotidie a 5*; *Tu es Petrus a 6.*

F0055 Argo MCPS 410 149-2. CD. *Palestrina: Mass & Motet "Tu es Petrus." Victoria. Mass & Motet "O Quam Gloriosum."* Choir of King's College, Cambridge. Stephen Cleobury. 1984 (rec. March 1983). Booklet (7pp) contains notes by John Whenham in English, French, German; Latin texts with English translations [originally issued on LP as Argo 410 149-1ZH in 1984; also on cassette Argo 410 149-4ZH; also issued on CD as London 433 914–2].

Contains mass *Missa Tu es Petrus a 6* [4:36 (*Kyrie*); 5:05 (*Gloria*); 8:34 (*Credo*); 2:38 (*Sanctus*); 3:08 (*Benedictus*); 2:37 (*Agnus Dei I*); 2:41 (*Agnus Dei II*); motet *Tu es Petrus a 6* [3:50]

F0056 Argo RG 186. LP. *Missa Aeterna Christi Munera.* The Renaissance Singers. Michael Howard. 1959 (rec. 1959, Church of St. Philip Neri, Arundel). Recording contains hymn *Aeterna Christi munera* (Amen to Plainsong II), antiphon *Vos qui reliquistis* with Benedictus sung to Plainsong II, with organ versets by Jean Titelouze [also listed as ZRG 5186].

Contains mass *Missa Aeterna Christi munera a 4.*

F0057 Argo ZK 4. LP. *Palestrina. Stabat Mater. [Additional motets]* Choir of King's College, Cambridge. David Willcocks. 1964. Liner notes by Robin Golding [also issued as Argo ZRG 5398].

Contains motets *Senex puerum portabat a 5*; *Hodie beata virgo a 5*; *Stabat Mater a 8*; magnificat *Magnificat primi toni a 8*; litany *Litaniae de Beata Virgine Maria a 8* [first of two 8-part settings for double choir].

F0058 Argo ZK 69. LP. *Palestrina/Veni Sponsa Christi.* Choir of St. John's College, Cambridge. George Guest. 1968 [also issued as Argo ZRG 578].

Contains mass *Missa Veni sponsa Christi a 4* [24.00]; motets *Veni sponsa Christi a 4* [3.05]; *Exsultate Deo a 5* [2.25]; hymns *In adventu Domini [Conditor alme siderum]* [6.45]; *Jesu rex admirabilis* [1.45]; magnificat *Magnificat sexti toni* [12.10]. Additional contents: plainchant antiphon *Veni sponsa Christi* [0.45].

F0059 Argo ZRG 690. LP. *Missa Assumpta est Maria*. Choir of St. John's College, Cambridge. George Guest. 1972. Notes by Alec Robertson.

Contains masses *Missa Assumpta est Maria a 6*; *Missa Brevis a 4*. Additional contents: plainchant antiphon *Assumpta est Maria*.

F0060 Ariola XA 28 152 K. LP. *Jubilate Deo.* Regensburger Domspatzen. Theobald Schrems. ca. 1959. Notes include Latin text with German translation; RCA Victor LM 2855 has texts with English translations on sleeve [also listed as Eurodisc 70 172 KK and S 70 173 KK in 1963; RCA Victor LM 2855 in 1965; Cetra KK 70 172 and SKK 70 173].

Contains motets *Dum complerentur a 6*; *Tu es Petrus a 6*; lamentation *Feria VI in Parasceve.*

F0061 Arion ARN 30 B 142. LP. *Messes des Paroisses avant Vatican II.* Ensemble Polyphonique de Montparnasse. Gaston Litaize. 1970s.

Contains mass *Missa Ad fugam* [*Kyrie* and *Gloria* only].

F0062 Arion ARN 68 274. CD. *Impropères du vendredi saint. Quatre Motets.* Concinité de Louvain Choir. Karel Aerts. 1994. Program notes (23pp) by Joël-Marie Fouquet and Karel Arts, English translation by Mary Pardoe. French and English texts and summaries included [previously listed as Arion 38423, LP issued 1978].

Contains motets *Ave regina coelorum* [6:21]; *Adoramus te Christe* [2:20]; *Pueri Hebraeorum* [3:16]; *Jesu Rex admirabilis* [3:14]; lamentation *Impropères du vendredi saint* [Improperia for Good Friday] [26:26].

F0063 Ars Musici AM 0946-2. CD. *Musik am Prager Hof Kaiser Rudolfs II.* Dialogo Musicale. Leo Meilink. 1992.

Contains madrigal *Vestiva i colli a 5* [3.55]. Additional contents: Philipp de Monte, mass *Missa sex vocum supra "Vestiva i colli"* [24.30].

F0064 Ars Nova VST 6003. LP. // Solisti del Gruppo Strumentale "V.L. Campi" di Piacenza. Giuseppe Zanaboni. Before 1981.

Contains ricercar *Ricercar del primo tuono a 4.*

F0065 Ars Nova VST 6007. LP. *8 Ricercari sopra li toni a quattro.* Complesso

Veneziano Strumenti Antichi. Pietro Verando. ca. 1968 [also listed VPC 1507].
Ricercar *Ricercari 1–8.*

F0066 Ars Nova VST 6043. LP. // I Madrigalisti di Genova. Leopoldo Gamberini. Before 1981.
Contains madrigal *Chiare, fresche e dolci acque a 4.*

F0067 Ars Nova VST 6095. LP. // I Madrigalisti di Genova. Leopoldo Gamberini. Before 1981.
Contains motets *Popule meus; Sicut cervus a 4.*

F0068 Ars Nova VST 6121. LP. // Budapest Madrigal Singers. Ferenc Szekeres. Before 1981.
Contains motet *Jesu rex admirabilis a 3.*

F0069 Ars Vivendi 2100203. CD. *La bella ninfa. Madrigale.* Hallenser Madrigalisten. 1990.
Contains madrigal *Vaghi fiori a 4* [2:02].

F0070 ASV Quicksilva QS 6086. CD. *Missa Papae Marcelli; Stabat Mater; 3 Motets. Palestrina.* Pro Cantione Antiqua. Bruno Turner. 1992. Program notes by Bruno Turner [orig. recorded 1978; previously issued on LPs from Nonesuch 71407 (1982); Musical Heritage Society 4608 (1980); also issued on Enigma K53560; Hispavox S90 109; ASV 2009].
Contains mass *Missa Papae Marcelli* [30:53]; motets *Peccantem me quotidie* [4:32]; *Dominus Jesus in qua nocte* [4:44]; *Alma Redemptoris Mater* [2:29]; *Stabat Mater* [9:27].

F0071 Bach Guild [Vanguard] BG 623. LP. *Italian Music of the Renaissance/Sacred and Secular.* Choir and Soloists of Polifonica Ambrosiana. Mons. Giuseppe Biella. 1962. Liner notes in Italian with English translation by E. Rella.
Contains mass *Missa Aeterna Christi munera a 4* [*Sanctus, Benedictus* only].

F0072 Bach Guild [Vanguard] BG 5059. LP. *Song of Songs.* Prague Madrigal Choir. Miroslav Venhoda. 1963 (rec. Baumgartner Hall, Vienna). Based on performance edition prepared by Venhoda from Haberl ed. vol. 4 [reissued as HM-9 SD ca.1972].
Contains motets from Book IV (1583) [21 of the 29 motets] [51:30 total].

F0073 BBC Artium CD 572. CD. *The Pontifical High Mass of St. Sylvester.* William Byrd Choir. Gavin Turner. 1985 (rec. December 31, 1984, Sistine Chapel, Rome). "A reconstruction of the Mass as it might have been conducted in the Sistine Chapel, Rome, in 1613." Plainchant from the Tridentine rite with Soriano's arrangement for double choir of Palestrina's *Missa Papae Marcelli.* "This performance was broadcast on BBC Radio 3 on 31 December 1984 as part of the series 'The Octave of the Nativity.' " Program notes (16pp) by Hugh Keyte, Jerome Roche, and Nick Sandon. Texts with English translations.
Contains mass *Missa Papae Marcelli a 8* [arranged by Soriano].

F0074 Bongiovanni GB 5544-2/5545-2. CD (2). *Giovanni Pierluigi da Palestrina. Messe mantovane vol. I.* Solisti della Cappella Musicale di San Petronio, Nova Schola Gregoriana. Sergio Vartolo. 1995. Liner notes (14pp) by Paola Besutti.

Contains masses *Missa in festis Apostolorum I a 5*; *Missa in festis Apostolorum II a 5*; *Missa in semiduplicibus majoribus I a 5*; *Missa in semiduplicibus majoribus II a 5*; *Missa Sine nomine a 5.*

F0075 Bongiovanni GB 5556-57-2. CD. *Giovanni Pierluigi da Palestrina. Messe mantovane vol. II.* Cappella Musicale di S. Petronio (soloists Renzo Bez [alto], Vincenzo di Donato [tenor], Furio Zanasi [tenor], Sergio Foresti [bass], Alessandro Carmignani [sgr], Michel van Goethem [sgr], Liuwe Tamminga [organ]). Sergio Vartolo. 1995, Verona Cathedral.

Contains masses *Missa De beata Virgine I*; *Missa De beata Virgine II*; *Missa De beata Virgine III.*

F0076 Bongiovanni GB 5558. CD. *Giovanni Pierluigi da Palestrina. Messe mantovane vol. III.* Cappella Musicale di S. Petronio (soloists, Liuwe Tamminga [organ]). Sergio Vartolo. 1996.

Contains masses *Missa In duplicibus minoribus I*; *Missa In duplicibus minoribus II.*

F0077 Brunswick 50125. 12-inch 78 rpm // Società Polifonica Romana/Roman Polyphonic Choir (Vatican Choirs). Raffaele Casimiri. ca.1928 [*Laudate Dominum* a probable reissue of Parlophone R20001; see item F0333].

Contains offertory motets *Exaltabo te, Domine*; *Laudate Dominum.*

F0078 Brunswick 50126. 12-inch 78 rpm // Società Polifonica Romana/Roman Polyphonic Choir (Vatican Choirs). Raffaele Casimiri. ca. 1928 [also listed as Brunswick A 5047].

Contains motet *Alleluia! Tulerunt Dominum a 5.*

F0079 Brunswick 50127. 12-inch 78 rpm // Società Polifonica Romana Romana/Roman Polyphonic Choir (Vatican Choirs). Raffaele Casimiri. ca. 1928.

Contains offertory motet *Improperium exspectavit a 5.*

F0080 Brunswick 50128. 12-inch 78 rpm // Società Polifonica Romana/Roman Polyphonic Choir (Vatican Choirs). Raffaele Casimiri. ca.1928 [also listed as Brunswick A 5046].

Contains mass *Missa Papae Marcelli a 6* [*Credo* only].

F0081 Brunswick Album X. 12-inch 78 rpm. *Selected Musical Gems by the Roman Polyphonic Society.* Società Polifonica Romana/Roman Polyphonic Choir (Vatican Choirs). Raffaele Casimiri. ca. 1928 [collected version of Brunswick 50125–50128].

F0082 Cambridge CRC 101. 10-inch LP. *Palestrina. Supplicationes. Victoria. Lassus. Byrd.* Harvard Glee Club. G. Wallace Woodworth. 1952 (rec. April 29, 1952 at Busch-Reisinger Musuem, Harvard University). Latin texts with English translation on record sleeve [also listed as TV 18377/8].

Contains motets *Confitemini Domino*; *Adoramus te, Christe* [attribution to Palestrina doubtful; probably by Anerio]; litany *Supplicationes ad Beatae Mariae Virginis* [Hab. XXVI, ii. No.1].

F0083 Cambridge CRS 202. LP. *Chansons and Motets*. Harvard Glee Club, Radcliffe Choral Society; Daniel Pinkham [organ]. G. Wallace Woodworth. ca. 1953–1955.
Contains mass *Missa O admirabile commercium* [*Benedictus* only].

F0084 Cambridge CRS 405. LP. *Sacred Polyphony.* Harvard Glee Club, Radcliffe Choral Society. G. Wallace Woodworth. 1958. Texts with English translation included.
Contans *Litaniae* [unspecified].

F0085 Camerata LPM 30 038. LP. // Hannover Solistenvereinigung. Garbers. Before 1981.
Contains *Missa Papae Marcelli a 6* [*Kyrie* only].

F0086 Camerata LPM 30 055. LP. *Italienische Chormusik.* Alsfelder Vokalensemble. Wolfgang Helbich. Before 1984.
Contains motet *Salve regina*; magnificat *Magnificat septimi toni.*

F0087 Capitol P 8126. LP. *Missa Papae Marcelli.* Roger Wagner Chorale. Roger Wagner. ca. 1950–1951 [also listed as Decca CTL 7010].
Contains mass *Missa Papae Marcelli a 6.*

F0088 Capitol P 8365. LP. *Roger Wagner Chorale*. Roger Wagner Chorale. Roger Wagner. 1957.
Contains motet *Tu es Petrus a 6* [arr. Roger Wagner].

F0089 Carisch BCA 7012. LP. *Antologia Sonora della Musica Italiana. Volume 4: Polifonia Sacra nel Rinascimento.* Coro Polifonico Romano. Gastone Tosato. ca. 1950. Liner notes in Italian and English by Luigi Colacicchi; sleeve lists primary musical sources for recorded works.
Contains mass *Missa Dies sanctificatus a 4* [*Benedictus* only]; motets *Dies sanctificatus a 4*; *Regina coeli a 4*; *O bone Jesu a 6*; improperia *Popule meus* [for 1573].

F0090 Carisch BCA 7013. LP. *Antologia Sonora della Musica Italiana. Volume 5: Polifonia Profana nel Rinascimento.* I Madrigalisti Milanesi. Renato Fait. ca. 1952. Liner notes in Italian and English by Riccardo Allorto. Italian texts of selections provided.
Contains madrigal *I vaghi fiori e l'amorose fronde a 4.*

F0091 Carus CAR 53 118. LP. *Palestrina. Bruckner: Motetten.* Limburger Domsingknaben. Mathias Breitschaft. ca. 1977 [also listed as FSM 53118].
Contains motets *Ad te levavi a 5*; *Dextera Domini a 5*; *Dum complerentur a 6*; *Hodie Christus natus est a 8*; *Laudate Dominum*; *Tu es Petrus a 6*; *Terra tremuit a 5*; lamentation *Lamentatio* [for Holy Saturday].

F0092 Carus CAR 63 107. LP. *Limburger Domsingknaben singen zur Weihnacht.* Limburger Domsingknaben. Mathias Breitschaft. Before 1984 [also listed as FSM 63107].

Contains motet *Ad te levavi a 5.*

F0093 CBC MVCD [Musica Viva] 1067. CD. *The Glory of Palestrina.* Elmer Iseler Singers. Elmer Iseler. 1994 (rec. Church of the Transfiguration, Markham, Ontario). On this recording, plainchant propers for the Feast of the Ascension (introit, offertory, communion) are interpolated into the performance of the polyphonic mass. Booklet (23pp) contains program notes by Lino Bianchi in English and French; texts provided with translations into English and French.

Contains mass *MissaAscendo ad Patrem* (*Kyrie* [3:21]; *Gloria* [4:52]; *Credo* [7:42]; *Sanctus* [4:37]; *Agnus Dei I* and *II* [2:22]); motets *Ascendo ad Patrem* [3:32]; *Quem vidistis, pastores* [3:38]; *Surge illuminare Jerusalem* [2:59]; *Assumpta est Maria* [2:37]; *Stabat Mater* [8:22]; magnificat *Magnificat Primi toni* [8:22].

F0094 CBC MVCD [Musica Viva] 1121. CD. *Heavenly Spheres.* Le Studio de Musique Ancienne de Montréal. Christopher Jackson. 1998 [rec. February 11–13, 1997, Chapelle du Grand Seminaire, Montreal]. Program notes (16pp) in English and French.

Contains motets *Salve Regina* [5:06]; *Beatus Laurentius* [3:38]; litany *Litaniae de Beata Virgine Maria a 6* [6:02].

F0095 CBC Transcriptions SM 86. LP. *Missa Brevis.* Tudor Singers of Montreal. Wayne Riddell. 1969.

Contains mass *Missa Brevis a 4* [24:07].

F0096 Centaur CRC 2303. CD. *Music for the Christmas Season.* Chicago A Cappella. Jonathan Miller. 1996 (rec. March 2–3, 1996 at St. Giles Episcopal Church, Northbrook, Illinois).

Contains mass *Missa O magnum mysterium a 6*; motets *O magnum mysterium a 6*; *Jubilate Deo universa terra a 5*; hymns *A solis ortus cardine*; *Christe redemptor omnium*; *Hostes Herodes impie.*

F0097 Chandos 0617. CD. *Palestrina: Music for Maundy Thursday.* Musica Contexta. 1998 (rec. October 23–25, 1997, All Hallows Church, Gospel Oak, London). Relevant plainchant and antiphons also interpolated on this recording.

Contains lamentations *Lamentation I* [8:11]; *Responsory I* [2:47]; *Lamentation II* [10:37]; *Responsory II* [2:57]; *Lamentation III* [8:39]; *Responsory III* [5:18]; *Benedictus for Holy Week* [8:07]; *Miserere mei* [10:59][Total timing 59:33].

F0098 Chanticleer CR 8801. CD. *Anniversary Album 1978–1988.* Chanticleer. Joseph Jennings. 1988.

Contains motet *Ave Regina coelorum* [3:42].

F0099 Christophorus 4005. CD. *Motetten der italienischen Renaissance.* Isaak Ensemble Heidelberg (Eva Lebherz-Valentin [sop], Arno Paduch [cornetto], Petra Manz-Bauer [viol], Andreas Grossmann [positive organ], Eva Schildkniecht [harpsichord]). 1999 [rec. June 1992; orig. released 1993; reissued 1999].

Contains motet *Introduxit me rex* [diminutions by Bassano].

F0100 Christophorus SCGLX 73 839. LP. // Kammerchor Leonhard Lechner. Willi Seebacher. 1960s.
Contains madrigal *Quando dal terzo cielo a 6.*

F0101 Christophorus SCGLX 73 910. LP. *O Freude über Freud. Festliche Weihnachtsmusik des 16. und 17. Jahrhunderts.* Musica Antiqua Wien, Wiener Motettenchor. Bernhard Klebel. ca. 1962.
Contains motets *Ave Maria*; *Hodie Christus natus est.*

F0102 Christophorus SCGLX 73 945. LP. *Musica Papale.* Musica Antiqua Wien, Wiener Motettenchor. Bernhard Klebel. ca. 1981.
Contains mass *Missa Papae Marcelli a 6* [*Credo* only].

F0103 Christophorus SCGLX 73 952. LP. *Missa Papae Marcelli. Canticum canticorum.* Wiener Motettenchor. Bernhard Klebel. 1980 [also released as CD 74512; Mass also released on Christschall 74512].
Contains mass *Missa Papae Marcelli* [26:28]; motets [from *Canticum canticorum*] *Osculetur me a 5; Nigra sum a 5; Vineam meam a 5; Si ignoras te a 5; Tota pulchra es a 5; Vulnerasti cor meum a 5; Dilectus meus a 5; Pulchra es a 5; Veni veni dilecti mi a 5* [22:46 total].

F0104 Christschall 115. 10-inch 78 rpm // Staatliche Vokalkappelle an der Allerheiligen-Hofkirche, München. Alfons Singer. ca. 1930.
Contains motet *Jubilate Deo a 8.*

F0105 Christschall 325B. 12-inch 78 rpm [2 sides]. // Lassus Vocal Quartet, Speyer. No director listed. ca. 1951–1952.
Contains magnificat, unspecified.

F0106 Classics for Pleasure [EMI] CDM 64045. CD. *Missa Hodie Christus natus est. Six Motets.* Choir of King's College, Cambridge. Philip Ledger. 1970s.
Contains mass *Missa Hodie Christus natus est a 8*; motets *Canite tuba a 5*; *Ave Maria a 5*; *Tui sunt coeli a 5*; *Jubilate Deo a 5*; *O magnum mysterium a 6.*

F0107 Classics for Pleasure [EMI] CFP 2180. CD. *Allegri. Lassus. Palestrina.* Choir of St. John's College, Cambridge. George Guest. 1991 (rec. July 1990, St. John's College Chapel, Cambridge) [also listed as EMI Eminence CDM 7 64115 2; CD-EMX 2180].
Contains mass *Veni sponsa Christi a 4*; motet *Veni sponsa Christi a 4.*

F0108 Claves D8206. LP. *Musiche Veneziane*. Teresa Berganza, instrumental ensemble. 1982.
Contains madrigal *Vestiva i colli a 5* [arranged].

F0109 Collegium COL CD 116. CD. *Ave gracia plena. Music in Honour of the Virgin Mary.* The Cambridge Singers. John Rutter. 1992. Program notes by John Rutter; texts with English translations in booklet.
Contains motet *Stabat Mater a 8.*

F0110 Collegium COLCD 122. CD. *The Song of Songs. Motecta ex Cantico Canticorum.* Cambridge Singers. John Rutter. 1994 (rec. November 1993, Lyndhurst Hall, London). Contains liner booklet (15pp) with notes by John Rutter; Latin texts with English translations. Contains motets *Canticum canticorum*, complete (29 motets) [total 69:02].

F0111 Collegium COLCD 124. CD. *Images of Christ.* Cambridge Singers. John Rutter. 1995 [also listed as cassette COLC 124].
Contains motet *Ascendo ad Patrem a 5*; *Improperia.*

F0112 Collins Classics 15092. CD. *Renaissance Masterpieces, vol. IV: Rome.* Choir of New College, Oxford. Edward Higginbottom. 1997 (rec. July 21–23, 1997, New College Chapel, Oxford).
Contains *Victimae paschali laudes* [4:02]; *Magnificat* [5:29]; *Ninc dimittis* [3:54]; *Dum complerentur* [6:02]; *Ad Dominum cum tribularer* [5:01]; *Stabat Mater* [9:19]; *Alma Redemptoris Mater* [2:44]; *Recordare* [9:41]; *Ad te levavi oculos meos* [6:31]; *Veni Sancte Spiritus* [3:41]

F0113 Collins Classics 50092. CD. *Palestrina. Missa Papae Marcelli. Stabat Mater. Allegri Miserere. Lotti Crucifixus.* The Sixteen. Harry Christophers. 1990 (rec. November 1989, St. Jude's Church, London). Notes in insert by Ivan Moody.
Contains mass *Missa Papae Marcelli* [3:56 (*Kyrie*); 5:47 (*Gloria*); 8:30 (*Credo*); 6:06 (*Sanctus-Benedictus*); 3:15 (*Agnus Dei I*); 3:35 (*Agnus Dei II*) [31:09 total]; motet *Stabat mater* [9:19].

F0114 Collins Classisc 70212. CD. *A Renaissance Anthology.* The Sixteen. Harry Christophers. 1990 [partial reissue of Collins 50092].
Contains mass *Missa Papae Marcelli a 6.*

F0115 Columbia 33CX1567. 12-inch LP. *Church Music.* Netherlands Chamber Choir. Felix de Nobel. 1958. Program notes (8pp) by Jeremy Noble; Latin and Italian texts with English translations on sleeve insert [some items also issued in 7-inch 45 rpm format as 8216 SEG but withdrawn by 1965; also issued as Angel S-35667, *Motets*].
Contains motets *Sicut cervus a 4; O beata et gloriosa Trinitas a 5; Adoramus te Christe a 4*; *Stabat Mater a 8*; madrigal *Soave fia il morir a 5.*

F0116 Columbia 4970. 10-inch 78 rpm // London Catholic Choir. No director listed. Before 1936.
Contains hymn *Veni creator spiritus.*

F0117 Columbia 5711. 10-inch 78 rpm (1/2 side). *Columbia History of Music. Volume I.* Westminster Choir. Sir Richard Terry. Before 1930. Series editor: Dr. Percy Scholes [also issued as part of Columbia set M 231].
Contains motet *Nunc dimittis a 4* [with free falsobordone].

F0118 Columbia 5712. 10-inch 78 rpm. Westminster Choir. Sir Richard Terry. March 1927. Series editor: Dr. Percy Scholes [also issued as part of Columbia set M 231, *Columbia History of Music. Volume I*].
Contains mass *Missa Papae Marcelli a 6* [*Sanctus* only].

F0119 Columbia D 11053. 12-inch 78 rpm // Antwerp "Caecilia" Choir. de Vocht. Before 1936.
Contains mass *Missa Papae Marcelli a 6* [*Sanctus* only].

F0120 Columbia D 17146. 10-inch 78 rpm // Westminster Abbey Choir [men]. Dr. Ernest Bullock. Before 1936 [withdrawn mid-1940s] [also issued as Columbia DB 1836].
Contains offertory motet *Super flumina Babylonis a 5.*

F0121 Columbia D 17193. 12-inch 78 rpm // Amsterdam "Bel Canto" Choir. Alphons Vranken. Before 1936.
Contains motet *Sicut cervus a 4.*

F0122 Columbia D 17194. 12-inch 78 rpm // Amsterdam "Bel Canto" Choir. Alphons Vranken. Before 1936.
Contains motets *Veni veni dilecte mi a 5*; *Vox dilecti mei a 5.*

F0123 Columbia D 17195. 12-inch 78 rpm // Amsterdam "Bel Canto" Choir. Alphons Vranken. Before 1936.
Contains mass *Missa Jesu nostra redemptio* [*Benedictus* and *Hosanna* only]; motet *Hodie Christus natus est a 8.*

F0124 Columbia D 696863/5D. 12-inch 78 rpm // Madrigal Singers. Lehman Engel. ca. 1940 [issued as set M299, 6 sides].
Contains *Missa Brevis a 4.*

F0125 Columbia D 72351D. 12-inch 78 rpm // De Pauer Infantry Chorus. De Pauer. Before 1936 [recording included in set MM 709].
Contains motets *O bone Jesu; Adoramus te Christe a 4* [attribution doubtful].

F0126 Columbia DFX 180 [Columbia-France]. 12-inch 78 rpm // Lyons Cathedral Choir. L. Vietti. Before 1936.
Contains mass *Missa Papae Marcelli* [*Benedictus* only].

F0127 Columbia LCX 21. 12-inch 78 rpm // Dayton Westminster Choir. John Finlay Williamson. Before 1936.
Contains offertory motet *Exaltabo te Domine a 5.*

F0128 Columbia ML 4144. LP. // De Pauer Infantry Chorus. De Pauer. ca. 1950–1951 [recording included in set CM-709, before 1948; also includes reissue of Columbia D 72351D].
Contains motets *Adoramus te* [attribution doubtful; prob. by F. Rosselli]; *O bone Jesu.*

F0129 Columbia RFX 56 [Columbia-France]. 12-inch 78 rpm // Strasbourg Cathedral Choir. Alphonse Hoch. Pre-1930/ca. 1938 [indications that this is an electric rerecording of an existing acoustic disc. This issue dated ca. 1938].
Contains motet *O bone Jesu.*

F0130 Columbia RG 16171 [Columbia-Spain]. 12-inch 78 rpm // Comillas Schola Cantorum. No director listed. ca. 1950–1951.
Contains motet *Exsultate Deo a 5.*

F0131 Columbia RG 16173 [Columbia-Spain]. 12-inch 78 rpm [2 sides]. // Comillas Schola Cantorum. No director listed. ca. 1950–1951.
Contains motet from Lamentations, *Matribus suis dixerunt.*

F0132 Columbia RS 577 [Columbia-Spain]. 12-inch 78 rpm // Orfeón Domosstiarra. S. Estraola. Before 1936 [also issued as American Columbia 3779X].
Contains motet *Exsultate Deo a 5.*

F0133 Columbia Special Products CSP P6 16401. LP (6). *Music. A Listener's Introduction.* Various performers, compilation made 1983. Designed to accompany Kenneth Levy's textbook of the same name [individual discs labeled 16402–16407. Palestrina selection is on 16402, derived from EMI recording of 1972, reproduced by permission]. Choir of King's College Chapel, Cambridge. David Willcocks.
Contains mass *Missa Papae Marcelli* [*Kyrie* only] [3:54].

F0134 Columbia University 103/104. 10-inch 78 rpm (2). *Early Liturgical Music.* Columbia University Choir. Lowell P. Beveridge. ca. 1940.
Contains motet *Exaltabo te Domine a 5.*

F0135 Concert Hall Society CHC 44. LP. // Dessoff Choir. Paul Boepple. 1952. Program notes and texts on sleeve [also listed as Nixa CLP 4].
Contains motet *Assumpta est Maria a 6.*

F0136 Concert Hall Society CHS 1100. LP. // Trapp Family Singers. Franz Wasner. ca. 1938–1939.
Contains motet *O bone Jesu a 4.*

F0137 Concert Hall Society CHS 1231. LP. *Sacred Music.* Dessoff Choir. Paul Boepple. 1956. Program notes by Paul Boepple; Latin texts with English translations on sleeve.
Contains mass *Missa Assumpta est Maria a 6*; motet *Stabat Mater a 8*; magnificat *Magnificat primi toni.*

F0138 Counterpoint [Esoteric] CPT 546. LP. *The Renaissance Chorus. Fifteenth and Sixteenth Century Motets.* The Renaissance Chorus. Harold Brown. 1956. Sleeve notes by Franzi Ascher [also issued as CPT 5546].
Contains motet *Exultate Deo a 5.*

F0139 Counterpoint [Esoteric] CPT 5602. LP. *Music of Palestrina.* Dessoff Choirs. Paul Boepple. 1964.
Contains motets *Exultate Deo a 5*; *Exaltabo te a 5*; *Surge illuminare Jerusalem a 8*: *Sicut cervus a 4*; *Veni sponsa Christi a 4*; hymns *Ave maris stella* [2 verses]; *Salvete flos martyrum*; lamentations *Lamentations, Book I: Lamed. Matribus suis*; magnificat *Magnificat quarti toni.*

F0140 Crossroads 22 16 0186. LP. *The Song of Songs.* Slovak Philharmonic Chorus. Ján María Dobrodinský. 1968. Program notes by Phyllis Mason [a Supraphon series].

Motets [all from Book IV, all a 5] *Osculetur me; Trahe me; Nigra sum; Si ignoras te; Pulchrae sunt genuae tuae; Fasciculus myrrhae; Vulnerasti cor meum; Sicut lilium; Introduxit me rex; Laeva ejus; Vox dilecti mei; Surge amica mea; Dilectus meus mihi; Surgam et circuibo; Dilectus meus descendit; Pulchra es amica mea; Quae est ista; Duo ubera tua; Quam pulchra es; Veni veni dilecti mi.*

F0141 Da Camera Magna SM 94054. LP. *Palestrina. Missa Sine Nomine. Motette. Ave Maria. Quattuor Antiphonae.* Schola Cantorum St. Foillan. Wilhelm Eschweiler. 1977. Anonymous notes in German and English on sleeve. The four Marian antiphons are *a voci pari*.

Contains mass *Missa Sine nomine a 4* [Mantuan, no *Credo*] [15:01]; motets *Alma Redemptoris Mater* [6:10]; *Ave Regina coelorum* [6:22]; *Regina coeli laetare* [6:25]; *Salve Regina* [7:24]; *Ave Maria a 4* [3:47].

F0142 Danica DCD 8163. CD. *Missa Papae Marcelli.* Copenhagen Boys' Choir. Ebbe Munk. 1995 [rec. February 1995].

Contains mass *Missa Papae Marcelli a 6*; motets "for the major festivals of the church year" [unspecified in source].

F0143 Decca LXT 2945. LP. *Choral Music of the 13th to the 16th Centuries.* Quartetto Polifonico Italiano. No director listed. 1954. Notes by Alec Robertson [also issued as London LL 995 and as LL 5359].

Contains motets *Hodie Christus natus est* [arranged Casimiri for single 4-part choir]; magnificat *Magnificat quarti toni* [arranged Casimiri]; Improperia *Popule meus* [arranged Terni]; hymn *Pange lingua gloriosi* [arranged Terni]; litany *Litaniae de BVM . . . Ave de coelis.*

F0144 Decca 433 678-2. LP. *Missa Assumpta est Maria.* Choir of St. John's College, Cambridge. George Guest. 1968 and 1972. [The present item may be a partial reissue of Argo ZK69, with the *Missa Assumpta est Maria* rec. and added in 1972 for this recording. *Missa Veni sponsa Christi* reissued on CD as EMI Eminence CD-EMX 2180 in 1991.]

Contains masses *Missa Veni sponsa Christi a 4*; *Missa Assumpta est Maria a 6*; motet *Veni sponsa Christi a 4*; magnificat *Magnificat VI toni.*

F0145 Decca 94 054. LP. *Palestrina. Werke für Männerchor.* Schola Cantorum St. Folian, Aachen. Wilhelm Eschweiler. ca. 1978.

Contains mass *Missa Sine nomine (Missa Mantovana)*; motets *Alma redemptoris mater a 4*; *Ave Maria a 4*; *Ave regina coelorum a 4* [a voci pari]; *Regina coeli laetare a 4*; *Salve regina a 4.*

F0146 Delos DE 3138. CD. *Ave Maria.* Ascension Music Chorus [Voices of Ascension]. Dennis Keene. 1993 [also issued on cassette CS3138].

Contains motet *Alma redemptoris mater a 4.*

F0147 Delos DE 3165. CD. *Beyond Chant: Mysteries of the Renaissance.* Voices of

Ascension. Dennis Keene. 1994. Program notes by Dennis Keene.
Contains motets *Sicut cervus a 4*; *Jesu rex admirabilis a 3*; *Exsultate Deo a 5*; *Exaltabo te a 5.*

F0148 Delos DE 3174. CD. *Voices of Ascension. From Chant to Renaissance*. Voices of Ascension. Dennis Keene. 1995. Program notes by Dennis Keene.
Contains motets *Surge illuminare a 8*; *Sitivit anima mea a 4*; *Hodie Christus natus est a 8*; *Ascendo ad Patrem a 5.*

F0149 Delos DE 3210. CD. *Prince of Music. The Greatest Choral Music of Palestrina.* Voices of Ascension. Dennis Keene. 1997.
Contains mass: *Missa Papae Marcelli a 6*; motets *Tu es Petrus a 6; Dum complerentur a 6; O Domine Jesu Christe a 4; Super flumina Babylonis a 4; Canite tuba a 5; Peccantem me quotidie a 5; Alma Redemptoris Mater; Sicut cervus a 4* [secunda pars *Sitivit anima mea*]; *Secundum multitudinem a 6*; *Rorate coeli a 5* [secunda pars C*anite tuba*].

F0150 Delos DE 3227. CD. *Visions of Heaven*. Voices of Ascension. Dennis Keene. 1996.
Contains motet *Jesu rex admirabilis a 3.*

F0151 Delos DE 3511. CD. *Horizons—A Musical Journey.* Voices of Ascension. Dennis Keene. 1995.
Contains motet *Sicut cervus a 4.*

F0152 Delyse ECB 3147. LP. *Choral Recital.* RHOS Male Choir. G. Williams. 1958.
Containts motet *Adoramus te Christe* [ed. G. Williams].

F0153 Discourses ABM 20. LP. *Missa "Tu es Petrus."* Choir of the London Oratory. John Hoban. 1975. Notes by Geoffrey Sharp.
Contains mass *Missa Tu es Petrus a 6*; motet *Tu es Petrus a 6.*

F0154 Durium SA 113. 12-inch 78 rpm. // [title]. Madrigalisti Milanesi. Renato Fait. ca. 1950 [reissued on Colosseum CLPS 1027, LP ca. 1952].
Contains motet *Tristis est anima mea a 4.*

F0155 ECM 1653. CD. *In Paradisum: Music of Victoria and Palestrina.* Hilliard Ensemble. Paul Hillier. 2000. Program notes by Ivan Moody.
Contains motets *Heu mihi Domine a 4*; *Domine quando veneris a 4*; *Libera me Domine a 5*; *Ad Dominum cum tribularer a 4.*

F0156 Eco [Mixtur] MXT Eco 576. LP. *Le Cappelle Musicali alla Rassegna Internazionale di Loreto.* Various performers: for the Palestrina selection, Aachener Domchor. Numerous directors listed. Before 1979.
Contains motet *Haec dies quam fecit Dominus a 6.*

F0157 Eco [Mixtur] MXT Eco 592. LP. *Corali del mondo a Loreto 1975.* Corale Città di Parma. Various directors. 1975.
Contains motet *Dum aurora finem daret a 4.*

F0158 Educo ECM 4003. LP. *Plainchant and Polyphony.* Choir of the Abbey and Seminary of Mount Angel, Father David Nicholson; Portland Symphonic Choir, C. Robert Zimmerman. 1956.
Contains magnificat *Magnificat octavi toni.*

F0159 Electrola STE 60602. 10-inch LP. *Missa Papae Marcelli.* Chor der St.-Hedwigs-Kathedrale Berlin. Karl Forster. 1964 [also issued on 12-inch LP as HMV ASD 569; and ALP 2019].
Contains mass *Missa Papae Marcelli a 6.*

F0160 EMI 063 02113. LP. *Palestrina.* Choir of King's College, Cambridge. David Willcocks. 1960s [also issued as EMI CSD 1237; Seraphim S-60187; reissue on EMI 137 154 555–3 (2)].
Contains masses *Missa brevis a 4; Missa Papae Marcelli a 6.*

F0161 EMI 065 03272. LP. *Missa Hodie Christus Natus Est. Six Motets.* Choir of King's College, Cambridge. Philip Ledger. 1970s [also issued as EMI ASD 3559 and on CD as CDM 7 64045 2].
Contains mass *Missa Hodie Christus natus est a 8*; motets *Hodie Christus natus est; Canite tuba in Sion; Ave Maria; Tu sunt coeli; Jubilate Deo; O magnum mysterium.*

F0162 EMI 065 99 685. LP. *Palestrina. Missa Tu es Petrus.* Tölzer Knabenchor. Gerhard Schmidt-Gaden. 1970s.
Contains mass *Missa Tu es Petrus a 8*; motets *Ave Maria; Quam pulchri sunt a 4; Tu es Petrus a 6.*

F0163 EMI 067 43 029. LP. *Palestrina. Missa Ave Maria.* Choir of King's College, Cambridge. Philip Ledger. 1982.
Contains mass *Missa Ave Maria a 6.*

F0164 EMI 137 154 555-3. LP (2). *Palestrina: Messen und Motetten.* Choir of King's College, Cambridge. Philip Ledger (*), David Willcocks (#). Before 1984 [a combined reissue of previous releases].
Contains masses *Missa brevis*#; *Missa Hodie Christus natus est**; *Missa Papae Marcelli*#; motets *Ave Maria**; *Canite tuba**; *Hodie Christus natus est**; *Jubilate Deo**; *O magnum mysterium**; *Tui sunt coeli**.

F0165 EMI ASD 3955. LP. *Palestrina. Missa Ave Maria in Six Parts.* Choir of King's College, Cambridge. Philip Ledger. 1982. Liner notes by Mary Berry and Iain Fenlon. Latin texts with English translations provided. In this performance, post-Tridentine plainchant Mass propers (Introit, Gradual, Tract, Communion) are interpolated as appropriate. The offertory is Palestrina's (polyphonic) *Ave Maria a 5* found in vol. IX, 13, of the Haberl edition.
Contains mass *Missa Ave Maria a 6*; motet *Ave Maria a 5* [IX, 13].

F0166 EMI CDC 7 47528 2. CD. *Palestrina. Missa Papae Marcelli. Motetten: Tu es Petrus, Laudate Dominum u.a.* Regensburger Domspatzen. Georg Ratzinger.

1986 (rec. Pfarrkirche S. Albertus Magnus). Contains booklet (12 pp) with notes by Karin Andrae in German, English, French. Latin texts provided.

Contains mass *Missa Papae Marcelli a 6* [4:00 (*Kyrie*); 5:47 (*Gloria*); 8:58 (*Credo*); 3:42 (*Sanctus*) ; 2:54 (*Agnus Dei I*); 2:30 (*Agnus Dei II*)]; motets *Rorate coeli a 5* [3.35]; *Hodie Christus natus est* a 8 [2.27]; *Pueri Hebraeorum a 4* [2.00]; *Terra tremuit a 5* [2.20]; *Ascendit Deus a 5* [2.08]; *Dum complerentur a 6* [3.06]; *Dum ergo essent a 6* [2.30]; *Ego sum panis vivus a 4* [3.04]; *Tu es Petrus a 6* [7.10]; *Laudate Dominum a 8* [2.58].

F0167 EMI CDC 7 49619 2. CD. *Procession with Carols on Advent Sunday.* Choir of King's College, Cambridge. Philip Ledger. 1981 (rec. December 20–21, 1979, King's College, Cambridge). Notes by Michael Till with texts of the service.

Contains "I Look From Afar" [adaptation of Palestrina] [2:49].

F0168 EMI Classics CDC 7 54455. CD. *Palestrina/Bach. Missa Sine nomine.* Concerto Palatino. Bruce Dickey. 1991 (rec. June 1991 at Doopgezinde Gemeente Kerk, Haarlem). The mass is performed in the arrangement made by Johann Sebastian Bach, with instrumental doublings and added continuo parts. Program notes by Bruce Dickey in English, French, German; texts with translations into English, French, German.

Contains mass *Missa Sine nomine a 6* [arr. J. S. Bach] [26:00].

F0169 EMI Classics CDK 65339. CD. *Baroque. Palestrina. Monteverdi. [Vol.7].* Choir of King's College, Cambridge. David Willcocks, Philip Ledger, et al. 1970, Chapel of King's College, Cambridge.

Contains mass *Missa Papae Marcelli a 6.*

F0170 EMI Classics CDZ 69703. CD. *Assumpta est Maria.* Clare College Choir, Cambridge. Timothy Brown. 1996 (rec. January 1996, Lady Chapel, Ely Cathedral).

Contains mass *Missa Assumpta est Maria a 6* [29:40]; motets *Assumpta est Maria* [7:19]; *Ave Maria* [3:33]; *Beata es* [2:56]; *Virgo Maria* [2:56]; *Hodie gloriosa semper Virgo Maria* [4:39]; *Regina coeli* [6:22]; magnificat *Magnificat septimi toni* [12:53].

F0171 EMI Reflexe CDC 7 47699 2. CD. *Musica della Cappella Sistina/Music of the Sistine Chapel.* Taverner Consort. Andrew Parrott. 1987 (rec. January 1986). Some works performed with embellishments. Program notes by Hugh Keyte in English, French, German. Texts provided, with translations in English, French, German [also issued as Virgin Veritas 61309 (CD); HMV 27 0565 1 (LP); *Stabat Mater* also reissued on Virgin Classics 45272 2].

Contains motets *Stabat mater a 8* [11.04]; *O beata et benedicta et gloriosa Trinitas a 5* [7.21]; *Jubilate Deo a 8* [4.11]; *Dum complerentur dies Pentecostes* [5.49]. Additional content includes Gregorio Allegri, *Miserere a 9* [13.20]; Cristóbal de Morales, *Lamentabatur Jacob a 5* [10.30]; Josquin Desprez, *Pater noster/Ave Maria* [8.35].

F0172 EMI Reflexe CDC 7 49010 2. CD (2). *Palestrina. Motettorum liber quartus quinque vocibus ex canticis canticorum. Madrigali spirituali.* Hilliard Ensemble.

Paul Hillier. 1986 (rec. November 18–23, 1984, London). Booklet (27pp) contains program notes by Bruno Turner in English, German, French; texts provided, with translations into English, German, French [also issued as Virgin ZDMB 61164 and Virgin Veritas 61168].

Contains motets, all a 5, *Osculetur me* [2.51]; *Trahe me post te* [2.32]; *Nigra sum, sed formosa* [3.10]; *Vineam meam non custodivi* [2.09]; *Si ignoras te* [2.43]; *Pulchrae sunt genae tuae* [2.51]; *Fasciculus myrrhae* [2.20]; *Ecce tu pulcher es* [2.30]; *Tota pulchra es* [2.13]; *Vulnerasti cor meum* [2.50]; *Sicut lilium inter spinas* [2.56]; *Introduxit me rex* [2.21]; *Laeva eius* [2.33]; *Vox dilecti mei* [2.05]; *Surge, propera amica mea* [2.16]; *Surge, amica mea* [2.33]; *Dilectus meus mihi* [2.31]; *Surgam et circuibo civitatem* [1.57]; *Adiuro vos, filiae Jerusalem* [3.25]; *Caput eius* [2.52]; *Dilectus meus descendit* [2.29]; *Pulchra es, amica mea* [2.37]; *Quae est ista* [2.24]; *Descendit in hortum meum* [2.45]; *Quam pulchri sunt* [2.40]; *Duo ubera tua* [3.40]; *Quam pulchra es* [3.00]; *Guttur sum* [2.44]; *Veni, veni dilecte mi* [2.54] [76:00 total]. Spiritual madrigals *Vergine bella* [3.34]; *Vergine saggia* [3.19]; *Vergine pura* [3.31]; *Vergine santa* [3.54]; *Vergine sol'al mondo* [4.17]; *Vergine chiara* [3.19]; *Vergine, quante lagrim'ho già sparte* [3.38]; *Vergine, tal è terra* [4.03] [31:00 total].

F0173 EMI SLS 5047(3). LP. // Choir of King's College, Cambridge. David Willcocks. 1960s.

Contains mass *Missa Brevis a 4*; motet *Haec dies a 6.*

F0174 Epic LC 3045. LP. *Choral Music from the Lowlands. Fifteenth and Sixteenth Centuries.* Netherlands Chamber Choir. Felix de Nobel. ca. 1955. Program notes by Klaus George Roy on sleeve.

Contains mass *Missa Papae Marcelli a 6.*

F0175 Epic LC 3359. LP. *Missa Brevis. Missa ad fugam.* Netherlands Chamber Choir. Felix de Nobel. 1957. Program notes by Allen C. Lannon on sleeve.

Contains masses *Missa Brevis a 4*; *Missa ad fugam a 4.*

F0176 Erasmus WHV 013. CD. *Palestrina. Stabat Mater.* Koorproject Rotterdam. Maarten Michielsen. 1990.

Contains mass *Missa Sine nomine a 6*; motet *Stabat Mater a 8.*

F0177 Erasmus WVH 042. CD. *Requiem.* Cappella "Palestrina." Maarten Michielsen. ca. 1990.

Contains mass *Missa pro defunctis.*

F0178 Erasmus WVH 121. CD. *Missa Lauda Sion for Four Voices.* Cappella "Palestrina." Maarten Michielsen. 1993 (rec. Rotterdam, August 1993).

Contains mass *Missa Lauda Sion a 4.*

F0179 Erato 9070-3. LP (4) [Four-volume multicomposer anthology]. Ensemble Philippe Caillard. Philippe Caillard. 1972.

Includes a rerelease of Erato 9502, item F0180.

F0180 Erato 9502. LP. *Palestrina. Missa Aeterna Christi Munera. Motets.* Ensemble Philippe Caillard. Philippe Caillard. 1969 [also listed as Erato EPR 15516].
Contains mass *Missa Aeterna Christi munera a 4*; motets *Tu es Petrus a 6; Hodie Christus natus est a 8; Tribulationes a 5; Peccavimus a 5; Sicut cervus a 5; Exultate Deo a 5*; magnificat *Magnificat sexti toni.*

F0181 Erato LDE 1001. 7-inch LP 33-1/3 rpm. *Polyphonic Motets of the XVIth Century.* Petits Chanteurs de la Renaissance. Pagot, Noyre. ca. 1953–1955 [also as LP Erato EJA 11; also in Haydn Society HS 9007].
Contains motet *Ego sum panis vivus* [cond. Noyre].

F0182 Everest SDBR 3174/3. LP. *Plainsong to Polyphony.* Choir of the Carmelite Priory. John McCarthy. 1967. Texts with English translations enclosed.
Contains masses *Missa Aeterna Christi munera a 4* [*Kyrie* only]; *Missa Ecce sacerdos magnus* [*Kyrie* only]; *Missa Lauda Sion a 4* [*Benedictus* only]; *Magnificat octavi toni.*

F0183 Everest SDBR 3193. LP. *The Sistine Choir in Concert at the Vatican.* Sistine Choir. Domenico Bartolucci. 1967.
Contains mass movement (unspecified *Benedictus*).

F0184 Festival 70-202. 10-inch LP. *Pre-Baroque Sacred Music.* Harvard University Chorus, Radcliffe Choral Society. Russell. ca. 1950–1951.
Contains magnificat *Magnificat quarti toni.*

F0185 FGLP 1028 FG [distributed by AudioSource]. LP. *The Candomino Choir.* Candomino Choir. Tauno Satomaa. 1983 (rec. November 13–15, 1982, Espoo, Finland). Program notes (12pp) by Juha Hovinen, in Finnish with English and German translation; Latin texts with English, German, Finnish translations inserted into sleeve.
Contains mass *Missa brevis a 4.*

F0186 Fonè 90 F 20/1-90F 20/2. CD (2). *Motetti. Madrigali spirituali.* Coro Polifonico Turritano. Antonio Sanna. 1996. Program notes by Antonio Ligios ca. 1990.
Contains masses *Missa "de Feria"*; *Missa Ut re mi fa sol la*; *Missa Brevis*; motets *Ave Maria; Adoramus te Christe; Pueri Hebraeorum; Domine quando pavesco; Hodie Christus natus est; Jubilate Deo; Quam pulchri sunt; Duo ubera tua; Quam pulchra es; Exsultate Deo; Stabat Mater; In festo unius martyris*; magnificat *Magnificat octavi toni*; spiritual madrigals *Figlio immortal d'immortal Padre; E se ma voi di qua giù son grate; Hor tu sol che di vivi almi splendori; Dammi scala del ciel e del ciel porta; E se fur già de le mie mani immonde; Vello di Gedeon, cui Dio sì largo; Novella aurora che nascend'allegri.*

F0187 Fonit LPU 008. LP. *Missa Assumpta est Maria.* Dessoff Choirs. Paul Boepple. Early 1960s. Texts with English translations included [also issued as Rarities Collection 008].
Contains mass *Missa Assumpta est Maria a 6*; motet *Stabat Mater a 8*; magnificat *Magnificat primi toni.*

F0188 Fonit LPZ 2021. LP. *Coro Franco Maria Saraceni degli Universitari di Roma.* Coro Franco Maria Saraceni degli Universitari di Roma. Fausto Alberto Razzi. 1962.
Contains madrigal *La cruda mia nemica a 4.*

F0189 Fono FGLS 25-4326. 10-inch LP. *Musica nel Sanctuario-Basilica Madonna del Sasso.* Coro Palestrina di Locarno. Walter Rüsch. 1966.
Missa Qual è il più grande amor [*Sanctus* only].

F0190 Fono FSM 33 207 [Edition Brockhoff]. LP. *Alte Musik im Dom zu Münster.* Posaunenchor, Domchor und Schola Münster (Heinrich Stockhorst [organ]). Hubert Leiwering. Before 1984.
Contains motets *Ecce veniet; Fratres ego enim accepi.*

F0191 Forlane 16771. CD. // Maîtrise des Hauts-de-Seine. 1997 (rec. Feb., April, Oct. 1997, Église Saint-Louis à Garches).
Contains motet *Sicut cervus a 4* [secunda pars *Sitivit anima mea*].

F0192 Fabbri SdM-008. 7-inch LP. *La Scuola Romana: Palestrina*. Performers not identified. 1964.
Contains masses *Missa Papae Marcelli a 6* [*Gloria* only]; *Missa Assumpta est Maria a 6* [*Benedictus* only]; motets *Super flumina Babylonis*; *Tota pulchra es.*

F0193 Fabbri SdM-150. 7-inch LP. *Il Madrigale.* Choral Ensemble. Renato Fait [for work named below]. 1964.
Contains madrigal *I vaghi fiori a 5.*

F0194 Gimell CDGIM 001. CD. *Palestrina Masses. Missa Benedicta es.* The Tallis Scholars. Peter Phillips. 1986 (orig. rec. 1981, Chapel of Merton College, Oxford). Liner notes by Peter Philips [originally issued on LP as GIM 1585–01] [the Josquin motet is the model on which the Palestrina mass is based].
Contains mass *Missa Benedicta es* [41:15]. Additional material includes plainchant, *Benedicta es* [2:24]; Josquin des Pres, motet, *Benedicta es* [6:55].

F0195 Gimell CDGIM 003. CD. *Palestrina Masses. Missa Nigra Sum.* The Tallis Scholars. Peter Phillips. 1986. Liner notes (2pp) by Peter Phillips [originally issued as LP 1585-03 in 1983].
Contains mass *Missa Nigra sum a 5* [35.06] [not based on Palestrina's own motet]. Additional content includes plainchant *Nigra sum* [1.19]; Jean Lhéritier, motet *Nigra sum* [5.05]; Tomas Luis da Victoria, motet *Nigra sum* [3.59]; De Silva, motet *Nigra sum* [1.46].

F0196 Gimell CDGIM 008. CD. *Palestrina Masses. Missa brevis. Missa Nasce la gioja mia.* The Tallis Scholars. Peter Phillips. 1986 (rec. Merton College Chapel). Program notes by Peter Phillips in English, French, German, Italian; the Italian text of the madrigal is provided with translations into English, French, and German.
Contains masses *Missa Brevis* [22:00]; *Missa Nasce la gioja mia* [25:00]. Additional content includes Primavera, madrigal *Nasce la gioja mia* [2:30].

F0197 Gimell CDGIM 020. CD. *Palestrina. Missa Assumpta est Maria. Missa Sicut Lilium.* The Tallis Scholars. Peter Phillips. 1989 (rec. Church of St. Peter and St. Paul, Norfolk). Booklet (23pp) contains program notes by Peter Phillips in English, French, Italian, German; texts provided with translations into English, French, Italian, German [previously issued as 1585T-20].
Contains masses *Missa Assumpta est Maria a 6; Missa Sicut lilium a 5*; motets *Assumpta est Maria a 6; Sicut lilium inter spinas a 5.*

F0198 Gimell CDGIM 339. CD. *Miserere.* The Tallis Scholars. Peter Phillips. 1985 (rec. 1980, Chapel of Merton College, Oxford). Program notes by Peter Phillips [issued as Angel RL 32122 in 1980, also as Classics for Pleasure 40339].
Contains mass *Missa Papae Marcelli a 6* [36:43].

F0199 Gimell CDGIM 994. CD. *The Tallis Scholars Live in Rome.* The Tallis Scholars. Peter Phillips. 1994 (rec. February 2–4, 1994, Basilica of S. Maria Maggiore, Rome). Recording of a concert marking the quatercentenary of Palestrina's death. Contains program notes in English, French, German; Italian; provides texts with English, French, and Italian translations.
Contains mass *Missa Papae Marcelli a 6* [32:22]; motets *Stabat Mater* [9:39]; *Surge, illuminare* [3:03]*; Alma redemptoris mater* [3:06]*; Nunc dimittis* [4:34]; magnificat *Magnificat primi toni* (2) [6:27].

F0200 Gimell CDGIMB 400. CD (4). *The Palestrina 400 Collection.* The Tallis Scholars. Peter Phillips. 1993 (discs orig. issued 1983–1989) [a compilation of issues GIM 001, GIM 003, GIM 008, GIM 020, items F0194, F0195, F0196, and F0197].

F0201 Giulia GS 201010. CD. *Il vero modo di diminuir. Virtuoso Music from 16th Century Italy for Cornetto, Organ and Harpsichord.* Doron David Sherwin [cornetto], Andrea Marcon [organ, harpsichord]. 1991. Program notes (20pp) by Doron Sherwin in English with German, French, Italian translations.
Contains motets *Fuit homo missus a Deo* [divisions by D. Sherwin] [4:37]; *Introduxit me Rex* [divisions by G. Bassano] [3:52].

F0202 Gramophone [HMV] AB 559 [HMV-Spain]. 12-inch 78 rpm // Barcelona "Orféo Català" Choir. Luis Millet. ca. 1930.
Contains mass *Missa Papae Marcelli a 6* [*Credo* only].

F0203 Gramophone [HMV] AF 523 [HMV-Spain]. 12-inch 78 rpm // Capilla de Música de Montserrat. David Pujol. 1943.
Contains motet *Ego sum panis vivus a 4* [Hab.V].

F0204 Gramophone [HMV] C 1473/6. 12-inch 78 rpm (4 discs) [electrical]. // Westminster Cathedral Choir. Sir Richard Terry (rec. 17 March 1927) [also issued as EH 163/6; Victor 35941/4].
Contains mass *Missa Papae Marcelli a 6* [omits *Agnus Dei I*].

F0205 Gramophone C 3914. 12-inch 78 rpm // Westminster Cathedral Choir. George Malcolm. Before 1936.
Contains hymn *Pange lingua gloriosi.*

F0206 Gramophone [HMV] D 336 and D 338, 12-inch 80 [*sic*] rpm [acoustic]. // Westminster Cathedral Choir. Sir Richard Terry (rec. May 1909, London; withdrawn by 1936) [HMV reissue of single-sided discs 04781, 04783, 04784].
Contains mass *Missa Aeterna Christi munera a 4* [*Kyrie, Gloria, Sanctus, Agnus Dei*].

F0207 Gramophone [HMV] D 826. 12-inch 78 rpm [acoustic]. // Sistine Chapel Choir. Baron Rudolf Kanzler. ca. 1904 [withdrawn before 1936].
Contains motets *Ave Maria a 4*; *Sicut cervus a 4.*

F0208 Gramophone [HMV] D 1647. 12-inch 78 rpm // Dayton Westminster Choir. John Finlay Williamson. Before 1936 [also issued as Gramophone EJ 430].
Contains motet *Exsultate Deo a 5.*

F0209 Gramophone [HMV] DB 1570. 12-inch 78 rpm //Cappella Sistina Choir. Antonio Rella. Before 1935 [part of series DB 1569/72, set GM-139, *Polyphonic Church Music*].
Contains motet *Sicut cervus a 4.*

F0210 Gramophone [HMV] DB 1571. 12-inch 78 rpm. *Polyphonic Church Music.* Cappella Sistina Choir. Antonio Rella. Before 1935 [original recording made ca. 1924] [part of set DB 1569/72; set GM-139; also issued as Victor 7813].
Contains motet *Super flumina Babylonis*; Improperia *Popule meus.*

F0211 Gramophone [HMV] DB 4896/7. 12-inch 78 rpm. *Polyphonic Church Music.* Choeur de la Cathédrale de Dijon. Joseph Samson. Before 1936 [part of series DB 4893/7, set GM-189; issued also as Victor 11680/81, from series 11677/81, set M212].
Mass: *Missa Assumpta est Maria* [*Kyrie, Sanctus, Benedictus, Hosanna, Agnus Dei*].

F0212 Gramophone [HMV] DB 21050. 12-inch 78 rpm // Cappella Sistina Choir. Domenico Bartolucci. 1950. Note indicates that this recording was made at the ceremony of the opening of the Holy Door at St. Peter's Basilica for the Jubilee Year of 1950.
Containts motets *Jubilate Deo a 8*; *O bone Jesu* [version unspecified].

F0213 Gramophone [HMV] DB 21140/2. 12-inch 78 rpm (3). // Cappella Sistina Choir [Domenico Bartolucci?]. ca. 1950–1951.
Contains mass *Missa O admirabile commercium a 5* [*Gloria, Sanctus, Benedictus* only].

F0214 Gramophone [HMV] E 336. 10-inch 78 rpm [acoustic]. // Alessandro Moreschi, Sistine Choir members. Baron Rudof Kanzler. 1904 [issue of Black & Tan 54788, matrix 2202b; see Opal 823, item F0323].
Contains madrigal *La cruda mia nemica a 4* [2:33].

F0215 Gramophone [HMV] EG 3431 [Electrola/HMV-Germany]. 10-inch 78 rpm // Regensburger Domchor. Theobald Schrems. Before 1936.
Contains mass *Missa Lauda Sion a 4* [*Benedictus* only].

F0216 Gramophone [HMV] EG 6812 [Electrola/ HMV-Germany]. 10-inch 78 rpm // Regensburger Domchor. Theobald Schrems. ca. 1942–1948.
Contains mass *Missa Papae Marcelli a 6* [*Sanctus* only].

F0217 Gramophone [HMV] EJ 129 [HMV/Germany]. 12-inch 78 rpm // Berlin Staats- und Domchor. Rüdel. Before 1936 [also issued as Victor 9250. This recording was also issued as Parlophone R 1021; Brunswick 30727; Odeon O-4305; and American Decca 20161, on 10-inch 78 rpm disc, as part of the *Two Thousand Years of Music* series, ed. Curt Sachs, Parlophone 1016/27; Brunswick 30722/33; Odeon O-4300/11; American Decca 20156/67, set P11, also as LP set DX 106].
Contains mass *Missa Papae Marcelli a 6* [*Sanctus* only].

F0218 Gramophone [HMV] EJ 130 [Electrola/HMV-Germany]. 12-inch 78 rpm // Berlin Staats- und Domchor. Rüdel. Before 1936.
Contains mass *Missa Papae Marcelli a 6* [*Benedictus* only].

F0219 Gramophone [HMV] GSC 56. 12-inch 78 rpm. *Choral Music of the Renaissance.* Danish Radio Madrigal Choir. Mogens Wöldike. ca. 1950 [part of series GSC 53/8, set GSC 9, Gramophone Shop Celebrities].
Contains motet *Super flumina Babylonis.*

F0220 Gramophone [HMV] GSC 57. 12-inch 78 rpm. *Choral Music of the Renaissance.* Danish Radio Madrigal Choir. Mogens Wöldike. ca. 1950 [part of series GSC 53/8, set GSC 9, Gramophone Shop Celebrities].
Contains motet *Dies sanctificatus a 4.*

F0221 Gramophone [HMV] GSC 58. 12-inch 78 rpm *Choral Music of the Renaissance.* Danish Radio Madrigal Choir. Mogens Wöldike. ca. 1950 [part of series GSC 53/8, set GSC 9, Gramophone Shop Celebrities].
Contains mass *Missa Aeterna Christi munera a 4* [*Agnus Dei I and II* only].

F0222 Gramophone GY 212 [HMV-Spain]. 10-inch 78 rpm // Montserrat Monastery Choir. David Pujol. 1940s.
Contains motet *Exsultate Deo a 5.*

F0223 Gramophone [HMV] HMS 35. 12-inch 78 rpm. *History of Music in Sound. IV. The Age of Humanism.* Brompton Oratory Choir. Henry Washington. 1953. Text (64pp booklet) by Gerald Abraham and Jack Westrup [pub. New York: Oxford University Press, 1953; Palestrina references pp.27–29. Includes numerous musical examples, Latin texts and English translations. Originally side 8 in a set of 13 discs; the present material reissued on LP as HMV HLP8; RCA Victor LM 6029, in series 6028–6029. Musical examples on Side 2, band 1a and 1b].
Contains mass *Missa Brevis* [*Agnus Dei II a 5* only]; *Missa Aeterna Christi munera* [*Sanctus* only].

F0224 Gramophone K 7378 [HMV-France]. 10-inch 78 rpm // La Manécanterie des Petits Chanteurs à la Croix de Bois. No director listed. France, before 1936 [also issued as Japanese Victor JA 688].
Contains motet *Alma redemptoris mater a 4* [Hab. V].

F0225 Gramophone K 7558 [HMV-France]. 10-inch 78 rpm // La Manécanterie des Petits Chanteurs à la Croix de Bois. No director listed. France, before 1936.
Contains motet *Sicut cervus a 4.*

F0226 Gramophone Z 187 [HMV-Scandinavia]. 12-inch 78 rpm // Palestrina Choir. Mogens Wöldike. Before 1936.
Contains motet *Sicut cervus a 4.*

F0227 Gregorian Institute of America GIOA CA-1. LP. *Cathedral Choirs of America: The Choir of Sacred Heart Cathedral, Newark, New Jersey.* Sacred Heart Cathedral Choir. John M. Oates. 1950s.
Contains motets *Adoramus te Christe a 4*; *O Domine Jesu Christe a 4.*

F0228 Gregorian Institute of America GIOA EL-17-19. LP (3). *Thirteen Centuries of Christian Choral Art.* Peloquin Chorale. Alexander Peloquin. 1959.
Contains mass *Missa Brevis a 4* [*Sanctus* only].

F0229 Gregorian Institute of America GIOA EL-30. LP. *Choir of the Pontifical North American College, Rome.* Pontifical North American College. Antonio Martorell. 1950s.
Contains motet *Ave Maria a 4.*

F0230 Gregorian Institute of America GIOA set PM 1. 12-inch 78 rpm. *Polyphonic Masters of the XVIth Century.* Gregorian Institute Choir. Vitry. 1948 [reissued on LP as GIOA PM-LP 1 ca. 1953–1955].
Contains offertory motet *Laudate Dominum a 5*; lamentations responsory *O vos omnes.*

F0231 Harmonia Mundi 25162. 10-inch LP. *Gloria in excelsis Deo. Advent und Weihnacht in Dom zu Münster.* Instrumental ensemble, Domchor Münster. Hubert Leiwering. 1963.
Contains motet *Ecce veniet dies illa a 8.*

F0232 Harmonia Mundi 30510. LP. *Masses and Motets.* Les Chanteurs de St.-Eustache. Père Émile Martin. 1967. Program notes by Chris Nelson on Odyssey reissue [reissued on Odyssey 32 16 0122].
Contains masses *Missa Ascendo ad patrem a 5; Missa In festis apostolorum I a 5*; motets *Surge amica mea a 5; Cantantibus organis a 5.*

F0233 Harmonia Mundi BMG 0542 77317-2. CD. *Missa in duplicibus minoribus. Lamentazioni. Motettes.* Maîtrise de Garçons de Colmar, Ensemble Gilles Binchois; Cantus Figuratus, Schola Cantorum Basliensis. Dominique Vellard. 1994. Liner notes by Horst Leuchtmann.
Contains mass *Missa in duplicibus minoribus II a 5*; motets *Ave regina coelorum; Gloriosi principes terrae*; lamentations *Lamentations of Jeremiah I–III.*

F0234 Harmonia Mundi HMC 901388. CD. *Missa Viri Galilaei. Motet Viri Galilaei. Magnificat prini toni.* Ensemble Vocale Européen de la Chapelle Royale, Ensemble Organum. Philippe Herreweghe, Marcel Pérès. 1992 (rec. June 5–7, 1991,

L'abbaye aux Dames, Saintes). Program notes in French with English and German translations; Latin texts with English, French, German translations.
Contains mass *Missa Viri Galilei* [40:40]; motet *Viri Galilei* [4:42]; magnificat *Magnificat primi toni* [11:56].

F0235 Harmonia Mundi HMF 221. LP. *Monteverdi: Messe a 4.* Deller Consort, Clemencic Consort (Robert Elliott [organ]). Alfred Deller, Rene Clemencic. 1978 [also issued as Ars Nova VST 6081].
Contains motet *Ave verum corpus.*

F0236 Harmonia Mundi 1C 065-99 601. LP. *Ave Maria Kaiserin. Musik im Dom zu Aachen.* Aachen Cathedral Choir. Günther Pohl. 1972. Program notes by "A. B." in German, English, and French; Latin texts included.
Contains motet *Terra tremuit a 5.*

F0237 Harmonia Mundi 1C 0655-99 685. LP. *Missa Tu es Petrus & Motetten.* Tölzer Knabenchor. Gerhard Schmidt-Gaden. 1974 (rec. Pfarrkirche, Langgreis). Anonymous liner notes in German and English. Latin texts for motets provided [also listed as Harmonia Mundi HMI 73–078; BASF HM 25 22061 3].
Contains mass *Missa Tu es Petrus a 6*; motet *Ave Maria; Quam pulchri sunt a 5; Tu es Petrus a 6.*

F0238 Harmonia Mundi 1C 165-99 895/1C 165-99 896. LP (2). *Virtuoso Verziehungskunst um 1600.* Schola Cantorum Basiliensis. 1980 (re. Kirche Rothenfluh, Basel, Switzerland). Texts of vocal works provided in the original languages (Italian, Latin).
Contains motet *Pulchra es amica mea* [arr. Rognoni-Taeggio]; madrigal *Io son ferito* [arr. Bassano].

F0239 Haydn Society HSL 2072. LP. *Masterpieces of Music Before 1750.* Various: for Palestrina selections, Copenhagen Men and Boy's Choir. Moller. ca. 1953–1955 [part of set HSL 2071/3 (HSL-B); also issued on Erato LDE 3018/9, *Histoire de la musique vocale].*
Contains mass *Missa Veni sponsa Christi* [*Agnus Dei I* only].

F0240 Herald 173. CD. *Ave virgo gloriosa.* Cardiff Metropolitan Cathedral Choir. David Neville. 1995.
Contains motets *Dum complerentur dies Pentecostes a 6; Sicut cervus a 4.*

F0241 HMV/His Masters Voice ASD 568. LP. *Carols.* Royal Choral Society. Malcolm Sargent. 1963 [also issued as ALP 2018].
Contains motet *Adoramus te Christe a 4.*

F0242 HMV/His Masters Voice ASD 641. LP. *Music of Byrd and His Contemporaries.* Choir of King's College, Cambridge. David Willcocks. 1965 [also issued on Electrola SME 914 69; and as ALP 2094; also issued also on LP Classics for Pleasure CFP 4144881 (cassette TC-CFP4481, CD as CFP 4481)].
Contains motets *Tu es Petrus a 6; Haec dies quam fecit Dominus a 6.*

F0243 Homochord 4-2941. 12-inch 78 rpm // Munich Cathedral Choir. Berberich. German, before 1936.
Contains motet *Dum complerentur a 6.*

F0244 Hungaroton SLPX 11328. LP. *Missa Sine nomine (Missa Mantovana)*. Györ Girls' Choir. Imre Kalman, Miklos Szabo. 1970s. Program notes by István Barna [also listed as Qualiton SLPX 11328].
Contains mass *Missa sine nomine ("Missa Mantovana")*; motets *Confitemini Domino; Adoramus te Christe; Gloriosi principes terrae; Alma redemptoris mater; Ave regina caelorum; Salve regina; Ave Maria; Sub tuum praesidium; Pueri Hebraeorum; Surrexit pastor bonus; Haec dies.*

F0245 Hungaroton SLPX 11491/3. LP (3). *Musical Life in Old Hungary from the 13th to the 18th Centuries. From the Early Era of Statehood to the Flowering of Transylvania.* Various soloists, Musica Antiqua Wien. Bernhard Klebel [1970s].
Contains motet *Laetus Hyperboream a 5.*

F0246 Hungaroton SLPX 11669/70. LP (2). *The Collection of Bartfa—16th–17th Century Hungarian Music.* Primavera Quintet (Erika Sziklai [sop], Livia Budai [alt]), Camerata Hungarica. Laszlo Czidra. 1970s. Program notes by Z. Falvy in Hungarian with English, German, Russian translations.
Contains madrigal *Vestiva i colli a 5.*

F0247 Hungaroton SLPX 11937. LP. *Magnificat.* Györ Girls' Choir. Miklos Szabo. 1978. Texts included.
Contains magnificat *Magnificat quarti toni* [9:40].

F0248 Hungaroton LPX 11979 and SPLX 11979. LP. *Giovanni Pierluigi da Palestrina. Missa "De Beata Virgine."* Choeur des Jeunesses Musicales de Hongrie. Gábor Ugrin. 1979. Booklet (19pp) with notes by István Homolya in English, German, and French [reissued on CD as HCD 12921, with Claudio Monteverdi, *Sacrae Cantiunculae*].
Contains mass *Missa de Beata Virgine a 6* [2:18 (*Kyrie*); 5:36 (*Gloria*); 8:56 (*Credo*); 4:05 (*Sanctus*); 3:03 (*Benedictus*); 5:55 (*Agnus Dei I* and *II*)]; motets [on LP version] *Sicut cervus a 4*; *Dum aurora finem daret a 4.*

F0249 Hungaroton SLPX 12184. LP. *Baroque Chamber Music.* Various instrumentalists. 1984.
Contains madrigal *Vestiva i colli* [4:52].

F0250 Hyperion CDA 66266. CD. *Palestrina. Missa Papae Marcelli. Missa Brevis.* Choir of Westminster Cathedral. David Hill. 1988 (rec. June 4–6, 1987, Westminster Cathedral). Program notes by Ivan Moody [also issued on Hyperion cassette KA 66266].
Contains masses *Missa Papae Marcelli* [*Kyrie* 4:28; *Gloria* 6:23; *Credo* 9:43; *Sanctus* 3:50; *Benedictus* 4:07; *Agnus Dei I* 4:59; Agnus Dei II 5:01]; *Missa Brevis* [*Kyrie* 3:09; *Gloria* 3:27; *Credo* 6:23; *Sanctus* 3:06; *Benedictus* 3:06; *Agnus Dei* I 4:00; *Agnus Dei II* 5:20].

F0251 Hyperion CDA 66316. CD. *Palestrina. Missa O Rex Gloriae. Missa Viri Galilei.* Westminster Cathedral Choir. James O'Donnell. 1989 (rec. June 22–24, 1988, Westminster Cathedral, London). Program notes by Ivan Moody; texts provided with English translations [also issued on Hyperion cassette KA 66316].

Contains masses *Missa O Rex Gloriae* [24:00]; *Missa Viri Galilaei* [34:00]; motets *O rex gloriae* [3:33]; *Viri Galilaei* [2:58; secunda pars *Ascendit Deus* 3:04].

F0252 Hyperion CDA 66364. CD. *Palestrina. Missae de Beata Virgine & Ave Maria.* Westminster Cathedral Choir. James O' Donnell. 1989 (rec. March 6–9, 1989). Program notes by Ivan Moody; texts provided with English translations [also issued on Hyperion cassette KA 66364].

Contains masses *De beata Virginea 6* (pub. 1570) [40.10]; *Ave Mariaa 4* [33.20].

F0253 Hyperion CDA 66490. CD. *Palestrina. Missa Aeterna Christi munera.* Westminster Cathedral Choir. James O'Donnell. 1991 (rec. February 12–15, 1991, Westminster Cathedral, London). Program notes by Bruno Turner in English, French, German; texts provided with English translations [also issued on cassette KA 66490].

Contains mass *Missa Aeterna Christi munera a 4*; motets *Sicut cervus a 4*; *Super flumina Babylonis a 4*; *Vidi turbam magnum a 6*; *Quae est ista a 5*; *Duo ubera tua a 5*; *Nigra sum, sed formosa a 5*; *Surge, amica mea a 5*; magnificat *Magnificat primi toni.*

F0254 Hyperion CDA 66733. CD. *Palestrina. Canticum Canticorum Salomonis. The Song of Songs.* Pro Cantione Antiqua. Bruno Turner. 1994 (rec. January 4–5, 1994). Program notes (19pp) in English, French, German by Bruno Turner; Latin texts with English translations.

Contains motets *Canticum canticorum*, complete (29 motets a 5).

F0255 Hyperion CDA 66850. CD. *Exultate Deo. Masterpieces of Sacred Polyphony.* Westminster Cathedral Choir, Joseph Cullen [organ]. James O' Donnell. 1995.

Contains motets *Sicut cervus a 4; Exultate Deo a 5; Ave verum corpus a 5.*

F0256 Hyperion CDA 66867. CD. *Holy Week at the Chapel of the Dukes of Braganza.* A Capella Portuguesa. Bernadette Nelson, Owen Rees. ca. 1996.

Contains motet *Fratres ego enim accepi Domino a 8.*

F0257 Hyperion CDA 66994. CD. *Advent at St. Paul's.* St. Paul's Cathedral Choir. John Scott. 1997 (rec. June 23–26, 1997, St. Paul's Cathedral, London).

Contains motet *Mattins responsory* ("after Palestrina") [3:13].

F0258 Hyperion CDA 67099. CD. *Missa Ecce ego Johannes.* Choir of Westminster Cathedral. James O'Donnell. 1997.

Contains mass *Missa Ecce ego Johannes*; motets *Tribulationes civitatum; Tu es Petrus; Peccantem me quotidie; Laudate pueri; Cantantibus organis*; magnificat *Magnificat quarti toni.*

F0259 Hyperion CDD 22028. CD (2). *Second Vespers for the Feast of Santa Barbara.* The Sixteen. Harry Christophers. 1988 (rec. March 28–30, 1988, St. Jude's on the Hill, Hampstead, London). Reconstruction by Graham Dixon of the Monteverdi

Vespers of 1610 as Second Vespers for the Feast of St. Barbara. Contains two sonatas from manuscript compiled in 1613 by Giovanni Amigone, and a Palestrina motet. Program notes (15pp) with texts and English translations [previously released as CDA 66311/2, also issued as cassettes KA 66311/2].
Contains motet *Gaude Barbara a 5.*

F0260 Istituto Internazionale del Disco IM 1001/IDIMS 6001. LP. *Missa Ut re mi fa sol la. Serie Cappella Sistina 1.* Coro della Cappella Sistina. Domenico Bartolucci. 1960s. Notes by Guido Pannain.
Contains masses *Missa Tu es Petrus a 6; Missa Ut re mi fa sol la a 6*; motets *Ad te levavi; Confitebor tibi Domine; Tu es Petrus a 6.*

F0261 Istituto Internazionale del Disco IM 1004/IDIMS 6004. LP. *Improperium. Missa Nigra sum. Serie Cappella Sistina 2.* Coro della Cappella Sistina [Collegio dei cappellani cantori]. Domenico Bartolucci. 1960s. Notes by L. Guadagnino.
Contains mass *Missa Nigra sum a 5*; offertory motet *Improperium expectavit a 5.*

F0262 Istituto Internazionale del Disco IM 1007. LP. *Offertori.* Coro della Cappella Sistina. Domenico Bartolucci. 1960s. Notes by L. Guadagnino.
Contains offertory motets [all a 5]: *Ad te levavi; Dextera Domini; Bonum est confiteri; Meditabor; Laudate Dominum; Confitebor; Terra tremuit; Angelus Domini; Precatus est Moyses; De profundis; Domine Deus; Exaltabo te.*

F0263 Istituto Internazionale del Disco IM 1010. LP. *Missa Papae Marcelli.* Coro della Cappella Sistina. Domenico Bartolucci. 1960s.
Contains mass *Missa Papae Marcelli a 6.*

F0264 JADC 114. CD (2). *Officium tenebrarum.* Cori Spezzati Vocal Ensemble (Harvé Lamy [tenor]). Olivier Opdebeeck. 1994 (rec. 1993, Collègiale Saint-Martin de Champeaux, France). Program notes in French, English, German, Spanish; Latin texts with French, English, Spanish translations. Lessons not set polyphonically by Palestrina are sung as plainchant [also listed as Champeaux CSM 0004].
Contains motet *Stabat Mater a 8*; lamentation *Lamentationes Hieremiae Prophetiae* [Lamentations, Book III, for Matins on Thursday, Friday and Saturday of Holy Week].

F0265 Jade JADC 28337-2. CD. *Canticum canticorum.* William Byrd Ensemble. William O'Reilly. 1995.
Contains motets *Canticum canticorum* (complete, 29 motets a 5).

F0266 Janus JAS 19004. LP. *Missa Brevis.* Le Quatuor Double. Yves Courville. 1965 (rec. Montreal February 20–21, 28, 1965). Program notes by Gilles Potvin [also listed as Pirouette JAS 19004].
Contains mass *Missa Brevis a 4.*

F0267 Kiwi LD-5. LP. *Sacred Polyphony of the XVI Century.* Choir of St. Mary of the Angels, Wellington. Maxwell Fernie. 1960s.

Contains masses *Missa Aeterna Christi munera a 4*; *Missa Brevis a 4*; motet *Diffusa est gratia a 5.*

F0268 Koch 7351. CD. *A Cappella from St. Thomas.* Choir of St. Thomas Church, New York. Gerre Hancock. 1980s.
Contains motets *Sicut cervus a 4*; *Exsultate Deo a 5.*

F0269 Linn Records CKD 052. CD. *The Golden Age, Volume 1: Europe.* Magnificat Ensemble. Philip Cave. 1995 (rec. November 1995, St. Jude's on the Hill, Hampstead).
Contains motet *Stabat Mater* [9:26].

F0270 London (Jubilee) 421 147-2. LP. *Allegri Miserere/Palestrina Stabat Mater.* Choir of King's College, Cambridge. Sir David Willcocks. 1963 (rec. August 1963, King's College Chapel) [also issued as Decca 421147–2 on LP, and on CD in 1988].
Contains motets *Stabat mater* a 8 [12.49]; *Hodie beata Virgo a 5* [4.21]; *Senex puerum portabat a 5* [4.59]; *Magnificat primi toni a 8* [6.12]; litany *Litaniae de BVM a 8* [15.46].

F0271 London OS 25118. LP. *Music for the Feast of Christmas.* Choristers of Ely Cathedral, Renaissance Singers. Michael Howard. 1960s.
Contains mass *Missa Dies sanctificatus a 4.*

F0272 Lumen 324 002. 12-inch 78 rpm // Paraphonistes de St. Jean-de-Matines. G. DeVan. Before 1942 [older numbering 32054].
Contains lamentation *Incipit oratio Jeremiae.*

F0273 Lyrichord LL 35. LP. *Motets for Christmas and Other Festivities.* Welch Chorale. James B. Welch. 1950. Program notes and texts on sleeve.
Contains motets *Hodie Christus natus est a 8; Rorate coeli desuper a 5; Dies sanctificatus a 4.*

F0274 Lyrichord LL 49. LP. *Giovanni Pierluigi Palestrina. Missa "Iste Confessor." Missa sine nomine (super modulum "Je suis désheritée").* Welch Chorale. James B. Welch. 1952. Text and English translation on sleeve [also released as Brunswick AXL 3016].
Contains masses *Missa Iste Confessor a 4*; *Missa Sine nomine a 4.*

F0275 Lyrichord LL 52. LP. *Motets of the Fifteenth and Sixteenth Centuries with Easter Themes.* Welch Chorale. James B. Welch. ca. 1954. Contains notes and English translations of texts.
Contains motets *Super flumina Babylonis a 4*; *Tu es Petrus a 6*; *Sicut cervus a 4*; *Haec dies quam fecit Dominus a 6.*

F0276 Lyrichord LLST 7247. LP. *Missa "Alleluya."* Wellesley Choir Singers. Peter Sipple (rec. 1976). Sleeve notes by Owen Jander.
Contains mass *Missa Già fu chi m'ebbe cara a 4*; madrigal *Già fu chi m'ebbe cara a 4.*

F0277 Lyrichord LLST 7249. LP. *Sing Joyfully.* St. Luke's Chapel of Men and Boys. Clifford Clark. ca. 1975. Compiled from tapes of live performances. Texts printed on sleeve.
Contains motet *Rorate coeli desuper a 5.*

F0278 Melodiya SM 020323/4. LP. // Tallinn Chamber Choir. ca. 1954.
Contains mass *Aeterna Christi munera a 4.*

F0279 Melodiya SM 02889/90. LP. // Chamber Choir "Ave Sol." ca. 1956.
Contains madrigal *I vaghi fior a 4.*

F0280 Mercury MG 10063. LP. *Sacred Music of the Renaissance.* Roman Vatican Choir. Msgr. Licinio Refice. 1947 [*Lamentations* are reissue of selection in SEVA 19; *Regina coeli* is from SEVA 18, which may be directed either by Refice or by Boezi].
Contains motets *Regina coeli laetare a 8; Super flumina Babylonis*; lamentations *Incipit oratio Jeremiae* [*Recordare; Aegyptae de dimus manum; Servi dominati sunt; Jerusalem*].

F0281 Meridian E4577069. LP. *Palestrina and His Successors.* Choir of St. John's College, Cambridge (Adrian Lucas [organ]). George Guest. 1982 (St. John's College, Cambridge). Program notes by Graham Dixon; texts provided with English translations.
Contains motet *Exsultate Deo* [2:33]; hymn *Pange lingua* [8:30].

F0282 Music Library Records ML 5001. LP. // *Stanford University Choir.* Stanford University Choir. No director listed. ca. 1950–1951.
Contains motet *Sicut cervus a 4.*

F0283 Music Library Records ML 7022. LP. *Madrigals and Motets.* Stanford University Chorus. Schmidt. ca. 1950–1955.
Contains motet *Super flumina Babylonis.*

F0284 Music Library Records MLR 7085. LP. *Motets and Carols.* Catawba Choir. Robert Weaver. 1950s.
Contains motet *Ad te levavi oculos meos a 4.*

F0285 Musical Heritage Society MHS 3291. LP. *Lamentations of Jeremiah.* Harvard Glee Club. F. John Adams. 1976 (rec. March/May 1974, St. Paul's Church, Cambridge, MA).
Contains lamentations *Lamentations of Jeremiah* [*Lamed; Matribus suis*].

F0286 Musical Heritage Society MHS 4850Z. LP. *Masters of the High Renaissance.* Pro Cantione Antiqua. Mark Brown. 1983. Contains anonymous notes; Latin texts with English translations.
Contains motet *Dies sanctificatus a 4.*

F0287 Musical Heritage Society MHS 6345. LP. *A Cappella Motets.* Philippe Caillard Vocal Ensemble. Philippe Caillard. 1966. Program notes by Bernard Vincent,

with English translation by Herman Adler on sleeve; Latin texts with English translations inserted [reissue of Erato LDE 3188].
Contains motet *Ego sum panis vivus a 4.*

F0288 Musique au Vatican 1116. 12-inch 78 rpm // Cappella Giulia Choir. Ernesto Boezi. Before 1948 [also listed as Odeon EMS 8].
Contains Improperia *Popule meus a 8* [2 sides].

F0289 Musique au Vatican 1162. 12-inch 78 rpm // Cappella Giulia. Ernesto Boezi. Before 1948 [from series MV 1159-1162; this disc also numbered Odeon EMS 3].
Contains motet *O quantus luctus hominum.*

F0290 Musique au Vatican 1186. 12-inch 78 rpm // Cappella Giulia. Monsignor Antonelli. Before 1948.
Contains motet *Pueri Hebraeorum a 4.*

F0291 Musique au Vatican 1187. 12-inch 78 rpm // Cappella Giulia. Ernesto Boezi. Before 1948.
Contains motet *Tota pulchra es a 5* [with Goudimel *Videntes stellam*; see SEMS 41, item F0385].

F0292 Musique au Vatican 1189. 12-inch 78 rpm // Cappella Giulia. Ernesto Boezi [also listed as Odeon EMS 38; on this release, *Introduxit me rex* is paired with Victoria's *O Domine Jesu*].
Contains motets *Improperium exspectavit a 5*; *Introduxit me rex in cellam a 5.*

Musique au Vatican—see also **SEMS**.

F0293 Muza N 0374. 7-inch 45 rpm *Crucifixus. Chor Chlopiecy I Muski Panstwowej Filharmonii Poznaniu* [Boys' and Men's Choir of the Philharmonia of Poznan]. Stefan Stuligrosz. 1960s.
Contains mass *Missa Papae Marcelli a 6* [*Kyrie*].

F0294 Muza SXL 0969. LP. *Renesansowe madrigaly I chansons.* Cantores Minores Wratislavienses. Edmund Kajdasz. 1970s.
Contains madrigals *I vaghi fior a 4*; *O che splendor a 4.*

F0295 Muza SXL 1146. LP. *Missa Papae Marcelli. Stabat Mater.* Cantores Minores Wratislavienses. Edmund Kajdasz. 1970s.
Contains mass *Missa Papae Marcelli a 6*; motet *Stabat Mater a 8.*

F0296 Muza SXL 1389. LP. *Missa Tu es Petrus.* Cantores Minores Wratislavienses. Edmund Kajdasz. 1970s.
Contains mass *Missa Tu es Petrus a 6.*

F0297 Muza XL 0164. LP. *Poznan Nightingales are Singing.* Boys' and Men's Choir of the Philharmonia of Poznan. Stefan Stuligrosz. 1960s.
Contains mass *Missa Papae Marcelli a 6* [*Sanctus*].

F0298 National Catholic Recordings NCR 1050. 12-inch 78 rpm // St. Francis de Sales Church Choir. No director listed [later 1930s].
Contains motet *O bone Jesu.*

F0299 Naxos 8.550572. CD. *Lesson I for Maundy Thursday.* Oxford Camerata. Jeremy Summerly. 1992.
Contains lamentations *Lesson I for Maundy Thursday*; *Lesson III for Maundy Thursday.*

F0300 Naxos 8.550573. CD. *Palestrina: Missa Papae Marcelli; Missa Aeterna Christi Munera.* Oxford Camerata. Jeremy Summerly. 1992 (rec. September 24–25, 1991; Dorchester Abbey, Oxfordshire). Liner notes (2pp.) by Jeremy Summerly.
Contains masses *Missa Papae Marcelli* [4:31; 5:30; 8:28; 8:49; 7:49]; *Missa Aeterna Christi munera* [2:07; 2:51; 5:05; 5:01; 4:53].

F0301 Naxos 8.550836. CD. *Early Music: Palestrina and Lassus.* Schola Cantorum of Oxford. Jeremy Summerly. 1993. Liner notes by Jeremy Summerly [also issued on cassette].
Contains mass *Missa Hodie Christus natus est a 8*; motet *Stabat mater a 8.*

F0302 Naxos 8.553238. CD. *Palestrina/Allegri: Choral Works.* Oxford Camerata (1), Schola Cantorum of Oxford (2). Jeremy Summerly. 1991 (1); 1993 (March 14–16) (2); Chapel of Hertford College, Oxford (2). Anonymous liner notes reprint those of Naxos 8.550573 (see item F0296) plus additional material on *Stabat mater* and Allegri's *Miserere*, which is also included here.
(1) *Missa Papae Marcelli* and *Missa Aeterna Christi munera* are apparently a reissue of Naxos 8.550573 (item F0300). (2*) Stabat mater* [9:14] is apparently a reissue of Naxos 8.550836 (item F0301) [cassette].

F0303 Naxos 8.553313. CD. *Palestrina. Missa de Beata Virgine.* Soloists of Cappella Musicale di S. Petronio di Bologna, Liuew Tamminga, organ. Sergio Vartolo. 1995.
Contains mass *Missa de Beata Virgine.*

F0304 Naxos 8.553314. CD. *Missa sine nomine, Missa L'homme armé, Three Motets.* Soloists of the Cappella Musicale di S. Petronio di Bologna; Liuwe Tamminga, organ. Sergio Vartolo. 1995 (rec. October 1995, Chiesa di S. Zeno a Cavalo, Verona).
Contains masses *Missa sine nomine a 4* (Not the mass a 6 as the cover indicates); *Missa L'homme armé a 4*; motets *Sicut cervus; Super flumina Babylonis*; *Peccantem me quotidie.*

F0305 Newport Classic NPD 85603. CD. *Musica Dei: God's Music.* Amor Artis Chamber Choir (Cynthia Richard Wallace [sop], Megan Friar [mezzo], Thom Baker [tenor], Richard Holmes [bass-bar]). Johannes Somary. 1994, St. Jean Baptiste Church, New York City.
Contains mass *Missa Regina coeli*; motets *Sicut cervus; Alma redemptoris mater; Surge, illuminare; Unus ex discipulis.*

F0306 Nimbus NI 1758. CD (5). *European Choral Music 1525–1751.* Christ Church Cathedral Choir, Oxford. Stephen Darlington.

An anthology compiled from individual Nimbus releases. See NI 5100, item F0307, and NI 5394, item F0308.

F0307 Nimbus NI 5100. CD. *Palestrina. Mass for Pentecost and Motets.* Christ Church Cathedral Choir, Oxford. Stephen Darlington. 1987 (rec. November 16–17, 1987, Dorchester Abbey, Oxfordshire). Program notes (14pp) notes by John Milsom, including Latin texts with English translations [also issued in NI 1758 (disc 2 of 5-disc set). On both releases, the *Missa Dum complerentur* is listed as the "Mass for Pentecost"].

Contains mass *Missa Dum complerentur* [33.40 total: 5:08; 6:50; 9:23; 4:06; 2:35; 2:41; 2:57]; motets *Super flumina Babylonis* [4.32]; *Exsultate Deo* [4.32]; *Sicut cervus* [3.23]; *O bone Jesu, exaudi me* [3.43]; *Dum complerentur dies Pentecostes* [6.41]

F0308 NI 5394. CD. *Palestrina. Missa O sacrum convivium.* Christ Church Cathedral Choir, Oxford. Stephen Darlington. 1993 (May 10–11). Liner notes by Andrew Carwood [also issued in NI 1758 (disc 3 of 5-disc set)].

Contains mass *Missa O sacrum convivium* [30:50 total: 3:41; 6:15; 8:08; 4:25; 3:20; 5:01]; motets *O sacrum convivium* [5:00]*; Coenantibus illis* [5:41]; magnificat *Magnificat sexti toni a 6* [11:48]. Additional contents include Morales, motet *O sacrum convivium* [4:40] (the model on which the Palestrina mass is based).

Nixa—see **Period**

F0309 Nonesuch 71407. LP. *Pope Marcellus Mass/Palestrina.* Pro Cantione Antiqua. Bruno Turner. 1978. Liner notes by Daniel Schillaci [recording made 1978 by P.C. A.; issued by Nonesuch 1982].

Contains mass *Missa Papae Marcelli a 6* [30:46]; motets *Dominus Jesus in qua nocte* [4:16]*; Alma redemptoris mater* [2:27]*; Peccantem me quotidie* [14:26]; *Stabat Mater* [9:25].

F0310 Nonesuch HC 3014 and HC-73014 A-F. LP (3). *Music at the Courts: Italy, Sweden, France. 16th to 18th Centuries.* Camerata Lutetiensis, Le Rondeau de Paris. 1967. Works performed by Camerata Lutetiensis on side 1 of set in arrangements for a set of viols. Detailed liner notes in English by Robert Erich Wolf.

Contains ricercari 1. Dorian [2:54]; 2. Hypodorian [2:36]; 3. Phrygian [3:31]; 4. Hypophrygian [2:59]; 5. Lydian [2:22]; 6. Hypolydian [3:39]; 7. Mixolydian [3:00]; 8. Hypomixolydian [3:21].

F0311 Novello NVLCD 102. CD. *Lamentations of Jeremiah.* Pro Cantione Antiqua. Bruno Turner. 1989 (rec. January 15–17, 1988, St. Alban's Church, Tooting, London.) Program notes by Bruno Turner. This disc is a recording based on manuscript in I-Rvat Cod. Ottobon. 3387. Latin texts with English translations included.

Contains Lamentations (complete).

F0312 Nuova Era 7257. CD. *Beata es Virgo Maria. Devozione mariana nel Rinascimento.* Corale Universitaria di Torino. Dario Tabbia. 1996 (rec. April to Novem-

ber, 1993, Chiesa della Misericordia, Turin). Latin texts with English, French, Italian trans. in container.
Contains magnificat *Magnificat quinti toni* no.2.

F0313 Odeon 80993. 10-inch 78 rpm // Sistine Choir. Raffaele Casimiri. Date not known; possibly a French or Italian issue associated with Casimiri Parlophone series of 1920s.
Contains motet *Sicut cervus a 4.*

F0314 Odeon EMS 1. 12-inch 78 rpm // Cappella Giulia Choir. Ernesto Boezi. ca. 1935.
Contains motet *Super flumina Babylonis a 4.*

F0315 Oiseau-Lyre CD 414 277-2OH. CD. // Amsterdam Loeki Stardust Quartet. 1991.
Contains ricercar *Ricercar del secondo tuono* [secundi toni, arranged].

F0316 Oiseau-Lyre CD 430 246-2. CD. *Italian Recorder Music.* Amsterdam Loeki Stardust Quartet. 1991. Notes by Clifford Bartlett.
Contains lamentation *Lamentationes Hieremiae* [arranged] [4:46].

F0317 Oiseau-Lyre OLS 153. LP. // Ambrosian Singers. John McCarthy. 1968.
Contains motets *Ad te levavi*; *Ave Maria.*

F0318 Oiseau-Lyre OL 269. LP. *Mass. Sine nomine. Mass. Ecce ego Joannes.* Carmelite Priory of London Choir. John McCarthy. 1964. Program notes by John Buttrey on sleeve.
Contains masses *Missa Ecce ego Joannes; Missa sine nomine (Je suis désheritée).*

F0319 Oiseau-Lyre OL 283 and **SOL 283**. LP. *Masters of the Renaissance. Victoria and Palestrina.* Choir of the Carmelite Priory of London (Henry Washington, organ). John McCarthy. 1965. Contains liner notes by John Buttrey.
Contains motets *Surge illuminare Jerusalem; Ave Regina a 4*; hymn *Veni Sancte Spiritus a 8*; magnificat *Magnificat primi toni.*

F0320 Oiseau-Lyre R 145. LP. *Music for Holy Week.* Ambrosian Singers. John McCarthy. 1968 (Also listed as Delyse DS3200).
Contains motets *Pueri Hebraeorum a 4; Improperia.*

F0321 Oiseau-Lyre SOL 293. LP. // Choir of the Carmelite Priory of London. John McCarthy. Mid-1960s.
Contains hymn *Veni sancte Spiritus.*

F0322 Oiseau-Lyre SOL 338-339. LP (2). *The Garden of Love. Palestrina: The Song of Songs.* Cantores in Ecclesia. Michael Howard. 1974. Liner notes by Michael Howard in English, French, German; texts of motets and translations into English, French, German provided.
Contains motets *Canticum canticorum*, complete (29 motets a 5).

F0323 Opal 823. LP. *Alessandro Moreschi. The Last Castrato. Complete Vatican Recordings.* Alessandro Moreschi, various soloists, Cappella Sistina Choir, others. Baron Kanzler and others. 1984. Collection of recordings made in 1902 and 1904 for the Red G & T and Black G & T labels (Victor production). Liner notes by John Wolfson and a historical article by Elsa Scammell. An issue of this recording was circulating in the 1920s and early 1930s but was apparently withdrawn before 1936 [see item F0214]. Moreschi sings the canto line, while three other singers (identities unknown but very likely from the Sistine Chapel) perform the other parts [also issued on CD as Opal 9823].

Contains madrigal *La cruda mia nemica a 4.*

F0324 Open University OUA 201. LP. *Renaissance Music.* The Linden Singers (Ursula Connors [sop], Elizabeth Harrison [sop], Jean Temperley [alt], Wynford Evans [ten], Ian Humphris [bar], John Huw Davies [bass]). Dinah Barsham. 1972. Recording which accompanied correspondence course material in Open University Arts Second Level course, *Renaissance and Reformation*, units 17–19, Renaissance Music.

Contains mass *Missa Aeterna Christi munera [Kyrie, Gloria, Sanctus, Benedictus, Hosanna* only].

F0325 Opus Musicum OM 101/03. LP. *Die Messe/The Mass.* Pro Musica Köln. Johannes Hömberg. 1978. Palestrina selection is on disc OM 102, side 1, band 1. Historical notes in German on the mass (14pp) by Johannes Hömberg, with English translation by A. C. Howie [stereo version OM 201/03].

Contains mass *Missa Assumpta est Maria a 6* [*Kyrie* only] [4:50].

F0326 Orfeo Records 1003. 12-inch 78 rpm // Trapp Chorus. No director listed [Franz Wasner?]. ca. 1951–1952.

Contains mass *Missa brevis a 4* [*Introit, Kyrie, Agnus Dei* only].

F0327 Oryx EXP 36. LP. *Sixteenth Century Music.* Les Petits Chanteurs de Mont-Royal. Leandre Brault. 1970 [also listed as Peerless EXP 36].

Contains mass *Missa Lauda Sion a 4* [*Sanctus* only]; motet *Praecatus est Moyses a 5.*

F0328 Overtone LP 4-5. LP. *Yale University Volumes I and II.* Yale University Music School Chorus. Paul Hindemith. 1953–1955.

Contains [Volume II] mass *Missa Sine nomine* [*Credo* only].

F0329 Paraclete/Gloria Dei Cantores GD CD 002. CD. *Gloriae Dei Cantores: Easter Day Mass.* Gloriae Dei Cantores (James E. Jordan [organ]). Elizabeth C. Patterson. 1996.

Contains mass *Missa Aeterna Christi munera a 4.*

F0330 Paraclete/Gloria Dei Cantores GDCD 013. *Prince of Music.* Gloriae Dei Cantores. Elizabeth Patterson [also issued on cassette GDC 013]. 1997.

Contains masses *Missa de beata Virgine II* [Mantuan]*; Missa Descendit angelus Domini*; motets *Super flumina Babylonis; Ad te levavi; Misereri nostri, Domine; Sicut cervus; Sitivit anima mea; Jubilate Deo.*

F0331 Parlophone E3185. 10-inch 78 rpm (1/2 side). // Westminster Cathedral Choir [Sir Richard Terry?]. Before 1936.
Contains motet *O salutaris hostia.*

F0332 Parlophone E10804. 12-inch 78 rpm // Chorus of La Scala, Milan. Vittorio Veneziani. Before 1936 [also listed as Odeon 123677].
Contains motet *Tenebrae factae sunt.*

F0333 Parlophone R20001. 12-inch 78 rpm [acoustic] // Sistine Chapel Choir. Raffaele Casimiri. 1920s [*Laudate Dominum* also issued Brunswick 50125, see item F0077].
Contains motets *Exultate Deo; Laudate Dominum.*

F0334 Parlophone R20002. 12-inch 78 rpm [acoustic]. // Sistine Chapel Choir. Raffaele Casimiri. 1920s.
Contains motets *Confitebor tibi Domine; Bonum est* [1 side each].

F0335 Parlophone R20004. 12-inch 78 rpm [acoustic]. // Sistine Chapel Choir. Raffaele Casimiri. 1920s.
Contains motet *Tribulationes civitatum* [secunda pars *Peccavimus*].

F0336 Parlophone R20006. 12-inch 78 rpm [acoustic]. // Sistine Chapel Choir. Raffaele Casimiri. 1920s.
Contains motet *Introduxit me rex.*

F0337 Parlophone RD 108. 10-inch 78 rpm // Turin Seminary Choir. Pistone. Date not known, before 1950 [Italian Cetra issue].
Contains motet *Hodie Christus natus est a 8* [III].

F0338 Parlophone RD 562. 12-inch 78 rpm Choir of the Accademia Santa Cecilia. Bonaventura Somma. ca. 1948 [older numbering PE 117].
Contains madrigal: *Ahi, che quest'occhi miei a 3.*

F0339 Pathé PA 2059.10-inch 78 rpm // Vienna Boy's Choir. Ferdinand Grossman. ca. 1950.
Contains motet *Salvator mundi a 4.*

F0340 Pathé PAT 63. 12-inch 78 rpm *Three Centuries of Organ Music.* André Marchal, Charles Hens et al. [organ]. Late 1930s [in series PAT 62/73].
Contains unspecified ricercar [perf. André Marchal].

F0341 Pathé PDT 95/9.12-inch 78 rpm // Les Chanteurs de St.-Eustache. Père Émile Martin. ca. 1942–1948 [set also associated with a spoken introduction, "Prestige de la messe" by Fr. Joseph Samson, on PDT 94. 10 sides in toto; reissued on LP as Pathé QTX 213; American Vox PTL 6790 ca. 1950–1951].
Contains mass *Missa Papae Marcelli a 6.*

F0342 Pathé PDT 220. 12-inch 78 rpm // Les Chanteurs de St.-Eustache. Père Émile Martin. ca. 1950.
Contains motet *Assumpta est Maria a 6.*

F0343 Pathé PDT 273. 12-inch 78 rpm // International Boys' Choir. Maillet. 1951. Note indicates this recording was made during mass at St. Peter's, Rome, on April 1, 1951; choir composed of about 3000 voices.
Containts motet *Sicut cervus a 4.*

F0344 Pathé X 93051. 12-inch 78 rpm (1/2 side). // Schola St. Léon IX de Nancy. Abbé Gaudard. Before 1936.
Contains motet *O bone Jesu a 6.*

F0345 Pathé X 93055. 12-inch 78 rpm // Schola St. Léon IX de Nancy. Abbé Gaudard. Before 1936.
Contains motet *Alma redemptoris mater.*

F0346 Pathé X 93085. 10-inch 78 rpm // Paris Teachers' Chorus. R. Ducasse. Before 1936.
Contains unspecified madrigal, sung in French.

F0347 Pavane ADW 7343. CD. *Russki Partes Choral Ensemble.* Russki Partes. Pekalitski. 1996.
Contains mass *Missa L'homme armé a 5*; madrigal *Alla riva del Tebro.*

F0348 Period/Nixa SPLP 513. LP. *A Concert of a Capella Music for Treble Voices.* Period Choral Society. Robert Strassburg. ca. 1953–1955. Some of these items are arranged for female voices only. Program notes, Latin texts with English translations on sleeve [also issued as Classic CLC 6138; Concerteum CPR 318].
Contains masses *Missa Descendit angelus Domini* [*Benedictus* only]; *Missa O rex gloriae* [*Crucifixus* only]; *Missa Sacerdotes Domini a 6* [*Pleni sunt coeli* only]; motets *Confitemini Domino; Hodie Christus natus est; Salve Regina a 5; Adoremus te Christe; Confitemini Domino; Jesu rex admirabilis a 3; Tua Jesu dilectio a 3*; magnificat *Magnificat quarti toni.*

F0349 Period/Nixa PLP 586. LP. *Old Italian Masters.* Flor Peeters [organ] [also issued as Contrepoint MC 20048; possibly reissued on Vanguard (1950s)].
Contains ricercar *Ricercare primi toni*.

F0350 Period PRST 2856. LP. // Coro della Cappella del Duomo di Treviso. Giovanni d'Alessi. 1950s.
Contains mass *Missa Sine nomine* ["*Je suis deshéritée*"].

F0351 Period SPL 597. LP. *Renaissance Music.* New York Primavera Singers. Noah Greenberg. 1954. Texts with English translations on sleeve; Dover reissue contains booklet with notes by Edward Lerner, as well as Latin texts and English translations [also issued as Contrepoint MC 20077; also as Dover HCR 5248 in 1965].
Contains motet *Assumpta est Maria* [4:25].

F0352 Period SPL 706. LP. *Tomas Louis de Victoria* [*sic*]. Sistine Chapel Choir. Domenico Bartolucci. 1954. Program notes by Bernard Lebow; Latin texts with English translations.
Contains motet *Sicut cervus a 4*; offertory *Improperium expectavit.*

F0353 Period SPL 744. LP. *Exaltabo te and Other Works*. Sistine Chapel Choir. Domenico Bartolucci. 1950s. Program notes by Bernard Lebow. Texts and English translations on sleeve.

Contains offertory motets (all a 5) *Exaltabo te; Bonum est confiteri; Laudate Dominum; Super flumina Babylonis; Pueri Hebraeorum*; motets *Dies sanctificatus; Popule meus* [Haberl XXXI 171–172]*; Tota pulchra es; Vox dilecti mei; Hodie Christus natus est; Tribulationes civitatum; Exsultate Deo.*

F0354 Philips A 00105L. LP. *Missa Papae Marcelli*. Netherlands Chamber Choir. Felix de Nobel. ca. 1951–1952 [reissued on Epic LC 3045 (ca. 1953–1955) as part of anthology].

Contains mass *Missa Papae Marcelli a 6.*

F0355 Philips A 00272L. LP. *Missa brevis. Missa ad fugam*. Netherlands Chamber Choir. Felix de Nobel. Early 1950s [reissued on Epic LC 3359].

Contains masses *Missa Ad fugam a 4; Missa Brevis a 4.*

F0356 Philips E 10003. 10-inch 78 rpm // Breda Choir. Before 1942.

Contains motet *Alleluia! Tulerunt Dominum.*

F0357 Philips NBL 5033. LP. *Palestrina Masses*. Netherlands Chamber Choir. Felix de Nobel. 1956 [see EPIC LC 3045 and EPIC LC 3359].

Contains masses *Missa Ad fugam a 4; Missa Brevis a 4; Missa Papae Marcelli a 6.*

F0358 Philips RGD 462862. CD (2). *The Best of the Renaissance. Tallis Scholars*. The Tallis Scholars. Peter Philips. 1999.

Contains mass *Missa Papae Marcelli a 6.*

F0359 Pierre Verany PVY 794041. CD. *Motets and Madrigals*. Akademia—Regional Vocal Ensemble de Champagne-Ardenne. Françoise Lasserre. 1994 (Convent of the Annunciation Dominican Church, Paris). Program notes (5pp) by Noel O'Regan.

Contains motets *Ave Maria; Salve Regina; Ave mundi spes; Ave regina coelorum; Alma redemptoris mater; Regina coeli laetare; Salve regina*; spiritual madrigals *Vergine bella; Vergine saggia; Vergine pura; Vergine santa; Vergine sola; Vergine chiara; Vergine, quante lagrime; Vergine, tale è terra*; magnificat *Magnificat primi toni.*

F0360 Pierre Verany PVY 795092. CD. *Giovanni Pierluigi da Palestrina. Canticum canticorum*. Akademia—Ensemble Vocal Regional de Champagne-Ardenne. Françoise Lasserre. 1995. Program notes (4pp) by Alain de Chambure.

Contains motets *Canticum canticorum* [complete, 29 motets a 5]

F0361 Pilz 44 2070 2. CD. *Famous a Capella Choruses*. Berlin Radio Choir. Dietrich Knothe. 1990s.

Contains mass *Missa Tu es Petrus a 6* [24:09].

F0362 Pleaides P 247-252. LP (12). *Historical Anthology of Music in Performance*. Various performers. 1969–1976 [recording of the *Historical Anthology of Music*, ed. Willi Apel].

Volume 6 (P251) contains mass *Missa Papae Marcelli* [*Agnus Dei I* only]; motet *Sicut cervus a 4*; madrigal *Alla riva del Tebro a 4*.

F0363 Polskie Nagrania PNCD 086. CD. // Cantores Minores Wratislavienses. Edmund Kajdasz. 1974 and 1976, Polish Radio Studio, Wroclaw [this version is apparently a reissue of performances on at least two LPs].

Contains masses *Missa Papae Marcelli a 6; Missa Tu es Petrus a 6*; motet *Tu es Petrus a 6*.

F0364 Polydor 22528. 10-inch 78 rpm // Paderborn Cathedral Choir. Gustav Schauerte. Before 1936.

Contains motet *O admirabile commercium a 5*.

F0365 Polydor 249 182. LP. *Advent mit dem Regensburger Domspatzen*. Regensburger Domspatzen. Hans Schrems. 1970s.

Contains mass *Missa Lauda Sion a 4* [*Benedictus* only].

F0366 [PRIVATE ISSUE] Benedictines of St. Benoit du Lac. Set III. 12-inch 78 rpm LP. [rereleased on LP MG1205?]. "Messe du Sacre Coeur." Probably released ca. 1950.

Contains motet *Jesu, rex admirabilis*; lamentation *Pars mea*.

F0367 [PRIVATE ISSUE] University of the South. LP. *University of the South*. University of the South Chorus. McConnell. ca. 1951–1952.

Contains hymn *Veni Creator Spritus a 4*.

F0368 RAI CT 7013-7014. LP [blank cover]. Coro di Roma della RAI, dir. Nino Antonellini [mass]; Coro di Torino della RAI, dir. Ruggero Maghini. 1970. Recording issued in conjunction with publication of the Bianchi/Fellerer biography *Palestrina* of 1971.

Contains mass *Missa Hodie Christus natus est a 8* [22:15]; motets [from *Canticum canticorum*, all a 5]: *Nigra sum; Vox dilecti mei; Dilectus meus mihi; Introduxit me rex; Vulnerasti cor meum; Surge amica mea* [18:10 total].

F0369 RCA RL 30 780 AS. LP. *Ein festliches Weihnachtkonzert aus dem Petersdom Rom*. Kammerorchester Rom, Chor der Cappella Sistina (Ingeborg Hallstein [sop], Flavio Benedetti Michelangeli [organ]). Quinzio Petrocchi, Domenico Bartolucci. Before 1984 [also issued on cassette RK 30 780 CT].

Contains motet *Hodie Christus natus est a 8*.

F0370 Regent REGFCM 103/4/5. CD (3). *Palestrina: Complete Four-Part Madrigals*. Consort Ars Music. Rafaello Monterosso. 1997.

Contains the complete production of four-part madrigals [including Book I (1555), Book II (1586), and the madrigals found in anthologies].

F0371 Renaissance X 55. LP. *The Choir of the Sistine Chapel*. Sistine Chapel Choir. Domenico Bartolucci. ca. 1950 [also issued on LP as Contrepoint MC 20066 ca. 1953–1955].

Contains motets *Dies sanctificatus; Exsultate Deo; Hodie Christus natus est; Pueri Hebraeorum; Super flumina Babylonis; Tribulationes; Peccavimus* [secunda pars of *Tribulationes*]; *Tota pulchra es; Vox dilecti mea; Bonum est confiteri; Exultabo te Domine; Laudate Dominum*; Improperia *Popule meus.*

F0372 Ricercar RIC 8029. CD. *Missa Assumpta est Maria. Motets.* La Chapelle Royale de Paris. Phillippe Herreweghe. 1980 (rec. July 14–16, 1980, Temple des Billettes, Paris). Liner notes by Philippe Beaussant and Jérome Lejeune [also listed as RIC 008, or as 241162].

Contains mass *Missa Assumpta est Maria* [24:00]; motets *O bone Jesu* [2:15]; *Peccantem me quotidie* [3:10]; *Ave Maria* [3:05]; *Sicut cervus* [2:16; secunda pars *Sitivit anima mea* 2:27]; *O beata et gloriosa Trinitas* [3:12; secunda pars *O vera summa* 2:55].

F0373 Ricercar RIC 152663. CD. *Motetti, Madrigali e Canzoni Francesi.* François Fauche [bass], Ensemble La Fenice (Jean Tubery [cornett/vornet muet/recorder], Christina Pluhar [triple harp], Matthias Spaeter [archlute], Jean-Marc Aymes [organ/harpsichord]). n.d. [Also numbered RIC 245132].

Contains madrigals *Io son ferito, ahi lasso; Vestiva i colli; Io son ferito; Vestiva i colli* [arranged]; ricercar *Ricercare*; motet *Pulchra es amica mea*; *Pulchra es amica mea* [arranged].

F0374 St. Olaf 3. LP. *St. Olaf Choir.* St. Olaf Choir. O.C. Christiansen. ca. 1950–1951.

Contains motet *Hodie Christus natus est.*

F0375 Sarx SX 010-2. CD. Giovanni Pierluigi da Palestrina. Missa Pro Defunctis. Motetti. Ars Cantica. Marco Berrini. 1995.

Contains motets *Domine, quando veneris; Commissa mea pavesco; Heu mihi Domine; Anima mea turbata est; Super flumina Babylonis; Ecce nunc benedicite; Ad te levavi oculos meos; Miserere nostri Domine; Ad Dominum cum tribularer; Sagittae potentis acutae; Fundamenta eius; Numquid Sion; Quia vidisti me, Thoma; Ego sum panis vivus; Sicut cervus* [secunda pars *Sitivit anima mea*]; mass *Pro defunctis* [Antiphona ad introitum; Kyrie; Gratualia; Tractus De profundis clamavi; Offertorium Domine Jesu Christe; Sanctus; Benedictus; Agnus Dei I, II, III].

F0376 Sarx SX026-2. CD. *Giovanni Pierluigi da Palestrina. Motecta Festorum Totius Anni [1].* Collegium Vocale "Nova Ars Cantandi." Giovanni Acciai. Late 1990s.

Contains motets (all *a 4*) *Dies sanctificatus* [3:02]; *Lapidabant Stephanum* [3:56]; *Valde honorandum est* [3:19]; *Magnum haereditatis mysterium* [3:27]; *Tribus miraculis* [3:56]; *Hodie beata virgo* [3:19]; *Jesus iunxit se* [3:56]; *O rex gloriae* [3:30]; *Loquebantur* [4:01]; *Benedicta sit* [3:51]; *Fuit homo* [3:19]; *Tu es pastor ovium* [3:15]; *Magnus Sanctus Paulus* [3:42]; *Surge propera* [3:28]; *Beatus Laurentius* [3:45]; *Quae est ista* [3:35].

F0377 Schwann SCH 317962. CD. [title]. Montserrat Capella, Montserrat Esolania. Ireneu Segarra. 1990s.

Contains mass *Missa De Beata Virgine a 6.*

F0378 Seraphim S-60187. LP. *Missa Papae Marcelli. Missa Brevis.* Choir of King's College, Cambridge. David Willcocks. 1972. Notes by Alec Robertson; texts provided with English translations [also issued as EMI CSD 1237; EMI 1C 063–02113].
Contains masses *Missa Papae Marcelli* [32:39]*; Missa Brevis* [25:00].

F0379 SEVA set 18. 10-inch 78 rpm // Vatican Singers. Ernesto Boezi. Date? [1948 source says Roman Vatican Choir—Refice].
Contains motet *Regina coeli a 8.*

F0380 SEVA set 19. 10-inch 78 rpm // Roman Vatican Singers. Licino Refice. Before 1948.
Contains lamentations *Incipit oratio Jeremiae.*

F0381 SEMS/Musique au Vatican 1. 12-inch 78 rpm // Cappella Giulia. Ernesto Boezi. ca. 1935.
Contains offertory motet *Super flumina Babylonis* [with Victoria *Tenebrae*, directed by Antonelli].

F0382 SEMS/Musique au Vatican 2. 12-inch 78 rpm // Cappella Giulia. Ernesto Boezi. ca. 1936–1942 [also listed as Odeon EMS 2].
Contains motet *Laudate pueri Dominum a 8.*

F0383 SEMS/Musique au Vatican 8. 12-inch 78 rpm // Cappella Giulia Choir. Ernesto Boezi. ca. 1936–1942.
Contains motet *Improperium exspectavit* [with Victoria *O vos omnes*].

F0384 SEMS 11/Musique au Vatican 1155. 12-inch 78 rpm // Cappella Giulia. Ernesto Boezi. ca. 1935 [also listed as Odeon EMS 11].
Contains motet *Tribulationes civitatum* [with secunda pars *Peccavimus*].

F0385 SEMS 13. 12-inch 78 rpm // Cappella Giulia Choir. Ernesto Boezi. Before 1942 [also listed as Odeon EMS 13].
Contains offertory motet *Bonum est confiteri a 5.*

F0386 SEMS/Musique au Vatican 16. 12-inch 78 rpm // Cappella Giulia Choir. Ernesto Boezi. Before 1942 [also listed as Odeon EMS 16].
Contains motet *Adoremus te Christe* [doubtful work].

F0387 SEMS 26/30. 12-inch 78 rpm [10 sides]. // Cappella Giulia Choir. Ernesto Boezi. ca. 1936–1942 [also listed as Odeon EMS 26/30].
Contains mass *Missa Papae Marcelli a 6.*

F0388 SEMS/Musique au Vatican 31. 12-inch 78 rpm // Cappella Giulia Choir. Ernesto Boezi. Before 1942 [also listed as Odeon EMS 31].
Contains motets *Alleluia. Tulerunt Dominum a 5*; *Laudate Dominum.*

F0389 SEMS/Musique au Vatican 35. 12-inch 78 rpm // Cappella Giulia Choir. Ernesto Boezi. Before 1942 [also listed as Odeon EMS 35].
Contains motet *Paucitas dierum a 5* [secunda pars *Manus tuae*].

F0390 SEMS 38. 12-inch 78 rpm // Cappella Giulia Choir. Ernesto Boezi. Before 1942.
Contains motet *Introduxit me rex* [with Victoria *O Domine Jesu*].

F0391 SEMS 41/Musique au Vatican 1187. 12-inch 78 rpm // Cappella Giulia. Ernesto Boezi. Before 1942 [also listed as Odeon EMS 41. NB: When *Tota pulchra es* was released as Odeon EMS 41, it was paired with *Exsultate Deo*; on the MV 1187 release, *Tota pulchra es* was paired with Goudimel's *Videntes stellam*].
Contains motets *Exsultate Deo a 5; Tota pulchra es a 5.*

F0392 SEMS 43. 12-inch 78 rpm // Cappella Giulia Choir. Ernesto Boezi. Before 1942.
Contains hymn *O felix anima a 3.*

F0393 SEMS/Musique au Vatican 44. 10-inch 78 rpm // Cappella Giulia. Ernesto Boezi. Before 1942 [also listed as Odeon EMS 44].
Contains motet *Vox dilecti mei a 5.*

F0394 SEMS 54. 10-inch 78 rpm // Cappella Giulia Choir. Ernesto Boezi. Before 1942 [also listed as Odeon EMS 54].
Contains offertory motet *Exaltabo te, Domine.*

F0395 SEMS/Musique au Vatican 1119. 12-inch 78 rpm // Madrigal Choir of the Schola Cantorum Pontificale. Mons. Antonelli. Before 1948.
Contains madrigal *I vaghi fiori e l'amorose fronde a 4.*

F0396 SEMS/Musique au Vatican 1146. 12-inch 78 rpm // Cappella Giulia. Mons. Antonelli [motet]; Ernesto Boezi [hymn]. Issued ca. 1942–1948; probably recorded by early 1930s.
Contains motet *Dies sanctificatus a 4*; hymn *Pange lingua gloriosi a 4.*

F0397 SEMS/Musique au Vatican 1156. 12-inch 78 rpm // Cappella Giulia Choir. Monsignor Antonelli. ca. 1935–1939.
Contains motet *Super flumina Babylonis a 4* [with Victoria *Tenebrae*].

F0398 SEMS/Musique au Vatican 1157. 12-inch 78 rpm // Cappella Giulia Choir. Monsignor Antonelli. ca. 1935.
Contains offertory motet *Laudate Dominum* [with Victoria *Caligaverunt*].

F0399 Sony Special Products A 324940. CD (3). *The Norton Recordings. Shorter Version.* Tallis Scholars. Peter Phillips. 1980 [selection under consideration derived from Gimell CDGIM 339, previously issued as Angel RL 32122].
Contains mass *Missa Papae Marcelli* [*Gloria* only] [CD1, track 13–14; also on cassette 1, A/6 section]

F0400 Sony Special Products A 720384. CD (3rd edition: 12 discs, 2 vols of 6 each). *A History of Western Music and the Norton Anthology of Western Music. Vol. 1.* Sound CDs to accompany the text of Donald Grout's and Claude V. Palisca's *A History of Western Music*, 5th edition (1996).
Contains mass *Missa Papae Marcelli* [*Credo* and *Agnus Dei I* only].

F0401 Stradivarius STR 33375. CD. *Giovanni Pierluigi da Palestrina. Ave maris stella.* Camerata Nova. Luigi Taglioni. 1996 (rec. September 19–22, 1996, Cripta della Casa Provincializia delle Suore "Ancelle della Carità," Rome). Notes (2pp) by Lino Bianchi, ca. 1986, and Matelda Viola (2pp) ca. 1996.

Contains motets *Ave Maria a 4* [3:19]; *Alma redemptoris mater* [secunda pars: *Tu quae genuisti*] [4:24]; *Veni sponsa Christi a 4* [2:57]; *Surge propera* [3:19]; *Quae est ista a 4* [8:58]; *Hodie beata Virgo* [3:23]; *Ave regina coelorum* [secunda pars: *Gaude virgo gloriosa*] [5:48]; *Ave Maria a 5*; magnificats *Magnificat quarti toni* [from Lateran codex 59] [9:51]; *Magnificat septimi toni* [from Magnificats, book III] [11:34]; hymn *Ave maris stella a 4* [6:50].

F0402 Stradivarius STR 33423. CD. *Palestrina: Missae ex Cipriano de Rore*. Delitiae Musicae. Marco Longhini. 1997 (rec. September 12–14, 1995, Church of S. Briccio di Lavagna, Verona). Program notes (5pp) by Marco Longhini.

Contains masses *Missa Quando lieta sperai; Missa Qual'è il più grande amore.* Additional contents include Rore madrigals *Quando lieta sperai* and *Qual'è il più grande amore.*

F0403 Stradivarius STR 33477. CD. *Palestrina: Missae ex Jacquet de Mantua.* Delitiae Musicae. Marco Longhini. 1997 (rec. August 27–29, 1997, Church of S. Briccio di Lavagna, Verona).

Contains masses *Missa Salvum me fac, Domine*; *Missa Aspice Domine*. Additional contents include Jacquet of Mantua motets *Salvum me fac, Domine* and *Aspice Domine.*

F0404 Stradivarius STR SIP 35. CD. *Sacred Polyphony of the Sixteenth Century.* Syntagma. Franco Monego.

Contains mass *Missa Brevis a 4.*

F0405 Studio SM 33-01. LP. *Monaco Cathedral Choir.* Monaco Cathedral Choir. H. Carol. ca. 1950–1951 [reissue of SM 61/4, 12-inch 78 rpm, 8 sides].

Contains motet *Improperium exspectavit.*

F0406 Studio SM 37-41.12-inch 78 rpm. *Polyphonic Church Music.* Choeur de la Cathédrale de Dijon. Joseph Samson. ca. 1950–1951 [part of set SM 37/41, 10 sides]; Palestrina on disk 39.] [Note: see F0445. F0406 may be an issue or reissue of F0445.]

Contains motet *Sicut cervus a 4*

F0407 Supraphon ARMU 005-2. CD. *Cantate Domino.* Chorus Kantilena, Brno State Philharmonic Orchestra Choir. Ivan Sedlacek. 1990s.

Contains motets *Ave regina coelorum a 4*; *Alma redemptoris mater* [number of parts not indicated].

F0408 Supraphon 31-0528-2. CD. *Ave Verum Corpus.* Bambini di Praga. Blanka Kulínsky, Bohumil Kulínsky. 2000 [rec. October 2000 in Prague].

Contains motet *Pueri Hebraeorum a 4* [1:32].

F0409 Supraphon SUAST 50578. LP. *Missa Papae Marcelli. Oratio Jeremiae. Paucitas dierum. Alleluia, Tulerunt Dominum.* Czech Philharmonic Chorus. Prague Madrigal Singers. Miroslav Venhoda. 1963 (rec. 1963, Church of the Virgin Mary, Prague) [also listed as Ariola XH28 841K (5); Parliament PLP 612].
Contains mass *Missa Papae Marcelli a 6*; motets *Alleluia! Tulerunt Dominum; Paucitas dierum*; lamentation *Oratio Jeremiae Prophetae.*

F0410 Supraphon SUAST 50775. LP. *The Song of Songs.* Slovak Philharmonic Chorus. Ján María Dobrodinský. 1968 [Crossroads 22160186, item F0140, presents a partial reissue of this recording, with 20 of the 29 motets plus notes in English].
Contains motets from *Canticum canticorum.*

F0411 Supraphon SUAST 50776. LP. *Missa Cantantibus organis, Caecilia.* Prague Madrigal Singers. Miroslav Venhoda. 1967. This is a recording of the complete mass, with each composer and his contribution designated.
Contains mass *Missa Cantantibus organis* [Palestrina's contribution is the *Et in terra pax*].

F0412 Supraphon SUP 11 0620-2 211. CD [reissue of an LP]. [title]. Czech Philharmonic Chorus. M. Bruni. 1975. Notes by Jaroslav Holocek.
Contains motet *Stabat mater a 8.*

F0413 Supraphon SUP 11 2137-2. CD. *Missa Papae Marcelli. Missa Hodie Christus natus est. Stabat mater.* Czech Philharmonic Chorus. Josef Veselka, [reissue of LP Supraphon 112.1807, rec. 1971, also listed as LP Ariola XH 28841 K(S)].
Contains mass *Hodie Christus natus est a 8* [36:00]; motet *Stabat Mater* [10:50]; improperia *Popule meus* [3:35].

F0414 Supraphon SUP 412 2141/42. LP (2). *Canticum Canticorum. The Song of Songs.* Czech Philharmonic Chorus. Josef Veselka. Late 1970s.
Contains motets of the *Canticum canticorum* (complete, 29 motets a 5).

F0415 Supraphon SUP 1412 2931/2932. LP (2). *Madrigals.* Czech Philharmonic Chorus. Josef Veselka. 1981 (rec. 1979). Texts on sleeve.
Contains madrigals *I vaghi fiori e l'amorose fronde a 4; Vestiva i colli a 5.*

F0416 Syrena 9473/74. 10-inch 78 rpm (4 sides). // Poznán Cathedral Choir. W. Gieburoskiego. Before 1936.
Contains motet *Stabat mater a 8* [1948 source says these are 12-inch discs].

F0417 Tactus TC 520001. CD. *Sacred Music Connected with St. Philip Neri.* Progetto Musica Vocal Ensemble, Progetto Musica Instrumental Ensemble. Giulio Monaco. 1995 (rec. March 1995, Santuario di Graglia).
Contains mass *Missa in minoribus duplicibus.*

F0418 Tactus TC 521601. CD. *Il primo libro di madrigali a quattro voci.* Concerto Italiano (G. Banditelli [sgr], C. Cavina [alto], S. Naglia [alto], G. Maletto [tenor], D. Carnovich [bass], A. Damiani [lute]). Rinaldo Alessandrini. 1992 (rec. December

4–7, 1992. Sala Bolognini del Convento di San Domenico, Bologna). Recording based on the 1596 edition of the madrigals, originally published in 1555. Program notes and texts in Italian, English, German, and French.

Contains madrigals [Book I, complete (30 works)]: *Deh, hor foss'io col vago della luna*; *S'il dissi mai, ch'io veng'in odio a quella*; *Queste saranno ben lagrime, e questi*; *Che no fia che giamai dal cor si sgombri*; *Rime, da i sospir miei nati e dal pianto*; *Lontan dalla mia diva*; *Nessun visse giamai più di me lieto*; *La ver l'aurora che si dolce l'aura*; *Chiara, si chiaro è de'vostr'occhi il sole*; *Chi stinguera il mio foco*; *Donna vostra mercede*; *Già fu chi m'ebbe cara e volentieri*; *Che debbo far, che mi consigli amore*; *Over de sensi è priva*; *Amor, fortuna e la mia mente schiva*; *Ne spero i dolci di tornin'in dietro*; *Gitene liete rime ov'or si siede*; *Mentr'a le dolci e le purpuree labbra*; *Amor che meco in quest'ombre ti stavi*; *Ecc'ove gionse prima e poi s'assise*; *Vaghi pensier che cosi passo passo*; *Mentre ch'al mar descenderanno i fiumi*; *Quai rime fur si chiare*; Sestina: *Ecc'oscurati i chiari raggi al sole*; *Rara beltà non mai piu vista in terra*; *Questo doglioso stil colmo di pianto*; *Mai fu piu crudo piu spietata morte*; *Privo di fed'oltra l'usato corso*; *Ma voi fioriti e honorati colli.*

F0419 Tactus TC 550201. CD. *Motetti madrigali et canzoni Francese di diversi eccellentissimi autori.* Musica Figurata. 1998 [rec. Pieve di S. Giovanni Battista, Saturnano-Pistoia].

Contains diminutions of motets *Introduxit me rex* [3:29]; *Pulchra es* [3:53]; *Tota pulchra es* [3:35]; *Fuit homo missus est* [5:45]; *Benedicta sit sancta Trinitas* [6:33]; *Ave Maria* [5:30].

F0420 Tactus TC 561901. CD. *Missa Loquebantur. Vespertina Psalmodia*. Stagione Armonica. Sergio Balestracci. 1998. Program notes in Italian by Sergio Balestracci (12pp) with English, French, German trans. in container.

Contains motet *Loquebantur in variis linguis.*

F0421 Tallis Choir TCD-03. CD. *The Music of Palestrina and Victoria.* The Tallis Choir [Toronto]. Peter Walker, Juergen Petrenko. 1991 (rec. May 1991, Grace Church-on-the-Hill, Toronto). Program notes in English; Latin text with English translations provided in box.

Contains motets *Assumpta est Maria* [5:57]; *Lauda Sion Salvatorem* [3:08]; *Stabat mater* [10:31]; *Haec dies* [1:46]; *Tu es Petrus a 6* [6:14]; *O magnum mysterium* [5:53].

F0422 Telarc TELA CD 80257. CD. *Royal Brass*. Empire Brass Quintet [also issued as cassette CS 30257]. 1990.

Contains ricercar *Ricercar del primo tuono* [arr. Empire Brass Quintet].

F0423 Teldec 4509-94561-2. CD. *Palestrina. Missa pro defunctis. Motets.* Chanticleer. Joseph Jennings. 1995 (rec. 1994, San Rafael, CA). Program notes by Stephen R. Miller (5pp) in English, French, and German; texts provided, with translations into English, French, German.

Contains mass *Missa pro defunctis* [21.14]; motets *Gaude gloriosa* [2.10]; *Salve regina a 5* [5.54]; *Pange lingua a 4* [7.31]; *O bone Jesu a 6* [3.02]; *Trahe me a 5* [2.34]; *Nigra sum, sed formosa* [3.13]; *Surge, propera* [2.20]; *Surge, amica mea* [2.33]; *Quam pulchra es* [2.47]; *Veni, dilecte mi* [2.34]; *Gaude, Barbara* [9.15].

F0424 Telefunken AS6 41036. LP. *Die Kleinorgel*. Albert de Klerk [chamber organ]. 1967 [also issued as SAWT 9409].
Contains ricercar *Ricercare primi toni* [arr. organ].

F0425 Telefunken AW6 42033. LP. *Recorder Music of Renaissance Italy*. Vienna Recorder Ensemble. 1977.
Contains two unspecified ricercari.

F0426 Turnabout 34309S. LP. *Palestrina. Missa de Beata Virgine. 3 Motets*. Spandauer Kantorei. Martin Behrmann. 1970. Liner notes by Egon Kenton [also listed as FSM 34 309. NB: *O magnum mysterium* also issued on Vox Cameo Classics 8839 in 1997].
Contains mass *Missa de Beata Virgine a 6* [31:44]; motets *Tu es Petrus a 6* [8:34]; *Lauda Sion salvatorem a 4* [3:54]; *O magnum mysterium a 6* [7:31].

F0427 Ultraphon AP 276. 10-inch 78 rpm // Choir of St. Nicolas Church, Freiburg. Bovet. Before 1935.
Contains mass *Missa Papae Marcelli a 6* [*Kyrie* only]; motet *Viri Galilaei* [arr. Bovet].

F0428 Unicorn UN LP 1013. LP. *Missa Veni sponsa Christi*. Vienna Kammerchor. Hans Gillesberger. 1955. Program notes by Klaus George Roy; Latin texts with English translations, on sleeve.
Contains mass *Missa Veni sponsa Christi a 4*; motet *Veni sponsa Christi a 4*.

F0429 United Artists UAL 7001. LP. *Leopold Stokowski Conducting the Symphony of the Air*. Symphony of the Air. Leopold Stokowski. Later 1950s.
Contains motet *Adoramus te Christe* [arrangement].

F0430 Urania US 57168. LP. *Madrigals and Motets. Thirteenth to Seventeenth Century*. Coro de Madrigalistas de Mexico. Luis Sandi. 1960s.
Contains motet *O quantus luctus*.

F0431 Veriton SXV 775. LP. Cantores Minores Wratislavienses. Edmund Kajdasz. 1970s.
Contains improperias *Cantica majoris hebdomadae: In monte Oliveti; Unus ex discipulis meis; Omnes amici mei; Tenebrae factae sunt; Ecce quomodo moritur; Popule meus; Crux fidelis; Vexilla regis; Adoramus te; O vos omnes*; lamentation *Lamentatio (Sabbato Sancto)*.

F0432 Victor 6442. 12-inch 78 rpm [acoustic]. // Sistine Chapel Choir. Antonio Rella. 1908.
Contains motet *Laudate Dominum quia benignus est*.

F0433 Victor 7812. 12-inch 78 rpm // Sistine Chapel Choir. Antonio Rella. ca. 1910 [also in set GM-139 and VM-182].
Contains motet *Sicut cervus a 4*.

F0434 Victor 7813. 12-inch 78 rpm // Sistine Chapel Choir. Antonio Rella. ca. 1910 [also issued in VM-182 and as Gramophone/HMV DB1571 in set GM-139].
Contains improperia *Populе meus*; [reverse side] motet *Super flumina Babylonis.*

F0435 Victor 9159. 12-inch 78 rpm // Maestri Cantori di Firenze. Sandro Benelli. Before 1936.
Contains motets *O bone Jesu a 4; Adoramus te Christe* [attribution to Palestrina doubtful].

F0436 Victor 13560. 12-inch 78 rpm *Medieval and Renaissance Choral Music.* Choir of the Pius X School of Liturgical Music. Mother G. Stevens. ca. 1940 [issued in 5–disc set M 739].
Contains motet *Pueri Hebraeorum a 4.*

F0437 Victor 15731. 12-inch 78 rpm // Pennsylvania University Choir. Harl McDonald. Before 1936 [withdrawn 1940s] [also issued as Gramophone EB 295].
Contains motet *O bone Jesu.*

F0438 Victor 17633. 12-inch 78 rpm // Augustana Choir. Henry Veld. ca. 1940.
Contains motet *Ecce quomodo moritur justus a 4* [actually by Ingegneri].

F0439 Victor 20410. 10-inch 78 rpm // Dayton Westminster Choir. John Finlay Williamson. Before 1936 [also issued as Gramophone EW 65].
Contain motet *Hodie Christus natus est a 8.*

F0440 Victor 20897. 10-inch 78 rpm (1/2 side). // Palestrina Choir. Nicola A. Montani. Before 1936.
Contains magnificat *Magnificat tertii toni* [*Gloria patri* only].

F0441 Victor 20898. 10-inch 78 rpm // Palestrina Choir. Nicola A. Montani. Before 1936.
Contains motet *Sicut cervus a 4*; improperia *Popule meus.*

F0442 Victor 21622. 10-inch 78 rpm // Palestrina Choir. Nicola A. Montani. Before 1936.
Contains motet *Adoramus te Christe* [attribution to Palestrina doubtful].

F0443 Victor 26782. 10-inch 78 rpm *Madrigals, Motets and Chansons.* Lee Jones Madrigal Singers. Lee Jones. ca. 1940 [issued in 4–disc set G 26].
Contains motet *Pater noster.*

F0444 Victor set E 101. LP. // Vocal Octet. No director listed. ca. 1950 [also issued as set WE 101, 45 rpm].
Contains motet *O bone Jesu.*

F0445 Victor set VM-212. Five 12-inch 78 rpm discs. *Dijon Cathedral Album.* Dijon Cathedral Choir. Joseph Samson. Before 1938. [May be identified with F0406] q.v.

F0446 Voce del Padrone/Odeon QBLP 5048. 10-inch LP. *Coro della Cappella Sistina.* Choir of the Sistine Chapel. Lorenzo Perosi. 1957.
Contains *Improperia*; motets *Sicut cervus a 4*; *Super flumina Babylonis.*

F0447 Vivarte 60660. CD. *Sing Choirs of Angels*. Malle Babbe Choir. Leny van Schaik. 1999 (rec. in Doopsgezinde Kerke, Haarlem).
Contains motet *Salve Regina* [2:11].

F0448 Vox PL 9740. LP. *Le Vergini. Stabat Mater. Super flumina Babylonis.* Choir of the Choral Academy, Lecco. Guido Camillucci. 1957.
Contains motets *Super flumina Babylonis* [3:00]; *Stabat mater a 8* [7:40]; spiritual madrigals *Vergine bella; Vergina saggia; Vergine pura; Vergina santa; Vergine sola; Vergine chiara; Vergine, quante lagrime; Vergine, tale è terra* [31:13 total].

F0449 Vox PL 10020. LP. *Missa Papae Marcelli. Missa Assumpta est Maria.* Pro Musica Choir, Vienna. Ferdinand Grossmann. 1956. Notes by Charles Stanley on sleeve.
Contains masses *Missa Papae Marcelli* [26:20]; *Missa Assumpta est Maria* [24:34].

F0450 Wealden WS 122. LP. // Choir of St. Mary's Parish Church, Woodford. Robert Munns. Before 1981.
Contains motet *Loquebantur variis linguis.*

F0451 Westminster W 9605. LP. *Missa Papae Marcelli.* Günther Theurig. Vienna Akademie Kammerchor. 1963. Text with English translation on sleeve.
Contains mass *Missa Papae Marcelli a 6* [38:33].

F0452 Westminster XWN 18632. LP. *Palestrina: Three Motets. Gallus. Ten Motets.* Vienna Akademie Kammerchor. Günther Theurig. Mid to late 1950s.
Contains motets *Stabat Mater*; *Pater noster*; *Super flumina Babylonis.*

F0453 Westminster XWN 18693. LP. *Missa Aeterna Christi munera.* Chanteurs de St.-Eustache. Père Émile Martin. 1959. Texts with English translation on sleeve.
Contains masses *Missa Aeterna Christi munera a 4*; *Missa Lauda Sion a 4.*

F0454 Westminster XWN 18836. LP. *Mass Pange Lingua. [Missa Assumpta est Maria].* Chanteurs de St.-Eustache. Père Émile Martin. 1959 [probably a reissue of recording of earlier (unknown) date; described on sleeve as "An Erato recording"]. Program notes by Philippe Caillard and J.F. Paillard, translated into English from original French; Latin texts with English translation on sleeve.
Contains mass *Missa Assumpta est Maria a 6.*

Appendix

This section contains recordings for which citations or contents, including main recording titles, could not be verified. It is understood that these citations may be incomplete or inaccurate, or that the titles either of the full recording or of the works reported to be by Palestrina are not accurately known.

Abbey LPB 816. LP. *In Quires and Places.* Choir of the Metropolitan Cathedral of Liverpool.
Palestrina work(s).

Alpha APR 306. [no further information.]
Motet *Haec dies quam fecit Dominus*

Argo R 1002. LP. Wesley Chapel Choir. Cleall.
Motet *Adoramus te Christe a 4.*

Capitol MC 20066. LP. Cappella Sistina Choir. Domenico Bartolucci. [This performance was probably issued on several other discs in the 1950s].
Motet *Tota pulchra es a 5.*

Hungaroton SLPX 12546. LP. Pecs Chamber Choir. Tillei.
Madrigal *I vaghi fiori e l'amorose fronde a 4.*

Melodiya D 027283/4. LP. Vocal Ensemble "Renaissance." ca. 1970.
Litany *Kyrie* [unspecified]; magnificat [unspecified].

Remington 199-167. Helsinki University Choir. Turunen.
Mass *Aeterna Christi munera a 4.*

Urania AP 276. Fribourg Choir.
Mass *Missa Papae Marcelli a 6* [*Kyrie* only].

Index of Titles and First Lines of Musical Works

Index of Names and Subjects